Rehabilitation Therapeutics of the Neurological Training

Wenru Zhao

Rehabilitation Therapeutics of the Neurological Training

Daoyin Technique in Chinese Medicine

PMPH PEOPLE'S MEDICAL PUBLISHING HOUSE Springer

Wenru Zhao
Neurological Training Rehabilitation
Research Room of Beijing Daxing
District Chinese and Western Medicine
Combined Hospital
Beijing
China

ISBN 978-981-13-0811-6 ISBN 978-981-13-0812-3 (eBook)
https://doi.org/10.1007/978-981-13-0812-3

Library of Congress Control Number: 2018956445

This Springer imprint is published by the registered company Springer Nature Singapore Pte Ltd.
The registered company address is: 152 Beach Road, #21-01/04 Gateway East, Singapore 189721, Singapore

I spent 4 years' day and night on this book. I spent three Spring Festivals and many weekends in my office. Rehabilitation Therapeutics of the Neurological Training : Daoyin Technique in Chinese Medicine *is finally completed. I enjoy myself for a while and am anxious about this book. Although this book is my painstaking effort for almost 20 years and is completed by my group, will it withstand the ordeal of time and tide? Is there any major regret and careless omission? In any case, who is coming will come.* Rehabilitation Therapeutics of the Neurological Training: Daoyin Technique:in Chinese Medicine *should be presented to the author sooner or later. This book should go through the test of time and tide, should be applied in clinic and should be discussed by the rehabilitation doctors.*

More than 10 years' clinical application proved that the therapeutic effect is good and the method is accepted by many patients, which make me feel comfortable. All these results give me courage. At least, this book serves as a modest spur to induce someone to come forward with his valuable. My purpose is to revive the old rehabilitation technique of Chinese nation to improve life quality of the disabled. I want to devote myself to rehabilitation medicine service. This book should receive the inspection and judgement of specialists, rehabilitation doctors, all sectors of society and the successors. This book may be only a start. After practice, modification, supplement and perfection, this book can be used to serve the disabled and benefit all mankind. That's what I want to and am happy to see.

When this book is going to be published, the most urgent thing I want to do is to thank the hospitals, companies and people that support and help me in the development of rehabilitation technique of neurological training and in the days of book writing. Since 2001, I came back to China and Xuanwu Hospital,

Beijing Municipal Rehabilitation Center, Tongren Hospital and National Research Center for Rehabilitation Technical Aids Affiliated Rehabilitation Hospital provide affordable conditions for the development of this technique, which play an important role in the early incubation and development of rehabilitation technique of neurological training. I want to thank the groups in different phases who don't give me up in the difficulties and who follow me and give up good pay and working condition regardless of hardship. They contribute to the development and progress of rehabilitation technique of neurological training and the development and application of rehabilitation enterprise.

It is estimable that Beijing Xingchengwanyou Science and Technology Ltd is the rehabilitation technological achievement transformation of neurological training. Since 2003, the company is leaded by general manager, senior engineer Hongquan Su, to raise money, prepare place, buy equipment and turn my thoughts into corollary equipment at any cost, because they are willing to try their best to develop corollary equipment of our own rehabilitation technique of functional training with proprietary intellectual property rights and contribute to the formation and industrialization development of this technique.

I want to thank the hospitals that recruit this technique. They take risks to recruit rehabilitation technique of neurological training for the local patients at first, broaden the clinical application range of this technique, and accelerate the pace of clinical verification and improved development. I want to thank the rehabilitation doctors, news media, all sectors of society, the patients and their family who accept and support rehabilitation technique of neurological training. They give me the courage and power to do further research on the rehabilitation technique of neurological training. I want to thank my family as well who support and understand me in these years.

With this, I realize that if neurological training has a little effect and contribution on the development and progress of rehabilitation medicine, it is the results of everyone's effort. Perhaps, the publishment of this book is only the start of the research work. My group and I will devote ourselves to the renaissance of rehabilitation technique in traditional Chinese medicine and progress of rehabilitation enterprise.

Beijing, China
28 July 2013

Preface

During the years I worked as an orthopedist specializing in the treatment and functional rehabilitation of spinal cord injury, I had the honor of studying in the department of physics and biophysics at the University of Salzburg for three years and then in the orthopedics and rehabilitation department of Jackson Memorial Medical Center at the University of Miami for three years. When I studied in the USA under the guidance of Professor Bernard S Brucker, I was brought into contact with the rehabilitation technique of electromyographic biofeedback and was immediately impressed. Since I returned to China in 2001, I have been dedicating myself to clinical practice, teaching, and research in the field of rehabilitation.

During the process of undertaking clinical rehabilitation, teaching, and research work, I truly realized the value and importance of rehabilitation work and recognized that rehabilitation medicine requires advanced technology and a wide breadth of knowledge. I realized that rehabilitation is a subject with practical value. When medicines, surgery, and other methods cannot recover lost motor function after an injury to the central nervous system, the method of rehabilitation training and rehabilitation medical engineering can remodel the disabled who have lost their self-help ability into those who have physical autonomy and are capable of taking care of themselves and returning to society. Rehabilitation medicine is a complicated and difficult cross-discipline subject, but it is a great way to help remodel people. All these aspects of rehabilitation medicine give me the passion and confidence to undertake rehabilitation medicine work.

I spent nineteen years, including six years in an elementary stage abroad and thirteen years' exploration at home, to develop a new rehabilitation technique that combines traditional Chinese and Western medicine. This technique's theoretical bases are CNS plasticity and functional reorganization and its training methods are neural potential development, motor program reestablishment, and motor pattern remodeling. The basic technique applied in these methods is a six-step Daoyin technique in traditional Chinese medicine of guiding collaterals through meridians to improve neural potential and recover functions of the nervous system; this process is also referred to as neurological training. Nine anatomical systems are controlled by nerves. Therefore, this technique can be widely applied. At present, using the six-step Daoyin technique, a series of therapeutic methods and corollary equipment have been in gradual development, which is called the rehabilitation therapy system of neurological training.

In the process of writing this book, I was supported by rehabilitation groups of neurological training and all sectors of society. I deliberated over the content of this book, simplified it by cutting out the superfluous, and strove for accuracy. However, my knowledge is limited and there may be some mistakes, so that I hope the reader will help me rectify them.

I hope this book can serve as a modest motivator to spur someone to come forward with their valuable contributions, so they can then activate the enthusiasm of medical workers for further exploration in this technique in order to improve it. In this way, the Daoyin technique from traditional Chinese medicine can then be spread worldwide.

Beijing, China
August 2013

Wenru Zhao
Zhaowenru

Acknowledgments

I spent four years, day and night, on this book. I spent three Spring Festivals and many weekends in my office. Now, *Rehabilitation Therapeutics of the Neurological Training: Daoyin Technique in Chinese Medicine* is finally completed. I enjoyed myself for a while and am anxious about this book. Although this book is the result of my painstaking effort for almost twenty years and is completed by my group, will it withstand the ordeal of time? Are there any mistakes or careless omissions? In any case, whatever happens, happens. *Rehabilitation Therapeutics of the Neurological Training: Daoyin Technique in Chinese Medicine* should be presented to the reader sooner or later. This book should go through the test of time, should be applied in clinic, and should be discussed by the rehabilitation doctors.

More than ten years' clinical application has proved that the therapeutic effect is good and the method is accepted by many patients, which made me feel comfortable. All these results gave me courage. At least, this book will serve as a modest motivation to encourage someone to come forward with their valuable ideas. My purpose is to revive an old rehabilitation technique of Chinese origin to improve the life quality of the disabled. I want to devote myself to rehabilitation medicine service. This book should receive the inspection and judgment of specialists, rehabilitation doctors, all sectors of society and their successors. This book may be only a start. After practice, modification, supplement, and perfection, this technique can hopefully be used to serve the disabled and benefit all mankind. That's what I want and would be happy to see.

When this book is published, the most important thing I want to do is to thank the hospitals, companies, and people that supported and helped me while I was developing this technique and during my days of book writing. In 2001, I returned to China. Xuanwu Hospital, Beijing Municipal Rehabilitation Center, Tongren Hospital, and the National Research Center for Rehabilitation Technical Aids Affiliated Rehabilitation Hospital provided affordable conditions for the development of this technique, which played an important role in the early incubation and development of rehabilitation technique of neurological training. I want to thank the groups in different phases who didn't give up on me despite the difficulties and who followed me and gave up good pay and working conditions regardless of hardship. They contributed to the development and progress of this rehabilitation technique.

My special thanks go to Beijing Xingchengwanyou Science and Technology Ltd., the transformation base for our technical achievement in neurological training and rehabilitation. Since 2003, the company has been led by general manager and senior engineer Hongquan Su. This company helped to raise money, prepare places, buy equipment, and turn my thoughts into corollary equipment at any cost, because they are willing to try their best to develop equipment for rehabilitation technique of functional training with proprietary intellectual property rights and contribute to the formation and industrialization development of this technique.

I want to thank the hospitals that adopted this technique. They took risks to adopt this technique for local patients at first, broaden the clinical application range of this technique, accelerate the pace of clinical verification, and contribute improvements and developments. I want to thank the rehabilitation doctors, news media, all sectors of society, the patients and their families who accepted and supported this technique. They gave me the courage and power to do further research on this rehabilitation technique of neurological training.

I want to thank my family as well, who has supported and understood me all these years.

With this, I realized that if neurological training has some impact or contribution to the development and progress of rehabilitation medicine, it is the result of everyone's effort.

Perhaps, the publication of this book is only the start of this research. My group and I will devote ourselves to the renaissance of rehabilitation technique in traditional Chinese medicine and progress of rehabilitation enterprise.

Contents

About the Author

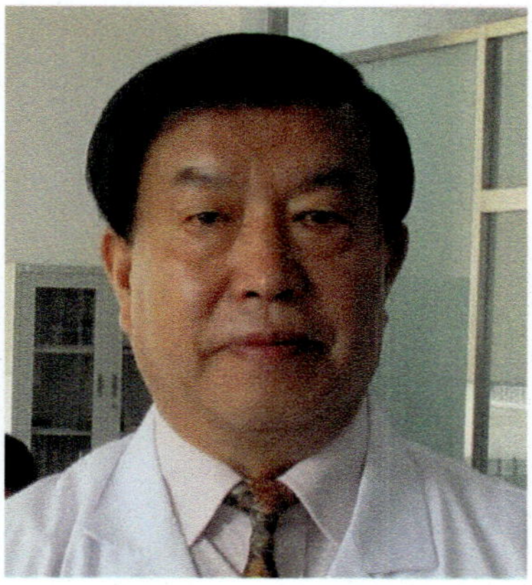

Wenru Zhao was born in November 1951 in the village of North Guanzhuang, located in Royang County of Hebei Province. He graduated from the medicine department of North China Coal Medical University in 1976. After graduation, he worked in the surgery department of his university's affiliated hospital. In 1986, he became a graduate student at Beijing Tuberculosis and Thoracic Neoplasms Institute, earning a master's degree in surgery. From 1995 to 2001, he went to Europe and America as a senior visiting scholar, which started his journey in the fields of clinical rehabilitation, teaching, and research.

He was the first president of the National Research Center for Rehabilitation Technical Aids Affiliated Rehabilitation Hospital. After being relieved of his office, he became the President Emeritus of this hospital and Chief Physician in rehabilitation. He was head of the department of functional therapy (rehabilitation) at Capital Medical University Xuanwu Hospital, vice president and director of the Rehabilitation Center of Neurological Training at Beijing Xishan Hospital, and the director of the Rehabilitation Center of Neurological Training of Capital Medical University Tongren Hospital. He worked in clinical practice, rehabilitation diagnosis and therapy, medical teaching, and research for 37 years. He founded the rehabilitation therapy system of neurological training. He is the chairman of a specialized committee called the Rehabilitation Medicine of Beijing Combination Society of Traditional Chinese and Western Medicine. He was a winner of a Prominent Achievement Award for master's degree recipients by the State Education Commission and Academic Degrees Committee of the State Council. Currently, he is involved in the National Key Technology R&D Program's "Three-stage Method and Corollary Equipment Research of Rehabilitation of Neurological Training of Motor Functions of Hemiplegic Lower Limbs."

Introduction

Traditional rehabilitation methods developed in the middle period of last century such as Bobath, Rood, Brunnstrom, PNF and motor relearning program (MRP), played an enlightened and foundation effect on rehabilitation in the long history of rehabilitation. However, the therapeutic effect is influenced because these methods are mainly passive movements, primary reflex and afferent stimulus. Therefore, it is extremely urgent to study the rehabilitation method that is better in accordance with the mechanism of motor functional recovery after CNS injury.

Neural potential development is the basis of promoting plasticity and functional reorganization of central nervous system. Six-step Daoyin technique in traditional Chinese medicine of guiding collaterals through meridians of complete active movement is accordance with rehabilitation method to develop brain potential. Daoyin feedback technique is an important method to reestablish motor program with a purpose through goal and motive mechanism and guided motor program signal real-timely detected and displayed. Effective restriction of unnecessary joint motion in limbs movements is the important segment to remodel motor pattern and is an essential process of transforming developed potential and reestablished motor program into actual motor function and life ability. The three-stage rehabilitation method of neurological training is the specific manifestation of clinical standard application of technique. A series of corollary equipment developed according to the methods is the important measures to implement the method correctly and realize the therapeutic effect. Accurate rehabilitation assessment, confirmation of main obstacles, formulation and selection of overall goal of rehabilitation, principle and specific method are essential rehabilitation strategy and tactics to obtain anticipated training effect.

This book is mainly used for clinical application and is to introduce basic mechanism, specific method and development of rehabilitation technique of neurological training. This book emphasizes on clinical indications, contraindications, announcements and rehabilitation dedicated device of neurological training. This book use easy, practical, understandable and simple description and illustration to analyze rehabilitation therapeutic technique of neurological training from the angle of integrated Chinese and Western medicines in order to make it practical. It is not only suitable for rehabilitation doctors and therapists in big hospitals, but also suitable for the doctors in community and village. For the teachers and students in medical school and physicians in other departments, the book has certain reference value. Therefore, rehabilitation medicine should run through therapy of all clinical departments and diseases.

We hope this book can serve as a modest spur to induce someone to come forward with his valuable contributions to encourage medical staffs, especially staffs in rehabilitation medicine to dig and learn the old rehabilitation technique in traditional Chinese medicine and its modern development in order to promote the renaissance of old rehabilitation technique and contribute to the development of rehabilitation medicine in worldwide.

Beijing, China
August 2013

1 Basic Theory of Neurological Training Rehabilitation

1.1 Abstract

1.1.1 The Mechanism of Recovering the Lost Motor Functions After CNS Injuries

Central nervous system (CNS) includes brain and spinal cord, which is the headquarters of somatic motor functions. Therefore, recovery of the central nervous system is prior to recovering the lost motor functions after central lesion.

Some experiments demonstrated that cells in CNS are not capable of regeneration, which is an unbridgeable obstacle for the mechanism of recovering the lost motor functions after central lesion. For a long time, it is widely believed in medical world that motor dysfunctions after real central lesion are unrecoverable and permanent motor function loss that due to degree and position of the injury is reasonable.

But the reality is not the case. For example, some patients and their family did not give up the treatment including rehabilitation training after central lesion. Some of them did not know the thesis that motor dysfunctions after central lesion are unrecoverable. Some of them were willing to receive treatment and keep doing exercise even they knew the thesis. It was beyond all expectations that a large number of them got improvements to varying degrees in motor function recovery. Thereafter, some researchers found that the lost motor functions after central lesion were partly recoverable through exercise. However, many medical scientists explained that the functions recovery was not due to brain cell regeneration and functions reorganizing on account of rehabilitation training, but due to the residual motor functions were improved by rehabilitation training.

For more than decade, both in animal experiments and in clinical practice, accumulating evidences showed that both in CNS of non-mammalian animals and mammalian animals, even in CNS of adult, there were structural plasticity change and functional reorganizing ability after central lesion. On the other hand, clinical and experimental study demonstrated that some parts of CNS were regenerative under certain circumstance. The regenerative ability was not good, but the regenerative parts could bine with targets properly. Therefore, the functions recovery after central lesion was possible. In the study of CNS, regeneration was widely accepted in the past few years and some related key factors were found. In the hypothesis of the functions recovery after central lesion, plasticity theory was the most widely focused and accepted.

Even the study about CNS regeneration and plasticity are under preliminary and insufficiency period, these results would shed light on the functions recovery after central lesion. At least these studies have proved irrecoverable functions after central lesion wrong and let the doctors and patients to understand the CNS function and the possibility of motor functions recovery after central lesion.

W. Zhao, *Rehabilitation Therapeutics of the Neurological Training*,
https://doi.org/10.1007/978-981-13-0812-3_1

1.1.1.1 Several Hypotheses of Functions Recovery After CNS Injuries

In the end of nineteenth century and 1930s, some researchers explained why the function was recoverable after central lesion. These hypotheses are as follows.

Hierarchical Re-representation Theory

Hierarchical re-representation theory was first proposed by Jackson in 1884 or so. He thought that the structures of nervous system were divided into different hierarchies from highest to lowest. Functions were not peculiar to one of the hierarchies, but one kind of functions could be represented repeatedly in different hierarchies. Superior hierarchy of the nervous system developed relatively late, was prone to be activated, regulated the functions fine and had inhibiting effect on inferior hierarchy of the nervous system. When the Superior hierarchies of the nervous system were injured, the inferior hierarchies of the nervous system were disinhibited and could accomplish or compensate the lost functions. Jackson's theory was the basis of neurological function compensatory principle.

Substitution or Vicarious Theory

Substitution or vicarious theory was first proposed by Mumk in 1881 or so. He thought that intact cortex could undertake the lost functions due to injury. The intact cortex should satisfy the following conditions. Firstly, the intact cortex was capable to accomplish the functions. Secondly, the intact cortex was under resting state. Thirdly, the intact cortex did nothing but undertaking the lost functions. These conditions seem not correct at present. However, Mumk's hypothesis became the forerunner of functional reorganization theory.

Diaschisis Theory

Diaschisis theory was first proposed by Monakow in 1914. He thought that partial brain tissues injury damaged the ability of other intact brain tissues that could receive normal afferent impulse from the injured parts. The other intact brain tissues would be into a specific "shock" phenomenon without receiving normal afferent impulse from the injured parts. Thereby, the functions and the morphology would be detached and this condition was called diaschisis. The intact brain tissues were in dysfunction and the symptoms would be watched. When the "shock" phenomenon disappeared, the functions of the intact brain tissues would be recovered. Later, the symptoms of partial brain tissues injury would be watched. The mechanism of the theory could be explained by the functional inhibition of metabolic remote area.

1.1.1.2 Brain Plasticity Theory

The mechanism of brain plasticity was related to many factors such as neurotomy, neurophysiology, neuropathology, neuroimmunology, neurochemistry and neuroelectricity.

In 1930, the students of Bltz firstly proposed the conception "plasticity of CNS". He thought that plasticity was an ability that could adapt to sudden change and deal with some kind of danger. The ability was the basis that CNS could reorganize to maintain proper functions structurally and functionally after central lesion. In the experiment, he observed the functional recovery of the amphibian without 1–2 limbs. He found that the animals could readjust to keep moving in a new way. However, he thought that the movements in a new way were the results of dynamic functional reorganization or adaption of CNS but not the regeneration. He thought that the functions recovery after central lesion was the results of functional reorganization of residual normal nervous tissues.

In 1969, the CNS functional reorganization theory was proposed and completed by Luria, Naydin, Tsvel, Kova and Vinarskaya. They realized that the residual parts of brain after injury could replace the lost functions in a new way through functional reorganization and thought that the functional reorganization was divided into two types, intra-system and inter-system. The intra-system mean that the compensation took place in the identical level or different level of the same system. For example, the lost functions were compensated by adjacent tissues of nidus or upper or lower tissues of nidus structurally. The inter-system mean that the lost functions were compensated by an entirely different system. For example, vision could be replaced by skin touch. Meanwhile, the compensation must be accomplished through specific rehabilitation training, which was also called retraining theory.

There are many ways to accomplish the functional reorganization after central lesion such as training, adjacent tissue compensation or offside tissue compensation, denervation supersensitivity, the axon collateral sprouting, latent pathway and enabled synapse and behavioral compensation. All these ways were known as the results of CNS functional reorganization.

Functional reorganization after compensation becomes the basis of the physiology, biochemistry or morphological changes of brain plasticity. After more than 40 years' experiments and clinical studies, brain plasticity theory was widely accepted by most researchers.

1.1.1.3 The Main Types and Mechanism of Brain Plasticity

CNS plasticity is that the nerve cells possessed with one kind of function can obtain other functions because of body functional requirements and the nervous system can adapt to new demands structurally and functionally through modifying itself. The higher the CNS plasticity is, the stronger the adaptability of the nerve cells is. The higher the CNS plasticity is, the easier the functional recovery after injury is. The experiments demonstrated that brain functional reorganization, enabled minor pathway and synapse sprouting were the significant manifestations of brain plasticity, which play important role in the recovery of the lost motor functions after central lesion [1].

Functional Reorganization of Cortex

When partial tissues responsible for the functional position were injured, the lost functions can transfer to the corresponding parts of contralateral hemisphere. In fact, nerve tissues of contralateral hemisphere replaced the injured nerve tissues because of the intrinsic factor (biological factor) or the external interference (treatment or rehabilitation training). Adjacent nerve tissues of injured parts replaced the injured nerve tissues to recover the lost functions.

Contralateral Transfer

The lost functions could transfer to the corresponding parts of contralateral hemisphere. The functions of the two parts were replaced and compensated each other.

Ipsilateral Functional Compensation

It is thought that cortical cells were not the same-size ratio with their dominant movements. It is a many-to-many way. The functions would not be totally lost even if the CNS cells were damaged. There were still a considerable amount of nerve cells in the periphery of the injured parts. The residual cells could reorganize through the intrinsic factor or the external interference to recover the lost functions.

Enabled Minor Pathway

Every nerve cell in CNS can communicate with other cells through synapses, which become the pathway for neural information conduction. However, most of the pathways are inhibited, dormant or activated alternatively. When the main neural pathway is damaged, the minor pathway will be enabled, but the functional differentiation is not elaborated.

Nerve Sprouting

The soma or proximal synapses that are damaged can lead to soma death. The proximal intact neuronal axons can communicate with targeted nervous tissues through nerve sprouting in order to replace the neuronal axons that lost functions.

Nerve sprouting includes regeneration sprouting and synapse sprouting. Regeneration sprouting means that disappeared synapse can be regenerative, but this kind is seldom. Synapse sprouting is common, which means dendrite or axon of normal neuron sprout to communicate with residual dendrite or axon of injured neurons and replace the lost functions. This is the morphological basis of functional recovery of central lesion, which indicates the functional compensation.

The subtypes of synapse sprouting.

Lateral Sprouting

Lateral sprouting means that there is lateral sprouting in nerve fiber, and then new axon sprouting is formed. Besides, there are new synaptic connection between the terminal and survival neurons or neurons surrounding injured region (see Fig. 1.1a). Lateral sprouting in nerve fiber can replace injured neurons to play roles.

Terminal Sprouting

Terminal sprouting means that there are some extensions in synaptic terminals of dead neurons. There are new synaptic connections between the extensions and normal neurons (see Fig. 1.1b). Terminal sprouting in nerve fiber can replace injured neurons to play roles.

Synapse Sprouting

Synapse sprouting means contact surface of synaptic terminals in dead neurons enlarge to increase the contact points. There are new synaptic connections between the contact surface and normal neurons. Neural information conduction pathway are built and synapse sprouting can replace injured neurons to play roles (see Fig. 1.1c).

In short, in all these three sprouting, there are new synaptic connections between dendrites and axons of dead neurons and normal neurons to replace injured neurons to play roles. Recent research indicated that the phenomenon extensively existed in CNS such as spinal cord, midbrain, cerebrum, epencephalon and thalamus. It is one of the mechanisms that underlie repairing injured neural networks. However, there are still some unsolved questions, such as the factors inducing sprouting and how to control the local condition of sprouting in order to facilitate the functional recovery. It is said that correct functional training (exercise stimulus) can induce sprouting to right direction. Conversely, incorrect functional training will mislead sprouting and hinder functional recovery.

1.1.1.4 Regeneration and Transplantation of Neural Cells

It is stated that neural cells are not regenerative after degeneration. Recent research demonstrated that neural stem cells in CNS had potential ability to differentiate into neurons and neurogliocytes, which was found in culture in vitro. This provided a new approach for treatment of nerve injury and retrogression.

1.1.1.5 Long-Term Potentiation (LTP)

Long-term potentiation means that synapses are in excitatory state for a long time after nervous centralis receive some kind of stimulus, which belongs to functional synaptic plasticity.

The mechanism of LTP may be related to increased presynaptic membrane neurotransmitter. Because LTP can influence synaptic plasticity and transmission efficiency, it is the basis of sensory memory. In addition to normal physiological conditions, LTP changes identically in pathologic conditions. Therefore, it is crucial for rehabilitation treatment, such as "objective-motive" active exercise training under the guidance of Daoyin technique in traditional Chinese medicine according to Meridian. It may be involved in inducing synaptic plasticity of LTP, which provides theoretical foundation for recovering motor functions.

1.1.1.6 Long-Term Depression (LTD)

Depression means the excitability of resting muscle is inhibited in one kind of movement, which guarantees the completion of the movement.

The functional nuclei that regulate muscular tension or coordinate voluntary movement are located in cerebellar cortex. This region is involved in united movement, motor plan and motor program compilation between this region and motor area, sensory area and association area of cerebrum. Through learning exquisite movements, a whole set of motor programs are formed in cerebellar cortex, which are based on local neuronal circuit of epencephalon and can combined with LTD of Purkinje cells. The axons of Purkinje cells are the only efferent fibers in cerebellar cortex, which can inhibit neuronal tonic firing of deep cerebellar nuclei such as roof nucleus, inter nuclei and dental nucleus. Purkinje cells can receive afferent signals simultaneously from climbing fibers and parallel fibers. Because the sensitivity of dendritic side to neurotransmitters is low, the time of the signal from parallel fibers is long. The conduction efficiency is low, which manifests as LTD. This is the characteristic synaptic plasticity of cerebellum.

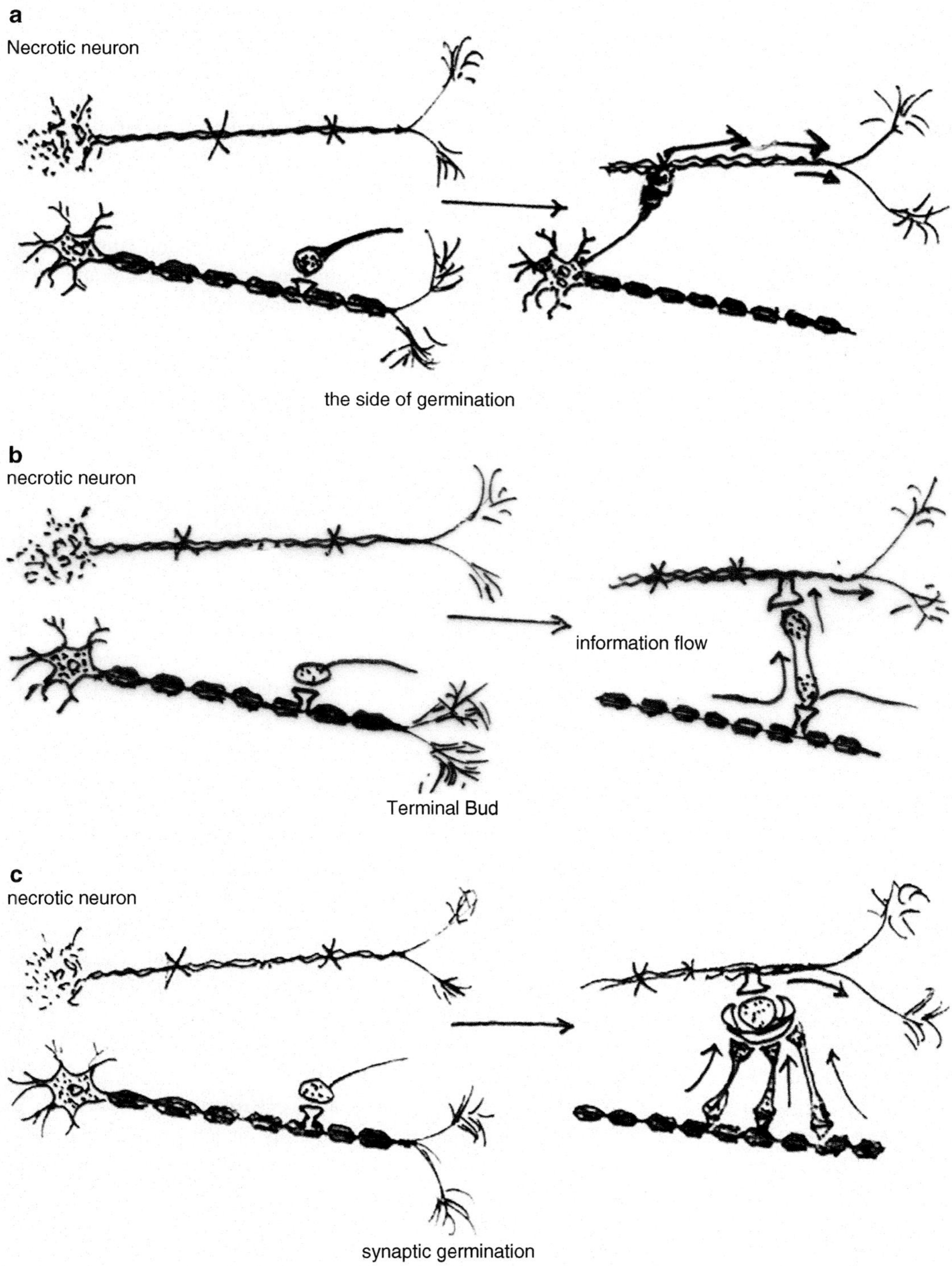

Fig. 1.1 (**a**) Lateral sprouting: new connection between new axons and normal neurons. (**b**) Terminal sprouting: new synaptic connection between new terminal extensions and normal axons. (**c**) Synaptic sprouting: increased contact points in synaptic terminals

The cause of this phenomenon is related to the low sensitivity of dendritic side to neurotransmitters. The reason why the functions of CNS are normal and are not disturbed by hyperexitation is related to LTD of Purkinje cells. This may be the theoretical basis of voluntary exercise therapy for myospasm.

In short, compensation and functional reorganization become the basis of physiology, biochemistry or morphological changes of brain plasticity. The mechanism of brain plasticity is related to neurotomy, neurophysiology, neuropathology, neuroimmunology, neurochemistry and neural electrical activities. For more than two decades, both in animal experiments and in clinical researches, brain plasticity is widely accepted by most researchers. Recently, some researchers pointed that the CNS plasticity conformed to "technical employ and dependence" principle, which meant voluntary exercise that had never been done could promote CNS plasticity. The voluntary exercise could be solidified through repeated training, which could lead to the redistribution and orientation of brain function division.

Therefore, Whether or not rehabilitation techniques to recover the lost functions after central lesion are effective, depend on whether or not the techniques could promote plasticity changes and functional reorganization of CNS and be employed in the voluntary exercise training of limbs dominated by brain. Although simple voluntary exercise training is merely to promote cells surrounding CNS injured area to play roles and replace the lost functions, the new activated cells can transform into cells with practical functions through further complicated training. However, this is the essential and important basis for the motor function recovery.

1.1.2 The State of Applied Rehabilitation Techniques at Domestic and Overseas at Present

Rehabilitation therapy is a new treatment that can facilitate functional rehabilitation in mind and body of patients and the disabled. It is a new technical specialty. Its objectives are to promote patients to recover the abilities of daily life, learning, work, labor and social life as much as possible and improve living quality. Therefore, it can alleviate the burden of family and society and help the patients integrate into society. Rehabilitation therapy includes many contents such as medical, professional, educational and social details. The scope of rehabilitation therapy includes naturopathy, occupational therapy, logotherapy, psychotherapy, rehabilitation engineering and traditional Chinese medicine therapy [2].

In tradition, rehabilitation medicine includes naturopathy and rehabilitation medicine. Physical medicine (physiotherapy) means that physical factors such as sound, light, electricity, magnetism, water, wax and thermodynamics act on human body to play a role in prevention and treatment of diseases through nerves, body fluids and endocrine. We do not discuss physical medicine in this book. Rehabilitation medicine is dependent on functional training to recover the lost functions maximally such as movements, speech, swallow, cognition, vision, defecation control and cardiopulmonary functions.

At present, rehabilitation techniques that were invented in the middle period of last century such as Bobath, Rood, Brunnstrom and so on, were still the main techniques of rehabilitation training at domestic and overseas and played important role in the foundation of medical rehabilitation philosophy and its clinical application. I think that the role of these rehabilitation techniques in promoting CNS plasticity remains unclear. Here are some characteristics and defects of these rehabilitation techniques.

1.1.2.1 Bobath Technique

Bobath technique is a rehabilitation training technique for child cerebral palsy and adult hemiplegia.

Mechanism

Bobath therapy was founded from the study of child cerebral palsy treatment, which based on neurodevelopment principle of exercise. Movement development is dynamic, sequential, from the head end to the tail end and from the proximal to the remote. Before children have consciousness, the movements are voluntary and then become adaptive and responsive.

Operational Approach

Through detailed assessment, the blastocolysis level could be found in sick child by Bobath therapy. In the next moment, the abnormal movements are inhibited and normal movements are promoted according to development sequence in order to recover motor functions ultimately. Therefore, Bobath therapy is also called neural development therapy (NDT). The specific methods are as follows:

Bobath Handshake

The patients are instructed to put the centre of the palm together with fingers crossed. Affected thumb is above unaffected thumb.

Reflex Inhibition Pattern

Hemiplegic paralytic upper limb of adult is passively in different positions such as abduction, extorsion, elbows extension, forearms supination, wrists and fingers stretch.

Key Points of Control

The patients are instructed to focus on the movements of these parts that include proximal parts such as neck, vertebral column, shoulder, pelvis, manubrium and scapula and distal parts such as toes, ankle, fingers and wrist. The abnormal motor pattern and muscle spasm can be changed by the movements of these parts.

Facilitation Technique

The voluntary movements can be induced by reflexes such as righting reflex, Protective reflection, and balance reflex and so on.

Proprioception and Skin Stimulus

The therapists use pat and load bearing to promote muscular tension and motion control.

The Evaluation of Bobath Therapy at Present

Vestibular stimulation method has a good effect on paralysis with sensory deprivation, which means that the patients are instructed to lie on or sit on the treatment ball and the whole body is moved by the therapeutic staff.

Limbs loads and compressing joints have a good effect on the patients.

Motor function recovery after CNS diseases should follow the principle of motor development sequence and the recovery is not mechanical.

It is groundless that the primary cause of the lost functions is low-level reflex release controlled by brainstem and spinal cord.

Some treatment theories proposed by Bobath according to Magnus' study. Magnus' concepts are dominant at that time, but not accepted by neurophysiologists these days. At present, it is thought that sensory afferent has no effect on motor control and the motor control is not dependent on reflex.

The spasm after CNS diseases is not the continuation of primitive reflex but the pathological irradiation of excitation.

It is groundless that head movements can dominate the movements of limbs. The experiments demonstrated that head movements cannot induce the movements of limbs.

In the treatment, both the passive inhibition and promotion exerted by the therapeutic staffs and the voluntary participation of the patients should be advocated.

It is difficulty to recover the motor coordination because of lacking the training without movements in active constrained movements.

1.1.2.2 Brunnstrom Technique

Brunnstrom technique is applied for assessment of paralysis after stroke and rehabilitation training.

Mechanism

Brunnstrom deemed that synergic movements and associative reaction are the inevitable process before normal voluntary movements recovery. This process is a part of the normal processes of functional recovery after stroke. In the early stage of recovery (Stage I to Stage III), the therapeutic staffs should help the patients to control and employ these patterns to acquire some movements. Once the synergic movements can be proceeded voluntarily, through corrective training, the wrong pattern can be got rid of and the normal pattern can be recovered.

The Main Methods of Brunnstrom Technique

Associative reaction, skin and noumenon stimulus can lead to mechanical synergic movements. In the basis of that, through the endeavor of exercise therapist and patients, semi-autonomous synergic movements will be accelerated and then the corrective and artificial training should be proceeded to separation movements.

In Brunnstrom therapy, limbs are used to complete myotatic reflex such as synergic movements, associative reaction, tonic neck reflex, asymmetrical tonic neck reflex, tonic labyrinthine reflex and tonic lumbar reflex with bridge type movements and passive movements. Rehabilitation methods are divided into six stages to induce autokinetic movements.

Assessment of Brunnstrom Therapy at Present

CNS promotion, peripheral and noumenon stimulus are comprehensively applied in Brunstrom method. From synergic movements to separate from synergic movements, it is useful for recovering the functions of limbs, wrists and fingers.

Bridge type movements can help the patients diagnosed of Cerebral Vascular Accident (CVA) to get rid of synergism of lower limbs, which is in favour of recovering the motor functions of lower limbs.

The six stages recovery assessment method of Brunnstrom is used extensively. Fugl—Meyer assessment method in the western world and Ueda Min method in the eastern world evolved from this.

Although Brunnstrom therapy is accepted by neurophysiologists, most rehabilitation therapists do not use it.

Brunnstrom therapy has no active restriction on unnecessary movements in the exercise. Therefore, it is unsatisfactory in recovering coordinative movements.

Although most rehabilitation therapists prefer Bobath therapy to Brunnstrom therapy, precise and long-term research done in 1990s showed that there was no significant difference between Bobath therapy and Brunnstrom therapy in treating adult hemiplegic paralysis.

1.1.2.3 Rood Technique

Mechanism

The basic viewpoint of Rood therapy is that motor pattern is developed from inherent basic reflex pattern. These patterns are constantly modified in usage and sensory stimulus until these patterns has ultimate control in conscious level of cerebral cortex. If proper stimulus is exerted to appropriate receptor, motor response will be induced reflectively and correct motor pattern will be achieved through repeated correct stimulus.

Principal Methods of Rood Technique

Stimulus

Skin and noumenon stimulus are used to facilitate or inhibit muscle contraction.

Load

When bearing load, pressure is given to the joint from two sides of the joint in order to promote deep postural muscle and inhibit muscle spasm.

Exercise

The proximity of burdened limbs is made to do some movements after bearing load.

Motor Control Training

Motor control training is completed according to motor control development sequence in Rood therapy.

The Assessment of Rood Therapy at Present

- The facilitation is conducted through skin stimulus, which is based on neurophysiology.
- The facilitation of freezing and brushing is effective during treatment process and 45–60 s after treatment. The effect of the brushing is better.
- In order to get the satisfying effect, the stimulus time should be long enough, but the effect does not last long after treatment.
- Proprioceptive Neuromuscular Facilitation (PNF) is further developed because of this technique.

- Skin stimulus is given first, and muscle contraction is given to facilitate the effect. It is wrong that the time interval is 30 min, because it is invalid when the time interval is more than 5 min.
- Unnecessary movements are not inhibited in this therapy. Therefore, the good coordinate exercise cannot be recovered.

1.1.2.4 Proprioceptive Neuromuscular Facilitation (PNF)

Mechanism

Research achievements are concluded from neurophysiology, motor learning and motor behavior.

Methods

Proprioceptive stimulus such as stretching, joint compress and traction and imposing resistance, spiral motor pattern and diagonal motor pattern are employed to facilitate motor functions recovery.

The detailed are as follows:

- Spiral and diagonal motor patterns includes 91 kinds of basic motor patterns. Most focus on the training mode that uninjured side movements induce injured side movements.
- Manipulative therapy technique: After stretching, resistance and synergic muscles contraction, antagonistic muscle contraction and motor neuron excitation threshold enhanced by stimulus are employed for suppressive therapy.
- Noumenon and skin stimulus: In PNF, only proper stimulus can induce correct motor direction. Noumenon sensory stimulus is given mainly through right palm. The secondary are skin stimulus such as hairbrush and temperature stimulus. In addition, moderate sound is prone to induce the activity of motor neuron. Soft sound can facilitate stabilization and big sound can facilitate movements.

The Assessments of PNF at Present

Positive Assessments

- True proprioception stimulus is finely used in this method.
- "Control-relax" training can enlarge joint range of motion confined by muscles contraction more rapidly and effectively than passive movements.
- Promotive motor pattern definitely accelerates muscles response.
- "Contraction-relax" and "Control-relax" both can enlarge ipsilateral joint range of motion. However, "Contraction-relax" training also can enlarge contralateral joint range of motion in case of contralateral amyotrophy.
- PNF can definitely increases the flexibility of shoulder, trunk and hamstring muscles.
- PNF can increase the excitability of spinal cord.
- Knees stretching may promote the excitability of vastus lateralis muscles.
- Joint compress transiently enhance the excitability of α spinal cord motor neurons.

Negative Assessments

- Overflow theory is groundless because strong contraction of healthy muscles promotes contraction of badly injured muscles through excitation diffusion.
- Diagonal motor has no promotive effect on quadriceps femoris.
- The theories of Magnus are no longer accepted by neurophysiologists nowadays.
- Similarly, this method cannot inhibit the unnecessary movements in the exercise. Therefore, it is difficult to achieve motor coordination.

1.1.2.5 Motor Relearning Program (MRP)

MRP means that motor functions recovery after central lesion is a relearning process, which takes advantage of learning and motive theory and the results from the research of human movement science and motor skills. On the premise of patients' subjective involvement and cognitive significance, according to information processing theory of motor learning and the method of modern motor learning, the patients are educated in order to recover the motor functions.

CNS is capable of reorganization and adaption. The therapy is a relearning process. Motor learning should be instructed using comprehensive scientific achievements and it is very important to master learn opportunity.

Mechanism Information Processing of Modern Motor Learning Should Be Fully Utilized in Motor Relearning

1. There are three elements in learning that may be used in relearning of stroke patients such as eliminating unnecessary muscle activity, using feedback to modify the movement output and obtaining improvements from practice.
2. There are two key components that must be considered when learning complicated motor skills such as what to learn and how to organize information correctly in order to complete assignments.
3. The importance of cognition should be emphasized. The reasons are as follows:
   (a) Two key components need cognition to be involved.
   (b) In order to recover as soon as possible, the patients should be instructed to recall the exercise and movements before injury in cognition in order to trigger the former and familiar motor program.
   (c) In the relearning, cognition is needed to control the unnecessary muscle movements in case of excessive movements.
   (d) In acquiring complicated motor skills, the cognition process is inevitable.
   (e) Memory is the storage and maintenance of post-learning experience. Learning is the premise of memory and memory is one of the important cognitive functions. Without bad cognition, learned experience and habits are hard to acquire and store.
4. In the early stage of motor skills learning, the patients should be instructed to be highly concentrated to acquire the message needed in processing behavior.
5. Because of the injury, information processing ability is limited. If the amount of information exceeds the ability of the patients, the behavior will break down. Therefore, therapists must control the balance between the mount of the information processing and the processing ability of the patients in order to move to the target step by step.
6. Therapy is not to strengthen the muscle but to enhance the motor control ability.
7. The patients should learn the meaningful daily functional movements but not the motor pattern.
8. Through motor analysis, therapists find the lost key movements of the patients, train the patients pertinently and practice the completed movements. According to the viewpoints of behavioral psychology, the therapists should not expect sudden turn up of complicated behaviors. Until all the details are correct, the final objective can be achieved through a series of staged half steps to move on.
9. The therapists should make full use of feedback, especially vision and verbal feedback, which can make the patients know the results of their behaviors, what is correct and what is incorrect.
10. Open loop training should be promoted, which means exercise should adapt to different circumstances but not confined in certain condition.

Training Methods and Techniques

1. The principles of training: According to the former theories and viewpoints, the principles of training are summarized as follows:
   (a) Even in the stage of totally unable voluntary movements, the patients should be instructed to do spiritual training according to the principles of MRP.
   (b) Before the training or at the beginning of the training, the patients are asked to recall the movements and activity they are able to do before injury in order to trigger the motor program that they mastered before.
   (c) The training should be started immediately after the patients in stable condition in case of extinction of acquired exercise habit and experience without repeated training and the learning of incorrect mode of activity.
   (d) Before training, sports science is used to analyze the detained exercise in order to find the mainly lost movements of the

patients, train them specifically and combine them to the whole functional activities.

(e) The control of the movements should be emphasized but not strengthening the muscle. The patients ought to practice daily functional activities objectively and practically to avoid the designed pattern or impractical training.

(f) In all the trainings, the patients are instructed to suppress unnecessary and excessive movements subjectively.

(g) Verbal tips and vision feedback are enhanced in the training to let the patients to know the results of their behaviors. The patients should be given feedback and encourage because of the correct behaviors. The incorrect behaviors should be modified subjectively and objectively. Therefore, PT technique is brought in.

(h) The training is transferred from subcortex to cortex. In the learning theory, the cognition stage with many mistakes is transferred to associative stage that is connected between external guidance and internal sensation. Finally, it will be transferred to auto-completed autonomous stage subconsciously. The mastered movements can be used in daily life.

2. Four steps of training
   - Analyzing the movements to find the mainly lost movements.
   - Practicing the lost movements.
   - Practicing the functional activities.
   - Transferring learned movements to the functional activities required for daily life.
3. The content of training includes seven aspects.
   - Functional training of upper limbs.
   - Functional training of mouth and face.
   - Training of sitting up at bedside.
   - Sitting balance training.
   - Standing and sitting up training.
   - Standing balance training.
   - Walking training.

The Assessments of MRP at Present

At present, therapists find that the effect of motor relearning program is good. However, there is no strict efficacy comparison between MRP and proprioceptive sensory neuromuscular promotion therapy or traditional exercise therapy. In addition, there is no active restriction on unnecessary movements in this method.

Although these therapies have already been accepted by most therapy centers at home and overseas, which are more and more widely used. However, the different perspectives are present in rehabilitation medicine at home and abroad. Scientists recognized that there were a lot of reserve of CNS cells and synapses and proper training could promote CNS plasticity in order to achieve functional reorganization. Scientists also found that the CNS plasticity and functional reorganization conformed to "skillful use and dependence" principle. At present, these theories are used to explain the mechanism of functional recovery of limbs movements after central lesion, but there is no obvious improvement in rehabilitation methods. Many scholars tried new rehabilitation treatment methods such as motor relearning program and constraint-induced movement therapy. Constraint-induced movement therapy is that uninjured side upper limb of the patients are tied up and are instructed to use injured upper limb to complete a certain movement. Because objective indicator of this method is not precisely quantified movement, exercise therapists can only tell the patients to use injured limbs to complete designed movements. When the patients fail to complete the movements because of the nonfunctional injured limbs, exercise therapists have no other choice. In addition, the patients try many times but still cannot complete the movement, which is thought that this part of functions cannot be recovered and the patients will lose confidence on rehabilitation training. When the patients are able to partly complete the movements and are instructed to complete designed movements required for multi-joint coordination exercise, functions of some paralyzed muscles are required to be compensated by other muscles, which will easily lead to abnormal motor pattern. Because the therapy is lack of pertinent strategy in motor program reconstruction and there is no way to actively confine the unnecessary movements in exercise, abnormal motor pattern will be intensified and will be difficulty to rectify after repeated trainings. Because of these defects, the therapy failed to be applied until now, which was developed in 1920s.

In recent years, some scientists proposed early, voluntary and intensified new rehabilitation theory and highlight the importance of voluntary movements. However, there was no improvement in the methods, which still are lack of the functions of promoting CNS plasticity and reorganization, the consciousness of motor program reconstruction and pertinent methods. Simple strengthening the muscle is the mainly training method, which is totally different from the training of CNS functional reorganization facilitated by motor program reconstruction and motor pattern remodeling. Muscular strength training is one kind of effect trainings and the results weakens or even disappear after stopping the training. For example, one was trained to lift 100 kg, but he did not lift it 1 year or more after stopping the training. On the contrary, motor program reconstruction training is one kind of established methodologies and its results will keep a long time after stopping the training. For example, once one learned cycling or swimming, he could not forget it 10 years after stopping cycling or swimming, which indicated the importance of CNS functional recovery and motor program reconstruction in rehabilitation therapy.

Motor relearning program was improved and advanced in theory. For example, Motor relearning program did not focus on strengthening muscles, but on motor control. It is necessary to learn the daily functional movements with practical significance and unnecessary movements in verbal and vision feedback and designed exercise but not the motor pattern. For example, without solid basis, there is no good effect when doing motor control and it is difficulty to exert functional movements with practical significance in the condition that it is unable to confine the unnecessary movements. In addition, it is scientific to learn motor pattern, because normal motor pattern is the basis of the daily functional movements with practical significance. For example, if the positions of hitting the ball when playing Ping-Pong game or swimming are not correct, it is hard to obtain good achievements and will influence the development from now on.

Rehabilitation methods are based on theory of traditional Chinese medicine, such as acupuncture and moxibustion, massage, cord embedding, main and collateral channels stimulus and Chinese herbal medicine. Modern medicine demonstrated that there were some certain regulating effects and rehabilitation efficacy in Chinese medicine rehabilitation therapy. Doctors of all dynasties summarized predecessor's experience and replenished and developed it in many different ways. There are a lot of content which are worth learning and promotion. It is closely related to modern psychotherapy, physical exercise therapy, naturopathy and information therapy and there is similarity between them, which is regarded as the comprehensive application of these therapies. From the origination, Chinese medicine rehabilitation therapy has close connection with Chinese traditional culture. Especially in the inheritance, the various factions summarized, replenished and developed it. The theory is extensive and profound, but inescapably mysterious, which is lack of definite concept. The principles are subjective abstract. Therefore, the application of Chinese medicine rehabilitation therapy is under restrictions. In addition, there is no objective indicator in the therapy and it is difficulty to be proved in basic research for application. Therefore, it is hard to be promoted in clinical rehabilitation.

In conclusion, it has been recognized that applied rehabilitation methods has no effect on promoting CNS functions recovery. Therefore, the scientists started to study the rehabilitation methods that can promote CNS functions reorganization. Although there is no improvement in specific methods and there are lack of ideas and specific methods to correct abnormal motor program and reconstruct normal motor program, the new "early, voluntary and intensified" rehabilitation is proposed. The importance of the rehabilitation is from voluntary movements to promoting CNS functions reorganization. Consequently, motor program reconstruction and CNS functions reorganization are important research directions of rehabilitation methods in the future.

Moreover, in the research and development of rehabilitation training equipment, there are many kinds of equipment, which is a general tendency to automation, large-size, complication and expensiveness. However, the equipment major in passive movements that means equipment helps people to do some movements and the movements substitution effect is strong, which go against the theory that CNS plasticity is based on the mechanism of skillful use and dependence. The equipment not only cannot actively recover the lost functions, but also bring out movements substitution effect, which will lead to muscle disuse and function decline, exactly as the case that special troops are capable of developing their potential and extraordinary abilities through scientific and tough training in specified conditions. The more automatic the rehabilitation equipment is, the stronger the movements substitution effect is and the weaker the effect of promoting CNS functions reorganization is. Therefore, it is more and more hopeless to recover the lost motor functions.

1.2 Theoretical Basis of Neurological Training Rehabilitation

The process of human movements is that the muscles orderly dominated by lower nerve center that is controlled by motor program of cortex motor center involved in joint motion contract and relax successively to generate coordination exercise and then complete specific functions. Motor pattern is the fundamental form for achieving the abilities of daily life. It can dominate muscles to complete multi-joint coordination exercise under the joint coordination of many axoneures. Motor program in the cortex motor center is the basis of motor pattern. High quality of human functional activities is dependent on the correct motor pattern. The formation of motor program is partly related to inherited development tendency, but most of them are acquired through learning.

Under the limitation of CNS cells regeneration, the lost motor functions after injury are mainly dependent on cells surrounding the injured are and are replaced by reserved signaling pathways, which mean that CNS plasticity is induced to achieve functional reorganization. Large CNS cells reserves are the basis of CNS plasticity and functional reorganization. The plasticity changes conform to the "skillful use and dependence" principle. Individually, only new voluntary movements (undone movements and unlearned movements) can lead to CNS plasticity and functional reorganization.

The training to recover lost motor functions after central lesion was divided in two stages (acute stage and chronic stage) and three steps. The principle is in order of difficulty and progressive. The first is to achieve CNS plasticity, which means inducing the activities of reserved nerve cells adjacent to injured area and starting to use reserved neural signaling pathway to replace the functions of injured nerve cells. During this process, "objective and motive", encourage and voluntary movements in imminent danger with protection play important roles, which are good methods and process to develop CNS potential. The motor program of joint motion dominated by brain is in real-time display when the patients do some joint movements. Subsequently disordered motor program can be corrected and normal motor program can be reconstructed through "objective and motive" mechanism, which are the essential part for the coordination of new activated neurons. Realizing coordinative movements of motor functions is based on reconstructing the motor program of joint movements. Proper exercise, constraining the model exercise without active movements and "objective and motive" mechanism are the effective methods for remodeling of motor pattern. The correct motor pattern is the premise and basis of activity of daily living and life quality improvement.

1.2.1 CNS Potential Development

The fundamental method to recover the lost functions after central lesion is to promote CNS plasticity in order to achieve functional reorganization through rehabilitation methods. The CNS plasticity conform to the principle "skillful use and dependence", which means voluntary limbs movements dominated by brain are able to promote CNS plasticity. The nature of rehabilitation methods is dependent on this. Rehabilitation training methods that conform to this principle are effective methods. Conversely, rehabilitation training methods that do not conform to this principle may have poor effect on therapeutic effect such as the training method major in passive movements.

Some experiments showed that there were plasticity changes in CNS. After craniotomy, electrostimulation was used to find the region responsible for the thumb flexion in the motor cortex of monkey and the region was removed. After the surgery, the ability of the thumb flexion was lost. However, 10 days after surgery, the power of gripping recovered to 90% of normal functions through training, which indicated that the functions of brain region responsible for the thumb flexion were replaced by that of other region. After the second craniotomy, the new cortex region responsible for the thumb flexion was found, which was located around the removed brain region in last surgery. The new cortex region responsible for the thumb flexion was removed and the ability of the thumb flexion was lost again. The power of gripping recovered through training, which indicated that the functions of new brain region responsible for the thumb flexion were replaced by that of other region. In order to exclude the possibility that the functional recovery is due to contralateral cortex compensation, after the surgery and before functional recovery, contralateral cortex region responsible for the thumb flexion was removed and the functions recovery of the thumb flexion dominated by original removed brain region was not influenced. These results further indicated that the functions of the original removed brain region were replaced by the adjacent brain region but not the contralateral cortex compensation.

Some scientists confirmed that one hemisphere can be compensated by the other hemisphere. One hemisphere of the monkey was removed, contralateral limbs were paralyzed, but the functions of contralateral paralyzed limbs were recovered again. These results indicated that uninjured side hemisphere replace the removed brain region to function, which was called contralateral transfer of brain functions.

Large CNS cells and signaling pathways reserves are the histological basis of CNS plasticity and potential ability. Inducing the functions of reserved CNS cells and signaling pathways is the basis of CNS functional reorganization. This training method can be used to develop CNS potentials.

CNS potentials should be developed under specific circumstance and using particular methods. The development of CNS potentials under natural conditions is limited. It is crucial that which kind of methods can induce the potential of human body to compensate the lost functions. At present, the development of human body potential focused on athletics, aerospace, work abilities and child intelligence development, which was seldom applied in medicine. English medical scientists in 1920s used constraint-induced movement therapy to promote the functions of paralyzed upper limbs in stroke patients. Uninjured side limbs were tied up and the patients were instructed to complete the designed movements using injured limbs. After a period of time, there was certain improvement in the functions of the injured limbs. If the patients are instructed to complete successive and complicated whole movements such as holding teacup, combing, fastening buttons and seating belt, which means the objective indicator of these movements is not exactly quantified, the physical therapists can only ask the patients to complete designed movements using injured limbs. However, if the patients cannot complete the movements because of the injured limbs, the physical therapists have no other therapies. In addition, the patients try many times but still cannot complete the movements. They will lose confidence and think that the functions cannot be recovered. If the patients are able to partly complete designed movements and are instructed to complete a designed movement required multi-joint coordination exercise, abnormal motor pattern will be induced because of the replacement of paralyzed muscles by other muscles. There is no pertinent method to reconstruct normal motor program. Therefore, abnormal motor pattern can be intensified and is difficulty to correct after repeated trainings. Because of these defects, the therapy has not been widely promoted and applied up to now.

The question is that which kind of methods can quickly induce the potential of human body to compensate the lost functions. In normal life, people can overcome difficulties and hardships using willpower. In dangerous condition, people can get through the difficulties through bursting into extraordinary ability. In specified conditions, tough training can lead a person to be a superman, such as the training of special troops of liberation army. These examples showed that human potentials can be induced through dangerous conditions such as willpower, goal, stimulus, misfortune, disaster and accident. These factors can promote the development of human potentials. The human potentials mainly are CNS potentials, because all the muscles are dominated by CNS. However, patients with hemiplegia and brain paralysis always have serious protopathy, such as hypertension, diabetes and heart disease. Therefore, under imminent danger, train may worsen the condition. Obviously, under imminent danger, the potentials development training cannot simply be employed in the rehabilitation of patients with central lesion.

Traditional rehabilitation methods mainly focus on passive movements. In training, there is no specific target of competition. Lack of "objective and motive" mechanism influences the effect of neuronal potentials development. For example, a high jumper practices high jump without cross-bar elevation. It is hard for him to increase the altitude of the jump. The cross-bar is the indicator of new jump altitude on the basis of training achievement in last jump. In order to jump over the new altitude, the high jumper needs to adjust mood, run-up speed, take-off distance, ground force and throw-over gesture to develop jump potential adequately. Then the jump altitude will be increased gradually. Passive movements are unable to develop potential.

Therefore, the patients should be enlightened and motivated to complete goal-oriented single movement, which is worth studying and looking for. In the process of movement completion, imminent danger condition without real threat will be constructed to develop CNS potential and recover the lost functions of the patients. In imminent danger, the patients are instructed to do goal-oriented voluntary movement, which is the good method for recovering the lost functions. Repeated trainings can transfer the functions in imminent danger into daily life abilities at ordinary times.

Regulation of movements based on regulation of mind and regulation of breathing is the basic technique of Daoyin technique in traditional Chinese medicine. The speech in Daoyin technique is able to enlighten and motivate human willpower commendably, which construct a safe "imminent danger" condition for functional rehabilitation. In modern opinion, the patients are instructed to concentrate to complete a designed movement and during this the therapists use Daoyin speech to create a condition of imminent danger, such as "Stand up, or you will fall down", "Hold up your body or you will crash" and so on. The therapists should encourage the patients maximally to complete the designed movements. When the movement is in the peak or holding weights, the patients should use willpower to hang on several seconds, such as "Hold on, 1, 2 and 3, you did great", "Hold on, 4, 5 and 6" and so on. In this process, the brain potential will be fully developed and utilized.

It must be emphasized that potential development is not muscular strength training but muscles capability training involved in joint motion dominated by CNS, which means that the functions of injured area are replaced by the nervous tissue surrounding the injured area through training. There is significant difference between recovering CNS functions and strengthening muscles.

1.2.2 Motor Program Reconstruction

Every movement of human body is dependent on the electrical signal from brain cells to muscles to drive and control. The signals are sent successively according to a certain proportion, such as

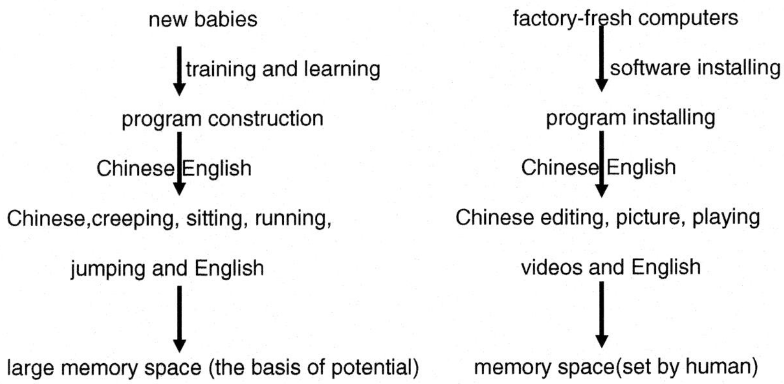
new babies
training and learning
program construction
Chinese English
Chinese,creeping, sitting, running,
jumping and English
large memory space (the basis of potential)
factory-fresh computers
software installing
program installing
Chinese English
Chinese editing, picture, playing
videos and English
memory space(set by human)

Fig. 1.2 The differences between human brain and computer

motor program. Motor program makes the human movements coordinative and orderly and makes it able to complete some certain movements. After central lesion, motor program will be damaged to varying degrees, because the formation of motor program is based on cells and signaling pathways. Damage of motor program can lead to motor dysfunction and abnormal motor pattern, which has a strong impact on life quality of the patients. In the process that CNS plasticity promotes functional reorganization and motor functions recovery, it is far from enough to develop CNS potential. It is essential to use methodology to make these new activated nerve cells function coordinately and orderly, which is the process of reconstructing motor program. Therefore, development of brain potential and reconstruction of normal motor program is the key of functional recovery after central lesion.

The motor programs of human cortex motor center are from two ways. The first is congenital, which is inherited from ancestors. Although it contributes seldom to the motor program, it can be used to obtain functions such as daily essential motor program including standing, walking, running and jumping. The second is acquired. Most of the motor programs are acquired through training. These motor programs must be constructed through learning and training after birth such as the specialized motor programs including swimming, cycling and somersault.

The nature of motor program is electrical signal orderly from cortex motor center to muscles involved in joint motion or multi-joint associated movement. If we compare human cortex motor center with computer, it is easy to understand what is motor program (Fig. 1.2). We found that there were many similarities between new born babies and factory-fresh computers. The factory-fresh computers have no functions but software installing. Unless you installed all kinds of software, you will not use the functions of the computer such as editing, reading pictures and playing videos. If the software is in English version, you can only edit English. If the software is in Chinese version, you can only edit Chinese. If the software is in Chinese-English version, you can switch the languages smoothly.

New born babies have nothing to do but sucking the breast, crying and screaming, defecating and flapping and kicking aimlessly, but the computer is able to learn and memorize just like the brain of babies. In the growing process of babies, it is easy to learn to sit up, creep and stand up. One year after birth, babies can learn to walk, run and jump. This is a process that a series of motor programs are constructed and perfected in the cortex motor center. Therefore, every voluntary movement should be dominated by motor program in cortex motor center. Voluntary motor pattern is dependent on the motor program is perfect or not.

Another example of daily motor program is robot. Robot is made from imitating human. In short, robot is composed of mechanical device, electromotor, power and Central Processing Unit (CPU). The software in CPU is the motor program of robot. The power turns the electromotor rotate and the rotation of the electromotor makes mechanical device function regularly.

And then the robot can be able to complete the designed movements. The key of this process is the motor program in CPU. Robot is less flexible than human and don't do some movements like human, because the software in robot is not the same perfect and precise as the motor program in human cortex motor center. However, this is a good example to demonstrate that there is motor program in human cortex motor center.

From above, we can conclude that what is motor program. Motor program in human cortex motor center is the same as computer program, which is a process that numerous motor neurons are instructed optionally or involuntarily to work coordinately and the electric signals are sent successively to muscles (initiative muscle, antagonistic muscle, synergistic muscle and neutralized muscle) involved in joint motion to varying degrees in order to complete muscle contraction, joint motion or multi-joint synergic movement essential for individual functions appropriately and opportunely.

After central lesion, the damage of motor program will lead to functions loss to varying degrees. Entire damage of motor program will lead to total functions loss. Some motor functions will be retained in part damage of motor program. Because the reserved signaling pathways between nerve cells are absent and the decreased synergistic effects of nerve cells lead to dyskinesia or abnormal motor pattern to varying degrees, the motor functions can be recovered through normal motor program reconstruction.

CNS of new born babies may be influenced by evolution of species, but has a tendency to develop naturally, which means that the abilities required for the survival of the species can be obtained through normal training. This is not always the case in reality, because the obtained functions tend to have a certain defect when it is not trained scientifically. In general conditions, human know nothing about whether their motor program is correct or incorrect. People may do not realize or understand why normal people have defects of motor pattern, because there are no tests and comparisons. The defects of motor pattern will lead to significant difference of motor abilities among individuals. For example, people are able to run, but there are significant differences of speed, duration and distance among individuals. This may be related to accuracy degree of running pattern. The formation of motor pattern is dominated by motor program in cortex motor center. The walking pattern of most people may be incorrect, because the degree of wear indicates the abnormal motor pattern. For example, someone's outside shoes wear out more quickly than others. Someone's inside shoes wear out more quickly than others. Moreover, heels of someone's shoes wear out more quickly than others. In addition, pigeon-toed and out-toeing walking pattern are abnormal motor pattern. If the abnormal motor patterns of these people can be corrected through scientific training, the athletic ability and performance will be increased.

Long-term abnormal motor patterns are caused by some reason such as restricted or compensatory abnormal motor patterns induced by muscle paralysis, joint damage or skeletal abnormality and related lesions. Long-term abnormal motor patterns can lead to formation of abnormal motor program in cortex motor center, which is the construction of abnormal motor pattern in rehabilitation medicine. Therefore, motor functions loss or abnormal motor functions induced by central lesion should be corrected through constructing normal motor programs on the basis of reconstructing or correcting disordered motor programs.

If the motor program has been constructed in cortex motor center and the cortex is damaged, there are differences between motor program reconstruction and the construction of motor program of new born babies. The brain of new born babies likes a blank sheet with natural development tendency, so the motor program is easy to be constructed. If the motor program has been constructed in cortex motor center and the cortex is damaged, it is difficulty to reconstruct the motor program, which is related to that the original signaling pathway is damaged. Like driving a nail into a plank, if the nail is driven slantingly, it is difficulty to be driven into the plank again after the nail is pulled out. Moreover, non-viable and non-apoptotic cells will influence the new intercellular signaling pathways. Therefore, reconstruction of normal motor program should be based on actual condition of abnormal motor program and be completed through targeted and repeated training.

The time spent in reconstructing motor program is related to evolution extent of species. The higher the evolution extent of species is, the longer reconstructing motor program takes, and the vice versa. For example, sheep can learn to walk and run several hours after birth, meanwhile people take a year or more to learn to walk and run. Therefore, reconstruction of human motor program is a relative long process. The patients are instructed on purpose to be trained in order to promote reconstruction of normal motor program. Ultimately, through repeated practical applied training, the motor program can be consolidated. Based on the fact, the course of rehabilitation training should take a lifelong time. If the patients want to be recovered within few days in hospital, it will have a strong impact on the therapy effect and destroy the patients' confidence.

However, how to construct the motor program in human brain?

In daily life, there is a truth that archery athlete aims at arrow target to practice archery so that degree of accuracy in archery can be increased. Otherwise, the degree of accuracy in archery cannot be increased without target. This is because archery is a motor program that is constructed in cortex motor center. Through repeated practice, the archery skill will be promoted continuously. When archery athlete aims at arrow target to practice archery, the first arrow may be shoot in the above of the bull's-eye. The archery result is sent to the brain and the brain will analyze numerous factors (altitude of arrow target, distance, wind direction, bow weight, arrow weight, arm strength and emotion) comprehensively. After calculation, the gesture of the second arrow can be decided such as lowering the arrowhead. The second arrow may be shoot in the below of the bull's-eye. The archery result is sent to the brain and the brain will know the arrowhead is too low. The gesture of the third arrow can be decided such as raising the arrowhead. The third arrow is shot in the bull's-eye. After repeated training, the speed and accuracy of the movements are controlled precisely by the brain so that the speed and accuracy of the movements will be increased. During this process, arrow target is the subjective indicator for illustration and feedback, which make the brain know the mistake, rectify it timely and set clear objective. Therefore, arrow target is essential external conditions for increasing the degree of accuracy in archery and constructing archery motor program. After repeated training, the motor program is consolidated.

The archery example showed that before reconstructing motor program, the motor program signals are transmitted real-timely from brain to muscles involved in joint motion during the process of voluntary movements. According to the practical condition of motor program, abnormal motor program can be rectified and normal motor program can be reconstructed.

1.2.3 Motor Pattern Remodeling

The development of CNS potential and reconstruction of motor program are not equal to practical motor functions. Through practical applied training, the motor functions can be transformed to daily life abilities. Just like a martial artist, the actual combat ability cannot be obtained merely through basic skills such as standing exercise, strength and speed training and martial arts repertoire such as shaolin boxing and Hung Ga. Only after basic skills and martial arts repertoire training, practical skill and tactic capability can be increased through exchanging experiences or fighting.

In the motor relearning program technique, the training of daily life practical functional activities should be emphasized, but not the designed patterns or impractical training. However, normal motor pattern is the best form for human to function. Abnormal motor pattern will influence the functions to varying degrees. Besides, the movements under long-term abnormal motor pattern can lead to complications. For example, the patients with hemiplegic circle gait have walking limitation, slow speed, increased energy consumption and falling injuries. Besides, walking under long-term hemiplegic circle gait may lead to disuse of hip flexors, bone and joint disease, pelvic obliquity and postural malformation, which have a strong impact on walking abilities and functions.

Normal motor patterns provide important guarantee for efficient functions and improvement of life quality. For example, in table tennis, method of holding tennis racket and posture of hitting the ball can directly decide the accuracy and quality of hitting the ball. The key points of deciding the accuracy are covering the ball using racket in 400 and swing of the racket to the direction of apex nasi. The waist drives the upper limbs to hit the ball, which is the key point of deciding the quality. Therefore, we can conclude the importance of normal motor pattern.

Motor program and motor pattern interact with each other and supplement each other. Motor pattern is the external manifestation of the motor program in cortex motor center. Motor pattern is dependent on motor program. Abnormal motor program definitely leads to abnormal motor pattern. On the contrary, abnormal motor pattern may lead to abnormal motor program through CNS plasticity. Therefore, after the construction of motor program, normal motor must be constructed in order to guarantee the normal function of motor program.

During the construction of motor program or after that, the keys of normal motor pattern remodeling are seizing the moment of motor pattern training and limiting the unnecessary movements in exercise.

The modes of abnormal motor pattern can be divided into three classes, such as abnormal motor pattern of upper limbs, abnormal motor pattern of trunk and abnormal motor pattern of lower limbs. Abnormal motor pattern of lower limbs indicates abnormal gait. At present, there are few methods to prevent and correct abnormal gait. The common methods include placing in good limbs position at early stage, constraint of walking out of bed, standing on correction board for foot drop, strephenopodia and strephexopodia, adorning orthotics, Bobath technique, Body Weight Support Treadmill Training (BWSTT) and the gait training instructed by the speech of exercise therapists [3]. Some reports showed that these methods have improvement effect on recovering walking abilities of hemiplegic patient and gait symmetry. There is no specific indication for these methods. Besides, corrective function of abnormal gait is decreased because the unnecessary movements in exercise cannot be constrained effectively. In addition, there is no constraint of exercise after training in all these methods. Out of training room, most patients still walk as original motor pattern, which is bad for decreasing the excitability of cortex abnormal motor center that means abnormal motor program cannot be rectified and there is no way to rectify the abnormal motor pattern. For example, a tobacco addict wants to quit smoking. In smoking cessation room, some methods are used to explain the smoking perniciousness to the smokers, but the tobacco addiction cannot be cut out after treatment, just as smoking habit and smoking desire.

In addition, there are short of dedicated device for gait training at home and abroad. Some scientists deemed that gait analysis system was an ideal gait assessment and training mode, but gait analysis system was only used for detecting gait, which provided scientific basis for clinical diagnosis and therapeutic regimen making. Gait analysis system was an equipment to assess the effect of gait training. When it was used for gait training, it had an impact on therapeutic effect because the unnecessary movements in exercise cannot be constrained effectively.

Training methods of preventing and rectifying abnormal gait at home and abroad at present are summarized, but the therapeutic effect is not entirely satisfactory. The reason is related to several factors:

- There is no systematic rehabilitation method for preventing and rectifying abnormal gait.
- The unnecessary movements in exercise cannot be constrained effectively, which is bad for reconstructing normal gait.
- There are no specific indications and contraindication of existing gait training methods.

- It is short of training equipment for rectifying abnormal gait and reconstructing normal gait.
- After training, the patients walk as original motor pattern and the excitability of abnormal motor center cannot be decreased, which is bad for constructing normal motor pattern.

The defects mentioned above have a strong impact on preventing and rectifying abnormal gait. Moreover, there are the same defects and deficiencies in preventing and rectifying abnormal motor pattern of upper limbs and trunk.

Considering that there is close connection between motor pattern and motor program, on the basis of rectifying abnormal motor pattern, it is an essential step to do the training of normal motor pattern remodeling. It is a step and target for rehabilitation training that must be taken seriously. During this process, except the designed restrictive targeted functional movements, functional movements training required for daily life should still be done and the unnecessary movements in exercise should be constrained effectively. After training, the patients should practice the movements maintained for a long time in daily life and restraint the unnecessary movements themselves.

1.3 The Principle and History of Daoyin Technique in Traditional Chinese Medicine (TCM)

1.3.1 The Principle of Daoyin Technique in Traditional Chinese Medicine

Daoyin technique in traditional Chinese medicine is an entirely voluntary movement on the basis of regulation of the mind and breathing, which integrate mind guidance, breath adjustment and body movement. It can regulate qi and blood, unblock the channel, coordinate viscera and recover body function, which is health maintenance and rehabilitation method of self-training. It was widely used in health maintenance and rehabilitation.

1.3.2 The History of Daoyin Technique in Traditional Chinese Medicine

The history of Daoyin technique in Chinese traditional medicine is very long, which can date back to the Spring and Autumn Period and the Warring States Period or even earlier time. Since the modern times, Daoyin technique in Chinese traditional medicine was seldom applied to clinic, but it was widely used in health maintenance such as five-animal boxing, eight trigrams boxing and Qigong, a system of deep breathing exercises. The ancient Daoyin technique in Chinese traditional medicine was able to spread in the world permanently, which had their reasons and practical application value. It is worth further researching and developing. Especially, there is a possibility that it can be used for modern rehabilitation clinic and benefiting the disabled and should be discussed deeply.

Some scientists deemed that Daoyin technique in Chinese traditional medicine originated from dance, which referred to the Old Stone Age at the earliest. It was closely related to later traditional therapies such as Daoyin, massage with hands and foots and traditional Chinese manipulation. The chapter of ancient music in *Mister Lv's Spring and Autumn Annals* was written in 239 A.D. The book recorded the dance with pertinent movements designed by tribal chiefs. The dance can regulate qi and blood, move muscles in exercise or work and resist lower limbs swelling, hindered joint motion and abasia induced by moisture. Therefore, in order to treat some rheumatism sore pain disease, the dance was used to regulate qi and blood to alleviate the disease. Daoyin was to move muscles and joints in exercise or work, which derived from dance movement. The early explanation of Daoyin was made by Wang Bing in Tang Dynasty who said "regulate qi in order to make your body peaceful and stretch your body in order to make it flexible".

Daoyin technique in the chapter of intention in Zhuangzi was called Taoyin. The ancient people thought it could free spirits and qi, keep fit and even prolong life. "exhale and inhale, exhale the old and inhale the new, stretch body like bears and birds. The people who did Daoyin and kept fit loved this, so did Peng Zu (The god of longevity in the ancient). This sentence depicted people who kept in good health liked to exhale the old and inhale the new with abdominal respiration and stretch body like bears and birds.

Because of the important effect of Daoyin in health care, after many weary centuries, Daoyin technique was developed slowly and was spread up to now with indomitable vitality. It got a great development and was applied to rehabilitation. In different dynasties, medical practitioners comprehended and applied Daoyin technique differently. However, in overall, it was upward developed slowly.

In the classics of traditional Chinese medicine Huangdi's Internal Classics during Qin and Han dynasty, several therapeutic methods are summarized, which derived from the ancient times and were effective. Daoyin was on the top of these methods. Daoyin technique was described as moving bones and joints in exercise or work in the book Suwen. Daoyin technique was used to treat callousness (symptoms of some diseases) in the book Lingshujing. If Daoyin technique was assisted with fire needle stimulation of ashi acupuncture point, it could recover sensory function. On the basis of hot compress and oral administration of medicine, if Daoyin technique was assisted with limbs exercise that can promote the circulation of qi, it can alleviate joints, soften ligaments and regulate heart and blood, which indicate the role of Daoyin technique in joint motion.

The book Synopsis of Golden Chamber written by Zhang Zhongjing in the Eastern Han Dynasty showed that Daoyin technique could promote the circulation of qi and blood and open the nine orifices in order to prevent diseases. When the limbs cannot be moved smoothly, Daoyin technique, expiration and inspiration, acupuncture and moxibustion and massage with paste preparation were used to open the nine orifices.

So far, the earliest book about Daoyin technique was Yinshu unearthed from Han dynasty tombs in Zhangjiashan Hubei province in 1983, which was written in the middle and late period of Warring States before 221 B.C. So far, the earliest book about illustration of Daoyin technique was Daoyintu unearthed from Mawangdui Han Dynasty Tomb in Changsha Hubei province in 1973 (Fig. 1.3). There is close connection between Yinshu and Daoyintu. Daoyintu illustrated Daoyin technique in the book Yinshu.

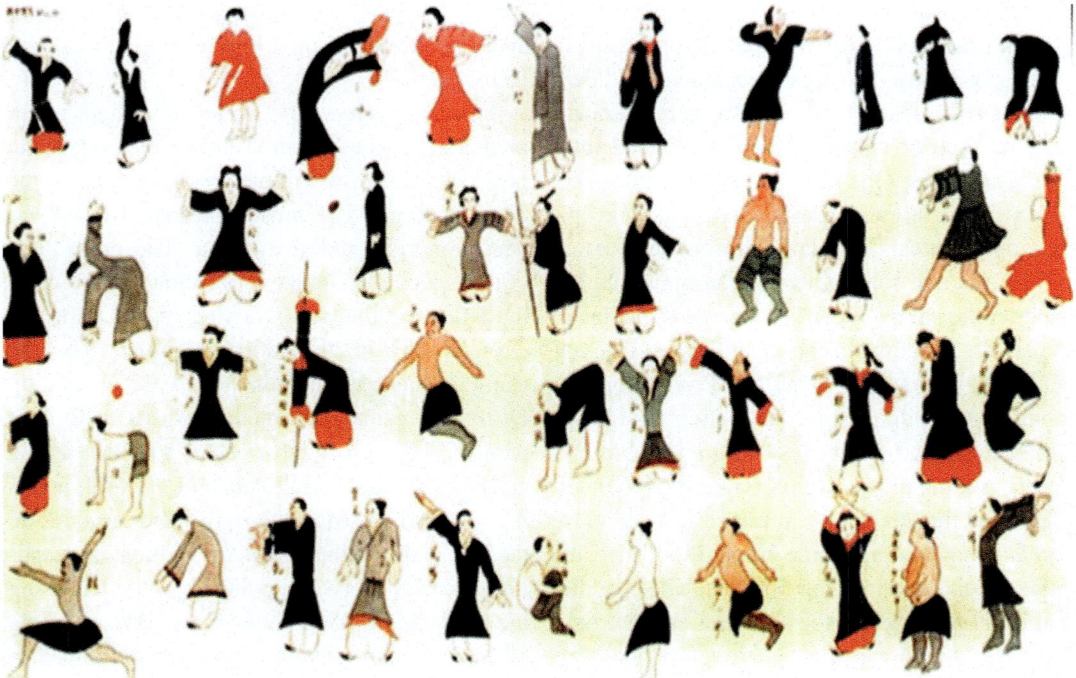

Fig. 1.3 Daoyintu unearthed from Mawangdui Han Dynasty Tomb in Changsha Hubei province in 1973

Operational methods include 68 kinds of Daoyin technique modes and 41 kinds of Daoyin therapeutic methods. *Daoyintu* illustrated Daoyin technique, which included 44 pictures. The pictures are different, which are divided into empty-handed and instrument-handed pictures. All of the pictures show whole movements with erect position.

In the clinic, the applications of Daoyin technique in different dynasties were not the same. For example, Daoyin technique to recover upper limbs functions in *Yinshu* is that uninjured side hands are used to grasp the injured side hands to stretch it towards the head. It can improve joint motion of injured side upper limbs and alleviate adhesion between muscles and joints to promote functional recovery. However, in the view of operation mode, it is a passive movement for the injured limbs. In fact, this is one part of the Daoyin technique. There are many operation modes in Daoyin technique, which are all voluntary movements good for functional recovery of lower limbs.

General Treatise on the Cause and Symptoms of Diseases [4] was written in 610 B.C. (Sui Dynasty), Daoyin technique was recorded to treat hemiplegia. Standing against the wall, holding the breathing and promoting the circulation of qi from head to foot are the specific procedures, which can be used to treat subcutaneous ulcer, hemia, stroke, hemiplegia and wandering arthritis. This type of technique can be divided into several subtypes. One subtype is that keeping the back straight, stretching foots and fingers, keeping mind calm, and entraining qi from head to ten toes of foot and soles. Qi can be confined in the center of the palm. Qi can be entrained from head to plantar Yongquan acupoint. This is Daoyin technique in standing position. Promoting the circulation of qi, inspire and expire slightly, inspire more and expire less with silent breathing are the main procedures. The circulation of qi is called that Qi can be entrained from head to plantar Yongquan acupoint. In addition, there is Daoyin technique in lying position. The specific method is making the toes upward and holding breathing, which can treat pain or numbness of waist and back, hemiplegia and make the ear hear something. The five sense organs (ears, eyes, lips, nose and tongue) should be often practiced in order to prevent diseases. This type of Daoyin technique can be used for rehabilitation training of the patients with conscious mind and stable condition. This is the precedent that early rehabilitation was used for preventing complications and promoting functional recovery.

During Song-Jin-Yuan Dynasty, Daoyin technique was developed for practice. One of the characteristics was that various kinds of Chinese meditations were developed on the basis of precedent Daoyin techniques. The book twenty-four Chinese meditations Daoyin techniques healing pictures wrote by Chen Tuan in Song Dynasty (A.D. 989), divided Chinese meditation into 24 kinds of movements and named them separately according to the 24 solar terms on the basis of correspondence between man and universe, five elements' motion and six kinds of natural factors and main and collateral channels theory. Every kind of methods based on viscera used Daoyin techniques to circulate main and collateral channels in order to prevent the diseases dominated by 12 meridians. Chinese meditations Daoyin techniques were definitely based on main and collateral channels theory for the first time, which had a great promoting effect on the development and enhancement of Chinese ancient Daoyin techniques.

Daoyin techniques included Slight heat method, Great heat method and the methods in the book Zhu Xian Daoyin pictures according to the 24 solar terms. The most representative method was immortal guiding method. The procedures of this specific method are as follows: pointing to the left using the hand, looking on the right and circulating Qi in 24 breaths; pointing to the right using the hand, looking on the left and circulating Qi in 24 breaths. This method was used to treat paralysis. The procedures of this specific method are as follows: standing, left foot forward, pointing to the right using the right hand, looking on the left and circulating Qi in 24 breaths; standing, right foot forward, pointing to the left using the left hand, looking on the right and circulating Qi in 24 breaths. This method was employed to circulate main and collateral channels and ease joint movement, which was known as one of the most effective methods for treating hemiplegia in ancient times.

Daoyin techniques in Qing Dynasty were simple and practical. The most representative Daoyin technique "Fen Xing Wai Gong Jue" was introduced in the book Shou Shi Chuan Zhen wrote in 1771. The procedures of this method are as follows: stand up, walk slowly, hold firmly with two hands; left foot forward, left hand swing forward and right hand swing back; right foot forward, right hand swing forward and left hand swing back; two foots cross forward, move forward dozens of steps and then move back dozens of steps; sit high and stretch the foots, twist the heels inward and then outside for 24 times.

The book dynamic exercise massage recipe was written in 1696 in Qing Dynasty, which combined Daoyin technique and massage to treat diseases. There were many methods such as acupoint selection, massage and Daoyin in this book, which were simple to use and had a unique curative effect on paralysis and chronic low back and leg pain. The correspondent static exercises were sedation, concentration, breathing modulation, licking the palate using tongue tip, omphaloskepsis, breathing slowly, rising the stomach and breathing rhythmically under resting state.

After the combination of dynamic exercise and static exercise, Daoyin techniques were developed to health maintenance and rehabilitation exercise method that could combine association of activity and inertia, association of insides and outsides, regulation of the mind and breathing and body movements.

In the view of modern medicine, Daoyin technique in Chinese is an important method to enlighten and arouse people to complete designed movements. The technique included static exercise with the breathing controlled by OBEs and dynamic exercise with OBEs, breathing and movements (imitation of various kinds of animals). Through regulation of the mind, regulation of breathing and regulation of movements, Daoyin technique could circulate main and collateral channels, regulate qi and blood, harmonize viscera, and strengthen the body resistance to eliminate pathogenic factors, strengthen homeostasis and have favorable influence on body metabolism to recover motor functions.

Modern medicine demonstrated that Daoyin technique was good for the regulation and rehabilitation of cardiovascular diseases, respiratory diseases, nervous system diseases, digestive system diseases and so on [5]. On the basis of precedent experience, doctors of all dynasties supplemented and developed it, which was worth considering and popularized. There are many relationships and similarities between Daoyin technique and modern psychotherapy, physical exercise therapy, naturopathy, information therapy and physiotherapy. Daoyin technique is the comprehensive application of all these therapies.

1.3.3 The Reason of Endangered Daoyin Technique in Traditional Chinese Medicine

From the birth of Daoyin technique, there was a close relationship between Daoyin techniques with Chinese traditional culture, especially during the development process. After the additions and deletions of doctors of all dynasties, the content of the theory was extensive and profound, but was with mystery inevitably, which were lack of definite concept and subjective and abstract. In addition, there are several defects and deficiencies.

From the documents of Daoyin technique in all dynasties, it was a self-exercise method to preserve one's health, which was appropriate for healthy person or sub-health person. It was difficulty to be applied for rehabilitation training of the disabled.

Although it could be applied for rehabilitation training of the diseases, the self-exercise way was its main method. The methods were all the bulk movements with complicated multi-joint movements, especially the 44 Daoyin pictures that were all bulk movements in standing position. It was not suitable for the disabled or the patients with more severe dyskinesia and the range of application was confined.

In the long development of Daoyin technique, there was no special equipment that cooperated with the application of Daoyin technique except some simple appliances such as sticks and swords. Without systematic basic theory and controlled clinical trial, even lack of clinical individual cases and specific objective indicator in treatment, the reliability of therapeutic effect of Daoyin technique was influenced.

In all ages, there were small changes in theories and methods of Daoyin techniques. Daoyin technique was developed slowly even stagnated without the promotion of modern theory of medicine. For these reasons, Daoyin technique was used for life cultivation and health preservation instead of clinical rehabilitation from Ming-Qing dynasty to modern times.

1.3.4 Basic Ideas of Renaissance of Daoyin Technique in Traditional Chinese Medicine

Daoyin technique in traditional Chinese medicine is a basic technique of regulation of movement on the basis of regulation of mind and breathing, which were all voluntary movement dominated by brain through using all the vigor. It was completely in conformity with "skillful use and dependence" principle. It was an important method instructed by modern medical theory to promote CNS plasticity and functional reorganization. Therefore, modernization and renaissance of Daoyin technique in traditional Chinese medicine should combine with modern medical theory form the aspects as follows. On the basis of inheritance of the precedent experience, it would contribute to the development of rehabilitation medicine in our country and even the world.

1. According to the rehabilitation principle from simple to complex, simplified and practical rehabilitation principle, and comprehensive rehabilitation principle, on the basis of inheritance of Daoyin technique in traditional Chinese medicine, through regulation of mind, breathing and movements, single multi-joint movement was transformed to the rehabilitation training technique from simple joint movement to multi-joint movement, which are applied to rehabilitation therapy of the patients with dyskinesia after central lesion.
2. According to the conditions required for clearing and activating the channels and collaterals and developing potential, Daoyin speeches are studied, which can inspire the patients, induce and create endangered circumstance. It is convenient for the therapists to instruct the patients to do rehabilitation training through Daoyin technique.
3. According to objective and motive, biofeedback and motor program theory, combined with advanced rehabilitation methods overseas and modern electronic technique, objective indicator of therapeutic effect of Daoyin technique are made to be in digital display and new rehabilitation therapy of traditional and western medicine is developed with the core technology of Daoyin technique. It is widely applied to rehabilitation training, which not only can reconstruct or enhance single muscle control signal, but also can be involved in reconstruction training of motor program of associated movements participated with several muscles.
4. Except for the motor functional rehabilitation, Daoyin technique in traditional Chinese medicine can be used in rehabilitation training method of other functions such as speech, swallow sphincter, cardio-pulmonary function, and vision, which becomes a series of rehabilitation treatment methods with the core technology of Daoyin technique.
5. A series of controlled clinical trial should be proceeded to demonstrate the therapeutic effect and study the mechanism. The indications and contraindications of Daoyin technique should be investigated to form a normalized and standard instruction, which lay the foundation of long-term development of Daoyin technique.
6. The characteristics of traditional Chinese medicine should be emphasized. We studied Daoyin technique throughout main and collateral channels and Daoyin methods with

virtual simulation through main and collateral channels pictures that are easy to be understood by the patients and to be popularized and applied. We also would verify the therapeutic effect.
7. We will develop the equipment applied for Daoyin technique in traditional Chinese medicine, because the equipment is important measure to ensure the correct methods and therapeutic effect. There are some kinds of training equipment used for developing potentials, reconstructing motor program and remodeling motor pattern of Daoyin technique. There are also some kinds of equipment used for gait training with unnecessary movements in balance training and active restriction movements.

Following the further study and the development of Daoyin technique, the application value will become increasingly higher and the application range will become more and more extensive, which will advance the development of rehabilitation medicine service.

1.4 Electromyographic Biofeedback

1.4.1 The Development History of Electromyographic Biofeedback Technique

The prototype of electromyographic biofeedback technique can be traced back to 1930, when Jacobson developed an instrument which could continuously detect the electromyographic signal, he found that the level of electromyographic signal could be influenced by cognitive activity, and therefore proposed progressive relaxation therapy based on this finding, which could be used for treatment of various mental and physical diseases such as hypertension etc. The modern sense of electromyographic biofeedback appeared in 1960s, Marinacci used electromyographic biofeedback technique to treat peripheral facial paralysis, sequela of polio paralysis and hemiplegia; Harrison and Mortensen used electromyographic biofeedback of the vision and audition signal to enhanced the patient control ability of tibialis anterior; Basmajian exhibited the clinical application of electromyographic technique in the recovery of neuromuscular system, the control of pain and the treatment of headache and so forth. In 1983, Wolf integrated electromyographic biofeedback technique into physical therapy, and used in the treatment of patients with hemiplegia and achieved a landmark result in the research of clinical effect. In the following 1990s and twenty-first century, electromyographic biofeedback technique was widely used in hemiplegia, paraplegia, cerebral palsy, disturbance of sphincter, headache, low back pain, and various wrist-hand functional disorders following the widely use of computer, it has become one of the effective treatments in the field of modern rehabilitation medicine.

1.4.2 The Principle and Clinical Application of Electromyographic Biofeedback Technique

1.4.2.1 Basic Concepts

The Definition of Biofeedback

In 2008, three internationally professional biofeedback organizations defined biofeedback together as follows: biofeedback is a process for the purpose of improving health conditions and functions, which urged individuals to learn how to change physiological activity. It uses delicate instruments to examine a variety of physiological activities including electroencephalogram, cardiac function, respiration, muscular activity, skin temperature, etc. These instruments can feedback this information to users accurately and quickly. The expression of the information often related to the change of thought, emotion, behavior promoted the change of physiological functions towards to the hopeful direction. After a period of training, these changes can be achieved without rely on instruments.

In brief, biofeedback is a method which can transform internal function changes which is unawareness by human beings under normal conditions, such as electromyographic, skin temperature, heart rate, blood pressure and so on, into audio-visual signals which can be awareness, and make patients to learn to control their involuntary functions according to these signals through guidance and self-training, and therefore used for prevention and treatment of diseases or rehabilitation training. To date, it has been reported in the literature that biofeedback has been used in the treatment of dozens of diseases such as tension-type headache, migraine, bronchial asthma, upper digestive tract ulcer, allergic colitis, hypertension, arrhythmia, etc. In the field of modern rehabilitation medicine, it is used in the treatment of cerebrovascular accident, spinal cord injury, cerebral palsy, spasm, flaccid paralysis, muscle disuse atrophy, pain syndrome, restricted joint range of motion, prosthetic function training, peripheral nerve injury, poisoning-induced nerve system diseases, etc.

Electromyographic Signal

It is traditionally believed that electromyographic signal is an electric signal which is produced by neuromuscular system activity under the quiet and contraction state of muscle, although this electric signal mainly derives from nerve or muscle requires further research to identity, in clinical, however, it is often regards the both as a whole, and is depicted various simple electromyographic signal as electromyography (EMG), EMG is also represents electromyographic signal. EMG is closely related with the functional status of neuromuscular system, it is an objective indicator which is used for clinical differential diagnosis of neurogenic and myogenic disorders, learning the location, degree and the status of functional repair, make rehabilitation treatment plan and evaluate the effect of rehabilitation training. In recent years, EMG is widely used in the fields of athletic training, biofeedback, gait analysis and artificial limb driving.

Principle of Electromyographic Biofeedback Technique

Electrographic biofeedback use EMG as its feedback information. The principle of which is take the recorded EMG through amplification, filtration, bidirectional rectification, integral, then use integrator voltage to drive display devices including voice, light, electric, digital, etc. Due to the proportional relationship between integrator voltage and muscular tension, people are able to directly observe the level of muscular tension or relaxation. Since skeletal muscle is under the control of voluntary nervous system, so the self-modulation of electromyographic is easy to learn, the therapeutic method is also easy to be accepted by patients, and the treatment effect is reliable, so electrographic biofeedback is one of the most widely used in clinical and the most successful feedback therapies.

1.4.2.2 Myoelectric Biofeedback Technique Principle

The feedback information of myoelectric biofeedback is illustrated by electromyography (EMG). Through amplification, filtering, bidirectional rectification and integration, integrator voltage driven display devices such as sound, light, electricity and digital to form EMG. Because of the direct ration relationship between integrator voltage and muscle tonus, the level of muscle tonus or relaxation can be directly observed. Because skeletal muscle is controlled by voluntary nervous system, myoelectric autogenous regulation is easy to learn. The therapeutic methods are easily accepted by the patients and the therapeutic effect is reliable. It is one of the most widely used and successful feedback therapies.

In a broad sense, the reason why the biofeedback technology is effective is that it is closely connected with the targeted training process under the mechanism of "objective and motive" and the study of "knowing defects and correct it". The study of "knowing defects and correct it" is similar with the archery training. The target can feed the results of archery back to the archer and the archer can ultimately increase the accuracy and reaction speed through correcting his own posture. The mechanism of "objective and motive" is a process of exceeding stated objective and developing own potential. Just like high jump, the cross-bar is the sign of altitude. If the jumper can jump over 1.4 m and the altitude of the cross-bar is 1.5 m, the jumper should exert run-up distance, speed, force, varied direction running during the way, take-off position, throw-over posture, mental state and courage to a certain extent in order to jump over the cross-bar. The exceeding 0.1 m is the result of developing potential. If there is no cross-bar, the jumping altitude may not be increased, because the potential of jumping cannot be developed.

In physiological mechanism, biofeedback technology can promote brain functions, because voluntary body movements are generated by nervous impulse signals from motor center in cortex to neuromuscular junction through nervous conduction pathway. The membrane permeability of nerve fiber can be changed and the internal flow of calcium ion will trigger exocytosis of synaptic vesicles. Therefore, acetyl choline is released from prejunctional membrane of neuromuscular junction and binds with receptor in endplate membrane through synaptic cleft to trigger endplate potential. Electrotonic potential can stimulate peripheral myolemma to generate action potential and muscle contraction will be induced. The normal physiological process originates from the transformation and transduction of primary electrical signal from brain cells, chemical signal and electrical signal. Primary electrical signal from brain cells in motor center of cortex can be transduced to stimulate muscle contraction and EMG. Therefore, EMG is the drive signal from brain to muscle, which can be consciously enhanced or attenuated by training. This is the basis of myoelectric biofeedback technique.

As for medical purposes, myoelectric biofeedback can be divided into three methods.

Feedback training of muscular flaccidity During treatment, according to the state of an illness, the therapists select the muscle, place the electrode, test EMG and instruct the patients to relax muscles absorbedly in accordance with the vision and sound signals transformed from EMG in order to achieve treatment goal.

Feedback training of muscular excitation the therapists place the electrode on the body surface of the muscle and instruct the patients to increase myoelectricity level absorbedly in accordance with the vision and sound signals transformed from EMG in order to enhance muscle force and recover motor function.

Sports coordination training.

1.4.2.3 Clinical Application of Myoelectric Biofeedback

Indications Myoelectric Biofeedback Can Be Widely Used to Treat Diseases of Different System

Tension Headache

Tension headache was induced by long-lasting muscular tension or blood vessel shrink in head, neck and shoulders. In clinic, mental factor usually induced muscular tension or blood vessel shrink in head, neck and shoulders that lead to local circulation disturbances and ischemia. The therapists not only instruct the patients to listen to themself and watch the abnormal EMG during treatment, but also let the patients to experience the normal EMG recorded before without headache and to compare the difference. The patients were encouraged to decrease the abnormal signal displayed by the biofeedback equipment through willpower.

Hemiplegia

Feedback training of muscular excitation can enhance muscle force and motor function. Similarly, feedback training of muscular flaccidity can be used to inhibit spasm as the circumstances may require.

Stammer

When speaking, masseter is in a relaxed state. However, the masseter is in a tension state when the patients with stammer start to say something, which is the reason of stammer. Myoelectric biofeedback can be used to treat stammer. When keeping silent, the patients should try to decrease the EMG of facial muscles, and then use this experience to control the EMG during speaking, and employ self-control behaviors to maintain the decreased physiologic electrical activity.

Bronchial Asthma
Mental stimulus is the important factor to induce asthma and aggravate it. Myoelectric biofeedback is combined with progressive relaxation training. The therapists place surface electrode on the forehead of the patients and read some warm and happy words silently in order to relax the patients' body and make their breath peaceful.

Emphysema
In patients with emphysema, diaphragm decreases, the movements are confined, residual volume increases and ventilation function declines. The electrode is placed on the body surface of rectus abdominis and musculus obliquus externus abdominis in order to train the patients' abdominal respiration and enlarge the range of motion of diaphragm.

Dysfunction of Oddi's Sphincter
The patients are trained to contract anal sphincter, urethral sphincter and pelvic floor muscle in order to control defecation and urination.

Hyperactivity
According to the EMG, once there is muscular tension signal, the children patients are trained to eliminate the tension signals.

Torticollis
The patients are instructed to enhance the muscle force of sternocleidomastoid in uninjured side. The therapists place the electrode on the body surface of sternocleidomastoid in uninjured side and let the patients flex the head to the shoulder in uninjured side and let the neck turn to offside. According to the feedback information from EMG, the patients know the enhancement extent of muscle force and will be more confident about the treatment. The therapists can decrease the tension of spasmodic muscle to relax spasmodic muscle.

Facial Paralysis
According to the dysfunction point, the therapists train frontalis, musculus risorius, orbicularis oculi muscle and orbicular muscle of mouth separately. The therapists train the patients to use sound to feedback information when the patients close their eyes so that the patients can receive information from EMG when closing their eyes.

Contraindications

Absolute Contraindications
Because myoelectricity myoelectric biofeedback has no effect on the patients' health and the patients do active training, there is no evident absolute contraindications.

Relative Contraindications
Skeleton and muscle diseases that can severely affect joint motion.

The patients with severe cognitive deficit or long-term administration of sedative, antidepressant and so on, or the patients who ignore instructions.

The patients are with skin damage, lesion and infection in the surface of training part so that the electrode cannot be placed.

Preparation Before Training

Understanding the Illness
Before training, the therapists should talk to the patients, know the mental and physiological status of them and do complete inspection of them. The therapists should know the disease characteristics, invalidism and recoverable extent. The therapists should evaluate the intelligence, audio-visual ability, attention and self-control comprehensively.

Training Environment
The training circumstance should be quiet, comfortable, air freshening and the room temperature should be 18–25 °C. The light should be dim and the furnishings should be clean and tidy. The therapists should reduce conversation and walking in the room. If possible, the training should be proceeded in a separate room in case of environmental disturbance.

Psychological Preparation
The therapists should specifically eliminate the patients' scrupulosity and explain the basic principle of myoelectric biofeedback, training methods, precautions and the purpose to the patients in

order to achieve self-control and self-regulation. The patients will be more confident about the treatment and place their hope on the therapeutic outcome.

Training Methods

The patients should be evaluated first. According to the dysfunction point, the therapists select the targeted muscles for training. The patients lie in a comfortable position. The therapist use 75% made of medicinal alcohol to disinfect the skin and put the electrodes on the surface skin of the training muscles with two main electrodes on both ends of the muscle belly and grounding electrode between the two main electrodes. The therapists let the patients to contract or relax the muscles actively and then instruct the patients to do feedback training of muscular excitation or feedback training of muscular flaccidity according to the feedback information from EMG.

For example, the problem of the patients with hemiplegia and pendency foot is pendency foot in injured side and weak muscle force of tibialis anterior muscle. Therefore, the therapists select tibialis anterior muscle as the targeted muscle. During training, the therapists place the electrodes on the surface skin of tibialis anterior muscle and ask the patients to do dorsiflexion of foot. The EMG will be showed on the fluorescent screen when active contraction of tibialis anterior muscle and the patients will know their shortcomings. In the next training, they will concentrate on the dorsiflexion of foot consciously and obtain lasting effect after repeated training.

1.4.3 Equipment Types of Myoelectric Biofeedback

1.4.3.1 Government Standard of Myoelectric Biofeedback

The Definition of Myoelectric Biofeedback Equipment

Myoelectricity is used as physiological information that can feed back to the patients for treating psychosomatic disorder and equipment of rehabilitation therapy through vision or audio.

Operating Conditions

- Environment temperature is 5–40 °C.
- Relative humidity is not more than 80%.
- Power supply should conform to the regulations as follows:
- alternating current supply: 220 ± 22 V (Volt), 50 ± 1 Hz.
- direct current supply: The voltage is no more than 60 V.

Property

- Range of measurement: 1 V to 999 μV.
- Maximum resolution (sensitivity): The minimum signal change detected by the equipment is less than 0.2 μV.
- Input noise: Less than 1 μV.
- Transmission bands: 120–1000 Hz (−3 dB).
- Differential-mode input impedance: More than 5 MΩ.
- Common mode rejection ratio: More than 100 dB.
- In the instruction book, the type of feedback signal should be described.
- When the EMG changes reach 0.2 μV, the feedback signal will change simultaneously.

In the myoelectric biofeedback equipment with computer, myoelectric measurement part should be isolated from computer and the computer should conform to relevant safety standards.

1.4.3.2 Electrode

The electrodes are used to measure and record the electrostatic phenomena of living body, which include microelectrode, surface electrode and needle electrode. Surface electrodes are usually used in myoelectric biofeedback. Biopotential is the potential difference between two electrodes, which can be conducted through the skin surface with one or two recording electrodes and a grounding electrode.

1.4.3.3 Neuroeducator III

1. Principle Neuroeducator III is one kind of myoelectric biofeedback equipment used for neurological training rehabilitation. The signal is extracted through root mean square of potential that is less than 0.2 μV noise level

and the bandwidth are 10–1000 Hz, which is obtained from analysis of surface electromyogram signal that is less than 140 dB. The signals are combined in order to exceed 0.1 s and are measured as μVs. The data of every one-tenth second at present is displayed on the color display in continuous curve (see Fig. 1.1). Myoelectric signals are presented to the patients in visual form. The equipment includes four signal channels that can be used to display four different myoelectric signals at the same time. Ag-AgCl surface electrode is used in this equipment.

2. Functions
   - Neuroeducator III includes many parameters that can be set up manually
   - Patient name and training part
   - Single screen or double-screen display
   - Screen time limit and potential upper bound
   - Curve color of myoelectric signals; altitude value and color of training goal line
   - Sound switch
   - Switch of electrocardio filtration system
   - Data storage and extraction

1.4.3.4 AM800 Therapeutic Equipment of Neural Network Reconstruction

AM800 can skillfully combine EMG and neuromuscular electrical stimulation, which can detect the extremely subtle EMG generated by nerve cells of the patients with stroke. When the EMG signal reach or exceed the setting domain of AM800, the equipment will emit electric stimulus and the patients will have a functional muscle contraction. The main effects are as follows:

- It is widely used for the hemiplegia patients after stroke to reconstruct cerebral neural network.
- Making the paralytic limbs to recover functions.
- Through cognitive re-learning, the residual nerve cells after stroke can regrow and reconstruct new neural network.
- Detecting the feedback of EMG and proceeding automatic electrical stimulation therapy.

1.4.3.5 Other Equipment of Myoelectric Biofeedback

There are other equipments of myoelectric biofeedback such as JD-2A myoelectric biofeedback equipment, ABD2100S myoelectric biofeedback equipment and so on. However, feedback information of most equipment is showed as number form, which is different from curve display that is visual and dynamic. The level of training target cannot be set in this equipment.

1.4.4 Advantages and Shortages of Myoelectric Biofeedback Technology

Biofeedback technology, especially myoelectric biofeedback had a prominent therapeutic effect on the contraction of voluntary muscles training, which was regarded as one of the new medical achievements in twentieth century.

The advantages of myoelectric biofeedback technology are as follows:

In myoelectric biofeedback technology, surface electrode or needle electrode can be used to transform imperceptible myoelectric signals into visual signal or auditory signal in real time. The signal can be used for precise judgment and provide scientific basis for pertinent therapeutic schedule. The patients will be more and more confident during treatment because of the improvement of training.

Comprehensive indications: Myoelectric biofeedback technology can be used for various diseases such as mental and psychological diseases, neuromuscular system diseases. It also can be used for excitation and flaccidity of palsy muscle, motor coordination training.

The training content should include mental regulation and encouraging words. The therapists should arouse the enthusiasm of the patients to achieve the required target, which is good for the motor function recovery on the basis of CNS function recovery.

Biofeedback signal (myoelectric signal) is in direct proportion to myodynamia within limits. Therefore, it can be used as the indicator of functional assessment.

Painless.

No time limit after injury.

Although some reports showed that biofeedback had good therapeutic effect, up to this day this technology was not widely popularized and applied, which was still not the main rehabilitation technology. The reasons are as follows:

The mechanism of biofeedback therapy is still unclear. That the feedback signal of the training is myoelectricity showed that myoelectric signals are generated from muscle contraction and the signal enhancement represent myodynamia strengthen. Because the therapists don't know that only recovery of CNS function can recover motor function, the training methods and time are unable to satisfy the demand of CNS plasticity and functional organization. The biofeedback therapy was applied incorrectly, which had a bad effect on the therapeutic effect. For example, some therapists used the equipment merely as electrical stimulation instrument and there were no mental regulation and encouraging words during treatment.

The therapeutic effect of biofeedback is exaggerated. For example, in Brucker myoelectric biofeedback therapy, there are 15 therapeutic times (one time a day) in one course of treatment and there are 50 min in every time. The total time in one course of treatment are 12.5 h, which go against the reality that reconstruction of motor function in higher evolved species take a long time. It is difficulty to improve lost motor functions after central lesion in this therapy. Even if there are therapeutic effects, it is hard to be consolidated in 15 therapeutic times (one time a day) in one course of treatment. The effects of this therapy were deemed to be not good over time.

Biofeedback technology failed to combine with other rehabilitation techniques. As an independent treatment item, the application of biofeedback technology cannot satisfy the demand of motor function recovery. Because recovering motor functions requires all-around training, only the muscle training is far from enough. In addition, there are no specific indications and contradictions in the application of biofeedback therapy.

Recently, myoelectric biofeedback tends to functional electric stimulus. Therefore, some biofeedback therapeutic equipments are with electric stimulus functions such as AM800 made in Denmark and homemade neural network reconstruction equipment. Because of the movement facilitation and movement substitution effect of electric stimulus, active movements will be reduced, which is adverse to neural potential development. In addition, the therapists don't realize reconstruction of motor program in the application of biofeedback therapy, which has a strong impact on therapeutic effects.

Limited training part: Myoelectric biofeedback therapy is dependent on surface electrode that receives the drive signal from brain to muscle. The electrode should be placed on the surface of trained muscle and it is difficult to treat the fine part such as hand, foot, rim of the eye and so on.

Patients' selectivity: the therapy required good compliance of patients and the patients should take part in the therapy actively. Therefore, it is not applied for the patients with severe dysgnosia or coma.

Even so, myoelectric biofeedback can provide real-time visual and audio feedback signals. Therefore, the patients can do the training with a purpose. When the signals are in comovement relationship with the drive signal from CNS to the joint muscle in the active joint motion, if the therapists use motor program to analyze the signals and use the method of abnormal motor program correction to reconstruct motor program, these will improve the CNS plasticity, functional reorganization and motor function recovery. These procedures are combined with other rehabilitation methods, which can be used for rehabilitation training, increase practical application and value of biofeedback and promote the development of rehabilitation medicine.

References

1. Bin G. Adams and Victor's principles of neurology. Beijing: People's Medical Publishing House; 2002. p. 53–5.
2. Hong D, editor. Rehabilitation medicine. Beijing: Peking University Medical Press; 2004. p. 26.
3. Duus P. Duus' Neurologisch-topische Diagnostik Anatomic Funktion Klinik. Beijing: Navy Press; 2000. Translated by Liu Zonghui, Hu Weiyi, Duan Guosheng
4. Guangdi D. Various pathogenic designate theory. Beijing: People's Medical Publishing House; 1993. p. 12.
5. Keji C. Traditional Chinese rehabilitation medicine. Beijing: People's Medical Publishing House; 1988. p. 170–1.

2 The Formation of Neurological Training Rehabilitation System

2.1 The Modernization of Daoyin Technique in Traditional Chinese Medicine

Although Daoyin technique has been developed for thousands of years and it contributed to the development of rehabilitation medicine of traditional Chinese medicine, ancient Daoyin technique in traditional Chinese medicine was short of vigor and substantial changes in the long development process. Especially, Daoyin technique does not combine with new medical theory and not advance with times. From orchestic Daoyin technique that focused on longevity to whole self-training way that focused on health maintenance and included eight trigrams boxing, five-animal boxing, shadowboxing and Qi gong, the progress of Daoyin technique is stuck and it is not applied for clinical rehabilitation.

Therefore, we should enlarge the application range and use value of Daoyin technique and should not stand still and refuse to make progress. We must combine Daoyin technique with modern medical theory and methods, improve it on the basis of inheritance and make Daoyin technique promote motor function recovery on the basis of CNS function recovery. Meanwhile, we start therapeutic effect validation and mechanism research, which will provide theoretical basis and clinic trial basis for long-term development and renaissance of Daoyin technique.

2.1.1 Theoretical Foundation of the Modernization of Daoyin Technique in Traditional Chinese Medicine

The meaning of rehabilitation is a process to recover original functions through various measures and means such as recreation, medical treatment, functional training and rehabilitation medicine engineering. In clinical rehabilitation, rehabilitation include exercise, cognition, speech and mentality, but usually point to motor function recovery. Motor function recovery includes nervous system dyskinesia, bone and joint dyskinesia and muscle injury dyskinesia. All tissues and organs of human body are possessed with huge functional reserve. It not only satisfies the demand of daily life, but also deals with contingencies. The basis of functional reserve is tissues and cells. For example, people can strengthen muscle force and endurance obviously through training. After training, people can complete unaccomplished movements before training and improve athletic performance, etc. Therefore, for the patients with hemiplegia or cerebral palsy after central damages, the lost functions can be recovered to varying degrees through proper rehabilitation training [1].

However, in the process of recovering and improving human functions, there is a common phenomenon that only active movements

W. Zhao, *Rehabilitation Therapeutics of the Neurological Training*,
https://doi.org/10.1007/978-981-13-0812-3_2

(especially the concentrated active movements) can recover and improve human functions. This is an undeniable fact in daily life. The reason why the active movements can improve functions is that active exercise conform to the "skillful use and dependence" principle that can promote CNS plasticity.

Not all the people that do active exercise are instructed by Daoyin technique. However, they all know they should concentrate on training, which is possessed with regulation of mind and breathing to a certain extent. Perhaps under correct Daoyin technique, active exercise can have better effect and the time spent is shorter. Basic technique that the regulation of movement is based on the regulation of mind and breathing is a completed method of concentration and active exercise training. Besides, the regulation of movement in Daoyin technique is in accordance to main and collateral channels. Therefore, Daoyin technique is a completed method of concentration and active exercise training with of traditional Chinese medicine characteristic. It is a scientific method that is completely in conformity with modern CNS plasticity and functional reorganization theory, which provides solid practice foundation and theoretical basis for modernization of Daoyin technique.

Short of the objective indicator of therapeutic effect is one of the key factors that influence the development of Daoyin technique. If there are objective indicators that can demonstrate the therapeutic effect of Daoyin technique, the therapists can set a target for the patients to catch up with and surpass and let the patients do targeted training. The objective indicator can improve the effect of Daoyin technique and make it become a training method that can be used in clinical rehabilitation.

In traditional Chinese medicine, brain is the house of mental activity, and in western medicine, brain is the advanced central nervous system that control general movements. Whether nerve in western or main and collateral channels in traditional Chinese medicine, the common point is that brain has a close relationship with body movements and brain is the highest center that control body movements. The difference between them is that in western medicine brain dominates the muscles responsible for body movements through neural electrical signal and in traditional Chinese medicine the house of mentality dominates body movements through Qi in main and collateral channels. Both the electric signals in western medicine and Qi in traditional Chinese medicine are one kind of messenger that transmits the signal from brain to muscles and are one kind of energy forms. If the house of mentality or brain is damaged, the cradle of messenger is damaged. Because the messenger is decreased or disappear, body movement may be lost to varying degrees. Now that both the electric signals and Qi are one kind of energy forms, they can be detected and received in real time, analyzed and demonstrated in a visual form. It provides theoretical basis and feasibility for realization of objective indicator of Daoyin technique.

2.1.2 The Formation and Specific Operational Approach of Six-Step Daoyin Technique

Although entirely active exercise guided by Daoyin technique can better promote motor function recovery after brain function reorganization. However, limited by the ancients' medical knowledge, the operating methods of Daoyin technique are whole movements such as immortal guiding and the zoomimic movements, which don't conform to the "from easy to difficulty and step by step" principle of rehabilitation training. It can influence the clinical use.

According to development of CNS potential and clearing and activating the channels and collaterals, ancient Daoyin technique was modified to six-step Daoyin technique, which was applied for rehabilitation training of single muscle contraction and single joint motion. Six-step Daoyin technique was not only used for patients with slight symptom, but also the patients with severe diseases. According to the pathway difference of the regulation of mind, Six-step Daoyin technique was divided into normal technique and six-step Daoyin technique guided by main and collateral channels. The two methods can be used separately or be used in combination in order to satisfy different clinical demands of the patients and avoid vanpidity of singular method in the training.

2.1.2.1 The Specific Procedures of Six-Step Daoyin Technique

The formation of six-step Daoyin technique is dependent on the basis of regulation of mind, breathing and movements. Motor imagery and imitation, concentration on one point, clearing and activating the channels and collaterals with sudden release of Qi, resistance exercise and speech inspirations, exploring the neural potentials are used in this technique. The rehabilitation principle is step by step and the specific procedures are as follows:

Motor Imagery and Imitation

The therapists explained the patients in detail and straightaway that electric signal were released by brain to control body movements and CNS functions recovery should be followed by lost motor functions after central damages. In the basis of characteristics of CNS function recovery, the therapists instructed the patients to do joint motion of uninjured side limbs (dorsiflexion of foot). Afterwards, the therapists let the patients to do the same joint motion of injured side limbs imitating the uninjured sides. The therapists should guide the patients to image the normal joint motion mode in injured side. Therefore, the correct motor imagery is constructed and the training content and the target are clear.

Setting Target

The therapists advised the patients to use "vigor" on the targeted muscles such as the tibialis anterior muscle in dorsiflexion of foot and triceps muscle of arm in elbow extension. One joint motion is done for each time and the target is one muscle. The principle should be from easy to difficulty and training the muscle one by one.

"Vigor" Assembly

In a warm, lucifugal and quiet room, through relaxing meditation, breathing regulation, the patients used mind to make the "vigor" and "Qi" concentrate on the muscle of joint motion through main and collateral channels. The therapists instructed the patients to be in a "Lock and Load" state. According to the main and collateral channels, this method is divided into the common method and the method of main and collateral channels.

1. The common method "vigor" assembly of six-step Daoyin technique

   On the basis of breathing regulation, ridding distraction and mental relaxation, the therapists instructed the patients (or the patients trained themselves) to concentrate and assemble "vigor" and "Qi" from the uninjured side limbs to injured side brain or to contralateral brain of the mobile joint. For example, if the patients want to exercise the left hip joint, they will assemble "vigor" to right brain. On the contrary, the patients will assemble "vigor" to left brain. Assembly of the "vigor" to the injured side brain can stimulate the injured side brain through the energy flow carried by "vigor" in order to promote resurgence of brain cells in penumbral area in which there are surviving cells around damage zone. The patients can actively concentrate on using injured side brain in order to promote the CNS plasticity and functional reorganization.
2. "Vigor" assembly of six-step Daoyin technique through main and collateral channels

   This method is divided into the dredging meridians through collaterals method and the dredging collaterals through meridians, which highlight the traditional Chinese medicine characteristics of six-step Daoyin technique. Dredging the main and collateral channels is similar with dredging a river. The water in the river likes the "Qi" in the main and collateral channels. Qi is the information flow between brain and viscera. If the river is stagnated, people cannot live without water. If the main and collateral channels are stagnated, the information cannot be exchanged and the viscera cannot work correctly. If the river can be dredged from two sides, the blockage will be loosened easily and be removed. The river is clear and can deliver water. The obstructed main and collateral channels can be dredged easily from two sides and recover the information conduction and exchange between brain and viscera.

According to the orientation of Qi in the main and collateral channels, Daoyin technique is divided into the dredging meridians through collaterals method and the dredging collaterals through meridians method. The dredging collaterals through meridians are based on the regulation mind and breathing. The patients are instructed to guide Qi to the targeted muscle and do joint motion. Afterwards, the patients guide Qi through meridians until the Qi is scattered in collaterals. On the contrary, the dredging meridians through collaterals method are based on the regulation of mind and breathing. The patients are instructed to guide Qi from the end of the collaterals to the targeted muscles and then do corresponding joint motion. Afterwards, the patients guide Qi through collaterals until the Qi is scattered in meridians.

However, whether the dredging meridians through collaterals method or the dredging collaterals through meridians method, they both are the process of clearing and activating the channels and collaterals dominated by brain. Through training, it can promote the ability of the brain to dominate the process of clearing and activating the channels and collaterals. This is similar with the process that training can promote CNS plasticity and functional reorganization in western medicine.

The two methods can be used alternatively in the training. Comparing the beginning of the meridians or the end of collaterals with the movable joint, if the distance between the movable joint and the beginning of meridians is shorter, the dredging collaterals through meridians method are used. If the distance between the movable joint and the end of collaterals is shorter, the dredging collaterals through meridians method are used. For example, in the training of elbow extension, the target is triceps muscle of arm, which belongs to the Tri-energizer Meridian of Hand-Shaoyang. Using mind, the patients are instructed to guide Qi from ulnar side of the third finger to the muscle belly of triceps muscle of arm through the reverse side of wrist and the space between radius and ulna of forearm. Qi is in a "Lock and Load" state and then into a cocking state. The conduction flow of joint motion through main and collateral channels is showed in Table 2.1 (Figs. 2.1, 2.2, 2.3, 2.4, 2.5, 2.6, 2.7, 2.8, 2.9, 2.10, and 2.11).

Trigger

The patients are instructed to regulate their breath and take a deep breath. Afterwards, the patients are guided to give out "vigor" to the targeted muscle suddenly. Contraction of the targeted muscle leads to corresponding joint motion such as dorsiflexion of foot and elbow extension. The patients concentrate on one muscle. There is a sentence in art of war that the army should attack one point with superior force in order to develop the function of Daoyin technique and achieve good effect.

Trigger is the important procedure of Daoyin technique. The patients are guided to release accumulative energy flow (Qi) to targeted muscle suddenly, which is vital for the CNS plasticity. Just as the process of pulling the trigger, the bullets are ejected from the bore with high energy and high initial velocity in order to hit the ulterior target easily.

The common Daoyin speeches are as follows:

- The therapists asked the patients: "Are you ready?"
- The patients say "Yes" or nodding.
- The therapists say "good, pay attention" and raise their voice suddenly (a powerful low voice) "Get up".
- The patients concentrate on the contraction of targeted muscle and lead the joint to the designed orientation.
- If the therapists instruct the patients torpidly and say "Get up" in a powerless low voice, the patients' enthusiasm and passion cannot be enlightened and the contraction of the targeted muscle and corresponding joint motion cannot be induced.

Table 2.1 The conduction flow of joint motion through main and collateral channels

Joint motion	The name of main and collateral channels	The beginning and the end
Shrug	The Small intestine Meridian of Hand-Taiyang	Contraction: outside of little finger (Shaoze)–ulnar side of palm (Qiangu)–capitulum ulnae (Yanglao)–elbow (Xiaohai)–shoulder joint (Jianzhen)–musculus levator scapulae Relaxation: musculus levator scapulae—the seventh cervical vertebra (Dazhui)–heart meridian—stomach (Zhongwan)–small intestine
Shoulder abduction	The Large Intestine Meridian of Hand-yangming	Contraction: the end of index finger (Shangyang)–radialis index finger (Erjian)–the space between the first metacarpal and the second metacarpal (hegu)–radialis forearm (Pianli)–outside of the elbow (Quchi)–outside of the upper arm (Binao)–deltoideus triangularis Relaxation: deltoideus triangularis—the seventh cervical vertebra (Dazhui)–supraclavicular fossa (Quepen)–lung meridians—large intestine
Elbow extension	The Tri-energizer Meridian of Hand-Shaoyang	Contraction: the end of the third finger (Guanchong)–the reverse side of wrist (Yangchi)–forearm (Waiguan)–the upper arm (triceps muscle of arm) Relaxation: triceps muscle of arm—shoulder (Jianliao)–the central region of mediastinum (Danzhong)–pericardium
Elbow flexion restoration	Lung channel of hand taiyin	Contraction: middle burner–stomach–lung–throat–oxter (Yunmen)–the upper arm (bicipital muscle of arm) Relaxation: bicipital muscle of arm—chelidon (Chize)–Yuji—the end of thumb (Shaoshang)
Wrist extension	The Tri-energizer Meridian of Hand-Shaoyang	Contraction: the end of the third finger (Guanchong)–the reverse side of wrist (Yangchi)–forearm (extensor carpi) Relaxation: extensor carpi—forearm (Waiguan)–shoulder (Jianliao)–the central region of mediastinum (Danzhong)–pericardium
Wrist flexion restoration	Pericardium channel of hand jueyin	Contraction: thorax cavity and pericardium—axilla (Tianchi)–the upper arm (Tianquan)–elbow center (Quze)–forearm (flexor muscle of wrist) Relaxation: flexor muscle of wrist—the centre of the palm (Laogong)–the end of the middle finger (Zhongchong)
Hip flection	The Stomach Meridian of Foot-yangming	Contraction: the side of ala nasi (Yingxiang)–inner canthus (Jingming)–upper teeth and ring lip (philtrum)–supraclavicular fossa (Quepen)–2.6 in. outside of ventrimeson (Guanmen)–groin (Qichong)–hip flexor Relaxation: Hip flexor—outside of tibia (Zusanli)–acrotarsium (Chongyang)–the inside of middle toe (Neiting)–outside of the second toe (Lidui)
Knee extension	The Stomach Meridian of Foot-yangming	Contraction: the side of ala nasi (Yingxiang)–inner canthus (Jingming)–upper teeth and ring lip (philtrum)–supraclavicular fossa (Quepen)–2.6 in. outside of ventrimeson (Guanmen)–groin (Qichong)–hip joint (Biguan)–the front of the thigh (quadriceps femoris) Relaxation: quadriceps femoris—outside of tibia (Zusanli)–acrotarsium (Chongyang)–the inside of middle toe (Neiting)–outside of the second toe (Lidui)
Strephexopodia	The Gallbladder Meridian of foot-Shaoyang	Contraction: outer canthus (tongziliao)–post aurem (Tianchong)–the seventh cervical vertebra (Dazhui)–oxter (Yuanye)–hip joint (Huantiao)–the outside of knee (Xiyangguan)–the outside of crus (peroneus longus and brevis muscles) Relaxation: peroneus longus and brevis muscles–lateral malleolus (Qiuxu)–acrotarsium—the outside of the fourth toe (Diwuhui)
Dorsiflexion of foot	The Stomach Meridian of Foot-yangming	Contraction: the side of ala nasi (Yingxiang)–inner canthus (Jingming)–upper teeth and ring lip (philtrum)–supraclavicular fossa (Quepen)–2.6 in. outside of ventrimeson (Guanmen)–groin (Qichong)–hip joint (Biguan)–the outside of tibia (Zusanli)–the front of crus (tibialis anterior muscle) Relaxation: tibialis anterior muscle—acrotarsium (Chongyang)–the inside of middle toe (Neiting)–outside of the second toe (Lidui)
Lumbodorsal muscle	The Urinary Bladder Meridian of Foot-Taiyang	Contraction: inner canthus (Jingming)–the top of the head (Tongtian)–Brain collaterals (Yuzhen)–the side of the seventh cervical vertebra (Dashu)–around the inside of the scapula–lumbodorsal muscle (Shenshu) Relaxation: lumbodorsal muscle (Shenshu)–kidney collateral

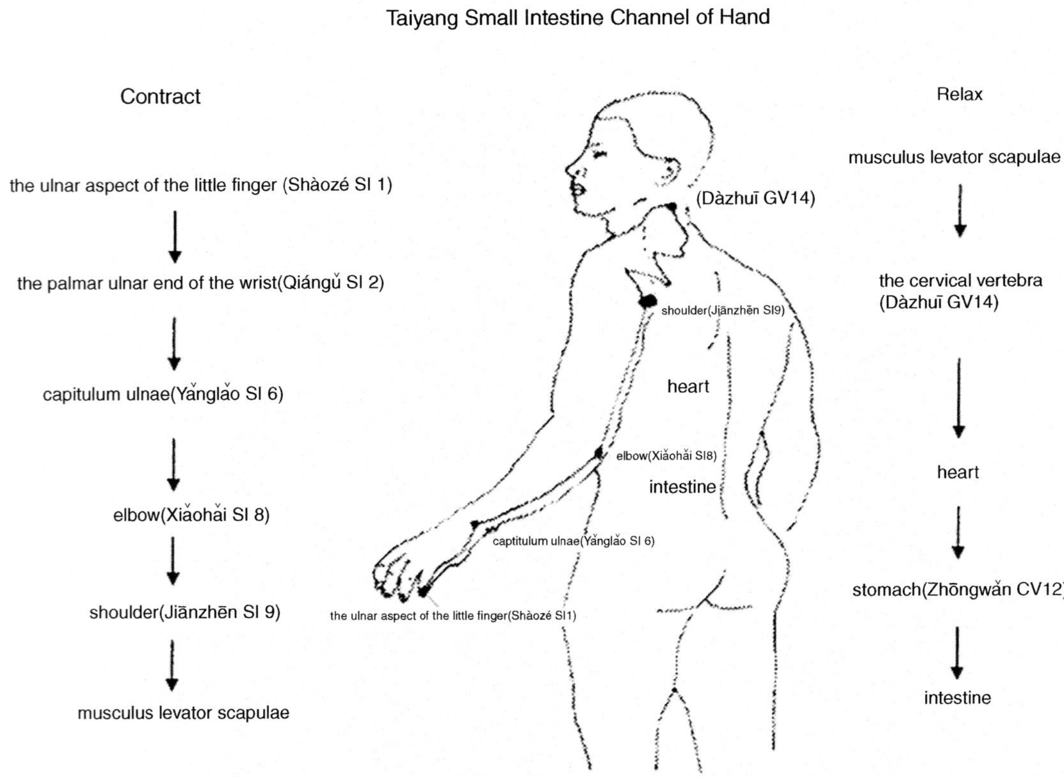

Fig. 2.1 Shrug of six-step of the dredging collaterals through meridians

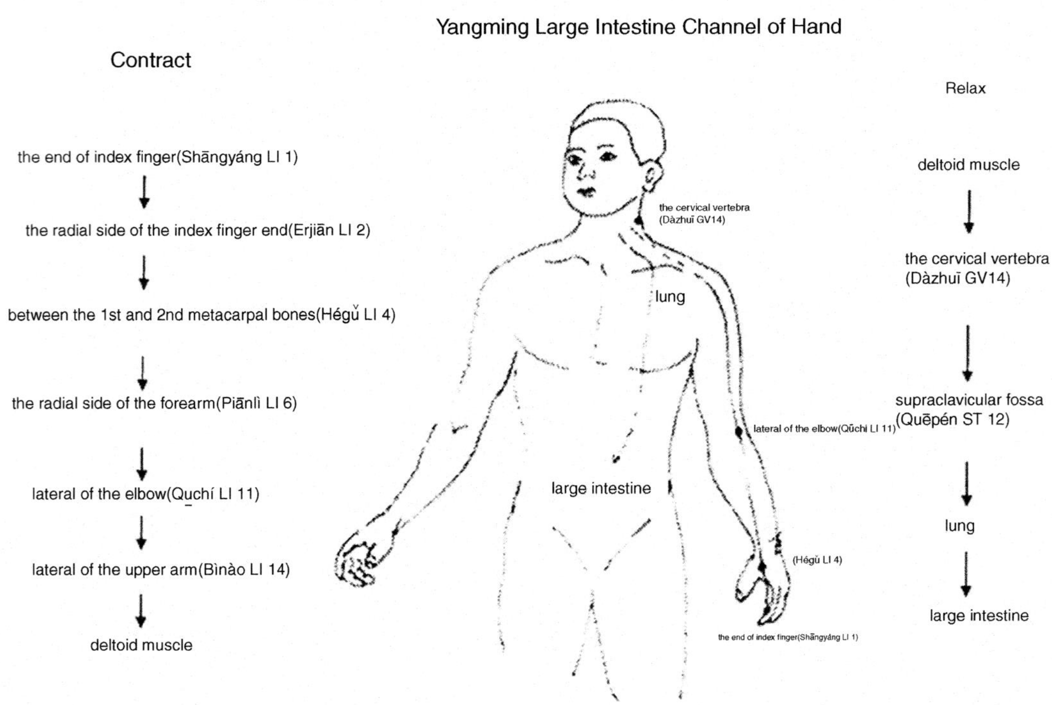

Fig. 2.2 Shoulder abduction of six-step of the dredging collaterals through meridians

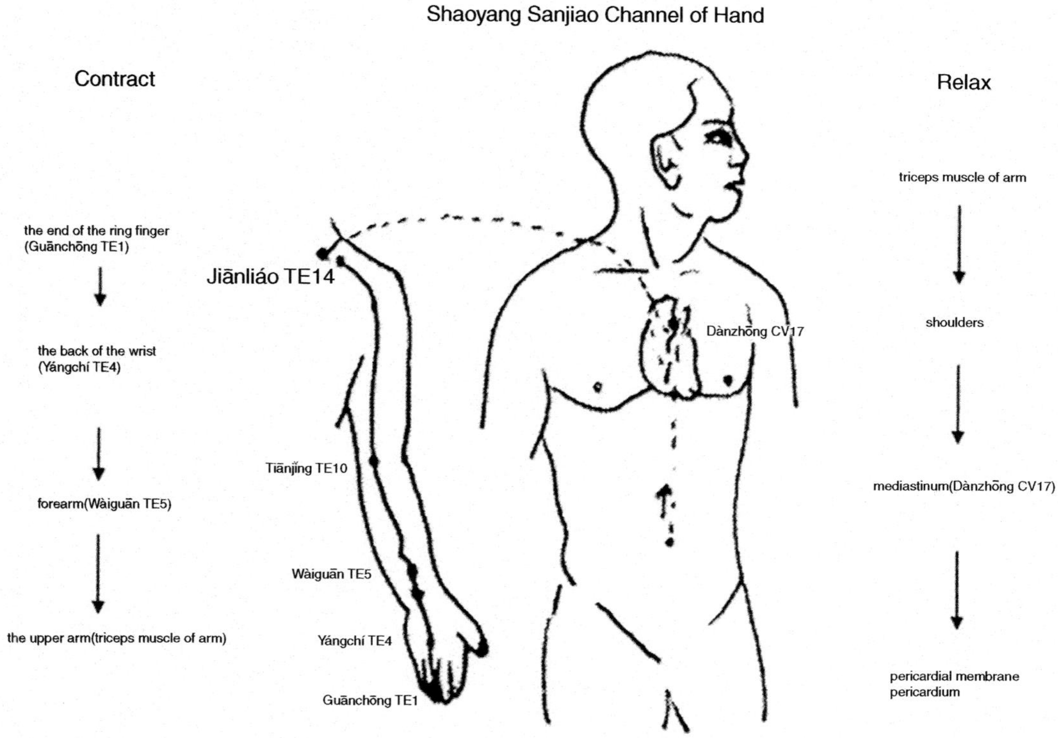

Fig. 2.3 Elbow extension of six-step of the dredging collaterals through meridians

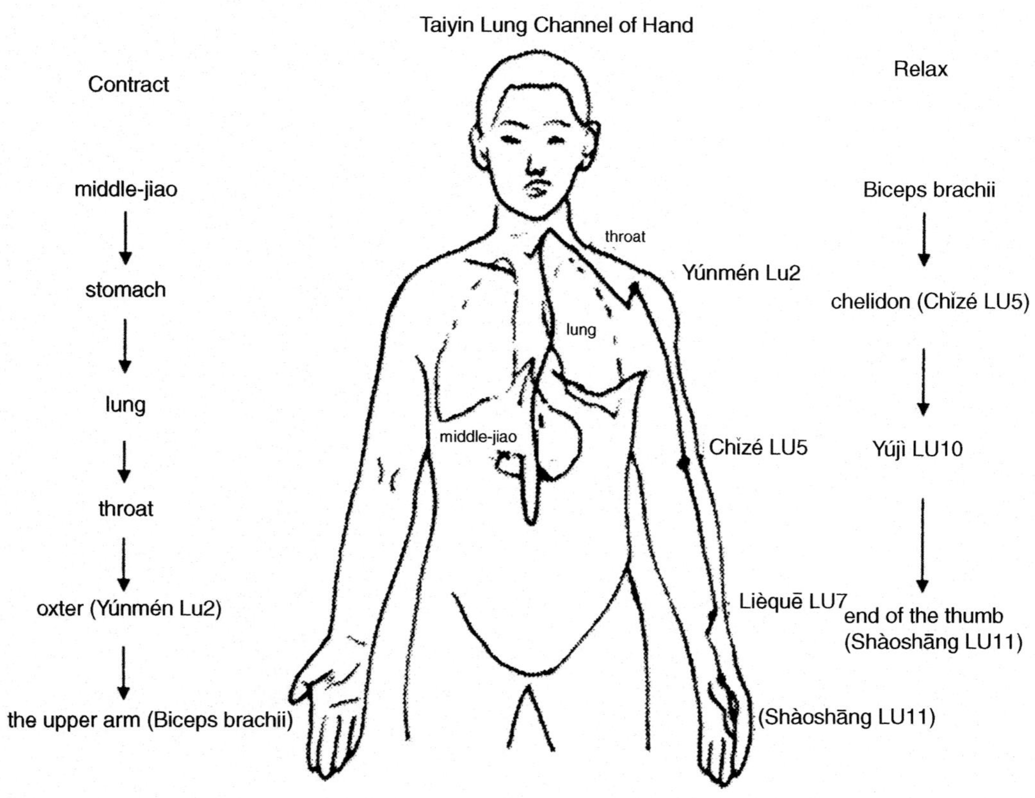

Fig. 2.4 Elbow flexion restoration six-step of the dredging collaterals through meridians

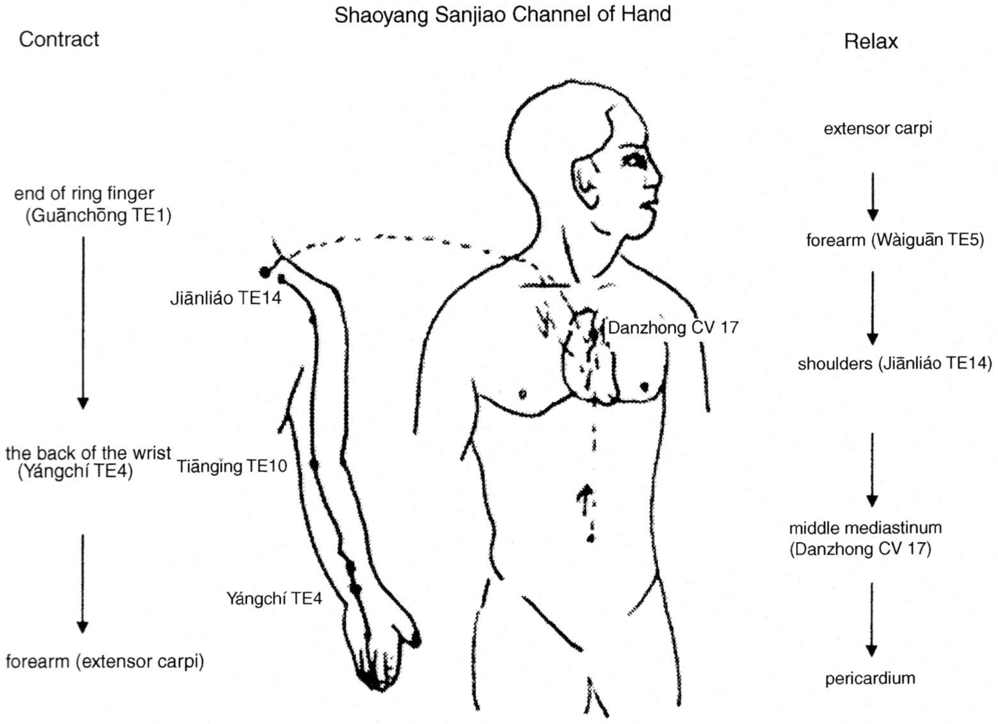

Fig. 2.5 Wrist extension of six-step of the dredging collaterals through meridians

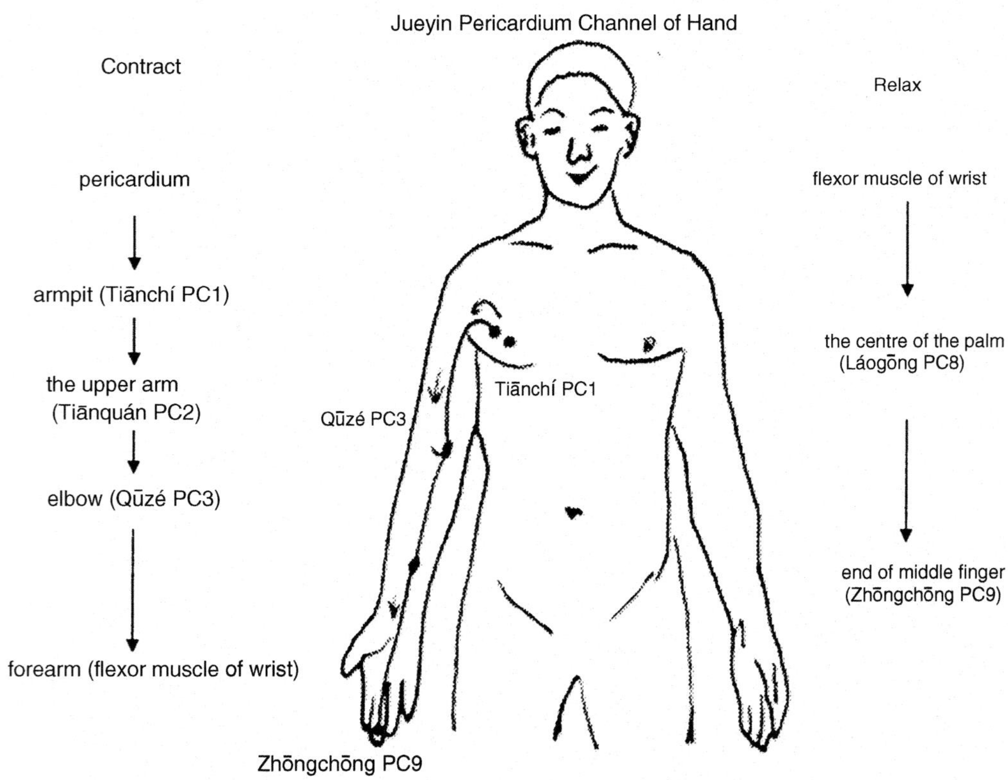

Fig. 2.6 Wrist flexion of restoration six-step of the dredging collaterals through meridians

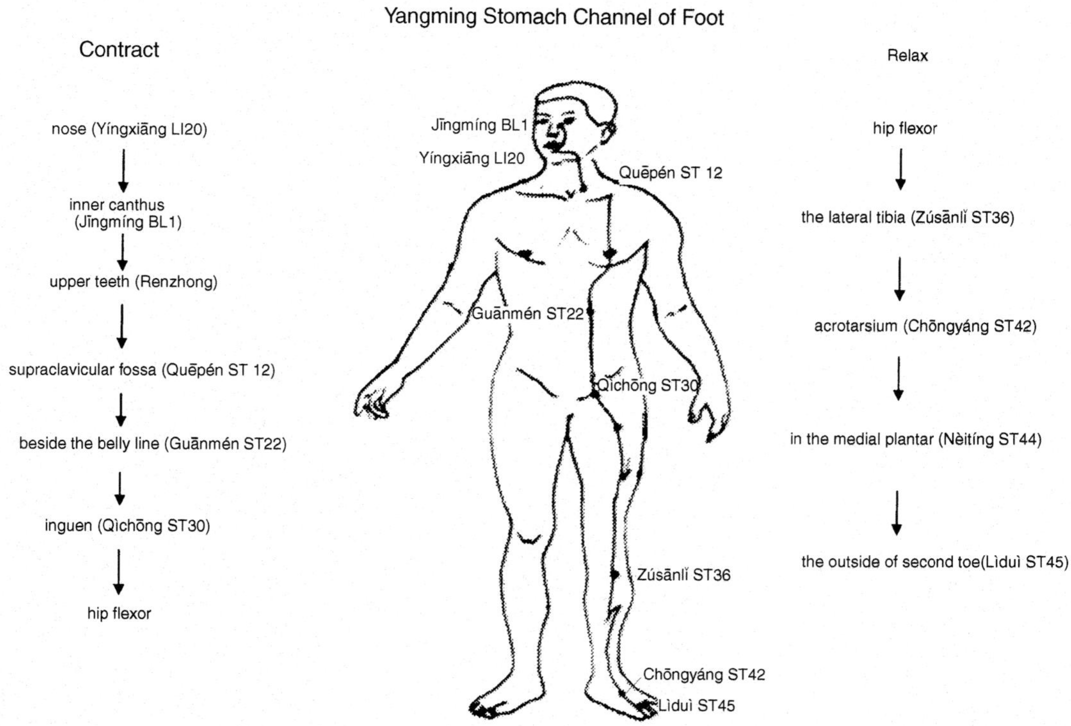

Fig. 2.7 Hip flection of six-step of the dredging collaterals through meridians

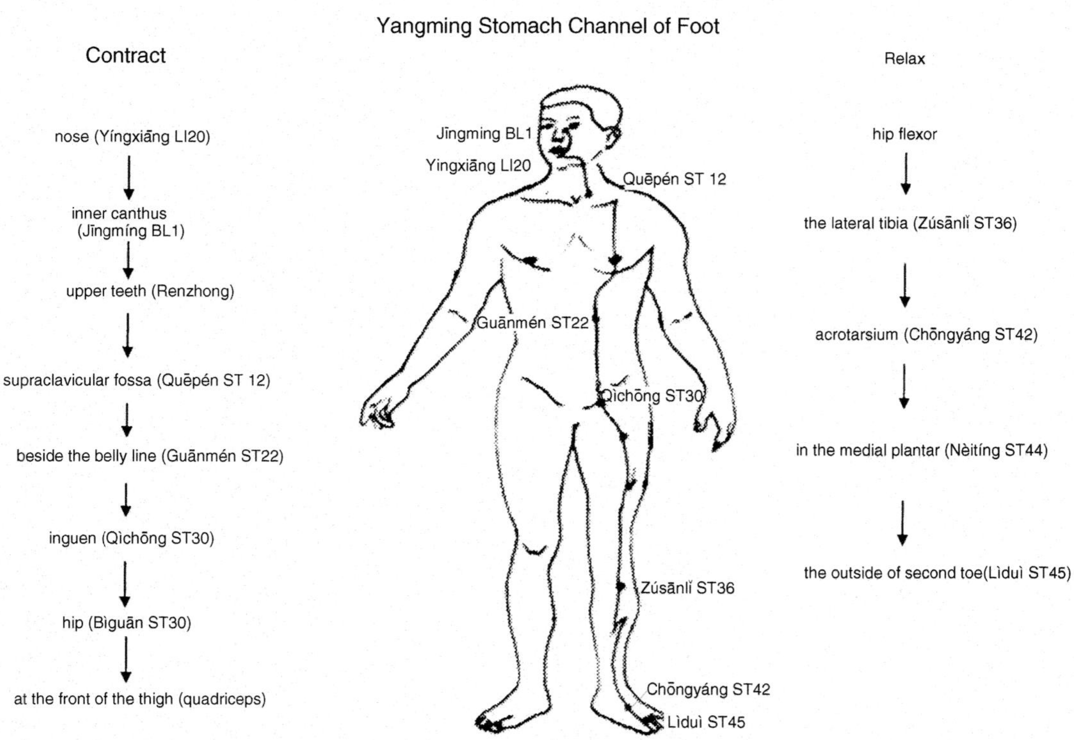

Fig. 2.8 Knee extension of six-step of the dredging collaterals through meridians

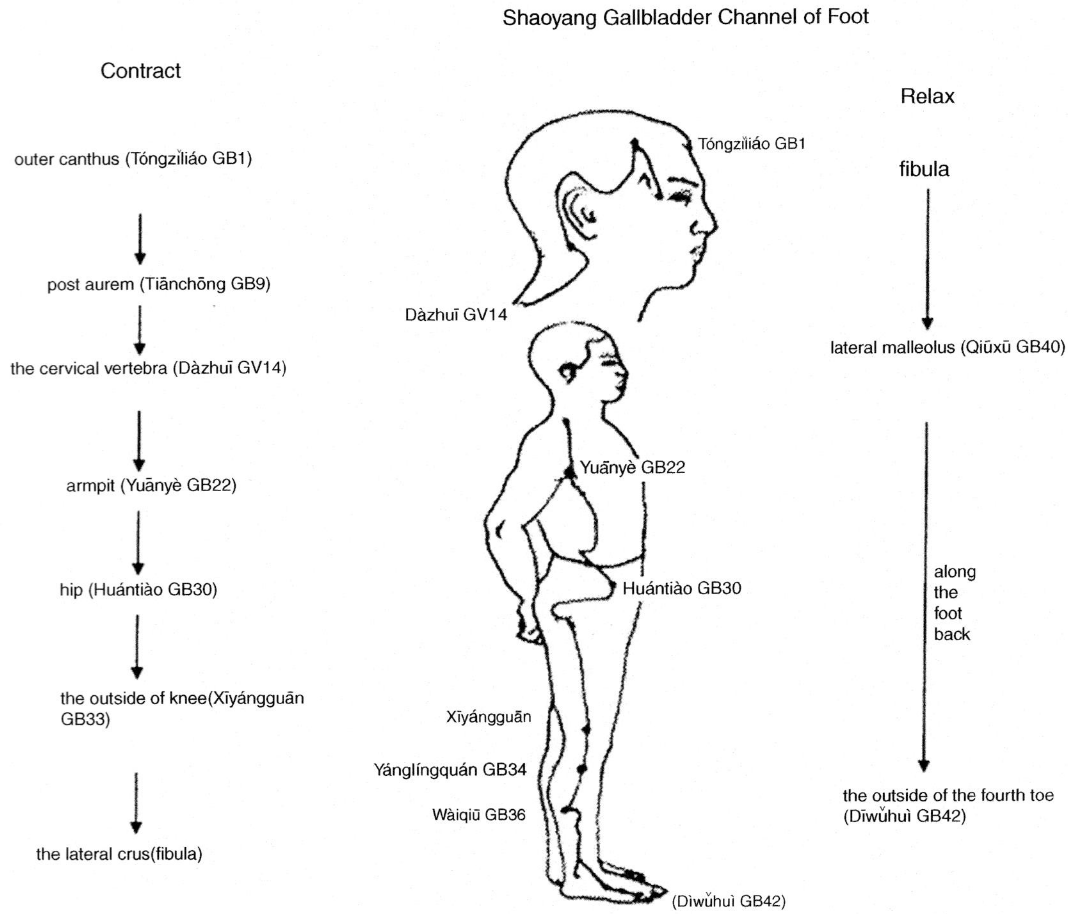

Fig. 2.9 Strephexopodia of six-step of the dredging collaterals through meridians

Insistence

The patients are instructed to induce muscle contraction and corresponding joint motion through trigger. Meanwhile, the therapists use hands to provide resistance on the orientation of the joint motion such as the metatarsophalangeal joints in dorsiflexion of foot and the rear side of forearm, even if the myodynamia is zero. The therapists let the patients to find the target and orientation of the released signal easily. The opportunity of exerting resistance is that the patients flex or extend the joint to the maximum angle. The strength of the exerted resistance is dependent on the intensity of the patients' myodynamia. The patients can resist the resistance and the joint motion angle cannot be reduced. When exerting resistance, the therapists encourage the patients to hold on for 6 s. This procedure can be completed using counting such as "one, two, three, you did great, four, five, six." When encouraging the patients, the therapists use words to create state of emergency such as "hold on or you will fall down" and "lift up or you will crash". The therapists encourage and urge the patients to complete the required joint motion. This process is essential for developing the neural potential. State of emergency can stimulate the patients into proximal response state. Under proximal response state, the strength of muscle power is six times of that in normal state. Proximal response state can improve myodynamia in different degree. The increase in the muscle power is related to the development of CNS potential. In addition, under the anti-resistance condition, the patients hold on one more second that is a process to develop a little more potential, activate more new brain cells and promote a little more recovery of motor function.

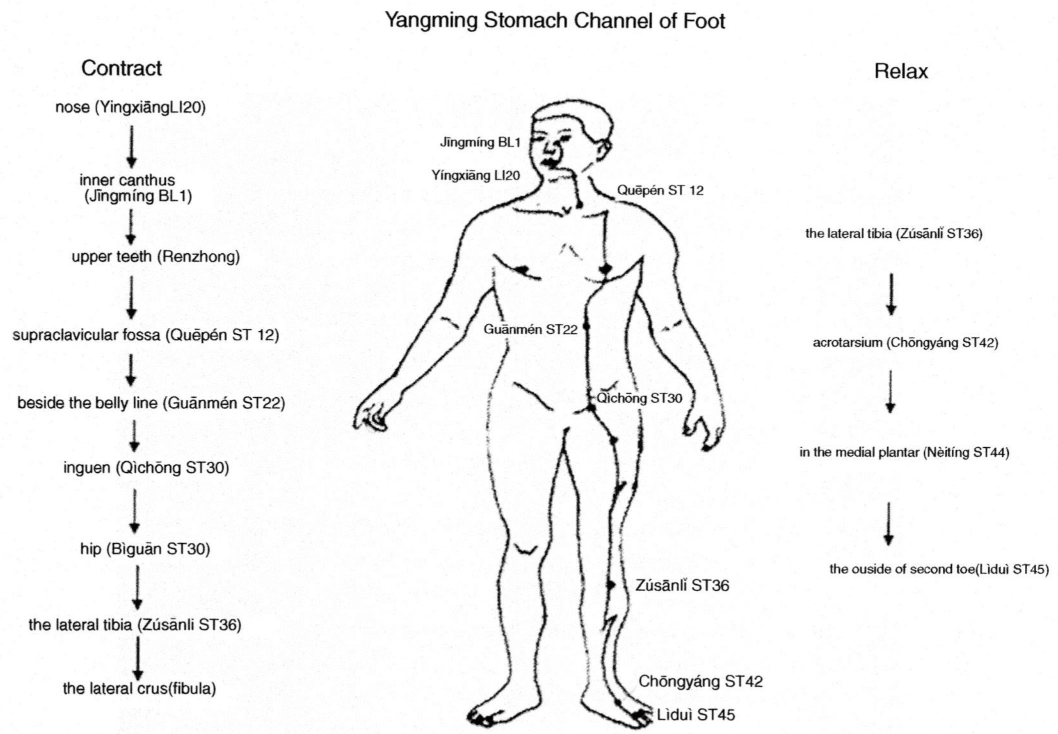

Fig. 2.10 Dorsiflexion of foot of six-step of the dredging collaterals through meridians

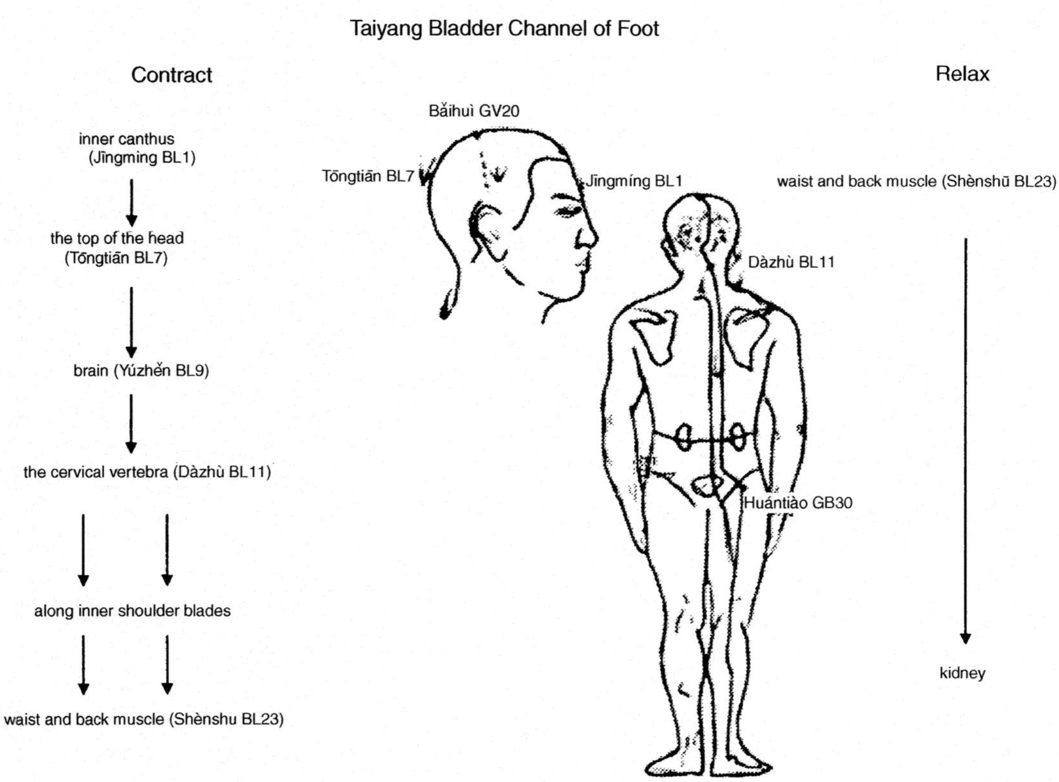

Fig. 2.11 Lumbodorsal muscle of six-step of the dredging collaterals through meridians.

Relaxation

Relaxation method is divided into the normal method and relaxation method of dredging collaterals through meridians.

1. The normal relaxation method
   After the end of movements, the therapists guide the patients to take a deep breath and breathe out quietly. The ratio of expiration time to inspiration time is 1:2. The patients keep relaxed wholeheartedly in order to allay tiredness and be beneficial to next movement.
2. After one time of Daoyin technique training, therapists are instructed to do joint motion passively and muscle massage in order to alleviate synarthrophysis and promote blood circulation of muscles. And then the patients will do the second training. The frequency of training is dependent on the patients' ability and 6–8 times per 15 min is appropriate.
   The relaxation method of dredging collaterals through meridians.
   After the anti-resistance movements, the therapists guide the patients to take a deep breath and during the slow expiration the patients can make Qi circulate in residual meridians. The ratio of expiration time to inspiration time is 1:2. The patients guide Qi to circulate in residual meridians and finally disperse in collaterals. For example, in the movement of elbow extension, after completion of anti-resistance, the patients are instructed to guide Qi along the shoulder to disperse in pericardium through Tanzhong. Qi in the relaxation method of dredging meridians through collaterals finally disperse in the beginning of the meridians.

2.1.3 Controlled Clinical Trial of Six-Step Daoyin Technique

2.1.3.1 Methods and Data

General Data and Grouping

From June 2006 to June 2008, in neurological training rehabilitation center of Beijing Tongren Hospital, we selected 60 stroke patients with hemiplegia and pendency foot. The medical history is from 1 to 5 years. The patients are divided into six step group and control group. There are 30 patients in each group.

1. Six-step group: There are 18 males and 12 females. The age range is from 35 to 76 years old. The mean age is 48.4 years old. The medical history is from 19 to 59 months. The mean medical history is 40 months.
2. Control group: There are 16 males and 14 females. The age range is from 34 to 71 years old. The mean age is 47.8 years old. The medical history is from 12 to 60 months. The mean medical history is 42 months.

Therapeutic Method

In six-step group, the six-step Daoyin technique is used to instruct the patients to do dorsiflexion of foot actively once a day. Every time takes 45 min and the total times are 30 times. In control group, dorsiflexion of foot promotion method of Brunnstrom is used in this training, which includes:

1. Bechterev/Marie-Foix reflection: The therapists press the patients' toes for plantar flexion in order to drag muscle spindle of plantar dorsiflexor. This reflection can induce dorsiflexion of toe, dorsiflexion of foot, kneebend and body bent at hips. The time of during is 15 min.
2. Finger percussion: The therapist use finger to rap lateral dorsum of foot quickly in order to facilitate ankle dorsiflexion. The time of during is 15 min.
3. Hairbrush stimulation: The therapist use hairbrush to stimulate lateral dorsum of foot. It takes 30 s once. It is enough to induce foot dorsiflexion reflex. The time of during is 15 min. Three kinds of treatments take 45 min (once a day, 30 days).

Functional Assessment

International universal Lovett MMT, ankle ROM and Fugl-Meyer are used for ankle dorsiflexion functional assessment method (zero: incapable of dorsiflexion actively; one point: partial dorsiflexion; two points: full dorsiflexion) and detection of electromyographic signal (Neuroeducator III produced by Therapeutic Alliances in America, 3 M Ag-AgCl surface electrode) in tibialis anterior muscle. The assessment should be proceeded before treatment and at the end of treatment.

Statistical Analysis

After the completion of all the experiments, Epidata 3.02 software is used to create database and all the data requires double entry and validation. SPSS 12.0 is used as statistical software for the comparison of functional assessment score within group before and after treatment and T-Test analysis of comparison between groups in control group and six-step group.

Results

Statistical analysis of four assessment indicators in six-step group demonstrated that there was significant difference between the data after treatment and that before treatment ($P < 0.01$). There was significant difference between the data of electromyographic signal after treatment and that before treatment in control group ($P < 0.05$). There was no significant difference in the data of other three indicators in control group ($P > 0.05$). Before treatment, there was no significant difference in comparison among groups of four indicators. There was significant difference of four indicators between control group and six-step group after treatment ($P < 0.01$, see Table 2.2).

Conclusion

Six-step Daoyin technique is an effective rehabilitation method that is in accordance with motor functions recovery mechanism after CNS damages.

Discussion

Necrocytosis of axoneuron can lead to dyskinesia of limbs. The key point of treatment is the functional recovery of axoneuron. Because the axoneuron is unable to regenerate itself, the lost functions after central damages should be compensated by the normal cells around the injured area. The standby conduction pathway is activated to replace the functions (development and utilization of neural potentials) of injured cells. The CNS contains great potentials that originate from numerous cells and synapses and is the basis of recovery of limbs motor functions through training after central damages. Therefore, development of neural potentials is the key of recovery of motor functions after central damages [2].

CNS potentials are the results of CNS plasticity and functional reorganization. However, the plasticity of nervous system is based on the "skillful use and dependence" principle, which means only active limbs movements can induce plasticity of motor cortex function and then improve the motor functions of limbs [3].

Traditional rehabilitation techniques that include Bobath, Rood and Brunnstrom are based on passive movement, primitive reflex and afferent stimulus. Reflex of lower nerve center such as myotatic reflex and tonic neck reflex are used to induce reflex movement of limbs, which is not in accordance with the "skillful use and dependence" principle required for plasticity of CNS functional reorganization. This may be the reason why the therapeutic effects of these rehabilitation methods are not satisfying. For example, foot drop of stroke patients with hemiplegia is

Table 2.2 Functional assessment comparison table of within group and between group before and after training ($\bar{x} \pm s$)

Assessment item	Group	Before training	After training	Within group *p*	Between group *p*
Myodynamia	Six-step group	1.32 ± 0.65	3.62 ± 1.21	<0.01	<0.01
	Control group	1.31 ± 0.47	2.13 ± 101	>0.05	
Myoelectric signal (μV)	Six-step group	26.18 ± 8.36	87.31 ± 23.66	<0.001	<0.05
	Control group	27.32 ± 10.54	43.18 ± 8.36	<0.05	
Joint range of motion (°)	Six-step group	9.23 ± 2.36	18.43 ± 2.68	<0.001	<0.01
	Control group	10.12 ± 2.36	13.47 ± 4.36	>0.05	
Fugl-Meyer	Six-step group	0.43 ± 0.50	1.7 ± 0.47	<0.001	<0.01
	Control group	0.50 ± 0.50	0.7 ± 0.47	>0.05	

due to the loss of voluntary movement functions of tibialis anterior muscle dominated by brain, myoparesis of tibialis anterior muscle and plantar flexion of shin and foot after contralateral motor center damages or conduction pathway damage. Therefore, the autokinetic movement of tibialis anterior muscle can be recovered only after recovery of functions of cortex motor center and conduction pathway. Afterwards, the dorsiflexion of foot can be recovered. Brunnstrom can induce dorsiflexion of toe, dorsiflexion of foot, knee-bend and body bent at hips through reflex. The reflex center is located in spinal cord. Just like knee jerk reflex through rapping patellar tendon, the effect on the cortex motor center is little. The unsatisfactory therapeutic effect of control group is due to lack of CNS plasticity and functional reorganization.

Daoyin technique in China is an important method to enlighten and motivate human willpower to complete designed movements in order to achieve functional rehabilitation. It has a long history. For the rehabilitation of apoplexy hemiplegia, the first volume of *General Treatise on the Cause and Symptoms of Diseases* written in Sui dynasty (B.C. 610) described four syndromes such as hemiplegia, disability of flexion and extension because of contracture of arms and legs, imbalance of hands and feet and phemilateral wind in wind disease that was related to sequela of apoplexy. There are more than 20 Daoyin techniques in this book include static exercise (breathing guided by spirit) and dynamic exercise supplemented by spirit, breathing and movements (imitation of all kinds of animals), which have good effect on dredging the channel, regulation of Qi and blood, balancing viscera, strengthening the body resistance to eliminate pathogenic factors, body steady state and metabolism through regulation of mind, breathing and movements. Modern medical research demonstrated that Daoyin technique has good regulative and rehabilitation effect on cardiovascular disease, respiratory disease, nervous system disease, digestive disease. Doctors of all dynasties supplemented and developed Daoyin technique from different aspects on the basis of experience of the predecessors. Many contents are worthy for reference and spreading. It has close relationship with modern psychotherapy, motorpathy, naturopathy and information therapy, which is the comprehensive application of all these therapies. From the birth of Daoyin technique, it is closely related to Chinese traditional culture, especially in the development. After additions, deletions and modifications by doctors of all dynasties, although the theory is extensive and profound, it is shrouded in mystery. Because it is short of definite concept, subjective and abstract, Daoyin technique is mainly used in life cultivation and health preservation but not in clinic from Ming and Qing Dynasties to modern times, which is endangered.

Daoyin technique can be used to instruct the patients to actively complete designed movement on the basis of regulation of mind and breathing. This process is in accordance with "skillful use and dependence" principle that can promote CNS plasticity. Therefore, Daoyin technique can better promote CNS functional reorganization and recovery of motor functions. However, the main training method of ancient Daoyin technique is to complete an integral movement such as immortal guiding and animal form, which is against the rehabilitation training principle of from the easy to the difficult and step by step. The patients cannot complete the movements because of the difficulty movements. After repeated failed training, the patients will lose confidence in rehabilitation.

Six-step Daoyin technique is based on the basic techniques of ancient Daoyin technique and is modified according to modern medical theory. After central damages, the functions training should focus on functional recovery of voluntary movements. In executing goal-directed complicated work, compilation of motor program and motor start are closely related to motor associated area. When the cortex motor center is damaged, this function can be destroyed to varying degrees and the recovery of the lost functions require reconstruction of this function. When starting a voluntary movement, the sporter should judge the primary objective and the position, decide the movement mode, time and speed, and then enter into critical state. Hereby, the first step of six-step Daoyin technique is motor imagery and imitation. The purpose of this step is to help the patients to construct the idea of voluntary movement, basic motor mode and orientation. Through regulation of mind and breathing, the patients get into critical state of exercise. On the basis of the targeted muscle, the patients are guided to send signal to the targeted muscle suddenly. The purpose of this method is to focus on one point with all power in order to achieve good effect. The purpose of holding on the counting method resistance is to let the patients find the target in brain. The counting method is used to instruct the patients to complete the training quantitatively in order to develop the neural potential of the patients. During the process, the therapists can encourage the patients and say "Stand up, or you will fall down" or "hold up, or you will crash" to create the dangerous atmosphere. The therapist should encourage the patients furthest to complete the designed movements by themselves. During this process, the neural potential of CNS and the functional reorganization can be developed well.

The electrical signal to activate and control muscle from brain is one kind of energy forms. Therefore, the process can motivate the energy flow of human body to promote CNS functional reorganization through CNS plasticity.

On the basis of regulation of mind and breathing, the regulation of movements in Daoyin technique can develop CNS neural potential and promote functional reorganization in order to recover paralyzed muscles dominated by autonomic nerve. The modernization development of Daoyin technique not only improve the therapeutic effect of rehabilitation, but also show the charm of ancient rehabilitation technique and contribute to rehabilitation medicine all over the world.

2.1.4 Clinical Indications and Cautions of Six-Step Daoyin Technique

2.1.4.1 Indications

Six-step Daoyin technique is a rehabilitation training mode during that the patients can do it themselves with guidance and instruction of the therapists. Because the method can focus on one muscle or one joint motion, it can be done lying in bed, sitting on a chair or wheelchair, or standing on the ground. Therefore, this method can be applied for the rehabilitation training of all motor dysfunctions, cognitive dysfunctions, visual dysfunctions, breathing dysfunctions, swallow dysfunctions and gatism. It can also be used in the rehabilitation training of scapulohumeral periarthritis, pain in waist and lower extremities, and muscles of bone and joint.

2.1.4.2 Contraindications

1. The patients with unstable vital signs.
2. This method should be used with caution in the patients with bone, joint and muscle injury and bad healing after surgery.
3. The patients with severe disturbance of consciousness or coma. (This method can be used with the help of equipment in the patients with stable vital signs.)

2.1.4.3 Cautions

1. Abiding by the principle of from the easy to the difficulty and step by step: The treatment should be started from single muscle and joint motion and then transited gradually to united movements with multiple muscles and joints.
2. Exerted resistance should be from weak to strong, especially in the patients with bone, joint and muscle injury and bad healing after surgery. The isometric muscular contraction should be done first in case of the wrong-orientation movement for bone, joint and muscle healing.
3. The application of Daoyin speeches. The therapists should use encouraging, inspiring words to create dangerous atmosphere. The critical words such as command and scold should be strictly prohibited. The therapists can only say how to do some movements better, but not say the patients do bad. The therapist must not show dissatisfied, impatient and disdainful expressions.
4. Special attention should be paid to the fact that Daoyin technique can guide Qi and recover CNS functions, but not strengthen the myodynamia. There is significant difference between the two.

2.1.5 The Application of Six-Step Daoyin Technique in Physical Therapy and Occupational Therapy

Six-step Daoyin technique can be employed for various kinds of rehabilitation training such as the development of neural potential, reconstruction of motor program and remodeling of motor pattern, whether using the normal method or the main and collateral channels method. According to free-hand training, equipment training and with or without therapists, six-step Daoyin technique can be divided into free-hand training, equipment training and self-training.

2.1.5.1 Non-instrumental Method of Six-Step Daoyin Technique

Non-instrumental method of six-step Daoyin technique is free-hand operational approach without any apparatus when the therapists treat the patients. The main contents include therapeutic schedule, mechanism explanation, six-step operating steps, Daoyin speeches and anti-resistance. The patients try not to use apparatus and the training should be done in a quiet, noiseless, lucifuge and warm room. It is also used in bedside rehabilitation training. The patients may lie in the bed, sit on a chair or stand on the ground, mostly sit on a chair.

Before training, according to the exercise prescription of the doctor, the therapists should do simple assessment and further understand the main dysfunction point. According to the principle of integrated planning, adjustment at any moment, supplementing the weak and attenuating the excited, the therapists determine the therapeutic schedule and objective of this treatment. The therapists usually stand in the paralyzed side of patients' limbs. The methods should be in accordance with the principle of from the easy to the difficulty and step by step. According to the different states of the patients' illness, there are difference in training method and training intensity. For the patients in convalescence with stable state and voluntary joint motion, the isotonic contraction training with resistance to muscles dominated by CNS can be given to the patients. For the patients lying in bed with severe condition, the isometric contraction training without resistance to muscles dominated by CNS can be given to the patients in order that rehabilitation training that includes cognitive disorder training and the training for coma patients can be given at early stage. The training forms free-hand six-step Daoyin techniques are as follows:

Active Range of Motion (ROM) Exercises

This training is appropriate for the patients in stable state of an illness and clear consciousness who can do voluntary joint motion completely or partially. In exerting resistance condition, the therapists employ six-step Daoyin technique to give voluntary joint motion training to the patients in proper position. The training should be given to the patients step by step and gradually increase the level of challenge.

Auxiliary Active Movements

This training is appropriate for the patients in stable state of an illness and clear consciousness who have active motor consciousness but cannot do voluntary joint motion. The therapists guide the patients to do joint motion with tooth and nail and help the patients to complete full-range joint motion. With the recovery of CNS functions and improvement of active movements ability, the therapists should reduce assistance gradually.

"Passive" ROM Exercises

This training is appropriate for the patients with stable vital signs, consciousness but not clear, cognitive dysfunction and without voluntary movements. This training should be carried out by two or more therapists. In special position, such as erect position, two therapists stand on the two sides of the patients. The two therapists help the patients to squat with protective belt for any contingency and the depth of squat (flexion angle of knee) is dependent on the step by step principle and the specific condition of the patients. When encouraging the patients with Daoyin speeches, the therapists help the patients to stand up. In the process of standing, the therapists can reduce auxiliary intensity suddenly. The patients are falling down non-autonomously. Meanwhile the therapists use Daoyin speeches to create dangerous atmosphere and help the patients to stand up again. Through repeated training, voluntary movements are induced in most patients. It is safer to do this training with electrocardiograph monitoring.

"Compulsive" ROM Exercises

In the condition of imperceptions and unwillingness, voluntary movements are induced in the patients in order to recover the patients' consciousness. It is appropriate for the coma patients with stable vital signs and good cardiovascular response. Before training, the patients should be trained to stand with the standing bed. When the patients can stand in 90° position for half an hour and the vital signs are stable, the training can be given to the patients. In addition, the training should be conducted with vital sign monitoring.

"Compulsive" ROM Exercises

During standing and squat training, there should be two or more therapists. The two therapists stand on the two sides of the patients and use protective belt to keep the patients safe. The training intensity should be in accordance with step by step principle and the specific condition of the patients. The procedures of the standing training are as follows: The depth of squat begins at 15° of the flexion angle of knee. On the basis of this, the depth of squat increases gradually. When encouraging the patients with Daoyin speeches, the therapists help the patients to stand up. In the process of standing, the therapists can reduce auxiliary intensity suddenly. The patients are falling down non-autonomously. Meanwhile the therapists use Daoyin speeches to create dangerous atmosphere and help the patients to stand up again. The procedures of the squat training are as follows: the therapist help the patients to squat slowly form the standing position. During the squat process, the therapists suddenly reduce the auxiliary power and encourage the patients to keep the body position in case to continue to squat.

Through repeated "compulsive" active movement training, the patients' motor responses are induced and the consciousness recovery of the patients is promoted. During this process, the therapists don't deem that the coma patients have no response to the training and should realize that no surface response don't equal to no deep response. It is a method to awake the coma patients and to prevent osteoporosis, myophagism and other complications.

The specific operational approaches of six-step Daoyin technique are introduced in the following pictures.

1. Six-step navigation physical therapy (SSNPT)
   - The normal method of NPT refers to Figs. 2.12, 2.13, 2.14, and 2.15.
   - The main and collateral channels method of NPT refers to Figs. 2.16, 2.17, 2.18, and 2.19.
2. Six-step navigation occupational therapy (NOT)
   - The normal method of NOT refers to Figs. 2.20, 2.21, 2.22, 2.23, 2.24, 2.25, 2.26, 2.27, 2.28, and 2.29.
   - The main and collateral channels method of NOT refers to Figs. 2.30, 2.31, 2.32, 2.33, 2.34, 2.35, and 2.36.

2.1.5.2 The Corollary Equipment Method

Corollary equipment is dedicated appliance and equipment for rehabilitation techniques, which

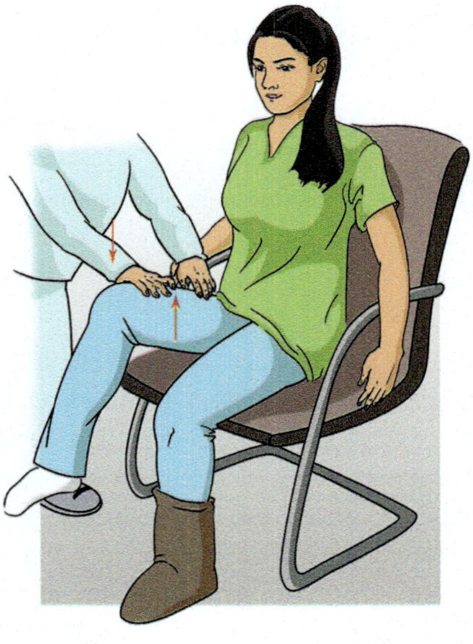

Fig. 2.12 Hip flection of the normal method

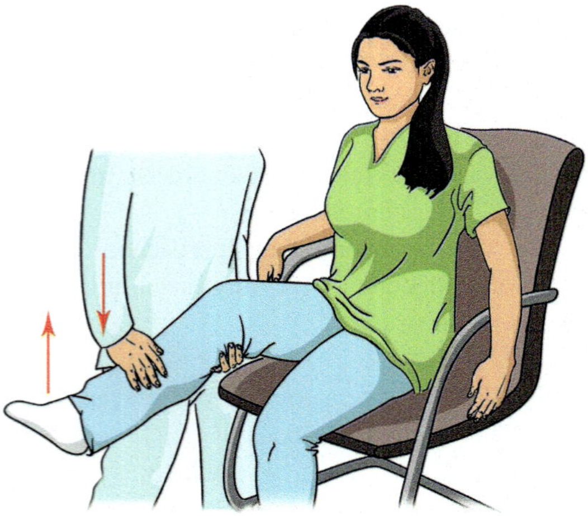

Fig. 2.13 Knee flection of the normal method

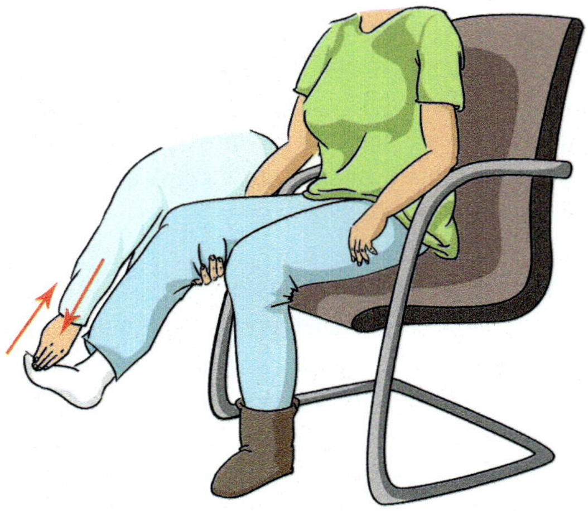

Fig. 2.15 Strephexopodia of the normal method

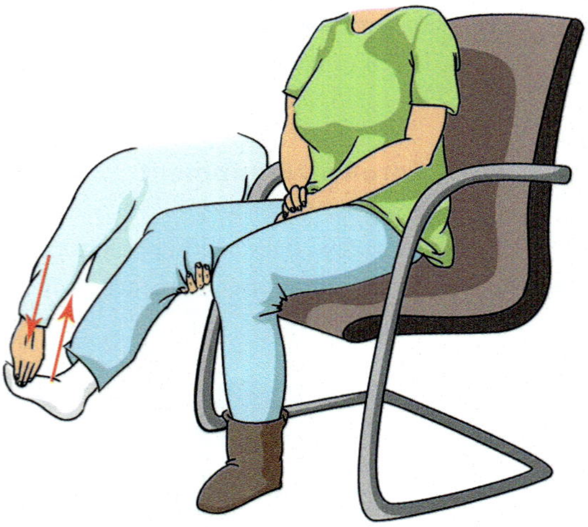

Fig. 2.14 Foot dorsiflexion of the normal method

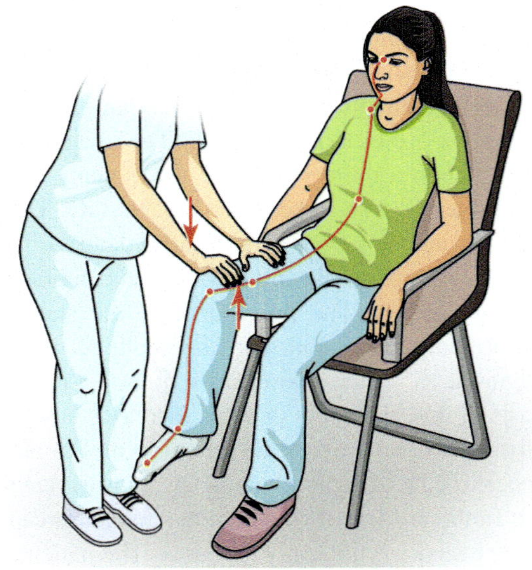

Fig. 2.16 Hip flection of the main and collateral channels method

are suitable for six-step Daoyin technique and neurological training (effect feedback technology of six-step Daoyin technique). The corollary equipment method is that the six-step Daoyin technique is carried out with corollary equipment. The objective of this method is to assure the correct application of this method and its effect. What calls for special attention is that the method plays a leading role in the process of rehabilitation training in spite of the important role of the equipment. The equipment plays a supporting role. We don't overemphasize the role of the equipment and should not chase the high-grade, precision and advanced equipment. The valuable rehabilitation training equipment is simple and is with good therapeutic effect, not the high degree of automation, expensiveness and large size.

The therapist or rehabilitation therapists with exquisite craft who understand six-step Daoyin technique and neurological training can achieve

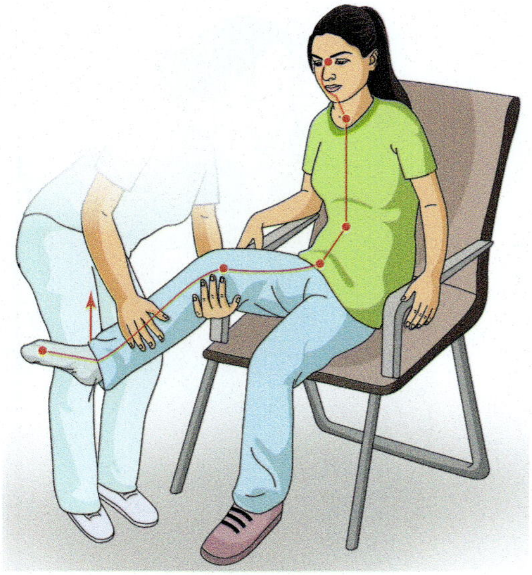

Fig. 2.17 Knee flection of the main and collateral channels method

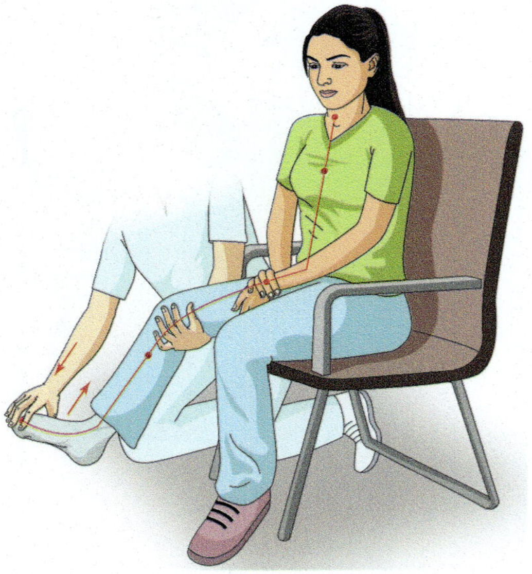

Fig. 2.18 Foot dorsiflexion of the main and collateral channels method

wonderful therapeutic effect without the corollary equipment. As a superb gongfu master without blade in hand can still beat the man with blade. In the contrary, a rehabilitation physician or therapist who doesn't understand six-step Daoyin technique well and doesn't apply the techniques appropriately cannot get good training effect, even they have many appliances.

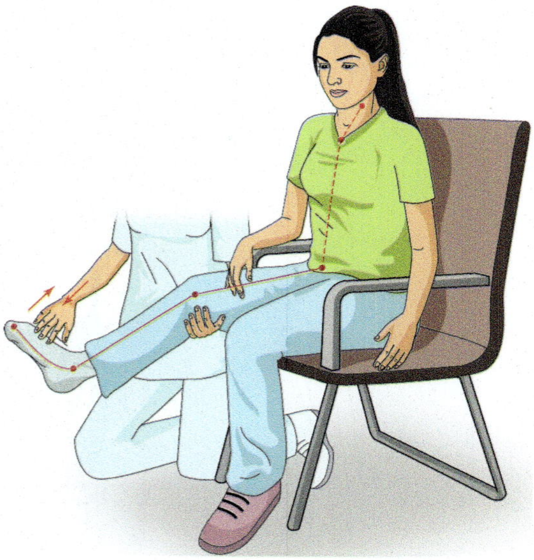

Fig. 2.19 Strephexopodia of the main and collateral channels method

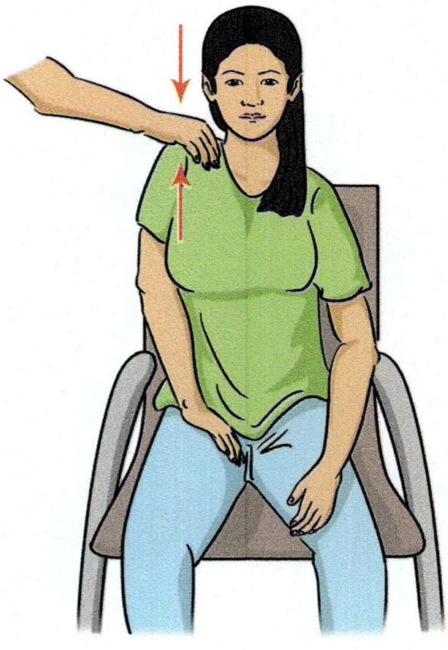

Fig. 2.20 Shrug of the normal method

2.1.5.3 Self-Training

Self-training is appropriate for the patients who received six-step Daoyin technique training or the self-training plan designed by rehabilitation physician of neurological training. The patients should be instructed by doctors or therapists. Self-training can be carried out in ward, parker or at home. The training can be carried out with

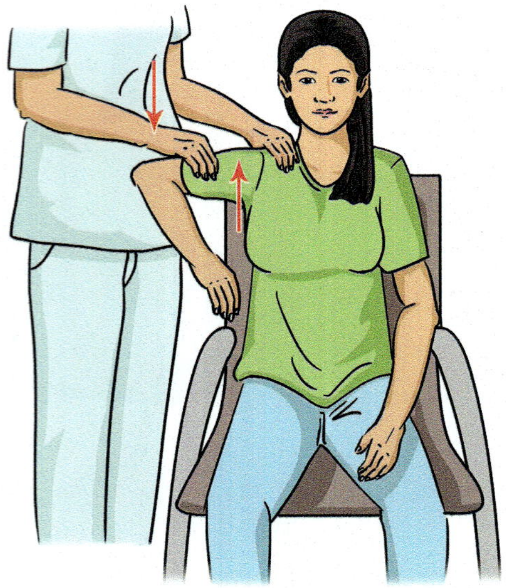

Fig. 2.21 Shoulder abduction of the normal method

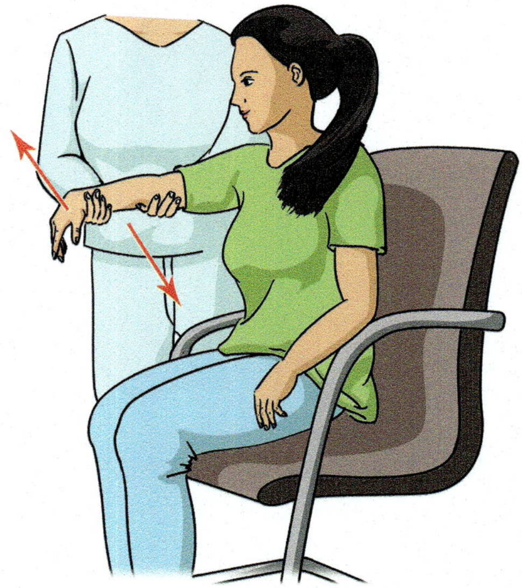

Fig. 2.23 Elbow flexion of the normal method

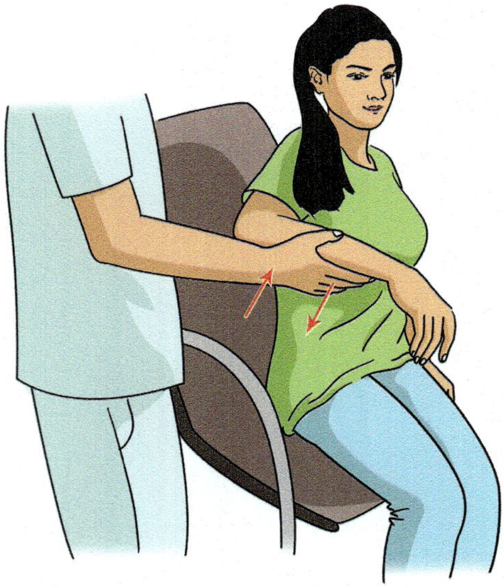

Fig. 2.22 Elbow extension of the normal method

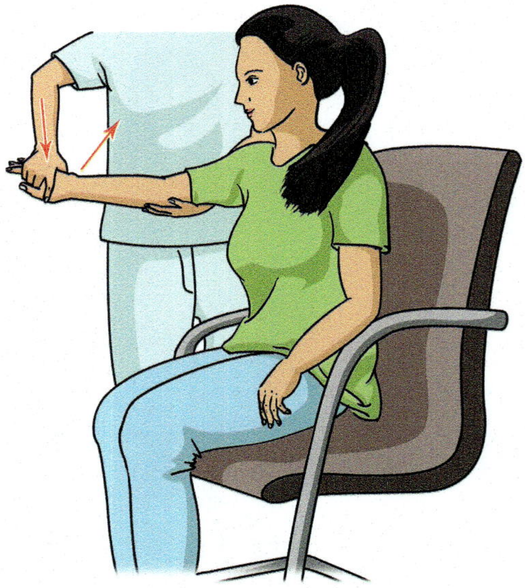

Fig. 2.24 Wrist extension of the normal method

multifunction training box guided by voice or video. The correctness and effect of self-training can be guaranteed by multifunction training box.

The common problems of self-training are that the patients cannot keep training frequently or the training method is wrong. Keep training is the important guarantee for maintaining functions and achieving therapeutic effects. The premise of keep training is the self-cognition of rehabilitation, perseverance and family monitoring. Quantitative index and training record are the effective measure to guarantee exercise. The bases of improving exercise effect are regular reexamination or contacting the training doctors, adjustment or modification of exercise project, and the correct application of the method.

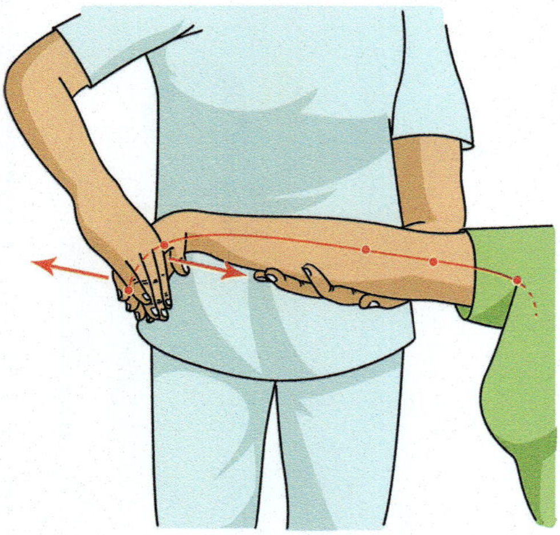

Fig. 2.25 Wrist flexion of the normal method

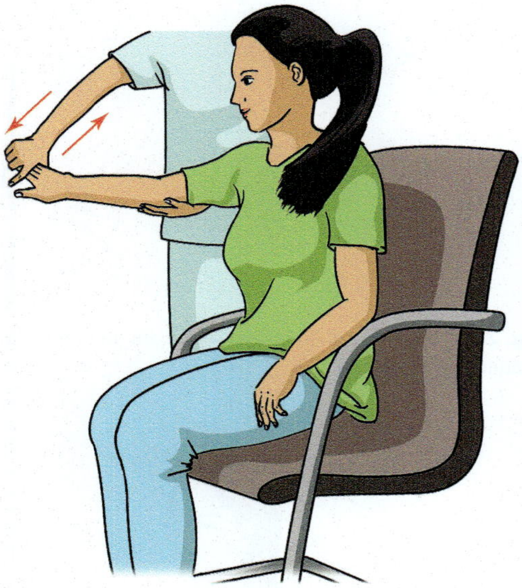

Fig. 2.26 Finger stretching of the normal method

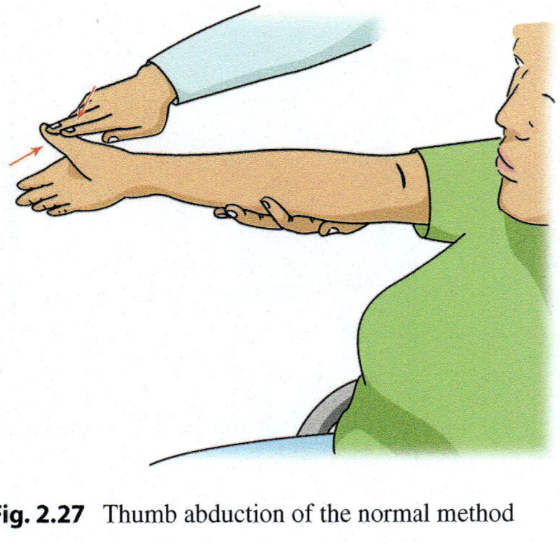

Fig. 2.27 Thumb abduction of the normal method

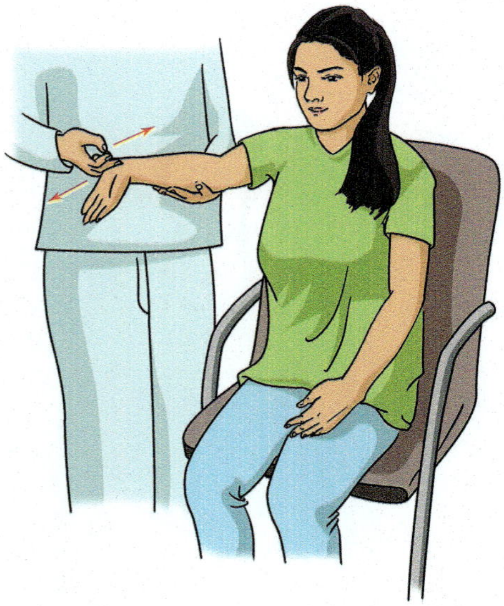

Fig. 2.28 Hallux flexion of the normal method

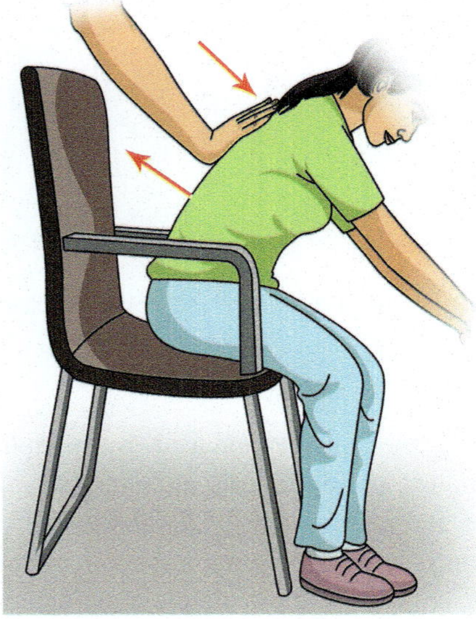

Fig. 2.29 Lumbus stretching of the normal method

2.1.6 The Application of Six-Step Daoyin Technique in Other Trainings

The basic techniques of six-step Daoyin technique are regulation of mind, breathing and movements. Six-step Daoyin technique not only can be used in motor function training such as hemiplegia, cerebral palsy, paraplegia, facial

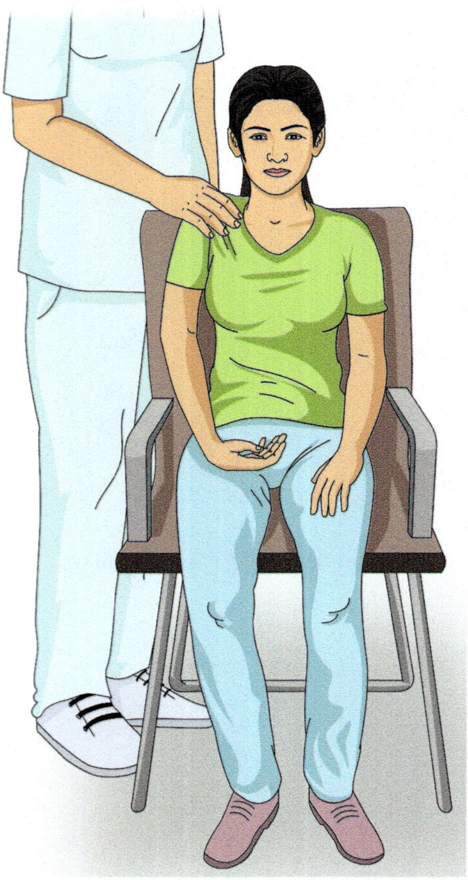

Fig. 2.30 Shrug of the main and collateral channels method

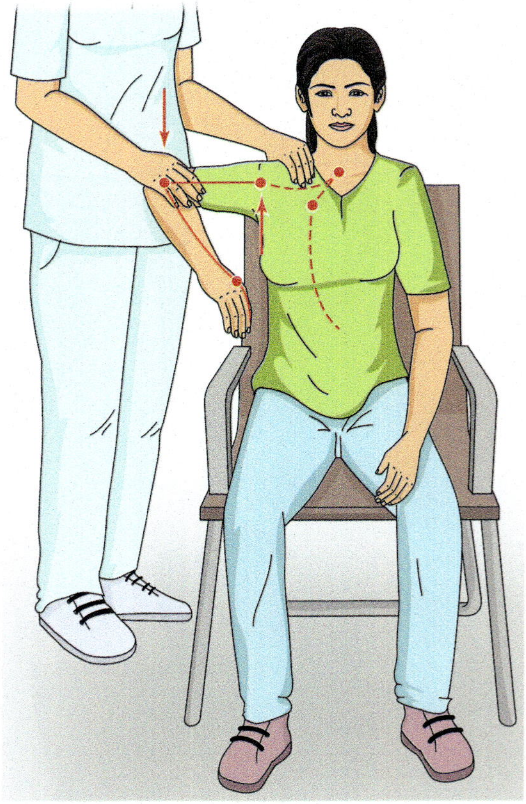

Fig. 2.31 Shoulder abduction of the main and collateral channels method

paralysis, monoplegia induced by peripheral nerve injury and dyskinesia after muscle injury of bone and joint, and also can be used in various aspects such as cognition, vision, audition, beauty, snore, swallow, diaphragm, sphincter and sub-health. The specific methods should be referred to individual chapters.

2.2 Therapeutic Methods of Neurological Training Rehabilitation

As previously mentioned, there is no regenerative ability in CNS cells. The lost functions after central damages are mainly dependent on nor-

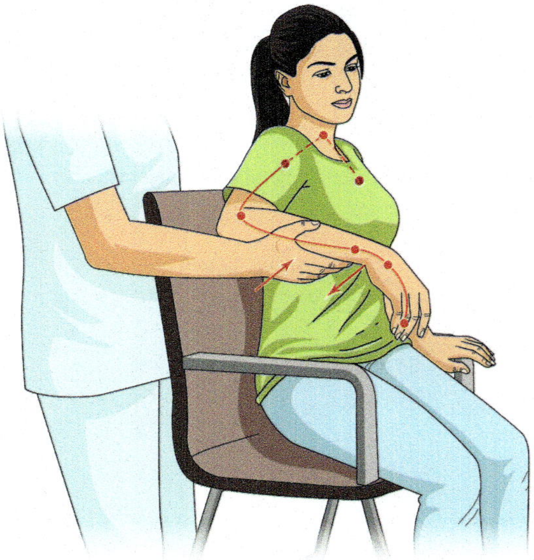

Fig. 2.32 Elbow extension of the main and collateral channels method

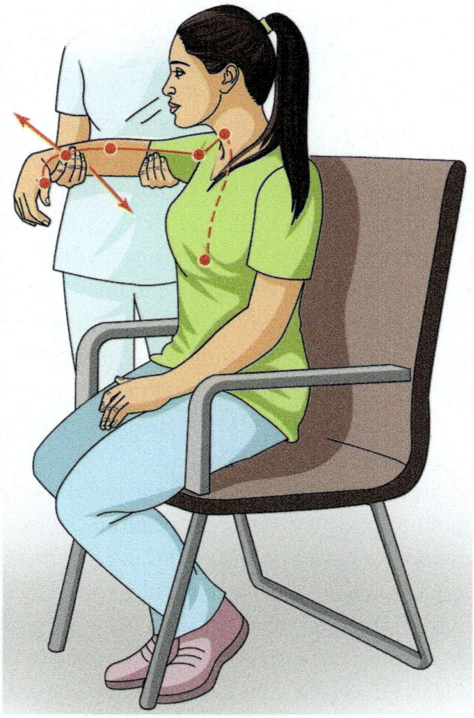

Fig. 2.33 Elbow flexion of the main and collateral channels method

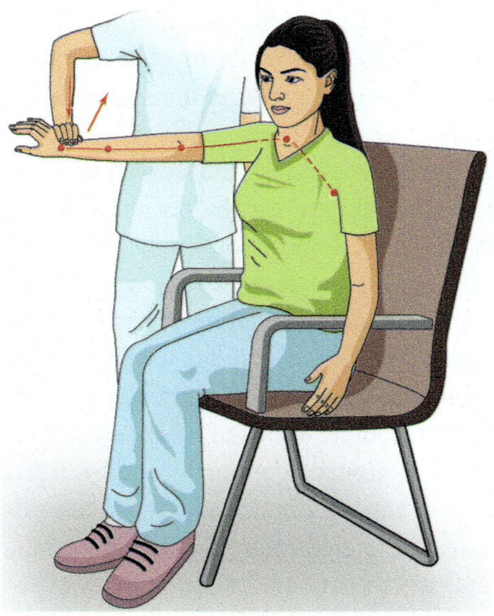

Fig. 2.34 Wrist extension of the main and collateral channels method

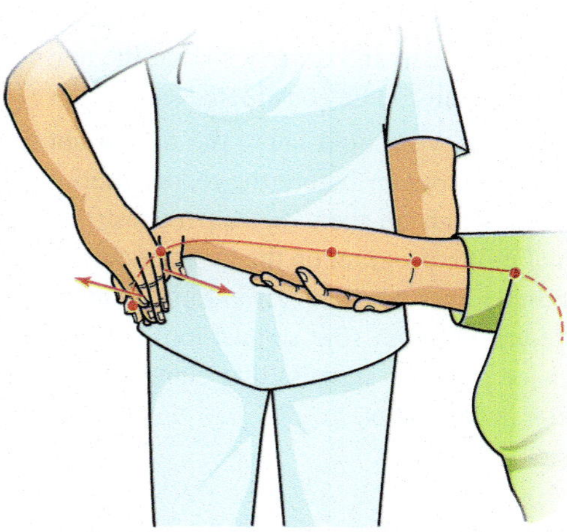

Fig. 2.35 Wrist flexion of the main and collateral channels method

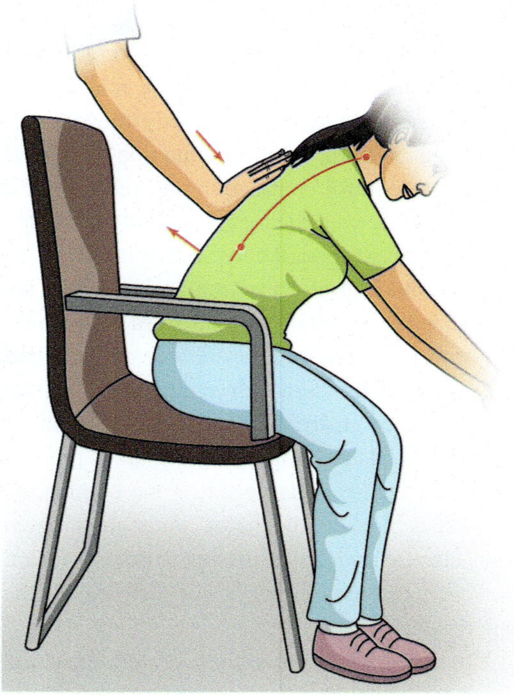

Fig. 2.36 Lumbus stretching of the main and collateral channels method

mal cells around the injured area or activation of spare conduction pathway to replace the functions of injured cells (development and utilization of CNS neural potential). Six-step Daoyin technique can develop the CNS neural potential better. However, developing neural potential is not enough. If the new activated cells should work coordinated and orderly, the motor functions can be recovered. The completion of one joint motion is the result of cooperation of many cells. One cell or one conduction pathway cannot complete the joint motion. The cells are trained to work coordinated and orderly so that the normal motor program can be constructed.

However, we should know the fact of abnormal motor program before the reconstruction of motor program an then we can reconstruct the normal motor program on the basis of correcting abnormal motor program. To do this, we must see the motor program (the acquisition and display of motor program signals) that control the joint motion in the cortex.

2.2.1 Acquisition of Motor Program Signal: Experimental Study on the Source of Surface Electromyogram Signal

After the injury of brain, spinal cord and nerve, it is known that the motor functions of limbs would be lost. Therefore, there is a close relationship between nervous system and body movements. In nervous system, the main function of central nerve is to control contraction and relaxation of muscles. Moreover, the main function of conduction tract and peripheral nerve is to transmit information from central nerve to muscles, which are recognized research result in modern medicine.

From the above mentioned, we can infer that the source of the signal detected in the muscle contraction by instrument is from cortex motor center, which is motor program signal. If the cortex motor center is damaged or the conduction pathway is blocked, the motor center cannot generate electrical signal even the muscle is intact. However, the hypothesis is not testified by the experiment.

Up to this day, the source of intramuscular electromyographic signal or surface electromyography signal (sEMG) still isn't identified. The sources of the two signals are mixed up and are controversial, but it is widely believed that the signal is due to electrical activity in muscle contraction. Therefore, it is called electromyography.

The source of EMG is a problem that must be clarified, because it is involved in the question that whether the motor program is existed, whether the motor program can be displayed and whether the functions of cortex motor center can be recovered or the limbs motor functions can be recovered through reconstructing normal motor program. If the EMG is generated by muscle contraction, signal amplification will lead to myodynamia enhancement. If the signal is from CNS, signal amplification will lead to CNS functions enhancement. There is significant difference between the training of simple enhancing muscle strength and the training of reconstructing motor program. Myodynamia training is a process of effect training. The effect will attenuate or disappear after training ceases. For example, a person who could lift 60 kg now can lift 100 kg through hard training, but cannot lift the same weight without training for one year or more. However, constructing motor program training is a process of established methodology. Unless the CNS is damaged severely, the effect will last a long time after training ceases. For example, once a person learned to ride a bike or swim, he can ride a bike or swim without training for 10 years. The example demonstrates that rehabilitation training should focus on brain functions recovery and reconstruction of motor program.

In order to clarify the question, we used animals in waken state to do mechanical stimulus experiment, which can rest the source and type of sEMG.

In previous studies, the researches on the source of sEMG are carried out through electrical stimulation. Some studies indicated that there was difference between sEMG signal detected through electrical stimulation of peripheral nerve and normal sEMG, which due to the interference of stimulative current that can hinder the analysis of signal resource. We used mechanical stimulus to induce voluntary contraction and reflex contraction of muscles in animals in waken state to exclude the interference of external stimulative current, which is good for the analysis of sEMG signal resource.

Thirty adult New Zealand rabbits (half males and half females) are used in our experiment. The rats were provided by Department of Laboratory Animal Science in Capital Medical University. The body weight is 2.15–2.60 kg and the average weight is 2.35 kg. We used Neuroeducator III, 3 M Ag-AgCl surface electrode that was produced by Therapeutic Alliances in America. Neuroeducator III was used to detect sEMG signal and record it. The signal is obtained from analysis of sEMG signal that is less than 140 dB. The root mean square of potential is less than 0.2 μV noise level and bandwidth is 10–1000 Hz. We combined during of sEMG signal to exceed 0.1 s and standard it as μVs. Meanwhile, the data in every one-tenth second is displayed in color display with continuous curve. The scan time limit of every screen is 20 s. The receive mode is ECG shielding signal. The data are stored for analysis.

We used hwato-med (0.35 mm × 13 mm) produced by Suzhou medical supplies limited company. We choose 1 cm above the trailing edge of heel with Achilles's tendon as the stimulating point. Acupuncture pin is inserted from 10 cm above the stimulating point until the acupuncture pin penetrates the tendon below the entry point. We observed whether the acupuncture pin can induce the contraction of musculus gastrocnemius and recorded the electrical signal.

The rabbit is fixed on the operation table. The surface skin is unhaired and the electrodes are placed around muscle belly. The first electrode is placed on the skin surface above the middle of the muscle belly that is 1 cm away from the muscle starting point. The second electrode is placed on the skin surface above the middle of the muscle belly that is 1 cm away from the muscle stopping point. Grounding electrode is placed between the two surface electrodes. The surface electrodes are linked to the first lead of Neuroeducator III the through wire. The procedures of the experiments are as follows: (1) In the waking state, the right Achilles's tendon is acupunctured to induce voluntary contraction of musculus gastrocnemius and the intensity and form of sEMG are detected in real-time. (2) Ischiadic nerve is detached. Midpoint of the line segment between ischial tuberosity and greater trochanter of femur is the mark. We cut open the back of the right thigh in length wise. One percentage lidocaine used for local infiltration, we cut open every layers below the skin, detach the tissues, find the ischiadic nerve and cut it off, put the distal end out of the incision and suture the incision. Achilles's tendon, distal ischiadic nerve stump, the right musculus gastrocnemius are separately stimulated. The contraction of musculus gastrocnemius is observed and the intensity and form of sEMG are detected in real-time. When the right ankle is passively moved, the contraction of musculus gastrocnemius is observed and the intensity and form of sEMG are detected in real-time. (3) The spinal cord is transected. The electrodes are placed in the skin surface of left musculus gastrocnemius and then are linked to the first lead of Neuroeducator III. 2 cm above the intercrestal line of pelvis, 1% lidocaine used for local anaesthesia, we cut open the middle of the back in length wise, detach the tissues layer by layer, expose the spine, cut off L2–L4 spinous process and vertebral plate, expose spinal cord, cut off spinal cord in L3 plane and suture the incision layer by layer. The left Achilles's tendon is stimulated to test the contraction of musculus gastrocnemius. The intensity and form of sEMG are detected in real-time. The rabbits are sacrificed using air embolism through rabbit's auricular vein.

The results: Thirty experiment animals were included in this experiment and the wave form, intensity and duration of the sEMG were detected for 180 times (Table 2.3).

Table 2.3 The detection result of electromyography signal of musculus gastrocnemius ($\bar{x} \pm s$)

	Normal state	Interruption of ischiadic nerve				Transected spinal cord
Items	Stimulation of Achilles's tendon	Stimulation of Achilles's tendon	Stimulation of nerve	Stimulation of muscle	Passive movement	Stimulation of Achilles's tendon
Signal strength (μV)	353.3 ± 96.1	0.3 ± 0.8	0.2 ± 0.4	5.0 ± 3.5	0.0 ± 0.0	27.9 ± 55.0
Wave form	Wide base random wave	Interference wave	Interference wave	Interference wave	No wave	Narrow base reflex wave
Wave length (s)	4	<0.5	<0.5	<0.5	0	<1

Our experiments demonstrated that the wave form of sEMG was high-strength wide base random wave when Achilles's tendon was stimulated and the voluntary contraction of musculus gastrocnemius was induced (Fig. 2.37). The wave length is 4 s. The joint is moved passively in order to pull the musculus gastrocnemius but cannot induce the muscle contraction. There is no sEMG signal received by the apparatus (Fig. 2.38). After transection of spinal cord, stimulating Achilles's tendon can induce reflex contraction of musculus gastrocnemius. At this moment, the low-intensity narrow base reflex wave can be received (Fig. 2.39) and the wave length is less than 1 s. After transection of ischiadic nerve, we stimulated Achilles's tendon, muscle and the distal end of transected nerve and cannot induce muscle contraction. However, we can receive weak irregular interference wave (Fig. 2.40, 2.41, and 2.42) and the wave length is less than 0.5 s.

The intensity of electrical signal (353.3 ± 96.1 μV) in voluntary contraction of musculus gastrocnemius is 12.7 times of that (27.9 ± 55.0 μV) in reflex contraction of musculus gastrocnemius after transection of spinal cord. The duration time is four times of that in reflex contraction. These evidences proved that the electrical signal received from skin surface of the muscle in voluntary contraction derived from high level motor center.

The cortex motor center generates nervous impulse signal. The signal reaches neuromuscular junction through neural conduction pathway step by step. The membrane permeability of neural fiber is changed, which induces inward flow of calcium ion. And then the exocytosis of synaptic vesicles is triggered and the acetyl choline are released from frontal membrane of neuromuscular junction. This is the process of the generation of voluntary movements. The acetyl choline can bind endplate receptors through synaptic cleft and induce endplate potential. Electrotonic potential can stimulate peripheral myolemma to produce action potential and induce muscle contraction. This is the process of the generation of voluntary movements. The physiological process is composed of the transformation and transduction of primary electrical signal to chemical signal and then to electrical signal. Conway and his colleagues detected the electrical signal of offside cortex motor center and EMG of extensor or flexor muscle of wrist and found that there were short-time low-frequency coherence between electrical signal and EMG in

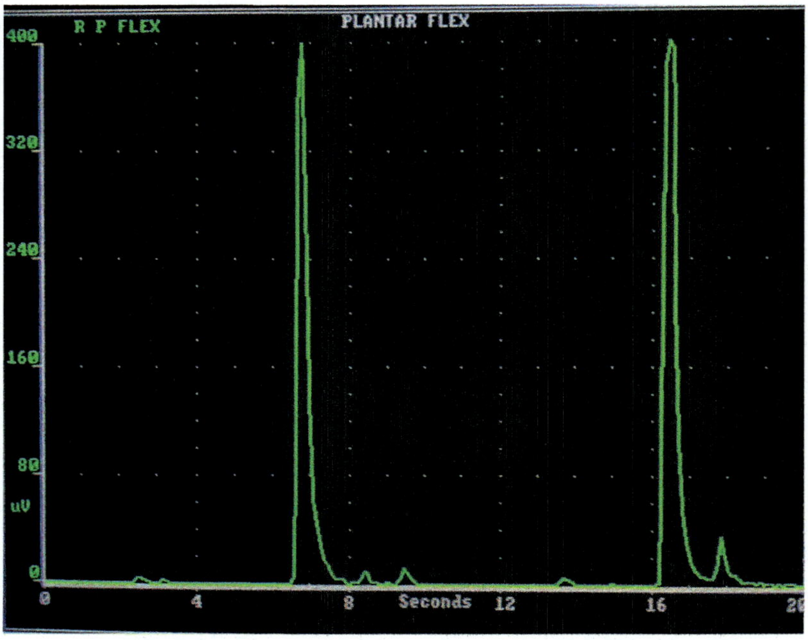

Fig. 2.37 The wave form of sEMG was high-strength wide base random wave when Achilles's tendon was stimulated and the voluntary contraction of musculus gastrocnemius was induced

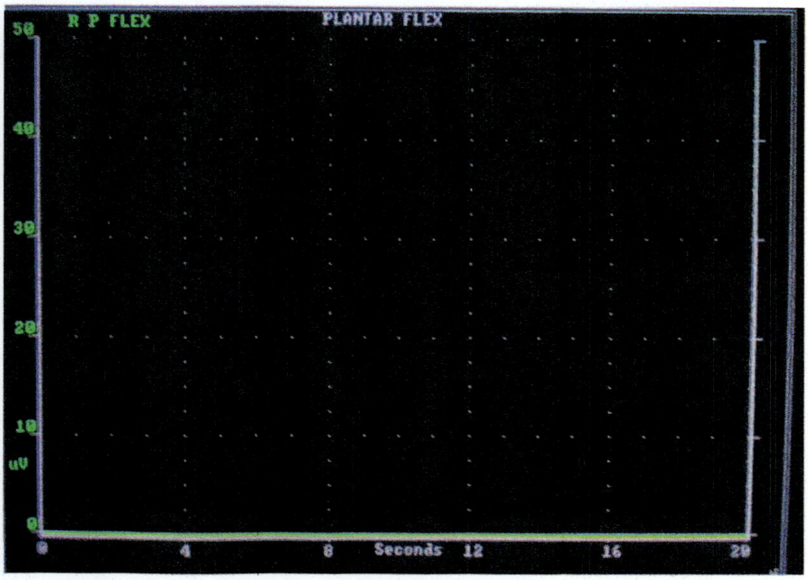

Fig. 2.38 The joint is moved passively in order to pull the musculus gastrocnemius but cannot induce the muscle contraction. There is no sEMG signal received by the apparatus

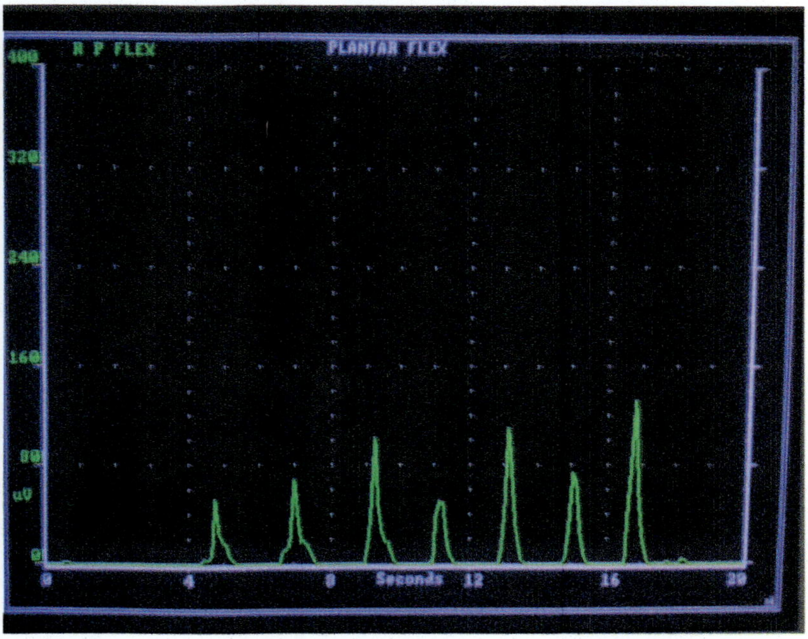

Fig. 2.39 After transection of spinal cord, stimulating Achilles's tendon can induce reflex contraction of musculus gastrocnemius. At this moment, the low-intensity narrow base reflex wave can be received

rapid active movement. According to the results, they inferred that low-frequency electrical signal of cortex motor center had some effects on the generation of EMG in rapid point-to-point wrist movements. EMG and brain electrical signal are used for controlling mechanical prosthesis and functional stimulation of paralytic limbs. Carmena and his colleagues used the brain electrical signals from cortex motor center of non-human primates to control the movements of mechanical arms successfully. In 1982, Graupe and his colleagues applied EMG for functional neuromuscular stimulation for the first time. He mapped the EMG obtained from upper trunk to functional neuromuscular stimulation signal and made the patients with paraplegia to walk.

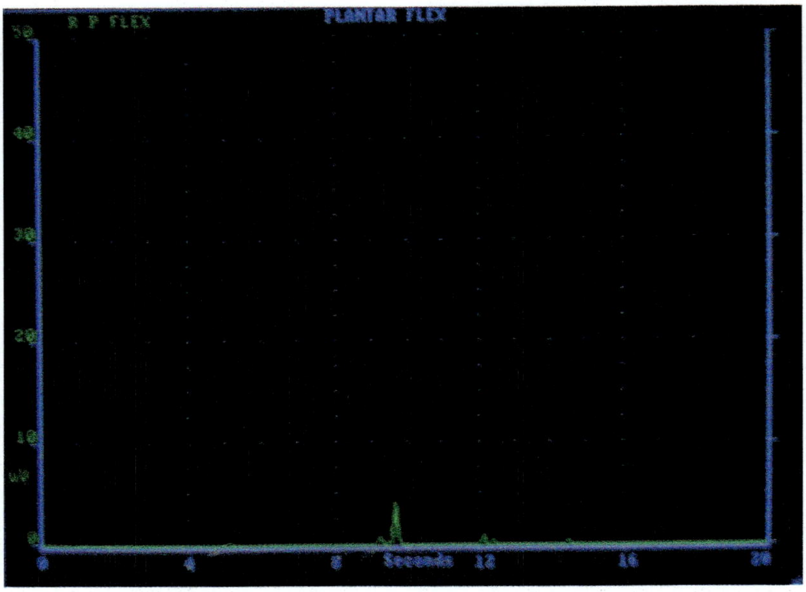

Fig. 2.40 After transection of ischiadic nerve, we stimulated Achilles's tendon and cannot induce muscle contraction. However, we can receive weak irregular interference wave

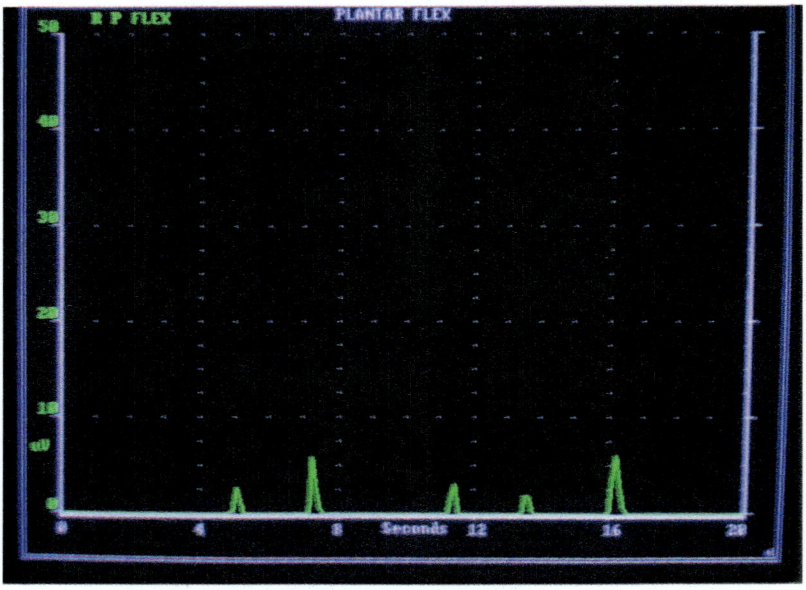

Fig. 2.41 After transection of ischiadic nerve, we stimulated muscle and cannot induce muscle contraction. However, we can receive weak irregular interference wave

Dyskinesia induced by central damages such as stroke, cerebral trauma and child cerebral palsy is due to irreversible damage to brain cells. There is no damage in the peripheral nerves and muscles of the patients and there are damages in the brain. We found in the clinic that the signal intensity from the skin surface of adult muscle is the same as that from the corresponding part in the child, but the myodynamia is significant different under the same electrical signal intensity. This phenomenon may be caused by the different volume and quality of child and adult. It is the difference between effectors but not the signal difference from motor cortex that drive the effectors. We inferred that the signal is form CNS to muscle but not generated by the muscle contraction.

In fact, the electrical signal received from muscle skin surface is generated before muscle

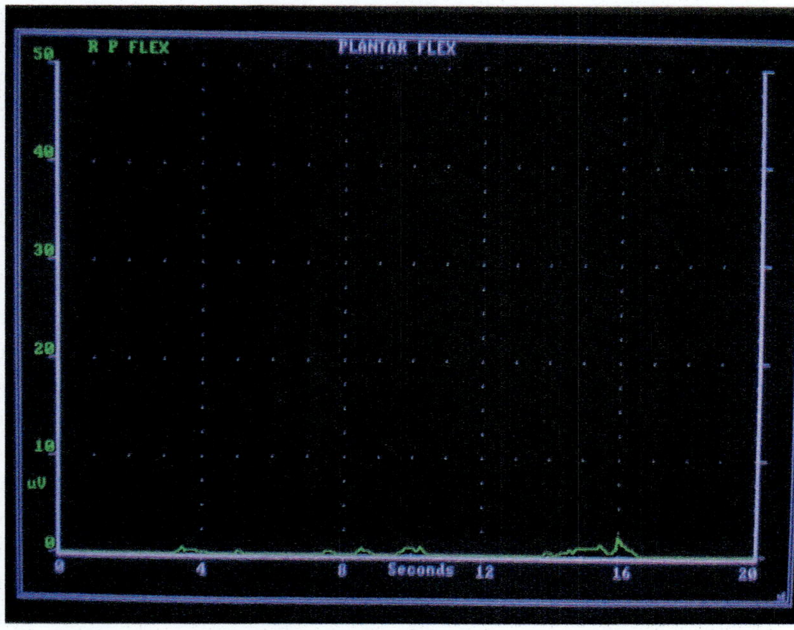

Fig. 2.42 After transection of ischiadic nerve, we stimulated the distal end of transected nerve and cannot induce muscle contraction. However, we can receive weak irregular interference wave

contraction, which is the control and drive signal from CNS to muscle. The intensity of this signal is not equal to myodynamia, but there is proportionality between the signal and myodynamia within limits.

We deem that there are two examples to prove the EMG is not directly from muscle contraction. The first is the generation of electrocardiosignal. The electrocardiosignal is from the atrionector located at the above of atrium dextrum. Atrionector can generate autorhythmic electrical excitation (electrical signal). This signal is conducted to atria myocardium and ventricular myocardium through atrioventricular bundle and ventricular Purkinje fibers and then induces the contraction of atria myocardium and ventricular myocardium. Electrocardiogram shows the conduction of autorhythmic electrical current in normal or abnormal atrial and ventricular tissue generated from atrionector but not from the contraction of atria myocardium and ventricular myocardium. When there is some kind of damages in atrioventricular tissue, autorhythmic electrical current may be influenced to varying degrees and the conduction is blocked, which can lead to systolic dysfunction of atria myocardium and ventricular myocardium. In clinic, the assessment and diagnosis of cardiac function can be detected with electrocardiogram.

On the other hand, the relationship between CNS and limbs movements can be explained using principle of automobilism. The "heart" of the automobile is the engine. The main component of the engine is internal combustion engine. Pulverization gasoline is combusted in the engine. The electric spark can light pulverization gasoline, which comes from automobile accumulator. Under the control of microcomputer, the drivers activate the ignitor and the power of ignition plug is on. When the ignition plug ejects electric spark, fuel injection nozzle in internal combustion engine start to eject gasoline and make it into spray pattern appropriate for burning. The heat from gasoline burning can move up the piston. The lifted piston can drive wheel move through conduction system and the car can move forward or backward.

Compared the relationship between CNS and limbs movements with principle of automobilism, the power is equal to human CNS and the electric wire is equal to nerve. Ignition plug is the same as neuromuscular junction. Burning of pulverization gasoline is the same as consumption of adenosine triphosphate (ATP) in muscle. The upward movement of cylinder plug is equal to muscle contraction. The conduction system is equal to joint motion. The axle drives the wheel to make the vehicle move forward, which is equal to the human movements driven by limbs.

One of the most important parts is piston movement after gasoline burning, which is the same as the process that electrical signals from CNS induce muscle contraction. It is an domino effect process that spark drives the cylinder plug move after gasoline burning. High heat energy make the cylinder plug move. During this process, the movement of cylinder plug is to make the wheel rotate but not to generate electricity. Unless the movement of cylinder plug drives specific power generation assembly such as thermoelectric generators, the electricity cannot be generated. In that case, the vehicles don't have power to move forward or backward. The result of consuming ATP is muscle contraction. The objective of muscle contraction is joint motion in order to make human body complete movements such as walking, running and jumping. It is a domino effect process but not the power generation process.

sEMG is one kind of quantitative index, which has clinical application value in the assessment of functional recovery of motor movements in the patients with CNS damages. There was no evidence to prove that the increase of sEMG can reflect the brain function recovery. We analyzed the source and type of sEMG through animal experiment and found that there was no sEMG in the process of the muscle traction by joint in passive movements. If the muscle is without innervation of peripheral nerve, the intensity of electrical signal induced by mechanical stimulation of peripheral nerve or muscle is low (less than 10 μV). The duration time is very short (less than 1 s). The weak electrical signals come from two ways. Firstly, the cell membrane permeability change after mechanical stimulation of nerve fiber or myofiber induces transfer of ions inside and outside of cell membrane. However, the potential difference generated by transfer of ions inside and outside of cell membrane cannot induce action potential and cannot induce voluntary contraction of muscle. Secondly, the sensitivity of signal receiving equipment is very high and it can receive cardiac electrical activity from the body surface. Although the ECG shielding system of the equipment was activated, it can received the low-intensity signal from the wire of the electrode on the skin surface and the signal was called interference wave by the author, which indicated that peripheral nerve and muscle are not the source of sEMG.

In the case the innervation of limbs were intact, Achilles's tendon was stimulated to induce the contraction of musculus gastrocnemius and the signal intensity was high (400 μV). The duration time is long (4 s). Although the reflex center that induced contraction reflex of musculus gastrocnemius was located in spinal cord, pain stimulation can induce avoidance reflex and brain dominated limbs to avoid pain stimulation. The voluntary contraction of musculus gastrocnemius could be induced so that the wave form was wide base random wave. After transection of spinal cord, we stimulated Achilles's tendon and detected low-intensity (less than 100 μV), short duration time (less than 1 s) electrical signal. This is because higher nerve center lost control of lower nerve center. In that case, the reflex was induced in spinal cord and the signals are only from motor neurons of anterior horn of the spinal cord. Therefore, the wave form was narrow base reflex wave. Just like the knee jerk reflex whose reflex center was in spinal cord, patellar tendon was knocked to induce involuntary and rapid knee jerk reflex.

We analyzed the experiment results and some phenomenon in life and deemed that electrical signals of muscle contraction received from skin surface mainly originated from cortex motor center. Simple peripheral nerve innervation, passive contraction of muscles and spinal reflex cannot induce electrical signals of voluntary contraction of muscles. Only the signals from brain to movements muscles through cascade conduction can induce electrical signals of voluntary contraction of muscles. Therefore, electrical signals received from skin surface on the part of muscles are the integrated electrical signal from higher nerve center and lower nerve center to muscles, mainly are electrical signals from higher nerve center.

Many muscles such as agonistic muscle, antagonistic muscle, synergic muscle and neutralized muscle are involved in the completion of a joint motion. Many joint motions are involved in a coordinate exercise of the limbs with practical functions. All the muscle that take part in the limbs movements are controlled by the electrical signals from CNS. These signals are released sequentially and proportionally in order to complete coordinated limbs movements. For the single joint motion, motor program means the ratio of signal intensity of agonistic muscle to the signal intensity of antagonistic muscle. The ratio of signal intensity of agonistic muscle to the signal intensity of antagonistic muscle is 10–1 in motor program of a normal joint motion. For the multi-joint coordinate exercise, motor program means the specified order of seniority of motor program in single joint motion. For example, in the motor program of walking, hip flexor of the "step forward" leg receive signals from cortex motor center firstly and the lower limbs step forward. Hamstring muscles receive signals from cortex motor center secondly to induce knee flexion. Tibialis anterior muscle receives signals from cortex motor center finally to induce foot dorsiflexion. These sequential and proportional signals from CNS are called motor program signals. Therefore, electrical signals of muscle contraction in joint motion and limbs movements are the motor program signals from CNS to muscles. This is different from the meaning of traditional EMG. Traditional EMG is the current generated by muscle contraction. However, motor program signals mean the electrical signals controlling or driving muscle contraction involved in joint motion but not the electrical signals generated by muscle contraction.

The relationship between myodynamia and motor program signals are mentioned before. The signal is in proportion to myodynamia within limits. The stronger the motor program signal is, the stronger the myodynamia is. Along with the increase of the motor program signal, the myodynamia is not increased proportional. The signal intensity of motor program in children and adults is 640–800 μV. The highest motor program signal of the person with strong myodynamia is less than 800 μV, but there is significant difference of myodynamia between the people with strong myodynamia and the people with weak myodynamia.

In clinical rehabilitation training, we found that the recovery of motor program signal is before the myodynamia recovery in the motor function recovery after CNS damages. This process took about 3 months or more. Long time muscle disuse induced amyotrophy. Although the signal was high, the effect of muscle contraction was weak. These results were published in Chinese Journal of Tissue Engineering Research [2011;15(46):8693–7].

2.2.2 The Role of "Objective and Motive" Mechanism in the Development of Human Potentials

Comfort and enjoyment are good intension and pursue in human life. Laziness many be the humanity, but the base of comfort and enjoyment is giving. You can get what you want only through giving. If a person has no plan, he idles away his time and does nothing day by day. Setting a goal can promote people to try their best. Setting a goal with some rewards and punishment can increase the work efficiency so that it can provide material basis for the people. Goal is the orientation and the motive of working. It can make people to complete the almost impossible task. Setting a goal promotes people to achieve or overfulfil the expectant indicator, which is called "objective and motive" mechanism and can promote human potentials effectively. The specific goal can be expressed by quantity, altitude, task and ability. In order to stimulate people's motive, the goal should be more clear and easier. The closer the relationship between the goal and the effect is, the more important the effect of potential development is.

"Objective and motive" mechanism can be applied for any area. It is said that the whole year's work depends on a good start in spring and the whole day's work depends on a good start in the morning, which demonstrates the importance of plan and goal. Our country sets Five-year Plan for development and lets the whole nation and various sectors step towards this goal. After eleven Five-year Plans, there were earth-shaking changes in China. If a primary school student can set a study goal very early by himself not by his parents, he may study very well. If he wants to enter into the top two schools (Tsinghua University and Peking University) in China and he does work hard, the chance to enter into Tsinghua University and Peking University is good.

"Objective and motive" mechanism was widely and necessarily applied for competitive sports training. For example, the cross-bar of jumper, the target of archery, target of shooting, weight of weightlifting and degrees of free exercises are all the goals of sports training. With these targets, the athletes can surpass them one by one through training and improve their competitiveness.

The training of recovery of motor function after CNS damages is a process of development of CNS potentials. Therefore, the training goals that are in accordance with "Objective and motive" mechanism, visualized, effective and practical can assure the effects of rehabilitation training.

2.2.3 The Display of Effect of Objective Indicators in Six-Step Daoyin Technique

Daoyin technique was invented 2000 years ago. Daoyin technique in modern times is seldom used in clinic, which may be due to lack of objective indicators in Daoyin technique. Therefore, the display and effect of objective indicators in Daoyin technique, especially the objective indicators in the application of Daoyin technique as adjuvant therapy, is the important symbol of development and renaissance of ancient Daoyin technique.

The display of effect of objective indicators in Daoyin technique is divided into different subtypes. The first is the objective indicator of long-term effect. At present, assessment methods of effect of rehabilitation therapy used at home and abroad are all the objective indicators of long-term effect. During the training process or after the training, the objective indicators of long-term effect such as myodynamia, ability of daily living, walking and balance ability can be obtained through international assessment methods, but these indicators can only assess the effects of rehabilitation training. Although the therapeutic schedule can be modified by this, these methods cannot be applied for direct adjuvant therapy. The second is that these indicators can be used as real-time display of objective indicators of direct adjuvant therapy. The effect of real-time display of effect of objective indicators is the same as target of the archery and cross-bar of jumping. These indicators can provide specific goals for the people who are trained and are good for timely adjustment of training scheme in order to do targeted training and promote training effect.

Six-step Daoyin technique can regulate the brain or the ability of muscle contraction dominated by CNS. This ability can be transmitted through motor program electrical signals sequentially and proportionally. This signal can be received from skin surface on the part of muscles through receiving equipment of electronic signal in real-time. The received signal is showed as waveform or sound in real-time, which is result feedback.

Feedback regulation is an important mechanism to achieve control and balance. This mechanism not only exists in human body, but also in daily life. The regulation of human endocrine, blood pressure and temperature are realized through feedback mechanism. The normal temperature of human body is around 37 °C. When the body temperature is less than 37 °C, excitability of thermogenic center in metathalamus increases, heat production increases, heat dissipation decreases, and the body temperature increases. On the contrary, when the body temperature is more than 37 °C, excitability of thermolytic center in anterior thalamus increases, heat production decreases, heat dissipation increases, and the body temperature decreases. On this account, body temperature can be maintained around 37 °C, which is good for the normal process of metabolism in vivo. The feedback mechanism is used in the equipment of maintaining environment temperature. If the room temperature is set to 24 °C, when the room temperature is lower than the setting temperature, the thermoreceptor of air-conditioner can detect the temperature change and the heating system of air-conditioner is activated to increase the temperature. When the room temperature reaches 24 °C, the heating system of air-conditioner stops. When the room temperature is higher than the setting temperature, the thermoreceptor of air-conditioner can detect the temperature change and the cooling system of air-conditioner is activated to decrease the temperature. Through repeated regulation, the room temperature is maintained around 24 °C.

It is observed from this process that feedback is the base of regulation. Without feedback, we cannot know the real-time situation and cannot analyze the correctness of the situation. Regulating system cannot adapt to the situation. Therefore, feedback and regulation are the process that we know what is correct and take steps to correct it with a purpose to achieve goals.

The real-time monitoring and display of motor program signal can be realized in six-step Daoyin technique, which is the combination of result feedback and regulation method. Through different lead receiving electrodes of signal monitoring equipment (four-lead in general), motor program signals from CNS to agonistic muscles or antagonistic muscles can be received separately when the patients are guided to do a joint motion and the signals from CNS to agonistic muscles of joint motion can be received in coordinated exercise for multiple joints. These two signals can be displayed real-timely in the fluorescent screen separately through curve form. Under the instruction of the therapists, the patients can be guided to do the training with a purpose. Real-time result feedback demonstrated that feedback not only let the therapists and the patients know existence, strength, right or wrong of motor program signals precisely to design correct therapeutic schedule and do targeted training, but also design different degree targets for the patients through software program of the equipment to use "objective and motive" mechanism to do the training of development of CNS potential.

For the patients who merely know whether the training can achieve the required goal, the sound feedback can be applied for meeting requirements. For example, in the training of elbow extension, signal intensity from CNS to triceps muscle of arm was 20 μV in last training and the setting goal required the patients to exceed this signal intensity in this training. Through the system settings of the equipment, when the signal exceeds 20 μV, the equipment makes a noise in order to let the patients know their progresses through hard work. However, the sound feedback is not precise and the sound is constant whether the value surpassing a goal is big or small. There is no visible and mobile curve surpassing the targeted horizontal line, which can motivate the patients to do their best. In addition, sound feedback is not appropriate for the training of regulation of proportion and intensity of motor program. For the patients with poor eyesight or blind person, compared with the training with no feedback, sound feedback is a more effective training method.

For correcting abnormal motor program and reconstructing normal motor program, visual feedback is a better method. When the patients are guided to do a joint motion, the equipment can detect motor program signal from CNS to agonistic muscles or antagonistic muscles and display it real-timely on fluorescent screen through curve form. According to the practical situation of motor program, the therapists can do various kinds of trainings such as the training of promoting agonistic muscle signal. Through the operating system of the equipment, the guided agonistic muscle signal last time is set as the baseline that should surpassed in this time. The guided antagonistic muscle signal last time is set as bottom line that should surpassed in this time (Fig. 2.43). During training process, the therapists use six-step Daoyin technique to guide the patients to surpass the baseline of agonistic muscle signal and bottom line of antagonistic muscle signal under the linear signal curve. Through motivated and targeted training, in the process of promoting motion signal gradually, the proportional motor program can be established.

The author combines six-step Daoyin technique with biological feedback technology to form rehabilitation method, which is called "Daoyin feedback technique in traditional Chinese medicine". Motor program signal is the objective feedback index of the effect of Daoyin

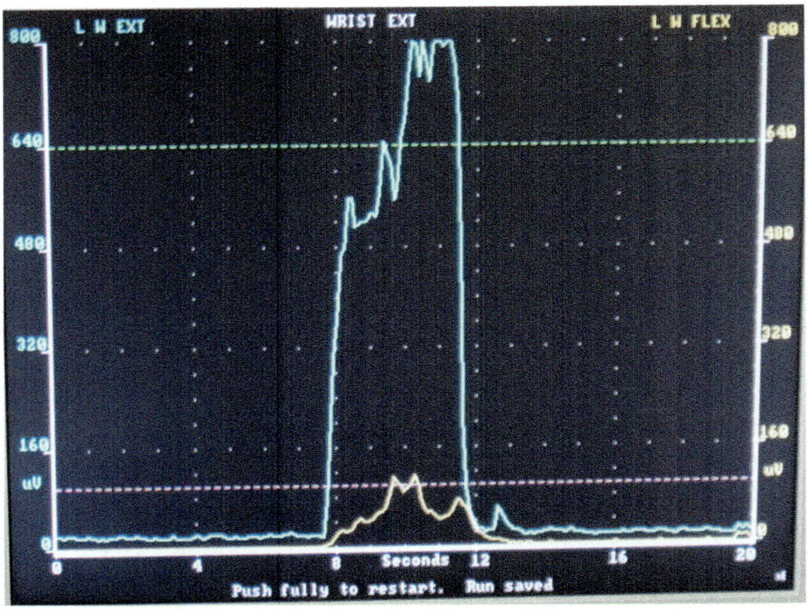

Fig. 2.43 Baseline setting in the training of reestablishing motor program

technique. Because continuous dynamic detection and real-time display in curve form are realized, the feedback effect of motor program signal is superior to that of target. Therefore, it is possible for targeted training of rehabilitation functional assessment, development of therapeutic schedule, establishment of surpassing and lowering target, development of CNS potential and reconstruction of motor program. It plays an indispensable role in development of CNS potential, implementation of reconstruction method of motor program and recovery of lost motor function. It can also open up a new way for modernization development and renaissance of Daoyin technique, establishment of new rehabilitation method.

2.2.4 The Origin and Definition of Neurological Training

Six-step Daoyin technique is applied in Daoyin feedback technique in traditional Chinese medicine. Qi is guided in this method and is used to dredge the channel and develop brain function, and then the brain or central nervous system is recovered. Therefore, the author called it neurological training. This technique is widely applied because every cell of nine anatomy systems is innervated by nerves. At present, on the basis of basic techniques of neurological training rehabilitation, the therapeutic methods are developed for motor function, cognition, vision, audition, swallow, sphincter, scapulohumeral periarthritis and Lumbago-leg pain. A series of techniques are formed to be used for almost all rehabilitation therapies. Therefore, it is called rehabilitation therapeutics system of neurological training. In this system, there are not only independent theory and rehabilitation method, but also a series of specific corollary equipment, which will be introduced in the following chapters.

The definition of rehabilitation technology of neurological training is that neurological training focus on rehabilitation techniques in traditional Chinese medicine with supplement of biological feedback technology and includes a series of new technologies in rehabilitation therapy that integrates traditional Chinese and western medicine. The basic theories of it are neural plasticity and motor program. The basic technique of it is Daoyin technique in order to clear and activate the channels and collaterals, develop brain functions. Modern electronic equipment are used to monitor the signal of potentials and the effect of Daoyin technique is displayed real-timely on fluorescent screen in curve form. Through feedback mechanism, the patients are instructed to regulate signal intensity with a purpose, adjust disorganized motor program and consolidate it, enhance myodynamia, remodel motor pattern with whole training, recover independent coordinated motor function and increase ability in daily life.

Daoyin technique is used in this therapy to develop neural potential, reconstruct motor program and remodel motor pattern, which plays an important therapeutic role. Motor program signal monitoring and real-time display of the effect of Daoyin technique provide the target required for promoting the effect of Daoyin technique through feedback mechanism, which plays a supportive therapeutic role.

Compared with traditional rehabilitation techniques, rehabilitation methods of neurological training focus on active movements and mainly act on CNS, but traditional rehabilitation techniques focus on lower nerve center and muscles. The comparison of the effect of the two methods is referred to Fig. 2.44.

2.2.5 Rectification of Abnormal Motor Program and Consolidation of Normal Motor Program

As what are mentioned before, muscles involved in single joint motion include agonistic muscle, antagonistic muscle, neutral muscle and synergic muscle. For the extension and flexion of joint, the movement muscles include simply agonistic muscle and antagonistic muscle. In elbow extension, triceps muscle of arm is the agonistic muscle and in elbow flexion bicipital muscle of arm is the agonistic muscle. Agonistic muscle is the main muscle to complete joint motion. The functions of antagonistic muscle are to maintain the stability of joint motion and prevent damage of excessive movement of joint.

The effect of agonistic muscle and antagonistic muscle on joint motion is the same as learning to ride a bike. The bikers are equal to agonistic muscles of joint. The people who uphold the bike are equal to antagonistic muscle. When riding, the bigger the difference between the force of pedaling and the force of upholding the bike

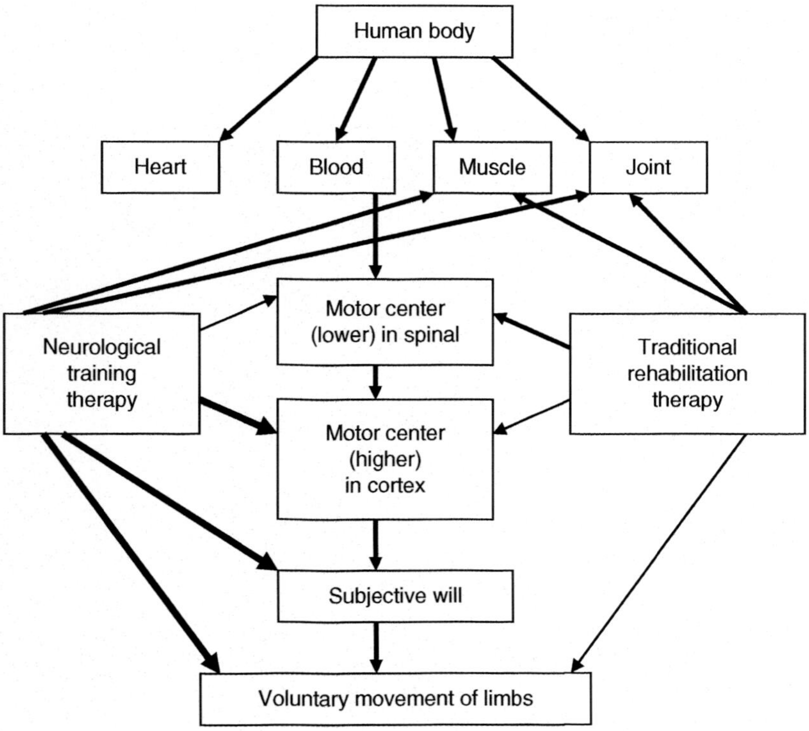

Fig. 2.44 Comparison of the effects of neurological training and traditional rehabilitation therapy

with backward traction is, the bigger the force of pedaling is and the faster the speed is. On the contrary, if the force of upholding the bike with backward traction is too big, the force of pedaling is becoming small and it is difficulty to ride a bike forward. Therefore, the proper proportion between the two forces is required to make the riding flexible and stable.

Joint motion is also the case. For the single joint motion, motor program center of single joint located in Brodmann 4 area gives out properly proportional motor program signal to be involved in the agonistic muscle and antagonistic muscle of joint motion, which is the important guarantee for flexibility and stability of joint motion. Through preliminary measurement, in joint motion of human body, the proper proportion of signal between agonistic muscle and antagonistic muscle is about 10–1. Motor program signal without this proportion is called disorganized motor program.

Accordance to the normal range of human motor program signal intensity (640–800 μV), when the signal intensity of agonistic muscle is 640 μV, the signal intensity of antagonistic muscle is 64 μV. On the basis of this, the more severely the proportion of motor program signal loses balance, the more difficulty the joint motion is. In the condition that the signal intensity of agonistic muscle keeps stable, the stronger the antagonistic muscle signal is, the more difficulty the joint motion is. When the proportion of motor program signal is inverted, the signal intensity of antagonistic muscle is stronger than the signal intensity of agonistic muscle. If the patients try to extend their elbows, because the signal form CNS to bicipital muscle of arm is stronger than the signal form CNS to triceps muscle of arm, the elbow extension cannot be completed, even there will be elbow flexion in the process of elbow extension.

Abnormal motor programs of single joint motion include following subtypes:

2.2.5.1 Subtype Accordance to the Signal Proportion and Intensity of Agonistic Muscle and Antagonistic Muscle

1. The type of no motor program signal: In severe CNS damages, neural cells that generate motor program signals or neural conduction pathways that conduct signals are destroyed severely and the muscles are completely paralyzed without motor program signals from the area of CNS damage to the muscles of joint motion in offside body part dominated by the area of CNS damage. There is no joint motion at last (Fig. 2.45). The type

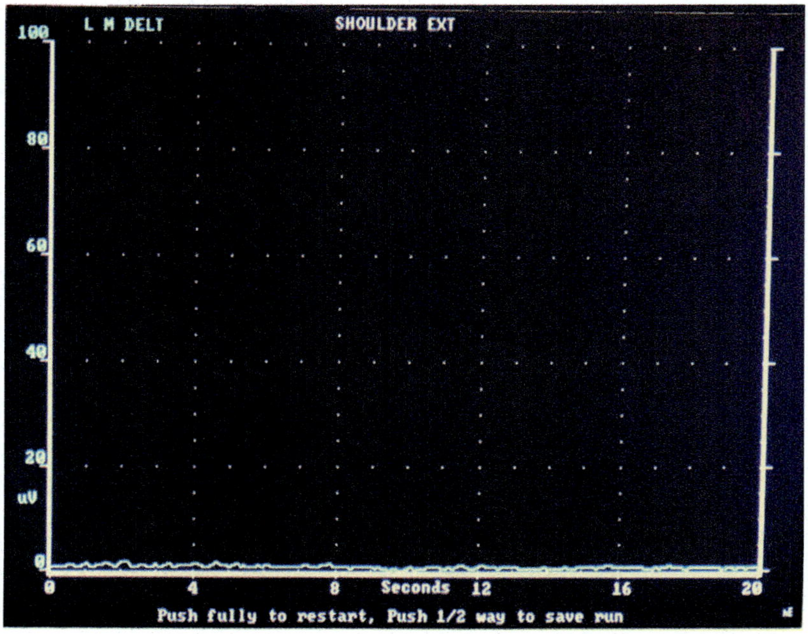

Fig. 2.45 The type of no motor program signal

of no motor program signal demonstrates that the CNS of the patients is damaged severely. It takes longer time to recover functions through rehabilitation training and there will be dyskinesia to some extent left.

2. The type of normal proportion of motor program signal with low intensity: This type of signal is commonly detected in the early period of CNS damages of the patients with paralyzed limbs who force themselves to do exercise such as the patients who don't walk out of bed without muscle spasm in upper limbs (Fig. 2.46). At this time, the patients are guided to do joint motion, when the joint of paralyzed side limbs can move, not only the motor program signal can be detected, but also the signal intensity proportion of agonistic muscle and antagonistic muscle usually is in a normal range, but the signal intensity will be decreased to some extent. This type of signal demonstrated that there were CNS damages, but there were still some normal neural tissue with functions. Because the patients don't force themselves to do joint motion too early, abnormal motor program is induced by that the function of paralyzed muscle is compensated by peripheral muscle. Through standard rehabilitation training such as three-stage method of neurological training introduced in this book, the patients with this type of signal can recover functions ideally and the abnormal motor pattern cannot be formed.

3. Disproportionality of motor program signal with low intensity: This type of signal is commonly detected in the early recovery period and medium recovery period of the patients with CNS damages (Fig. 2.47). Compensatory mechanism is activated and undead neural tissue in injured CNS area and around injured CNS area can replace the functions of injured neural tissue. However, because the time is not appropriate and the functions are not replaced completely, the signal intensity from CNS to the muscle of joint motion is weak. Moreover, there is no compatible ability of the compensated neural tissue. Therefore, the proportion of motor program signal to agonistic muscle and antagonistic muscle is disordered. There is more severe dyskinesia in the patients with this type of signal who has abnormal motor pattern. The therapy usually takes a long time. On the basis of developing neural potential, reestablishing motor program, restricting motor pattern training in unnecessary movements in exercise, there will be good functional recovery.

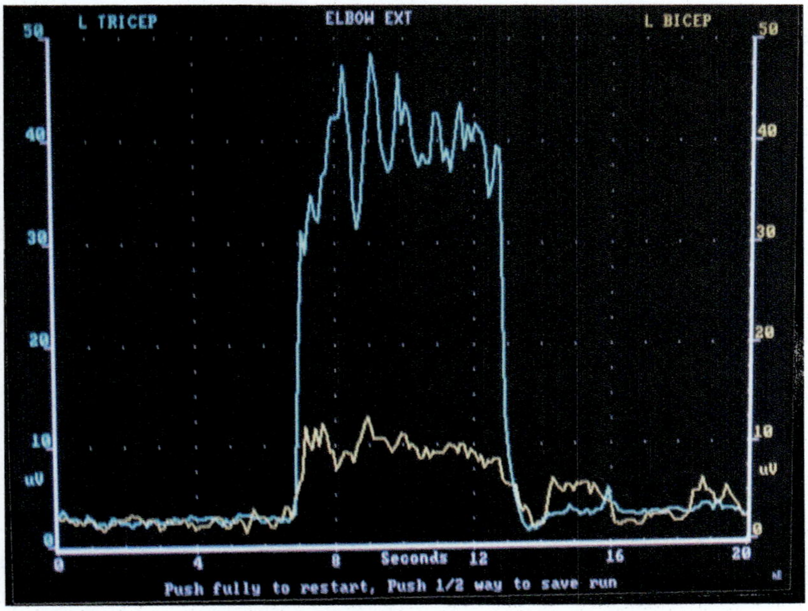

Fig. 2.46 The type of normal proportion of motor program signal with low intensity

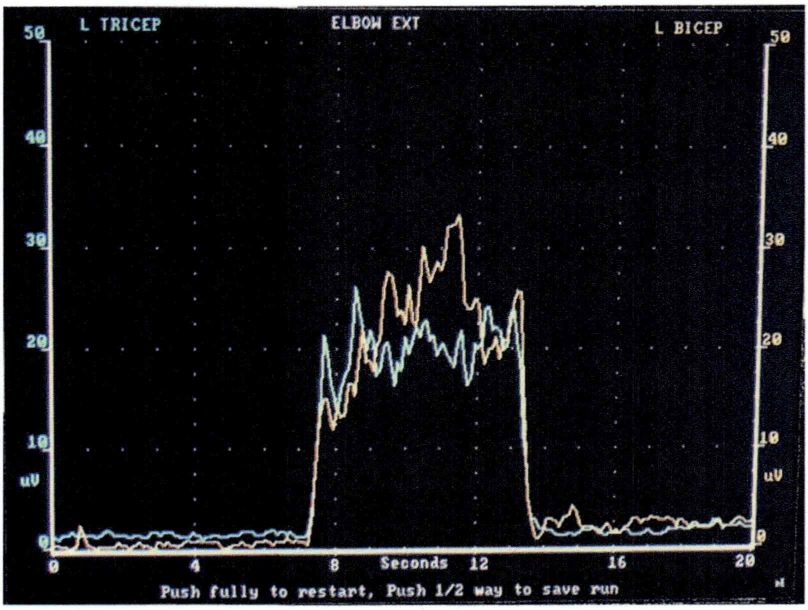

Fig. 2.47 Disproportionality of motor program signal with low intensity

4. Disproportionality of motor program signal with normal intensity: This type of signal is commonly detected in the late recovery period and sequelae period of the patients with CNS damages and without standard rehabilitation training (Fig. 2.48). Because of long medical history, the functions of neural tissues in injured penumbra are recovered. The functions can be replaced by the neural tissue around the injured area and distal area. Through neural plasticity, functional reorganization is realized, but the neural tissue and cells of functional reorganization without training are lack of compatible ability. Although the signal intensity of motor program is not low, the proportion is disordered. Therefore, the dyskinesia is still obvious. In allusion to these patients, the training of rectifying disordered motor program, reestablishing normal motor program and remodeling motor pattern can result in better effect.
5. Irregular proportionality of motor program signal with high baseline delay form: Normal motor program signals are in accordance with the law of "all or none" in action potential generation and conduction. The signal is conducted to corresponding muscle and induces the contraction of the muscle. After the completion of joint motion, the muscle relaxes. At this time, there is no motor program signal. Therefore, during resting stage (the muscle relax), the signal baseline of normal motor program is zero.

This type of signal is commonly detected in the recovery period of the patients with higher CNS damages (brain damages, Fig. 2.49). The functions of higher nerve center are not recovered, whose inhibitory effect on the lower nerve center is weak. Therefore, the excitability of lower nerve center is activated and continuous or frequent weak electrical signal can be released. Irregular signal curve constantly above zero baselines is generated. This type of signal may decrease the stimulus threshold of muscle excitability evidently and the muscles are always in tension state. With slight stimulus, the long-term contraction or spasm of the muscle can be induced and it is difficulty to recover to relaxed state.

The rehabilitation training principle of these patients should be put on the recovery of higher nerve center functions. Through the training of developing neural potential and reestablishing motor program, motor function can be better recovered. In addition, the training of relaxed muscle is essential. The prompt relaxation after muscle contraction is a process that higher nerve

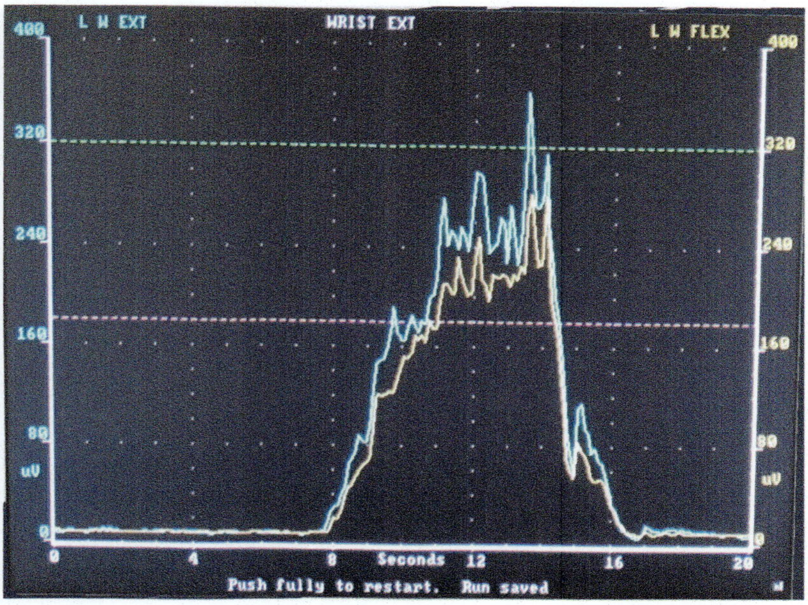

Fig. 2.48 Disproportionality of motor program signal with normal intensity

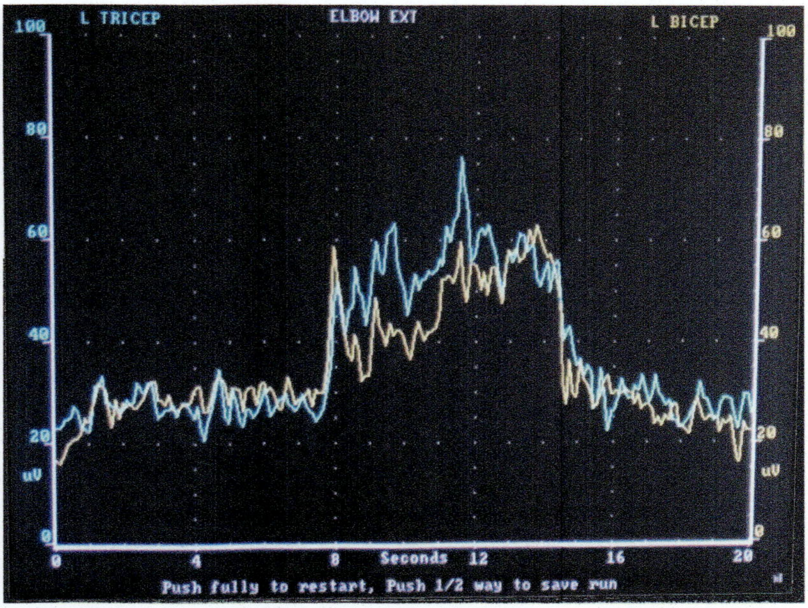

Fig. 2.49 Irregular proportionality of motor program signal with high baseline delay form

center controls lower nerve center and the recovery of higher nerve center functions.

Under the continuous detection and real-time display of motor program signal in neurological training equipment, the patients are guided to strengthen the agonistic muscle signal and attenuate antagonistic muscle signal in order to restore the normal proportion of 10–1. The abnormal motor program can be rectified gradually and will be consolidated through repeated training.

2.2.5.2 Classification of Signal Intensity of Agonistic Muscle

1. Abundant incremental type: This type of wave form is observed in the recovery period of the patients with lighter CNS damages. In every training, the signal intensity of agonistic muscle increases little by little (Fig. 2.50, 2.51, and 2.52). When the patients are guided to complete joint motion, the signal intensity of agonistic muscle can surpass the baseline last

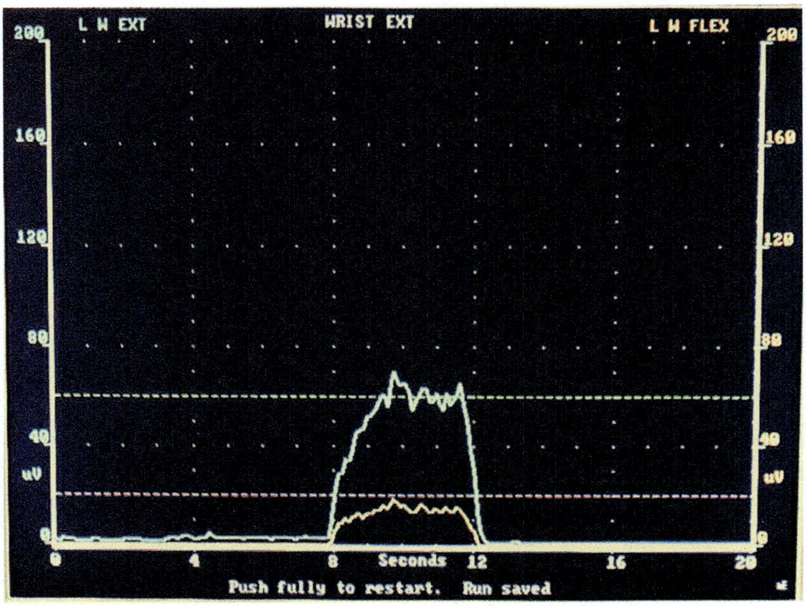

Fig. 2.50 Abundant incremental type I

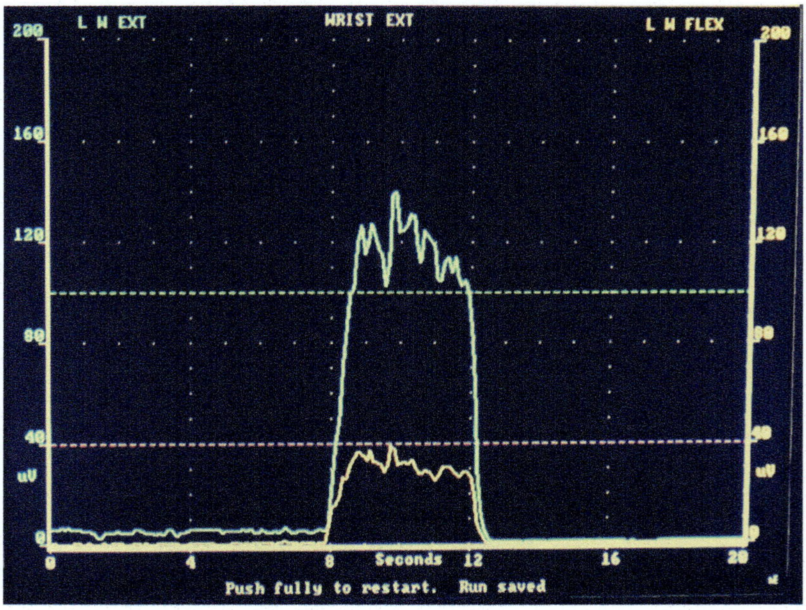

Fig. 2.51 Abundant incremental type II

time easily. The times can be reach five times or more, which make people think that the signal resource of motor program is abundant and inexhaustible. This type of signal demonstrated that the CNS damages were slight or the injuries were repaired even though the CNS damages were severe. The functional reorganization was realized, which indicated that the motor function recovery of the patients with this type of signal was ideal after training and its prognosis is good.

2. Exhausted decay type: The characteristic of this wave form is that motor program signal of agonistic muscle is strong in the first training and the signal intensity don't increase, but decrease in the following training. There is lacking in strength of agonistic muscle and make the people think that the signal resource

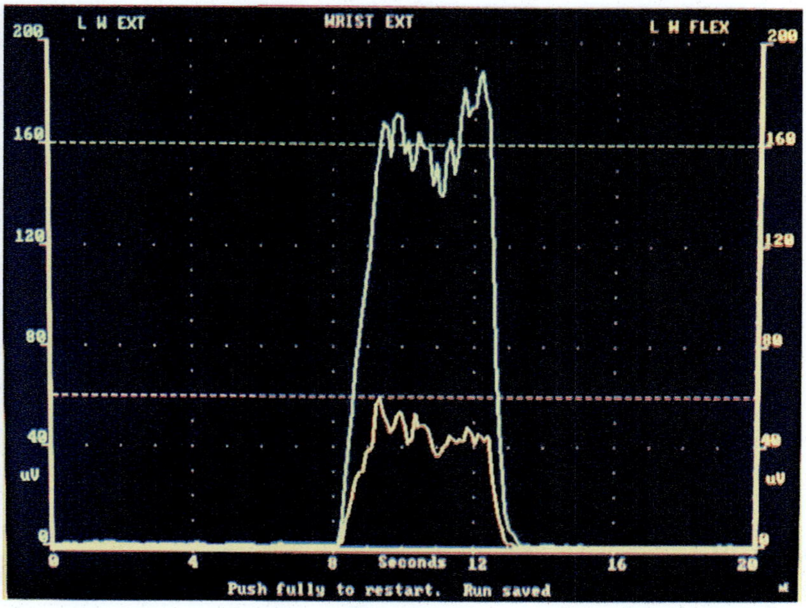

Fig. 2.52 Abundant incremental type III

is limited cannot be supplemented in time, which is called gradually exhausted decay type (Figs. 2.53, 2.54, and 2.55). This type of signal is commonly detected in the patients with motor neuron degeneration, complete peripheral nervous injury or incomplete peripheral nervous injury, which declared that the neural injury is severe or there is progressive neuropathy. The effect of rehabilitation therapy is not ideal and its prognosis is bad.

3. Initiating delay type: When the therapists guided the patients to do joint motion, the patients try to move joint with subjective consciousness after the instructions, but the signal from CNS to agonistic muscle is delayed and the corresponding joint motion is delayed accordingly (Fig. 2.56). Under normal circumstances, movements instructions are given to the patients and they try to move joint. Then there will be signal and joint motion soon.

   The reason of slow start of joint motion is due to the selection of motor program and disorder in the starting process, which is the result of cortex motor center damages. The other situation includes hypertonia of antagonistic muscle and severe disorder of motor program. The agonistic muscle can hardly drive joint motion.

   There is difficulty in single joint motion and snail pace of the patients with this type of signal. The key point of training is the starting speed training of motor program. Under no earth gravity circumstances, the patients are guided to give out motor program signal and induce corresponding joint motion. The time from giving out instruction to the appearance of motor program signal is defined as objective indicator. The patients are guided to try to shorten the starting time gradually.

4. Zero slow type: Under normal circumstances, after completion of active contraction, motor program signal should disappear immediately. The curve should return to Zero baseline (Fig. 2.57). When the patients complete joint motion, the therapists guided the patients to relax and the motor program signal stops, but the signal curve cannot decrease to zero immediately, but the process is slow (several minutes in some situation), which is called Zero slow type curve.

The generation of this type of signal is due to incompatible work of CNS cells. When the movements idea is formed, there are only partial cells that are activated and give out electrical signal in the corresponding cortex motor center,

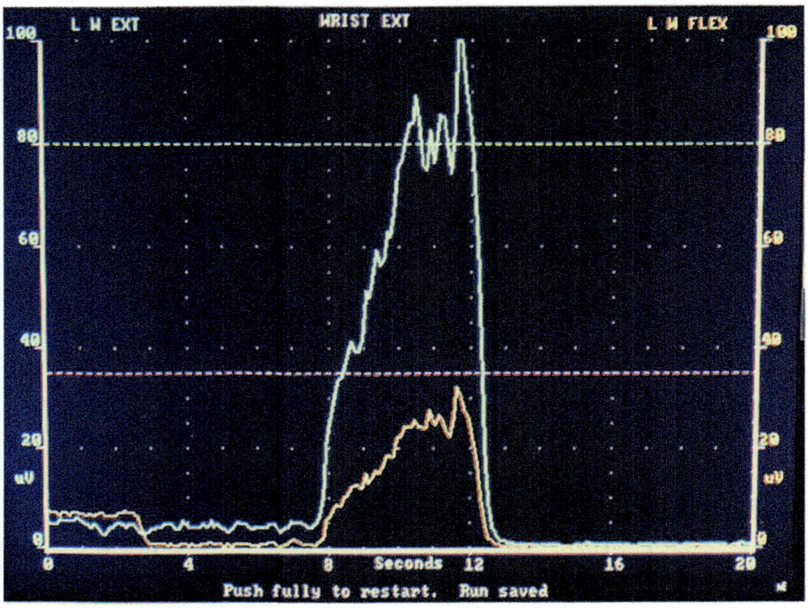

Fig. 2.53 Exhausted decay type I

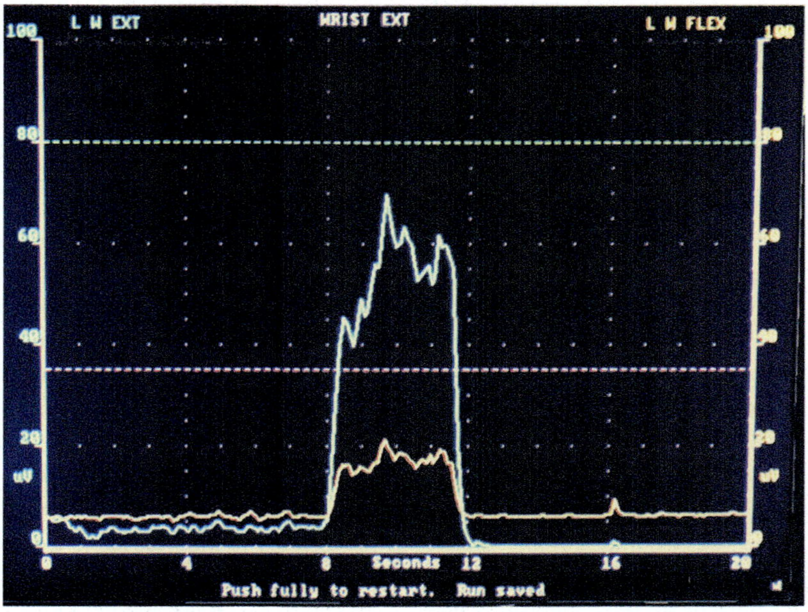

Fig. 2.54 Exhausted decay type II

whereas the other cells are not activated. When the previous cells gave out the signal, the other cells are activated. Therefore, in muscular flaccidity period, there are still signals from nerve cells to the muscles and the muscles are excited, even tension increasing and spasm. In other situation, after higher CNS damages, the excitability of lower CNS is released and the continuous signal can induce muscle spasm.

The training for this type of signal is relaxing training, whose objective is to develop CNS potentials and recover the ability that higher nerve center controls lower nerve center. The time of the process that the signal returns to zero is defined as objective indicator. Time limit in every screen is 40–60 s or the scan is continuous. The patients are guided to relax continuously until the signal returns to zero.

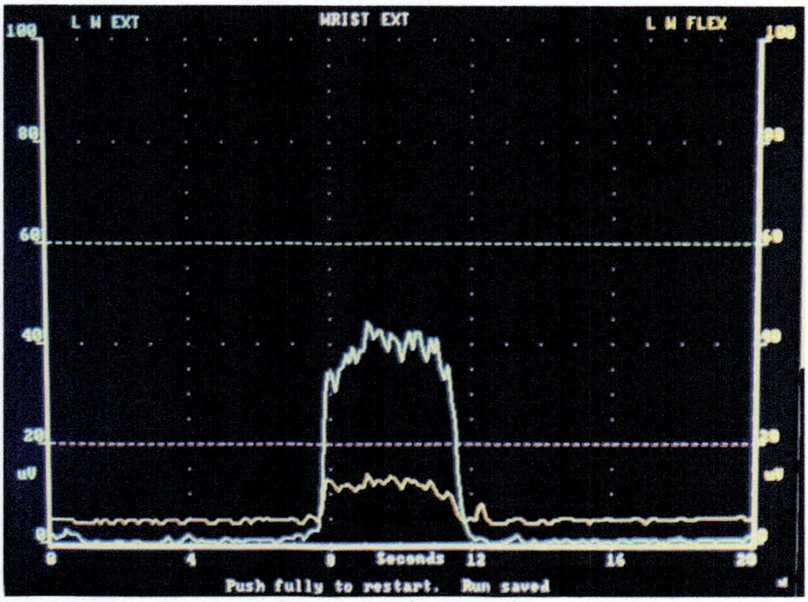

Fig. 2.55 Exhausted decay type III

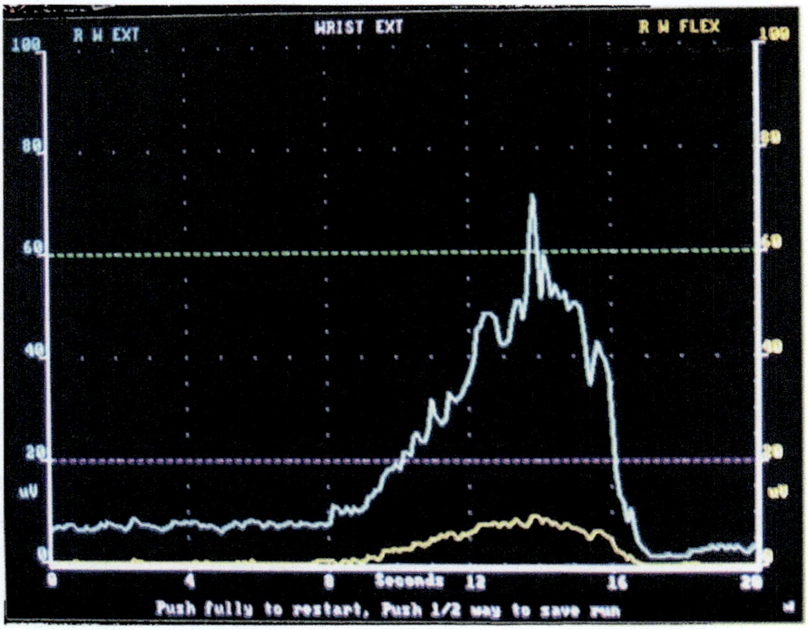

Fig. 2.56 Initiating delay type

The time of establishing or consolidating motor program is related to evolution extent of species. The higher the evolution extent is, the longer the time of establishing motor program takes. On the contrary, the time is shorter. For example, several hours after the birth of sheep, it can walk and run, whereas people need 1 year or more to learn to walk and run. When the motor program is already established in the motor center and the motor cortex is damaged, the process of motor program is complicated and takes more time.

Therefore, the process of reestablishing human motor program is relatively chronic. Repeated training is needed to reestablish motor program. After repeated basic training (3–6 months), the motor program is consolidated and the therapeu-

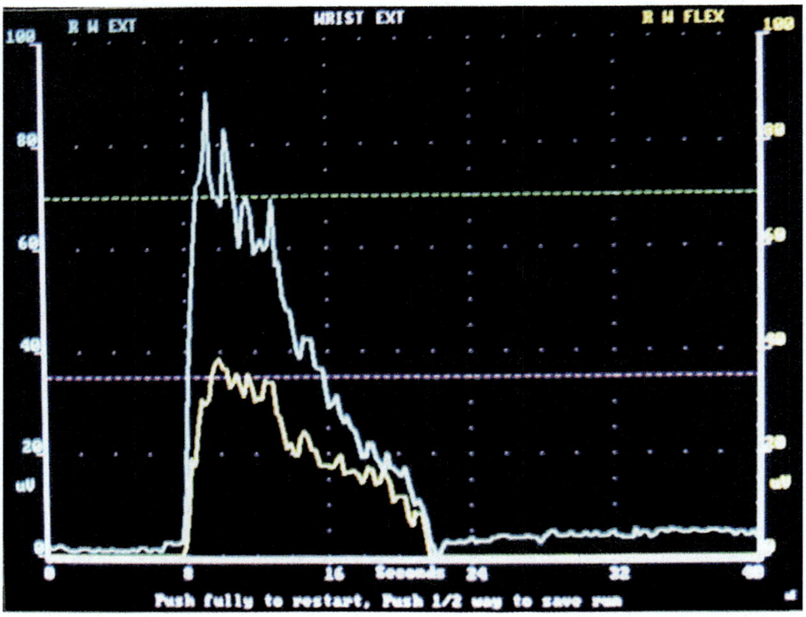

Fig. 2.57 Zero slow type

tic effects can be consolidated. After this, the functions can be maintained through continuous exercise.

Many patients and their relatives, even the doctors and the therapists, cannot understand the same training. There are examples that some skills are mastered through repeated training in daily life such as shooting and archery athletes. The shooters or archery athletes can enhance and keep the good score through shooting the target every day. This is a perfection, refinement and consolidation process of archery or shooting program.

2.2.6 Indications, Contraindications and Cautions of Rehabilitation Therapeutics Methods of Neurological Training

Neurological training is composed of a series of methods, which includes the training of dyskinesia induced by hemiplegia, paraplegia, cerebral palsy, facial paralysis, visual impairment, swallow, throat muscles, diaphragm and sphincter and training methods of cognition, speeches, beauty, scapulohumeral periarthritis, pain in waist and lower extremities and osteoarticular diseases. The indications and contradictions of all kinds of diseases are slightly different, but they are basically similar.

2.2.6.1 Indications

1. All kinds of diseases include hemiplegia, paraplegia, cerebral palsy, facial paralysis, peripheral nerve injury, visual impairment, swallow disorder, respiratory dysfunction, cognitive disorder, speech disorder, sphincter of Oddi dysfunction, scapulohumeral periarthritis, pain in waist and lower extremities and osteoarticular diseases.
2. The consciousness of the patients is clear.
3. There is no obvious disorder in cognitive function.

2.2.6.2 Contraindications

1. The patients with unstable vital signs in the early period of diseases, severe weakness or cachexia.
2. Subjective consciousness or active movement training may endanger the patients' life or worsen the condition of the patients, such as unstable state of hypertension or unhealed fracture in the early period of fracture fixation.
3. The patients with psychiatric disorders and incompatible with treatment.

4. In the patients with deep venous thrombosis and limbs swelling, active movement may make the embolus fall off.
5. The patients are in coma or serious cognitive disorders, who are not appropriate for reestablishing training through directly using motor program and need to develop training in advance.

2.2.6.3 Cautions

1. Choosing appropriate method according to different situations. In the therapeutic methods of neurological training, the therapy points in different stages are different. We should choose different methods according to different situations. For the patients with weak signals. The development of neural potential should be emphasized. The proportion of agonistic muscle signal and antagonistic muscle signal should not be overemphasized. Otherwise, the patients may feel depressed and then lose the confidence in the therapy because they cannot Meet the requirements. Meanwhile, these have an important effect on the development of neural potential. Just as in the difficulty times, it is unpractical to overemphasize nutrition structure. It is essential to eat full in order to save people's life. Under the sufficient life supply, it is able to lay emphasis on nutrition structure of eating. In the first stage of training, the reserved neural cells and conduction pathways should be activated firstly. Afterwards, the cells and pathway are cooperated to work together to reestablish motor program. If the new cells are not activated, the cooperative work will fail.
2. During training, the therapists should emphasize on the therapy methods and mechanisms, which include the relationship of brain and body movements, what's motor program signal and the functions of training. All these can motivate the patients and let the patients take part in the training and know their progress in the training.
3. The attitude of the training it is forbidden to show during dissatisfaction, impatience, the expressions, speeches and behaviors that can jeopardize the patients' self-respect during training, especially order speeches and scold speeches. The therapists should use negotiation, conciliation and induction to let the patients cooperate with the therapists.
4. The therapists should emphasize on the communication with the patients. Mission completed training should be avoided. At the end of the training, in allusion to the patients' problems, the therapists give the patients self-training tasks and inspect the tasks results the next day.

2.3 The Type and Methods of Establishing Coordinated Movement Procedure

2.3.1 The Significance of Establishing the Coordinated Movement Procedure in Recovering Coordinated Movement

As mentioned above, the movement procedure of the single joint is located in the area 4th of cortical motor, while the movement procedure of multi-joint coordinated movement is located in the area 6th of cortical motor [4]. Single joint activity is the basis of associated movement of limbs; single joint activity disorder can severely influence the coordinated movement of the multi-joint, and can even make the coordinated movement unable to be completed. Multi-joint coordinated movement is the complex form of the movement of limbs, while the flexible single joint activity is the highest movement form of the human body. For instance, it is hard for an ordinary people who have not been improved through training to carry out single activity of auricular and little finger, yet only may be achieved by special training.

However, a functional action which has a real meaning, such as walking, running, jumping, and picking up a cup and drinking and so on, must be the results of the coordinated movement of multi-joint, most of the single joint activities do not have practical function which can be used in daily life. Without the activity of single joint, however, the coordinated movement which is formed by multi-joint activity and has practical function is impossible. Therefore, both of them are essential and supplement each other, and they are one of the questions which must be putting a high value during rehabilitation training.

Multi-joint coordinated movement is the movement which is often referred to the involvement of whole limbs (such as upper limb or lower limb) or more joints, it is this movement which is governed by the most complex movement. Therefore, establish the movement procedure of multi-joint movement, must be based on the basis of established single joint movement procedure.

2.3.2 The Type and Methods of Reestablishing Coordinated Movement Procedure

Multi-joint coordinated movement is an activity which referred to two or more practical functional meaning joints. In the activities of practical daily life, the form of associated movement is produced by the need of practical work, it included many types, and without bounds. Such as back somersault, people without training may not be completed, while through training they can somersault 360, when through science and diligent long time training, they will have the ability to somersault 720 or more.

From the point of rehabilitation training, it is puts particular emphasis on the ability of restore the need of original daily life of patients. This ability can be roughly divided into multi-joint coordinated movement of upper limbs and lower limbs. Therefore, it can be trained by designed multi-joint coordinated movement. This is not request patients to movement which must be use this pattern in their future life, but the process which is training cortex motor center to coordinate each joint to take the coordinated movement for the need of daily life by different ways. Just as we have studied Advanced Mathematics in school, but we may not engage in the work which is related to mathematics after graduated. Maybe some people will think that that period of time is wasted, but this is not the case. Since learning is only one of the means and progresses of training, it is a progress of training the practical ability of the brain to discover, analyze and solve problems, but not what has learnt. Similarly, through the training of the movement procedure of designed multi-joint coordinated movement, training the brain's ability of integrated management and coordinate the movement of each joint, instead of trained to be an fixed, rigid single movement pattern.

Establishing a movement procedure of multi-joint coordinated movement needs based on the practical functional defects and daily life of the patients, for instance, upper limbs can take the training of procedural reestablish such as pick up a cup, drink water, brush teeth, tie a belt, fasten a button and so on; lower limbs can take the training of procedural reestablish such as squat, stand up, walk and reach a stage and so on (Table 2.4).

2.3.2.1 The Training of Reestablishing the Movement Procedure for Picking Up a Cup Multi-joint Coordinated Movement

This program can control the movements that require multi-joint to pick up a cup and grasp something through upper limbs. It is one of the essential basic movements in daily life. This movement can be divided into three joint motions, which include anteflexion of shoulder joint, extension of elbow joint and grabbing. Excessive dividing causes chaos and induces difficulty in analyzation and memorizing in the patients, and then the training effects can be influenced. During the motor program, anteflexion of shoulder joint, flexor digitorum after extension of elbow joint and finger and grasping should be done sequentially.

The therapists place the reception electrode of motor program signal on the skin surface of agonistic muscles in three groups separately, which include three electrodes of the first lead in anterior deltoideus triangularis, three electrodes of the second lead in triceps muscle of arm and three electrodes of the third lead in flexor digitorum. Every lead includes three electrodes. The first surface electrode is placed on the proximal end of muscle belly, the second electrode is placed on the distal end of muscle belly and the grounding

Table 2.4 Reestablishing multi-joint coordinated movement procedure, examples of the sequence of sent out signals

Name of the movements	Joint movement	Agonist	Sequence of sent out signals	Onset position of limbs
Pick up a cup	Shoulders extend forward	Anterior deltoid	1	Upper anatomic position
	Stretch the elbow	Triceps muscle	2	
	Bend fingers to grasp	Flexor of fingers	3	
Drink water	Bend fingers to grasp	Flexor of fingers	1	Sitting position
	Bend elbow	Bicipital muscle	2	Table plane
	Shoulders abduction	Middle deltoid	3	Grasp the cup
Comb hair	Bend elbow	Bicipital muscle	1	Sitting position
	Shoulders abduction upward	Levator scapulae	2	Table plane
	Shoulders downward	Pectoralis Major muscle	3	Grasp the comb
Squat	Bend hips	Hip flexors	1	Standing position
	Bend knees	Hamstrings	2	
	Body bend forward	Abdominal muscle	3	
Stand up	Extend knees	Quadriceps femoris muscle	1	Sitting position
	Extend hips	Gluteus maximus muscle	2	
	Body straighten	Psoas	3	
Walk	Move the centre of gravity to offside	Hip abductors	1	Standing position
	Bend hips	Hip flexors	2	
	Foot flexed	Tibialis anterior	3	

electrode is placed on the distal end of muscle belly (Fig. 2.58). Under real-time display of the signal circumstances, the therapists use Daoyin technique to guide the patients to give out the signals sequentially and do joint motion orderly. This training should be done slowly at first, and after proficiency it can be accelerated. The training can be done through picking up a teacup or grasping something.

2.3.2.2 The Training of Reestablishing Walking Motor Program

Walking is an important guarantee of the daily life quality. Abnormal walking is the resource of abnormal motor pattern of lower limbs such as circle gait, dragging gait and swaying gait. Therefore, walking training is the basic training to rectify the abnormal motor pattern of power limbs.

This movement can be simply divided into three joint motions, which include load bearing of offside lower limbs, hip flection and dorsiflexion of foot. During the motor program, load bearing of offside lower limbs, hip flection and dorsiflexion of foot should be done sequentially.

The therapists place the reception electrode of motor program signal on the skin surface of agonistic muscles in three groups separately, which include three electrodes of the first lead in offside hip abductors (contraction when the lower limbs bear load), three electrodes of the second lead in hip flection and three electrodes of the third lead in skin surface of tibialis anterior muscle. Every lead includes three electrodes. The first surface electrode is placed on the proximal end of muscle belly, the second electrode is placed on the distal end of muscle belly and the grounding electrode is placed between the first and the second (Fig. 2.59). Under real-time display of the signal circumstances, the therapists use Daoyin technique to guide the patients to give out the signals sequentially and do joint motion orderly. This training should be done slowly at first, and after proficiency it can be accelerated. The training can be done through walking training, but it should be monitored continuously under the neurological training equipment. The patients should do every joint motion under the signal program.

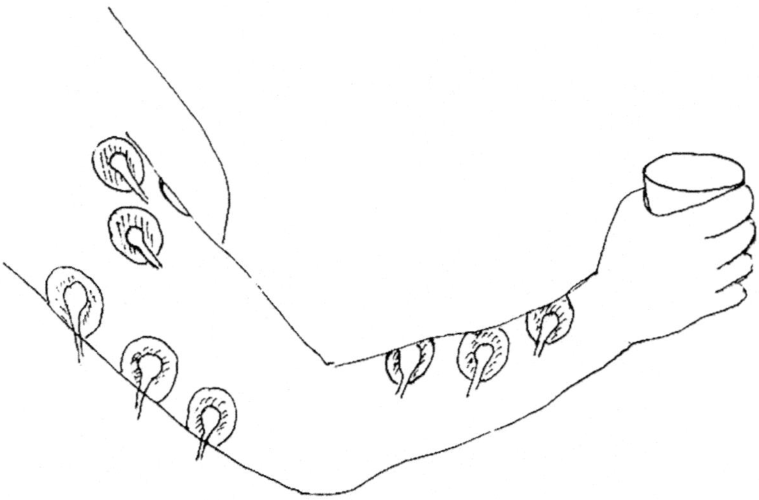

Fig. 2.58 The training of reestablishing motor program of multi-joint coordinated movement of picking teacup

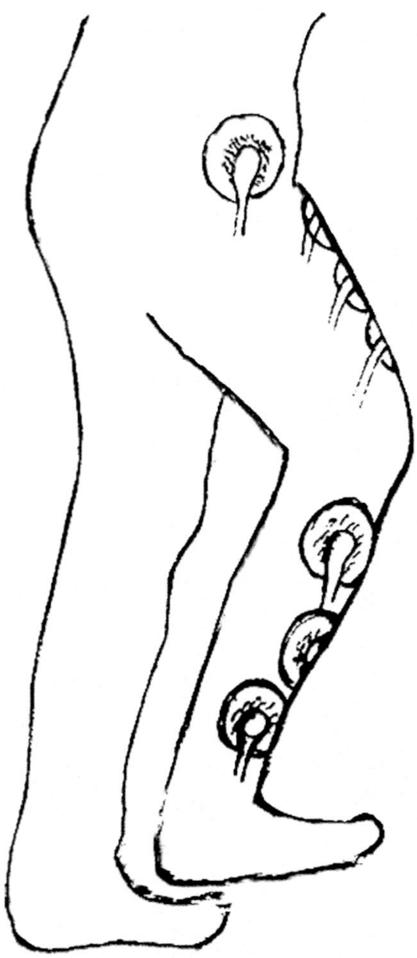

Fig. 2.59 The training of reestablishing walking motor program

2.3.3 Indications, Contraindications and Cautions of Reestablishing Multi-joint Coordinated Motor Program

2.3.3.1 Indications

1. The training can be done in the third period of rehabilitation therapeutics of neurological training.
2. Single joint motor program that control paralytic limbs is already established.
3. The patients are capable to complete full range joint motion autonomously.
4. Myodynamia of agonistic muscle is no less than III level (Lovett manual muscle test).
5. The patients with stable vital signs

2.3.3.2 Contraindications

1. The patients with infirmity and unstable vital signs.
2. The autonomous movements of joint are still not recovered. Motor program of single joint is still in chaos.
3. The range of whole joint motion that the patients can complete is less than 50%.
4. Myodynamia of agonistic muscle is less than III level (Lovett manual muscle test).
5. It is difficulty to recover normal motor pattern or it takes a long time. In the short term it is difficulty to be realized in the patients with severe syndromes.

2.3.3.3 Cautions

1. The training should be step by step. If it is difficulty for the patients to complete the motion require three joints, it is obliged to do united motor program training require two joints. With ability improvement, the patients can do the training that can reestablish motor program and require three or more joints.
2. Focus on preventing unnecessary joint motion in the early stage of training, in order to rectify abnormal motor program and effectively restrict unnecessary joint motion in the movements, weight reduction training equipment and motor pattern molding instrument can be used to help training.
3. Flexible adjustment the items of training can be decided according to physical situation of the patients.
4. Improve functional recovery of cortex motor center in the training: The therapists should establish multi-joint coordinated motor program training to recover the functions of cortex motor center, but not the stiff limbs motor pattern.
5. Monitoring and preventing excessive agonistic muscle involved in joint motion the numbers of monitoring parts should be less than three. Otherwise, there are too many curves in the screen, which can lead to visual confusion and affect the effect of training.

2.3.4 Clinical Application Study on Mechanism of Rehabilitation Therapeutics of Neurological Training

2.3.4.1 General Data and Inclusion Criteria

Form June of 2006 to June of 2008, we picked up 64 inpatients with Apoplexy hemiparalysis and restricted extension of the knee joint in rehabilitation centre of neurological training of Beijing Tongren Hospital. There is no criterion about sex and body side. There were 36 male patients and 28 female patients. The age is from 30 to 70 years old. The average age is 52.6 years old. In all the patients, there were 24 patients with cerebral hemorrhage and 40 patients with cerebral infarction. The course of disease is about 1–5 years and the average is 3.62 years.

Patients' inclusion criteria are as follows: (1) It is in accordance with the diagnostic criteria of national cerebrovascular disease conference in 1995. The cerebral hemorrhage and cerebral infarction are confirmed by CT or MRI in the patients with restricted extension of knee joint due to hemiplegia. (2) There is no significant dysgnosia (MMSE scores are no less than 20). (3) There is no severe adhesion of knee joint and the passive movement range is normal. (4) In the hospital, after traditional rehabilitation methods therapy, the patients' situation was not improved significantly.

Patients' exclusion criteria are as follows: (1) The patients are diagnosed with severe cardiac insufficiency, pulmonary insufficiency, liver insufficiency and renal insufficiency, severe infectious diseases, bone fracture and cachexy and they cannot do rehabilitation training. (2) The patients are diagnosed with severe cognitive disorder or they take medicine such as sedatives, antidepressants and diazepam in long term and cannot coordinate the treatment and influence electromyography inspectors. (3) The patients with frequent epileptic attack. (4) There are other diseases that can influence movements such as all kinds of myopathy, bone and joint injury and peripheral nerve injury. (5) The patients stop treatments for other reasons and cannot adhere to treatment for90 times.

2.3.4.2 Specific Methods of Rehabilitation Therapeutics of Neurological Training

In a warm, quiet, soundproof and lucifugal room, the patients sited in front of the screen. Neurological training equipment was used. 3 M Ag-AgCl surface electrode were placed on quadriceps femoris separately. The first electrode is placed on the skin surface of muscle belly in quadriceps femoris 6 cm above patella. The second electrode is placed 12 cm vertically above the first electrode. The grounding electrode is placed between the first and the second. The surface electrode is linked to the first lead of neurological training equipment through wire. 3 M Ag-AgCl surface electrode were placed on hamstring muscles separately. The first electrode is placed on the skin surface of muscle belly in hamstring muscles 2 cm above popliteal space. The second electrode is placed 6 cm vertically above the first electrode. The grounding electrode is placed between the first and the second. The surface electrode is linked to the third lead of neurological training equipment through wire. The therapists use six-step Daoyin technique to exert resistance in the orientation of joint motion and encourage the patients to try to extend knee for 15 min in sitting position, erect position and walking position actively. The highest signals gathered from motor center to quadriceps femoris and hamstring muscles for the first time are defined as the initial data. Two marked line are based on two signals. Daoyin technique is used to guide the patients to try to make the signal from CNS to quadriceps femoris surpass the baseline and the signal from CNS to hamstring muscles go below the baseline. During therapy, when the signal intensity reaches the summit, the therapists use words such as "Hold on, or you will fall down", "Hold higher, or your feet will touch the ground!" and "Climb over, or you will slip" to make the patients feel dangerous. The patients should make the signal from CNS to quadriceps femoris surpass the baseline as much as possible and decrease the signal intensity from CNS to hamstring muscles or don't increase the signal intensity. Afterwards, the new summit is defined ad baseline. The same method is used to guide the patients to go against resistance. The patients should try to make quadriceps femoris signal surpass new baseline and hamstring muscles signal go further below new baseline. The rest can be done in the same manner.

The training should be done 45 min one time and one course of treatment includes ninety training.

2.3.4.3 Assessment Method and Statistical Analysis

Lovett manual muscle test (Lovett MMT), range of motion (ROM) of knee joint, Fugl-Meyer lower extremity motor function assessment, sEMG intensity and proportion of quadriceps femoris and hamstring muscles signals are used in this experiment. At the beginning of therapy and at the end of the therapy, the assessment should be carried out and the data is collected [5].

The results of data are showed as Mean ± SD ($x \pm s$). SPSS 12.0 statistical software is used for statistical analysis. T test is used in mean comparison of two samples.

2.3.4.4 Results

We assess and analyze the myodynamia, active ROM of knee joint, Fugl-Meyer lower extremity motor function score and motor program signal before and after therapy of quadriceps femoris and hamstring muscles in 64 patients. The analysis results are showed in Table 2.5. There are significant differences in quadriceps femorismotor program signal intensity, myodynamia, Fugl-Meyer and active ROM of knee joint before and after therapy ($p < 0.01$). After therapy, myodynamia and signal intensity of hamstring muscles are higher than these before therapy, but there is no significant difference before therapy and after therapy ($p > 0.05$). Before therapy, signal intensity from cortex motor center to hamstring muscles is higher than that from cortex motor center to quadriceps femoris. The proportion between

Table 2.5 statistical analysis of function assessment data before and after therapy ($\bar{x} \pm s$)

Assessment items		Before therapy	After therapy	*P* value
Lovett MMT	Quadriceps femoris	2.67 ± 1.62	4.10 ± 0.62	<0.01
	Hamstring muscles	2.30 ± 1.17	3.82 ± 280.76	>0.05
Active ROM (°)		4.38 ± 2.36	28.80 ± 7.68	<0.01
Fugl-Meyer		15.71 ± 7.21	25.75 ± 6.30	<0.01
Motor program signal (μV)	Quadriceps femoris	42.13 ± 28.24	107.81 ± 50.63	<0.01
	Hamstring muscles	57.67 ± 34.17	62.13 ± 28.24	>0.05
	Differences	23.94 ± 20.30	56.88 ± 43.35	<0.01

them is 1.4 and 1. There are difficulties in extension of knee joint of limbs in hemiplegic side and rigidity or recurvatum in walking in the patients with this proportion. After therapy, signal intensity from cortex motor center to quadriceps femoris is increased. There is significant difference before therapy and after therapy ($p < 0.01$). Although signal intensity from cortex motor center to quadriceps femoris is increased, there is significant difference before therapy and after therapy ($p > 0.05$). After therapy, there is significant difference between signal of hamstring muscles and signal of quadriceps femoris ($p < 0.01$). The proportion between them is 1.4 and 1 before therapy and the proportion is improved to 1 and 4.1 after therapy, which is the main reason of substantial improvement of autonomic movements of knee joint.

2.3.4.5 Discussion

1. The coordinated and orderly collaboration of central nervous cells is the basis of motor function recovery. The completion of autonomic movement of any joint is the results of the coordinated and orderly collaboration of central nervous cells. Some research indicated that the number of central nervous cells required for fine movement is much larger than that for gross movement. For example, the number of motor center cells required for controlling a thumb is equal to that required for controlling an upper limb. The premise of numerous cells to complete a joint motion is the coordinated and orderly collaboration of them.

   Although central nervous cells are unable to regenerate, central nervous tissue is able to compensate the lost functions just as other tissues through CNS plasticity. The lost cells after CNS damages can be supplemented by the following several aspects in order to recover the original motor functions. (1) The undead cells in injured area and cells in penumbra area can recover functions with the changes of internal environment. (2) The normal cells around injured area can obtain the same functions as that of the injured cells through training. (3) Regenerated central nervous cells Because central nervous cells are unable to regenerate, there are seldom regenerated cells, which have little effect on the recovery of motor function. No matter which kind of cell, the cells should be cooperated to establish new connection in order to recover motor function because the relationship between cells is changed. Therefore, recovering the coordinated and orderly collaboration of cells is the basis of recovering motor function. The training of recovering the coordinated and orderly collaboration of cells is a process to reestablish motor program in motor center.
2. Human autonomic movements are dominated and controlled by motor program in cortex motor center. The motor programs in motor center are from two aspects. (a) The first is congenital, which is inherited from ancestors and account for a small fraction of total. (b) The second is acquired and account for a large fraction of total, which is acquired motor program through learning. Motor program is electrical signal from cortex motor center to single joint or multi-joint to complete all kinds of movements. if we compare cortex motor center and computers, we can better understand the motor program. There are many similarities between new born babies and factory-fresh computers. For example, there are only recognition and storage of software in factory-fresh computers without any other functions. Only the software are installed, the computers are possessed with various kinds of functions such as editing, mark identification and screening. If the installed software is English version, it is able to edit English. If the installed software is Chinese version, it is able to edit Chinese. If the English version and Chinese version are both installed, it is able to edit English and Chinese through switching. The new born babies cannot do nothing but sucking the breast, crying and moving without any purpose. However, the babies' brain has the same memory function with hard disk of computers. During the development, through learning, they can creep, sit and stand. They learnt to walk and

jump about 1 year after born. This is the process of motor program establishment and perfection. It seems that every autonomic movement must be dominated by motor program in cortex motor center. The norm of autonomic motor pattern is dependent on the perfection of motor program or not. The athletes can promote competitiveness through training, which may be related to the fact that the training improves motor program and enhance myodynamia.

3. Digital objective display of motor program signal is essential external condition for rectifying disordered motor program and reestablishing normal motor program. After central nervous cells damages, motor program can be destroyed to varying degrees. Totally destroy of motor program leads to completely lost of movement, partially destruction of movements or abnormal motor pattern due to short of cooperation of compensatory cells. In all these conditions, normal motor program should be reestablished.

Central nervous system of newborn babies may be influenced by evolution of species and is tend to normal development, which means common training can make the species are able to survive. This is not always the case. There are some defects in the abilities acquired without scientific training. Under general circumstance, people have no idea about whether their own motor pattern is normal or not. People may not realize or totally understand the defects of motor pattern in normal people. This is because there is no test and comparison. The defects of motor pattern can lead to difference of human athletic ability. For example, people are able to run, but there is difference in the running speed, running duration time and running distance. This may be related to the accuracy of motor program of individual running. However, the formation of motor pattern is dominated by motor program in cortex motor center. Therefore, central nerve damages can lead to motor function lost or abnormal motor function. Rectifying disordered motor program or reestablishing normal motor program is required to recover functions.

If the motor center where motor program has already established is destroyed, the reestablishment process and difficulty of motor program is different from the reestablishment process and difficulty of motor program in newborn babies. The brain of newborn babies is like a blank paper. With natural tropism, motor program is relatively easy to be established. In the damaged brain area where motor program has already been established, it is difficulty to reestablish motor program, which may be related to the damage of original conduction pathway between cells. Like driving a nail into a plank, if the nail is driven slantingly, it is difficulty to be driven into the plank again after the nail is pull out. Moreover, non-viable and non-apoptotic cells will influence the new intercellular signaling pathways. Therefore, reconstruction of normal motor program should be based on actual condition of abnormal motor program and be completed through targeted and repeated training.

In daily life, there is a truth that archery athlete aims at arrow target to practice archery so that degree of accuracy in archery can be increased. Otherwise, the degree of accuracy in archery cannot be increased without target. This is because archery is a motor program that is constructed in cortex motor center. Through repeated practice, the archery skill will be promoted continuously. When archery athlete aims at arrow target to practice archery, the first arrow may be shoot in the above of the bull's-eye. The archery result is sent to the brain and the brain will analyze numerous factors (altitude of arrow target, distance, wind direction, bow weight, arrow weight, arm strength and emotion) comprehensively. After calculation, the gesture of the second arrow can be decided such as lowering the arrowhead. The second arrow may be shoot in the below of the bull's-eye. The archery result is sent to the brain and the brain will know the arrowhead is too low. The gesture of the third arrow can be decided such as raising the arrowhead. The third arrow is shoot in the bull's-eye. After repeated training, the speed and accuracy of the movements are controlled precisely by the brain so that the speed and accuracy of the movements will be increased. During this process, arrow target is the subjective indicator for illustration and feedback, which make the brain know the mistake, rectify it timely and set clear objective. Therefore, arrow target is essential external conditions for increasing the degree of accuracy in archery and constructing archery motor program. After repeated training, the motor program is consolidated.

In the extension of joint motion in our research, normally strong signal is from brain to quadriceps femoris and the result is extension of knee joint. Meanwhile, weak signal is from brain to hamstring muscles to maintain fixed tension and increase stability of knee joint in extension of knee joint. After brain damages, in the abnormal motor program, except the weak signal intensity, the signal form brain to quadriceps femoris is the same strong as signal from brain to hamstring muscles or there is no significant difference between the two signals. Therefore, there is no extension of knee joint or it is difficulty to extend knee joint. It is essential to rectify disordered motor program and reestablish normal motor program in order to observe practical condition of motor program in extension of knee joint.

Daoyin feedback techniques in traditional Chinese medicine can guide the patients to extend knee joint actively, the movement results are detected by signal detection equipment and displayed on the screening in real-time. The dynamic continuous motor program feedback signals are provided to play a role that is more important than that of the target so that the training have a definite object in view training. Daoyin technique are used repeatedly to encourage the patients to promote signal intensity of agonistic muscle and lower signal intensity of antagonistic muscle in order to recover the normal proportion of the two signals and improve the function of extension of knee joint. Therefore, objective display of motor program signal of extension of knee joint is important external condition for reestablishment. Targeted repeated training is the important process to achieve reestablishment.

The time spent in reconstructing motor program is related to evolution extent of species. The higher the evolution extent of species is, the longer reconstructing motor program takes, and the vice versa. For example, sheep can learn to walk and run several hours after birth, meanwhile people take a year or more to learn to walk and run. Therefore, reconstruction of human motor program is a relative long process. Too short therapy course can lead to relapse of the disease, even futile treatment. If the patients want to be recovered within few days in hospital, it will have a bad impact on rehabilitation training effect. Through long-term clinical practice, the author found that obvious functional recovery of dyskinesia in lower limbs caused by central nervous damages took 3 months. However, for the upper limbs, especially hands, obvious functional recovery of dyskinesia took 6 months or more. Therefore, the author recommended that the therapy course of rehabilitation training is from 3 to 6 months. This is why we use 3 months and 90 times rehabilitation trainings as one therapy course.

4. In the Daoyin feedback technique in traditional Chinese medicine, Daoyin technique plays the main role in therapy. Effect display and signal feedback play an essential supporting role. In this therapy, Daoyin technique is used to develop CNS potential. Signal detection equipment display the Daoyin technique effect objectively and provide the surpassing target for the patients. Daoyin technique plays the main role in therapy. Effect display and signal feedback play an essential supporting role. However, without effective digital curve to display motor program, it can make the therapists don't know the specific circumstance of motor program exactly. And then there is no way to rectify and reestablish training. Therefore, training plays an essential role in reestablishment of the training.
5. "Neurological training" is the generalization of Daoyin feedback technique in traditional

Chinese medicine. Six-step Daoyin technique training is used for central nervous system, which means there is CNS plasticity induced by Daoyin training. Finally, functional reorganization is achieved and the lost motor function is recovered. Therefore, the author called it "neurological training" in order to emphasize the characteristics of rehabilitation in traditional Chinese medicine that are different from other rehabilitation therapy methods.

6. The key component of signal received from skin surface of muscle belly is motor program signal. Because of the complexity of neuromuscular system, anatomical and physiological characteristic of many related electromyography signal remains unclear. The source of signal received from skin surface of muscle is unknown. Whether it is the control signal or drive signal form cortex motor center to muscle or it is electrical signal generated by muscle? It is generally described as biological electrical signal of neuromuscular activities. Because the signal is received from skin surface of the muscle, it is called surface electromyography signal, which is composed of action potential of different motor unit. Motor unit is composed of a group of muscle fibers dominated by identical motor nerve.

The author detected electromyography signal of the patients with spinal shock and completely peripheral nerve injury and found that electromyography signal cannot be detected in passive muscle movement. Irregular electromyography signal induced by heteronomous spasm of muscle in spastic period may be from spinal cord motor neurons [6]. In clinic, the author found that the highest electrical signal received from skin surface of muscle in children and adults is less than 800 μV, but there is significant difference of myodynamia between children and adults with identical signal intensity. It is showed from one side that signal received from skin surface of muscle may be the drive signal from central nerves to muscle. The muscles involved in joint motion include agonistic muscle, antagonistic muscle, synergistic muscle and neutralized muscle. Agonistic muscle and antagonistic muscle play the main role in joint motion. Therefore, we select agonistic muscle and antagonistic muscle signals as the motor program signals that are from cortex and control the joint motion. The appropriate proportion of the two kinds of muscles is the basis of autonomous movements of joint. Signal intensity of motor program is in direct proportion to individual myodynamia. Its effect on joint motion is similar with pulling a cart. The force of pulling a cart is 100 N. If the assistant behind the cart do not push the cart forward, but pull back with 100 N force. The result is that the cart cannot move forward with the forces from two persons. The smaller the drag force of the assistant become, the bigger the difference between the forces from two persons is, the bigger the force of moving forward is. And then the cart can move forward. However, human joint motion requires certain tension of antagonistic muscle in order to keep the stability of joint motion. Therefore, in the joint motion, certain antagonistic muscle drive signal is from cortex motor center.

Appropriate difference in the intensity of command signal from motor center to agonistic muscle and antagonistic muscle involved in joint motion is the basis of joint flexible motion. Completion of a function requires many joints and muscles. It also requires motor center to give out command according to the sequence of joint motion, which is called motor program of coordinated movement. From this, during joint motion, the signal received from skin surface of muscle is drive signal from cortex motor center to muscle, but not generated by muscle contraction.

Our results showed that rehabilitation technology of Daoyin feedback in traditional Chinese medicine is an effective method to improve extension of knee joint in the patients with hemiplegic stroke, which can develop CNS potentials and promote reestablishment of motor program. It can provide experiment basis and theoretical basis for clinical application of new therapy and renaissance and modernization of Daoyin technique.

References

1. Hongshi M, editor. The theory and practice of rehabilitation medicine. Shanghai: Shanghai Scientific & Technical Publishers; 2000.
2. Shepherd GM. Neurobiology. Shanghai: Fudan University Press; 1992. Translated by Nanshan C. & Hongzuo A, DAI Hongzuo
3. Shifang Z. Research and rehabilitation of brain plasticity after cerebral apoplexy. Chin J Phys Med Rehabil. 2002;14(7):437–9.
4. Linying Z. The research progress and application of stroke rehabilitation technology. J Chin Clin Rehabil. 2004;8(34):7768–9.
5. Yulong W. Rehabilitation evaluation. Beijing: People's Health Publishing House; 2000. p. 88.
6. Wenru Z, Brucker BS, Xiuru W, et al. Application of myobiofeedback in the injury of old cervical spinal cord. J Chin Rehabil Med. 2003;18(2):91–3.

3 Neurological Training Methods of Developing Neural Potential

3.1 The Basis of Neural Potential

Limbs movements are meaningful functional movements through regular muscle contraction and relaxation dominated by cortex motor center of brain according to human willpower. After CNS damages, there is motor function lost to varying degrees. Because of low regeneration capacity of CNS, it is deemed for a long time that the possibility of recovering the lost motor functions after CNS damages is small, which make many patients lose hope on functional recovery.

With the control study and rise of rehabilitation method, we found that after CNS damages there are significant differences in functional recovery between the patients with rehabilitation therapy and the patients without rehabilitation therapy. The death rate decrease, functional recovery degree, decreased degree and the rate of going back to work of the patients with rehabilitation therapy are superior to these of the patients without rehabilitation therapy, which indicate that rehabilitation may recover the lost functions to varying degrees. In that way, after CNS damages, why the training can recover functions under the condition that CNS is lack of regeneration capacity and function cannot be recovered? This question deserves profound thinking and discuss.

Damage is an inevitable thing that is of frequent occurrence in daily life. The reason why human can live long is mainly related to three functions.

1. Adaption is an ability that people can change themselves to adapt the condition changes to survive when the external conditions or circumstance is changed. For example, people who lived in tropic move to cold north and they can increase their freeze resistance capability to adapt the cold environments in north.
2. Regeneration is an important mechanism of recovering functions after human tissues damages, which is the main route to recovery after many tissues damages and is also the measure to recover original function preferably. For example, the skin tissue of human body is damaged. Afterwards, new cells are generated through mitosis and regeneration of new vessels can recover the original function. However, the recovery ability is different in different tissue types. There is strong regeneration capacity in epithelial tissue, liver, spleen, skeleton and muscle. Whereas, regeneration capacity of central nervous tissues include spinal cord and brain tissue is very weak. For a long time, it is deemed that central nervous tissue is lack of regeneration capacity. That's why the lost function is had to be recovered after CNS damages. Some research in recent years demonstrated that there is regeneration capacity in CNS. However, the lost motor function after

W. Zhao, *Rehabilitation Therapeutics of the Neurological Training*,
https://doi.org/10.1007/978-981-13-0812-3_3

damages is seldom recovered if there is no intervention. Therefore, we deemed that regeneration capacity of CNS tissues has no effect on the functional recovery after CNS damages. In other words, it is far from satisfactory to recover motor function after CNS damages only through regeneration of neural tissues.

3. Compensation: When the tissue some part is damaged, under the effect of some factor, homogeneous tissue around the injured area or in distal part replace the functions of the injured tissue, which is called compensation. This capacity is very important for the tissue that lases functions and is with bad regeneration capacity. After acute stage, the compensatory capacity is high in the early stage of the disease and become less and less as time goes on. Therefore, after damages, the patients should begin rehabilitation training as early as possible. However, from the degree and quantity of compensation, the longer the time takes, the higher the compensatory is.

However, regardless of what kinds of functions and approaches, it is not practical to recover lost functions only through natural repair. Because there is limitation of repair capacity in self-repair ability and it is unable to recover the original functions. The repair time is long and it is easy to generate some complications such as abnormal motor pattern. Therefore, the method should be used to recover the lost functions. Especially for the CNS tissue with low regeneration capacity, it is a complicated question to recover its functions after damages, which is worth further research and investigation.

3.1.1 Theoretical Basis of Developing Potential

The function ability of human body can be improved or enhanced through special scientific training or under exceptional circumstances. Under normal circumstances, there is no improvement, but under exceptional circumstances, these functions can be boosted and beyond several times of original ability, which is called potential. The basis of potential is tissues and cells in reserve and the method of developing potential is that tissues and cells are trained to play their role sufficiently or extraordinarily.

The range of potential is wide, which includes motion, thinking, operation, memory, control and viscera function. These can be divided into several types:

1. Functional reserved type: This type means that tissues and cells are already able to play roles and they possess abundant functions after satisfying normal physiological activity and daily life movements. The effects of these functions include two ways. The first is to supplement additional functional requirements. When people increase activity level suddenly, the reserved functions should be activated. For example, there are 303 million alveoli and in normal circumstances 180 million alveoli are enough. However, when people do strenuous exercise, more alveoli should be activated, even all alveoli are activated. Myodynamia can be adjusted as required. People can lift 10 kg, and also can lift 50 kg or more without special training when it is necessary. The second is that when partial tissues are damaged and lose functions, the functions can be supplemented by reserved functions.
2. Efficiency improvement type: This type is based on the original functions that can be improved through training. The involved tissues don't certainly be increased. For example, Myodynamia can be adjusted as required. Through weight training, a person can lift 100 kg or more who can only lift 50 kg before. It is always the case for pulmonary function. Through diaphragm training, the contractility can be increased. During inspiration, the thorax volume increases obviously. Tidal volume increases obviously with enlargement of pulmonary alveoli in order to satisfy the demand for oxygen.

There are potentials in the flexibility of reaction and movements. Through training, people can react faster to external stimuli such as the reaction time of boxing and running starting, natural hitting reaction speed of playing ping-pong and the flexibility degree of human body. Through scientific training, these functions can be improved obviously.

3. Tissues reserved type: Tissues reserved type means that although some tissues are not possessed with some kind of function, they can acquire this kind of function through learning and training. This kind of function is stored in organs and human body in the form of tissues and cells before training.
4. Application form type: Application form is to promote efficiency through technical changes, which can be acquired through long-term training such as Taijiquan. The fighting skills of the person who practice Taijiquan for a long time may be increased obviously, but the myodynamia may not be increased obviously. There are some realms such as "Exerting force before the opponent and achievement before acting" and "one blow can put someone to death". Practice makes perfect, which means the functions can be perfected through repeated practice. Perfection belongs to one kind of application form potential. A surgeon can tie a knot, 30 knots for the beginner and 60–80 knots or more for the practician. Although there are the same amount of joints and muscles, the results can be different.
5. Compensatory type: Compensatory type potential means that when a part of function is lost, the homogeneous tissue around the injured area or in distal part replace the functions of the injured tissue.

   For nervous system and the muscles dominated by CNS, compensatory type potential is divided into neural compensatory potential and muscular compensatory potential. Neural compensatory potential can recover the function of its dominated muscles in order to recover the original functions of muscles. Therefore, it is in favor of recovering normal motor pattern. Muscular compensatory potential can make the limbs and joints to complete the same motor function movement, but it is prone to form abnormal motor pattern because of the compensation of other muscles. For example, when hip flexors are paralyzed because of neural injury or muscle injury and the hip cannot be flexed, hip abductors can make the hip flex slightly to let the lower limbs move forward in order to complete stepping forward, but the circle like abnormal gait pattern is formed. The patients with amputation of two upper limbs, through training of lower limbs and toes, can acquire the similar functions of upper limbs and hands. For example, the feet can be used to complete the functions of upper limbs and hands in normal state such as toothbrush, combing, eating and repairing watch. All these belong to muscular compensatory potential.

   Neural compensatory potential can be developed and utilized through nature and practice. Nature compensation is a process that tissues reestablish functions through self-adjusting ability after damages. The start of reestablishing this function may be through some kind of tendency induced by lesion area or inducing factor. The compensation take place in the early stage after damages and its effect may be limited. The other way is to promote central nervous cells to play compensatory role through active movement called "use" in order to achieve functional organization and recover the ability of control limbs and joint motion. This is the main measure to recover functions after central nervous damages. Its mechanism can be referred to the second section in Chap. 1.
6. Regeneration type: Regeneration potential is that after cells damages, homogenous cells around injured area generate new cells to recover tissues and functions through mitosis, which is the functions of most tissues and cells in human body. However, the regeneration capacity is greatly different in different tissues. For example, after epithelial tissue damages, in certain degree and area of damages, the original form and function can be recovered. Regeneration capacity of spleen and liver is remarkable too. Regeneration capacity of muscle is weak. Scar is easy to be formed through fiber tissue connection. Regeneration capacity of central nervous system is weak. Regeneration capacity doesn't play a leading role in the recovering motor functions of injured area.

In a word, although there is inter-related phenomenon in the potentials mentioned above with different forms, its basis is tissues and cells. Targeted measures should be adopted to promote development and utilization of these potentials in rehabilitation training in order to recover more lost motor and cognitive functions.

3.1.2 The Condition of Developing Potential

Development of potential not only requires special condition, but also requires the persons who were trained and were with preparation to apply and develop potential. The development degree is related to the adopted methods. For example, under dangerous circumstances, the persons without training or preparation lose their head, even lose motor and thinking functions. The result is that the persons not only cannot use development potential to cope with dangerous accident, but also lose the possessed capacity under normal circumstances. For the persons with training or preparation, they can be calm in the hour of peril and use their head in a crisis. The result is that on the basis of the original functions, they can motivate more functions to cope with an emergency and complete the mission or pull through difficulties.

In conclusion, there are several points in favor of developing potential.

3.1.2.1 Willingness of Active Participation

Potential development is a chronic and tough training process. Without the willingness of active participation of the patients, it is hard for the patients to persist and it is easy to be abandoned halfway. The patients will never achieve their objectives. If the patients understand the meaning of developing potential and its important effect and function on their future, the patients can take part in the training actively. Not only the patients can persist, but also the development effect is good. This requires the joint effort of the patients, relatives of the patients and doctors in order to achieve the objective that the patients take part in the training actively and voluntarily.

3.1.2.2 Definite Surpassing Target

Setting a definite surpassing target is the important measure to develop potential, recover and improve functions.

"Objective and motive" mechanism can be applied for any area. It is said that the whole year's work depends on a good start in spring and the whole day's work depends on a good start in the morning, which demonstrates the importance of plan and goal. Our country sets Five-year Plan for development and lets the whole nation and various sectors step towards this goal. After eleven Five-year Plans, there were earthshaking changes in China. If a primary school student can set a study goal very early by himself not by his parents, he may study very well. If he wants to enter into the top two schools (Tsinghua University and Peking University) in China and he does work hard, the chance to enter into Tsinghua University and Peking University is good. "Objective and motive" mechanism was widely and necessarily applied for competitive sports training. For example, the cross-bar of jumper, the target of archery, target of shooting, weight of weightlifting and degrees of free exercises are all the goals of sports training. With these targets, the athletes can surpass them one by one through training and improve their competitiveness.

For the patients who want to do rehabilitation training, the long-term target of rehabilitation can be set. However, it is practical to set immediate and definite surpassing targets such as the intensity of motor program signal, myodynamia, touching altitude, walking distance and the range of joint motion. Immediate target can be modified as needed. Exception of the training that the patients do, the patients achieve or surpass the target through hard work, can see their progress timely and is pleasure to receive further therapy. However, the target should be set reasonably. If the target is too high and the patients want to achieve it in a short time, it is difficulty for the patients to complete. There will be pessimistic mood of the patients that is bad for rehabilitation.

3.1.2.3 Satisfying the Requirements of Active Movement

Use means that brain controls body movements and active use is the most fundamental measure to develop potential. Unless satisfying the requirements of active movement, it is hard to promote CNS plasticity and achieve functional reorganization finally.

There is a good example about the training of special troops. Special troops are capable of developing their potential and extraordinary abilities through scientific and tough training in specified conditions such as severe cold, the intense heat of summer, extreme climate and conditions with wire entanglement and mire. In competitive sports, good achievement can be obtained through scientific and planned active movement training.

There are also ways to promote competitive sports performance through electrical stimulus and illegal drugs, which have side effects. Electrical stimulus can stimulate the excitability of muscles, but the reflex arc is located in spinal cord and it has no effect on recovering higher neural center because it is afferent stimulus. Therefore, electrical stimulus can maintain muscle tension, increase blood supply of muscle and promote muscle contractility, which belong to efficiency training. However, drugs can increase the nutrition supply of muscle and promote the excitability of nervous system abnormally and temporally just like the patients with manic psychosis. Drugs can make the body to exert ability abnormally. However, all these cannot recover normal active movement completed with muscles dominated by CNS. Moreover, illegal drugs can harm human body and it is forbidden in rehabilitation training.

For example, in our daily life, if we learn cycling and swimming, it is practical to use electrical stimulus, drugs, acupuncture and massage, because these methods are not in accordance with motor relearning mechanism. Only through practical training, we can learn riding and swimming, because riding and swimming are active movements, which conform to the requirements of promoting CNS potential development. We can increase the technical level of riding and swimming, if we can do planned scientific training.

Passive movement is a process that the people are driven by other people or equipment to move. Because the patients don't use their brains to complete or try to complete one limb movement or trunk movement, it has no effect on developing potential. Therefore, the main function of passive movement is to prevent adhesion of joints, muscles, tissues, contracture of tendon and play a supportive therapeutic role in recovery of motor function actively.

3.1.2.4 Methods to Motivate People into "Reactive State"

In dangerous emergency state, for a person who is with good psychological quality, deal with affairs smoothly and is bridle-wise can enter into full alert, concentrated and competent state immediately in order to deal with dangerous reactive state. Some research showed that in this state myodynamia of human body is six times of that in normal state. Enormous energy is activated to cope with dangerous factors and get through the difficulty.

The method that is effective to motivate human body into reactive state is creating imminent danger state by all means such as scenario simulation and speech intimidation. For the patients with rehabilitation training, if the created imminent danger state is too severe, the accident can be induced, because most patients with limb paralysis due to stroke are associated with hypertension and diabetes. Therefore, it is necessary to investigate and find the training method to create imminent danger sate and not to induce accident, which is good for the patients [1–5].

The therapists should make the patients to see and feel safe when the patients receive training. They must exactly know there is no danger such as falling down and bumping in any training to what extent, which is the fundamental measure to eliminate or alleviate the scruple of the patients. Additionally, creating strict quantitative imminent danger state has no harm and side effect on the patients in developing potential. The author called this safe imminent danger state.

In the premise of ensuring safety, creating imminent danger state is an important procedure to guarantee the effect of potential development.

With respect to the effect of potential development, the effect of imminent danger state is better than that of "Simple endeavor". The former is that the patients without any preparation are forced by emergency situation to motivate their own potentials to cope with accidents, whereas the latter is that the patients consciously try to complete some kind of unaccomplished mission such as lifting 100 kg. Imminent danger state can make human body try to motivate itself and overcome the adverse factors. If human body cannot overcome the adverse factors, it is possible that there is some kind of result that has adverse effects on human body or influences human body irreversibly. Afterward, human body enters into "reactive state" immediately in order to motivate all the powers to cope with dangerous factors at the utmost. During this process, the embodied potentials are developed and utilized maximally. In the simple endavour state, the patients know exactly mission for fulfillment and there is no harm to themselves even complete it or not. The patients just try to complete it and cannot enter into "reactive state" very well, which can influence the effect and degree of potential development.

There are many ways to create imminent danger state. During training, the therapists can use them flexibly. As mentioned above, scenario simulation and speech intimidation are used to create imminent danger state. This method has effect on potential development, but the effect is not ideal in the training without practical movements. For example, in the process of active movement training, sudden "zero gravity" or sudden reduction of assisted force with scenario simulation and speech stimulation are used to compel the patients to enter into "reactive state" in order to improve the effect of potential development.

3.1.2.5 From Easy to Difficulty and Step by Step

Rehabilitation training is a chronic even life-long process. The problem usually in clinic is that the patients and relatives of the patients cannot keep rehabilitation training for some reasons such as lack of self-confidence or money. They always doubt, give up or take a negative altitude on that they can recover their functions through rehabilitation training. They even cannot keep training for a complete course of treatment. Because of this, they usually give up without accomplishing anything or halfway. The patients usually think that there is no treatment value for further rehabilitation and then they give up rehabilitation training. Therefore, it is important to restore their confidence to rehabilitation. The most effective method to restore confidence is that they can see their progress through training.

In order to increase the confidence of the patients to rehabilitation, it is necessary to let the patients see their own progress in rehabilitation training timely. In the process of rehabilitation training, the therapist should let the patients feel that they have access to functional improvement and complete rehabilitation training easily if they try. Therefore, on the basis of detailed functional assessment, designed rehabilitation training program should conform to the principle "from easy to difficulty and step by step", which means simpler training method is adopted. The training should be started from the part where the functions are easy to be improved in and then transited to the part where the functions are hard to be improved with high intensity and complicated methods. The parts of training are generally from trunk to lower limbs, and to upper limbs and hands; from single joint detached movement to multi-joint associated movement. In the training methods, potential development, reestablishment of motor program and remodeling of motor pattern are sequentially done during training. For example, the patients are unable to sit independently. Potential development training of lumbodorsal muscles should be done firstly. Through the training for 2–3 weeks, the patients can be able to sit independently. The patients see with their own eyes and be keenly aware of the effect of training. And then their confidence will be increase greatly and they want to take part in the subsequent training actively, which can further promote the training effect. Afterward, the training of lower limbs and upper limbs can be started.

Progressive potential development is an important guarantee for the smooth training and to prevent fear of the patients to difficulty, which is creating "minor imminent danger state". The therapist let the patients do potential development training positively and relaxedly and the training effect will be better. For example, the author classify the potential development training of lower limbs to six grades (30° per grade) according to flexion angle of knee joint. From low angle, with the help of the therapists and according to the progress condition of the patients, the difficulty is increased gradually and the assisted force is decreased gradually. Whether the training is in the starting grade or the ending grade, the therapists can decrease the assisted force suddenly in the training process and say "Stand up, or you will fall down" "Hold on, or you will bump", which can motivate the potential of the patients and they can sit up independently.

3.1.2.6 Appropriate Physical State

The premise that training can improve motor function, cognitive state and memory ability is good physical states include stable vital signs, acid-base balance, fluid balance, electrolyte balance in vivo and stable functions of all viscera that include stability of diet, sleep and defecation. Appropriate physical state not only is good for the training safety, but also can have good effect on training because the patients are with abundant vigor and physical power and can coordinate with the training.

3.1.2.7 Secure Safeguard Procedures

Preventing the accident in the training is a special problem that we need to pay attention to. According to the specific condition of the patients, feasible safeguard procedures are adopted in order to eliminate the hidden danger and the fear and panic of the patients. Specific corollary equipment neurological training is equipped with weight loss system. On the one hand, this system can reduce the patients' weight to varying degrees through regulating tractive force as the patients need in order to make the patients are capable of sitting up and walking. On the other hand, suspension function of weight loss system can assure the patients not to fall down or bump so that it plays a safety protection role.

In addition, for the patients with unstable state of an illness or severe cardiovascular diseases, the training should be done under electrocardiograph monitoring to know the change of cardiac function timely in order to find the problem and deal with it and make rehabilitation training safe and stable.

3.2 The Application of Six-Step Daoyin Technique in Potential Development

3.2.1 Clearing and Activating the Channels and Collaterals of Daoyin Technique

The study about Chinese Qigong demonstrated that nervous system can influence human functions through regular and conscious exercise and the practitioners can possess the capacity that people without exercise cannot have. Some research indicated that consciousness or idea are closely related to the integration of high-grade part in nervous system and can control and regulate organ activities and turn them into material strength of muscle movement.

Daoyin technique in traditional Chinese medicine can enlighten and motivate human willpower. The regulation of movement is based on the regulation of mind and breathing, which means the patients use brain to control limbs movements and employ Daoyin speeches to create state of emergency without risk in order to achieve functional rehabilitation. However, Daoyin technique in all dynasties attached most importance to whole movement of self-exercise and cannot be directly used for rehabilitation of the patients with obvious dyskinesia of limbs. Because it is short of definite concept, subjective and abstract, Daoyin technique is mainly used in life cultivation and health preservation but not in clinic, which is endangered in modern times.

Six-step Daoyin technique in traditional Chinese medicine is the basic technique that inherited from ancient Daoyin technique in traditional Chinese medicine and is based on the regulation of mind, breathing and movements. It is divided into six steps. The strategy of it is that concentrating superiority in force to attack one spot. The patients are guided to do single joint motion. During this process, there are two characteristics. The first is the training of one muscle contraction. One muscle plays an important role in single joint motion, which is the contraction of agonistic muscle to complete joint motion. Compared with the whole movement (simultaneous multi-joint motion with one or more limbs) of human body, it is easy to be completed and produce a better effect. The second is the process of clearing and activating the channels and collaterals through concentrating superior energy. The process of regulation of mind and breathing is to concentrate all energy on brain. During this process, it not only can clear and activate the channels and collaterals, but also can make the muscles in stand-by condition. The patients are guided to use brain to control muscles suddenly, which means the patients use brain to control one muscle and concentrate superiority in force to attack one spot. It is prone to dredge the relationship between brain and muscle and has a better effect on developing brain potential and recovering lost motor function. The procedures of six-step Daoyin technique are as follows: the therapists exert resistance properly in the orientation of joint motion of the patients (metatarsophalangeal joints on instep of dorsiflexion of foot) in order to let the patients' brain to find the target that receive signals and the orientation of exerting. It is also the case when myodynamia is zero. In clinic, that myodynamia is zero is not equal to that the muscle is out of control. The research of the author indicated that the signal from central nerve to muscle is 360 times more sensitive than the muscle contraction assessed in clinic. Therefore, zero myodynamia is not equal to zero signals. The therapists encourage and urge the patients to complete the required joint motion. When exerting resistance, the therapists encourage the patients to hold on for 6 s. This procedure can be completed using counting such as "one, two, three, you did great, four, five, six." When encouraging the patients, the therapists use words to create state of emergency such as "hold on or you will fall down" and "lift up or you will crash" in order to develop the neural potential as much as possible.

During training, the signal intensity of agonistic muscle should be increased and the signal intensity of antagonistic muscle should be decreased in order to practice the ability of joint coordinated movement dominated by brain. This is the training process to reestablish motor program. Agonistic muscle and antagonistic muscle can switch roles in different joint motion. For example, in elbow extension of joint motion, triceps muscle of arm is agonistic muscle and bicipital muscle of arm is antagonistic muscle. While in elbow flexion joint motion, bicipital muscle of arm is agonistic muscle and triceps muscle of arm is antagonistic muscle.

The procedure of regulation of mind in normal Daoyin technique is not in accordance with the course of main and collateral channels. Although normal Daoyin technique can make the patients to concentrate on the training, the training degree of injured side brain is decreased due to voluntary movement, which has a certain effect on developing brain potential through Daoyin technique. Moreover, the traditional Chinese characteristics of Daoyin technique in traditional Chinese medicine are not prominent in normal Daoyin technique.

Main and collateral channels are the pathways where Qi and blood can circulate. Its functions include connecting visceras in vivo, connecting limbs in vitro, communicating all the limbs and bones, relating the five sense organs and nine orifices, regulating yin and yang, infiltrating and irrigating Qi and blood, moistening and nourishing the whole body, enriching yingqi and weiqi, defending exogenous pathogenic factors. Traditional Chinese medicine deemed that accumulated internal injury induce yin-yang disharmony, disordered Qi and blood, rise suddenly and sharply of the liver-yang, swirl of endogenous wind, exuberance of stagnated heat, phlegm and anger, fleeing in the meridians, impatency of brain and mind. Afterward, the patients suddenly faint and are in stroke hemiplegia. Li shizhen pointed out that brain is the headquarters of mind. The mind hidden in the five internal organs are all the concrete manifestations of mind in brain.

Thereout, we can tell the relationship between motor function and brain with main and collateral channels. Main and collateral channels like nerves. If the main and collateral channels are blocked, the signal of autokinetic movement dominated by brain cannot be conducted fluently, which can induce dyskinesia in corresponding body part. On the other hand, after brain damages, main and collateral channels are out of control, which is the fundamental factor to induce limbs dyskinesia.

The regulation of mind, breathing and movements of Daoyin technique in traditional Chinese medicine is to guide the patients to use mind to circulate Qi in main and collateral channels and use brain to control autonomous movement. Mind is the functional activity of brain. Qi is the messenger of brain regulating main and collateral channels. In brain, the patients use mind to circulate Qi to the muscle involved in joint motion through main and collateral channels in order to dredge the channels. Therefore, the messenger of brain controlling muscle timely and effectively delivers message to the muscle involved in joint motion and autonomous joint motion is induced. Afterward, Qi disperse in the main and collateral channels, which is a relaxed process and also the process of dredging brain, clearing the heart, enlightening the mind and activating collaterals. The process can promote brain potential development and functional reorganization. On the basis of the process, motor program can be reestablished and motor function can be recovered. It is scientific and important for the Daoyin rehabilitation technique in traditional Chinese medicine to recover the lost motor function after brain damages.

Therefore, in a word, regulation of mind is a process that brain give out movement messenger to clear and activate the channels and collaterals. Regulation of breathing is a process that brain is prepared to give out movement messenger. Regulation of movement is a process that movement messenger induces autonomous movement of joint from brain to the muscle involved in joint motion.

Many researchers use modern experiment methods to investigate the nature of main and collateral channels and found that main and collateral channels are a junction zone located in loose connective tissue. The content of interstitial fluid is high so that the physical property is low-resistance. And directional flow of interstitial fluid is closely related to propagated sensation along channel. Some research also indicated that main and collateral channels may be related to physiological information conduction system of stem cells over the entire body. Stem cells are activated to release cell active substance, which is related to nervous-endocrine-immune system and function together. If nervous-endocrine-immune system is damaged, stem cells system can compensate the lost functions or repair functions.

Dredging collaterals through meridians method is that mind regulates Qi from the beginning of main and collateral channels to agonistic muscle of movable joint. Afterward, brain gives out signal to activate joint motion. In the orientation of joint motion, according to the specific condition of the patients, the therapists exert resistance to develop potential fully. After completion of joint motion, the patients are still guided to relax themselves and use mind to regulate Qi along with residual main and collateral channels until Qi disperses in collaterals gradually.

According to the different orientation of Qi, dredging collaterals through meridians method is divided into "dredging collaterals through meridians" and "dredging meridians through collaterals". Its objective is to bring out clearing and activating the channels and collaterals of six-step Daoyin technique. Like a blocked pipeline, if we dredge from one side, plugging matter may be pushed to one side and become tighter. Therefore, it is uneasy to be loosen and hard to be dredged. If we dredge the pipeline from two sides, it is easy to be loosen and hard to be dredged (Fig. 3.1, 3.2, 3.3, and 3.4).

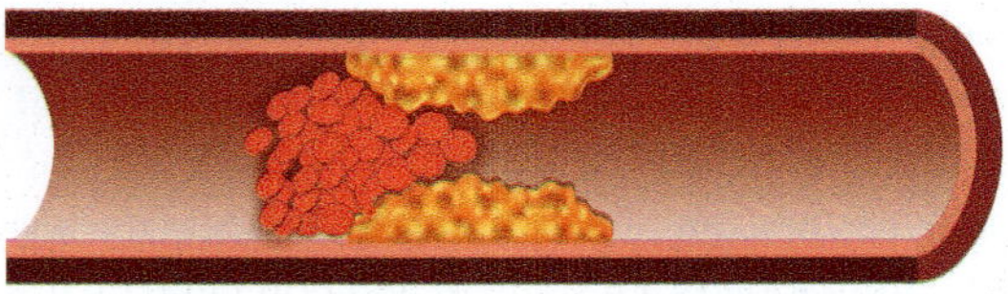

Fig. 3.1 Sketch map of stricture site in pipeline

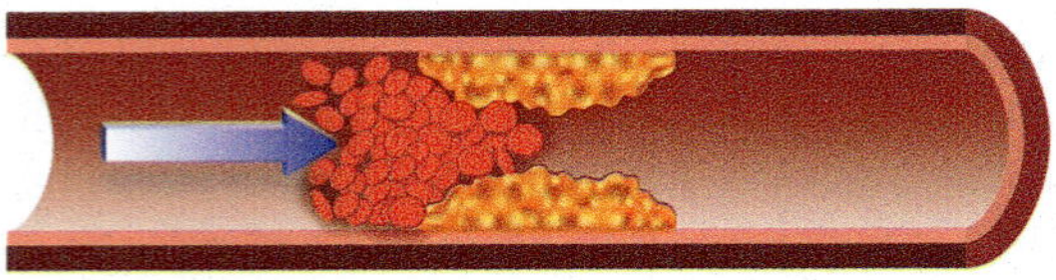

Fig. 3.2 Dredging along with flow direction

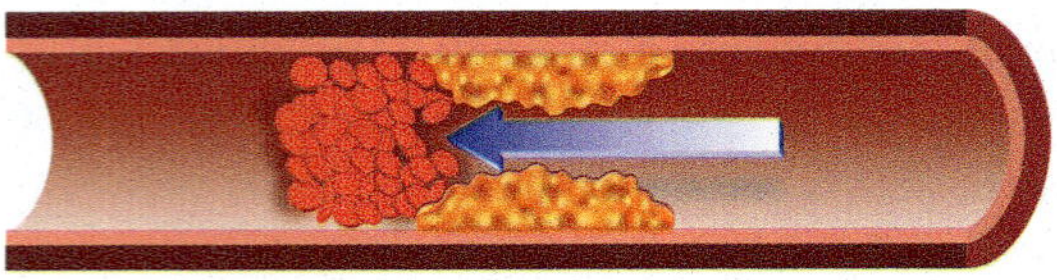

Fig. 3.3 Dredging against flow direction

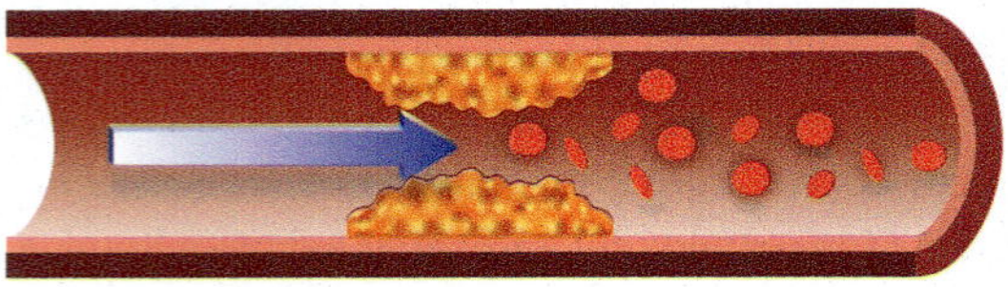

Fig. 3.4 Dredging along with flow direction once more

Dredging meridians through collaterals method is used to regulate mind and breathing. According to the route lead by animation spot of meridian points, the patients are guided to use mind to regulate Qi from the beginning of main and collateral channels to agonistic muscle of movable joint. Afterward, brain gives out signal to activate joint motion. In the orientation of joint motion, according to the specific condition of the patients, the therapists exert resistance to develop potential fully. (When myodynamia is zero, the resistance should be exerted because the resistance can increase muscle tone and make it easy for brain to find the orientation and induce muscle contraction.). After completion of joint motion, the patients are still guided to relax themselves and use mind to regulate Qi along with residual main and collateral channels until Qi disperses in meridians gradually.

Both dredging collaterals through meridians and dredging meridians through collaterals are the process that brain guides Qi to circulate in main and collateral channels and brain is used to dredge main and collateral channels. If the patients concentrate to a certain extent, during the circulation of Qi in main and collateral channels, the patients can feel slightly hot along main and collateral channels, especially the acupoint. In clinic, during the circulation of Qi in main and collateral channels, the muscle micro-contraction around main and collateral channels can be induced. Therefore, the process of dredging collaterals through meridians is also a process that cortex motor center controls muscle micro-contraction, which is good for promoting CNS plasticity.

Therefore, the two methods are used alternatively to clear and activate the channels and collaterals. The alternative times and time are mainly dependent on dredging collaterals through meridians with subsidiary role of dredging meridians through collaterals. We place dredging collaterals through meridians first and dredging meridians through collaterals second. The alternative ration of dredging collaterals through meridians and dredging meridians through collaterals is 3–1 to 5–1.

Therefore, according to main and collateral channels, Daoyin feedback rehabilitation technique is implemented to develop neural potential better, promote compensatory mechanism, repair injured brain, improve therapeutic effect of rehabilitation and recover lost motor function.

3.2.2 Classification of Potential Development Training

According to the rehabilitation training principle "from easy to difficulty and step by step", potential development training is implemented hierarchically in order to prevent the damages of bone, joint and muscle. There are postural hypotension and collapse due to high-intensity training, even life-threatening accident.

The classification of training refers to the angle of joint motion range change or the training time.

3.2.2.1 Classification Method of Joint Motion Range

Classification method refers to the angle of joint motion range change, which is appropriate for potential development training of upper and lower limbs.

The objective of upper and lower limbs potential development is to develop CNS potential that control muscle contraction of upper and lower limbs. However, the development of this potential can be realized only through active movement training of limbs. For example, six-step of dredging collaterals through meridians is used to lift and lower upper limbs, stand and sit down with lower limbs. Because the patients with different dyskinesia and lack of autonomic movement, they need to be helped to do active movement or compelled to do active movement in order to complete the designed movement. Therefore, it can promote the plasticity and functional reorganization of CNS that control upper and lower limbs.

During the process of potential development, the difficulty is related to the angle of joint flexion and moment of force. For standing up with lower limbs and pushing up with upper limbs, when the flexion range of joint motion is less than 90°, the larger the range is, the bigger the difficulty is. The littler the range is, the smaller the difficulty is. When the flexion range of joint motion is more than 90°, the larger the range is, the smaller the difficulty is. The littler the range is, the bigger the difficulty is. When the flexion range of joint motion is equal to 90°, the difficulty is the biggest. Similarly, for sitting down with lower limbs and pushing down with upper limbs, when the flexion range of joint motion is less than 90°, the larger the range is, the bigger the difficulty is. The littler the range is, the smaller the difficulty is. When the flexion range of joint motion is more than 90°, the larger the range is, the smaller the difficulty is. The littler the range is, the bigger the difficulty is. From the range of whole movement, whether in standing up, sitting down or pushing up, pushing down, the difficulty is in direct proportion to the range of joint motion. The larger the range of joint motion is, the bigger the difficulty is. Therefore, according to the angle in the range of joint motion, we assess the difficulty of the training. Thirty degrees are set as one coefficient of difficulty and there are six coefficient of difficulty, which is called six-level classification method of potential development training in lower limbs (Table 3.1).

The difficulty classification of potential development training in trunk.

When doing potential development training of trunk, the patients lie on the back and the sunk of lower waist in the training bed is used to regulate the difficulty of the training. The sunken depth of the training bed is training 18 cm, which is composed of three training stereoplasm sponge

Table 3.1 Six-level classification method of potential development training in lower limbs

Coefficient of difficulty	The degree of knee joint extension or flexion (0°)	Myodynamia	Vital signs	Supplementary measures	
				Weight loss (kg)	Exerting resistance (kg)
1	0–30°	0	Basically stable with weak constitution	One third to one fourth of body weight	Supplement wanted
2	30–60°	I	Stable with weak constitution	One fourth to one sixth of body weight	Supplement wanted
3	60–90°	I–II	Stable with weak constitution and autonomous joint motion	One fifth to one eighth of body weight	Supplement wanted
4	90–120°	II–III	Normal with full range autonomous joint motion	One eighth to one tenth of body weight	Exerting resistance when the range of knee joint is more than 90°
5	120–150°	III–IV	Normal with autonomous anti-resistance	5 kg	Exerting resistance when the range of knee joint is more than 90°
6	150–180°	IV–V	Normal with high anti-resistance	5 kg	Exerting resistance after beginning joint motion

Table 3.2 The classification of potential development training in trunk

Coefficient of difficulty	Cushion number	Myodynamia	Vital signs	Supplementary measures	
				Weight loss (kg)	Exerting resistance (kg)
1	3	0–II	Basically stable with weak constitution	One third to one fourth of body weight	Supplement wanted
2	2	III–IV	Stable with autonomous joint motion	One fourth to one sixth of body weight	Exerting slight resistance
3	1	IV–V	Normal with full range autonomous joint motion and anti-resistance	5 kg	Exerting resistance after beginning joint motion

Table 3.3 Classification method of potential development training time

Coefficient of difficulty	Time (min)	Vital signs	Supplementary measures
1	1–5	Basically stable with weak constitution	Supplement wanted
2	6–10	Stable with weak constitution, autonomous joint motion ans without anti-resistance	Supplement wanted
3	11–15	Stable with full range autonomous joint motion, weak constitution and autonomous anti-resistance	Normal, exerting resistance properly
4	16–20	Stable with strong anti-resistance	Exerting resistance after beginning joint motion

cushions that are 6 cm in depth. According to this depth, they are divided into three levels (Table 3.2). The more the cushion number is, the smaller the difficulty is and the less the cushion number is, the bigger the difficulty is.

3.2.2.2 Classification Method of Training Time

According to the training time and time interval between trainings, the classification method is appropriate for potential development training in all parts.

When the stamina of the patients is good, the time of potential development training is 30 min every time. In the middle of the training, the rib belts should be loosened to let the patients have a break for 1–2 times in case that the rib belts oppress the chest and influence breathing. The break takes 3–5 min every time and the training time is about 20 min. Every 5 min is a training magnitude and there are four levels. According to the specific condition of the patients, the training time can be adjusted (Table 3.3).

Potential development training requires 1–2 therapists and potential development training device is used to do the training. Potential development training device is equipped with weight loss system. According to vital signs of the patients such as breathing, blood pressure, pulse, body temperature, electrocardiogram and stamina, the therapists set the quantity of weight loss. According to the types of the training, the parts of exerting resistance are different. The part for exerting resistance of potential development training in upper limbs is shoulder-back. The therapists use sandbag or hands to exert resistance. The part for exerting resistance of potential development training in lower limbs is shoulder of the patients.

3.3 Clinical Indications and Cautions of Potential Development

3.3.1 Clinical Indications and Cautions of Upper Limbs Potential Development Training

3.3.1.1 Indications and Contraindications

1. Indications: Potential development training in upper limbs is appropriate for the training of dysfunctions in the patients in stable

condition with acute, chronic and obsolete hemiplegia, cerebral palsy, child cerebral palsy, complete or incomplete paraplegia, peripheral nerve injury, bone and joint muscles dysfunction after CNS and bone joint damages in order to recover autonomous motor function in upper limbs or prevent myophagism and osteoporosis.
2. Contraindications: Contraindications of potential development in upper limbs include the patients in acute stage with unstable condition, the patients in uncontrolled condition with severe hypertension and diabetes, the patients with severe heart disease, pulmonary dysfunction and low cardiovascular response capacity and the patients with subluxation of shoulder joint and severe dislocation in upper limbs.

3.3.1.2 Cautions

It is important for potential development training to keep the training safe. Moreover, there are other items. For the patients with weak constitution or long-term bedridden patients, the adaptive training should be done before this type of the training in order to increase the stress capability of the patients' angiocarpy. When the patients stand erectly for 30 min and blood pressure, pulse and electrocardiogram are stable, this type of the training should be done. The training should be step by step. The therapists regulate the training through changing the weight and training time. High training intensity should be avoided. During training, the enthusiasm of the patients and the training atmosphere should be fully activated. The therapists should use encouraging words and scolding and critical words should be avoided. Severe patients can do the training by cardiogram monitor and the disease condition should be watched carefully. If there is any problem, the training should be stopped immediately.

3.3.2 Clinical Indications and Cautions of Potential Development Training in Trunk

Potential development in trunk is the training that can be done while the patients lie in bed. There is no restrict requirement for the patients' constitution. The patients are capable of doing twin bridge training can use this training, but the vital signs of the patients should be watched carefully.

3.3.2.1 Indications and Contraindications

1. Indications: It is appropriate for the motor function recovery training of dysfunctions in the patients in stable condition with acute, chronic and obsolete hemiplegia, cerebral palsy, child cerebral palsy, complete or incomplete paraplegia, the patients with lumbodorsa injury or spinal postoperation dysfunction after CNS and bone joint damages.
2. Contraindications: Contraindications of potential development in upper limbs include the patients in acute stage with unstable condition, the patients in uncontrolled condition with severe hypertension and diabetes, the patients with severe heart disease, pulmonary dysfunction and low cardiovascular response capacity, the patients with unstable internal fixation and unhealed centrum after spinal operation and the patients with child cerebral palsy and congenital dislocation of hip joint.

3.3.2.2 Cautions

There are several items that should be paid attention to in potential development training in trunk. For the patients with weak constitution, the adaptive training should be done before this type of the training in order to increase the stress capability of the patients' angiocarpy. When the patients lie in bed and do twin bridge training five times and blood pressure, pulse and electrocardiogram are stable, this type of the training should be done. The training should be step by step. The therapists regulate the training through changing the weight and training time. High training intensity should be avoided. During training, the enthusiasm of the patients and the training atmosphere should be fully activated. The therapists should use encouraging words and scolding and critical words should be avoided. Severe patients can do the training by cardiogram monitor and the disease condition should be watched carefully. If there is any problem, the training should be stopped immediately.

3.3.3 Clinical Indications and Cautions of Potential Development Training in Lower Limbs

Potential development in lower limbs is one of the most applied neurological rehabilitation training in clinic. Not only there are many indications of this training, but also there is a good therapeutic effect. The patients who lose active movement completely can recover autonomous motor function of lower limbs to vary degrees in a short time.

3.3.3.1 Indications and Contraindications

1. Indications: Potential development training in lower limbs is appropriate for the training of dysfunctions in the patients in stable condition with acute, chronic and obsolete hemiplegia, cerebral palsy, child cerebral palsy, complete or incomplete paraplegia, peripheral nerve injury, bone and joint muscles dysfunction after CNS and bone joint damages. It is also appropriate for the patients whose lower limbs functions cannot be improved in traditional rehabilitation therapy.
2. Contraindications: Contraindications of potential development in upper limbs include the patients in acute stage with unstable condition, the patients in uncontrolled condition with severe hypertension and diabetes, the patients with severe heart disease, pulmonary dysfunction and low cardiovascular response capacity, the patients with dizziness and drop of blood pressure when standing up, the patients who stand erectly for 30 min but blood pressure, pulse and electrocardiogram are unstable and the patients with child cerebral palsy and congenital dislocation of hip joint.

3.3.3.2 Cautions

There are several items that should be paid attention to in potential development training in lower limbs. For the patients with weak constitution or long-term bedridden patients, the patients should do standing bed training before this type of the training in order to increase the stress capability of the patients' angiocarpy. When the patients stand erectly for 30 min and blood pressure, pulse and electrocardiogram are stable, this type of the training should be done. The training should be step by step. The therapists regulate the training through changing the weight and training time. High training intensity should be avoided. During training, the enthusiasm of the patients and the training atmosphere should be fully activated. The therapists should use encouraging words and scolding and critical words should be avoided. Severe patients can do the training by cardiogram monitor and the disease condition should be watched carefully. If there is any problem, the training should be stopped immediately. The application of Daoyin technique in the training should be emphasized. Daoyin technique is the main training method. Potential development training equipment of lower limbs is the assisted corollary equipment of Daoyin technique.

3.4 Clinical Experiment of Potential Development

3.4.1 The Development and Clinical Application of Potential Development Training Equipment of Upper Limbs

The upper limbs dysfunction after central nervous system damages is one of the difficulties in rehabilitation therapy. Although there are many therapies, the therapeutic effect is not ideal because of the simple training method and apparatus such as occupational therapy. The author develops potential development training equipment of upper limbs in order to promote upper limbs motor function recovery.

3.4.1.1 Materials and Methods

1. The constitution of potential development training equipment of upper limbs: Potential development training equipment of upper limbs is composed of hand expansion board, pedestal, limbs control training system, bearing supporting system, hammock and suspension

system, weight loss pulley system, weight loss sandbag or handle. Bearing supporting system is made of hot drawing welded steel tube whose diameter is 36 mm and thickness is 4 mm. The bend frame (120 cm × 180 cm) is connected to pedestal. The pedestal is made of the same tube. The superstratum of dual-tier framework (180 cm × 150 cm × 20 cm) is covered by aluminium alloy plate and compressed by spongy cushion whose thickness is 3 cm. In the middle of the top of braced frame, one corner and side wall, pulley is welding fixed. Steel wire whose diameter is 3 mm is used to connect hammock in frame and handle or weight loss sandbag hook in side wall. Hammock is fixed to the chest of the patients. The weight of weight loss sandbag includes 5, 10 and 20 kg. The quantity of weight loss can be regulated through changing the number and kind of sandbag. The therapists can grip the handle during training and regulate the quantity of weight loss through assisted force.

2. Training methods: The training methods are as follows:
   (a) Preparation before training: The patients dress hammock, put on hand expansion board, lie in push-up position, kneel on sponge cushion of pedestal. In this position, the patients' hands are exactly on the vertical surface weight loss pulley in the middle of the top of braced frame with the width same as shoulder. Hammock is connected to hook of weight loss system. The therapists stand on the injured side of the patients. According to sandbag in exercise prescription, the therapists can grip the handle during training and regulate the quantity of weight loss through assisted force.
   (b) Training: There are two kinds of training such as pushing up and down. Pushing-up training is defined as that the patients' upper is on flexed position of elbow joint and the patients move their body center to paralyzed side. The patients are guided to take a deep breathing, breathe out slowly, concentrate on deep inspiration and hold the breathing, and then concentrate on triceps muscle of arm in paralyzed side. During the slow pushing-up process, the patients should feel the contraction of triceps muscle of arm. When the patients cannot push up themselves, the therapists should help them. When the extension angle is more than 90°, the therapists reduce assisted force suitably according to the condition and use the words "push up, or you will fall; hold on, or you will bump" to create dangerous atmosphere. The therapist should encourage the patients to push up by themselves. Pushing-down training is defined as that the patients' upper is on extension position of elbow joint and the patients move their body center to paralyzed side. The patients are guided to take a deep breathing, breathe out and push down slowly. During the slow pushing-down process, the patients should feel the contraction of triceps muscle of arm. When the patients cannot push up themselves, the therapists should help them. When the extension angle is less than 90°, the therapists increase assisted force suitably according to the condition and use the words "push up, or you will fall; hold on, or you will bump" to create dangerous atmosphere. The therapist should encourage the patients to hold on in this position for 3–5 s.
   (c) Training time is 30 min every time and one time a day. One course of therapy includes 30 times. After one course of therapy, the therapist should assess the therapy effect and decide whether to do the next course of therapy or not.

3.4.1.2 Clinical Application

1. Clinical data: From April 2006 to October 2007, potential development training equipment was used to treat 56 patients with upper limbs motor dysfunction who are all the inpatients and outpatients in neurological rehabilitation training center in Beijing Tongren Hospital affiliated to Beijing's Capital Medical University. There are 42 males and

14 females. The age is from 18 to 62 years old. The average age is 41.33 years old. The shortest medical history lasts 6 months and the longest lasts 146 months. The average is 37 months. There are 29 patients with hemiplegia after cerebral infarction, 12 patients with hemiplegia after cerebral hemorrhage, ten patients with hemiplegia after brain damage and ten patients with spinal cord injury. There are 26 patients with right hemiplegia, 25 patients with left hemiplegia and five patients with dual bilateral limbs dysfunction.

2. Functional assessment and data analysis: Lovett MMT myodynam assessment, range of joint motion (ROM) and motor program electrical signal intensity are used as assessment methods. At the beginning of the training and the end of the therapy, the therapists assess myodynamia of triceps muscle of arm, autonomous range of joint motion and electrical signal intensity. SPSS12.0 statistical software is used for T test analysis. The results are referred to Table 3.4.
3. Results: Statistical analysis of assessment data and security of equipment are as follows:
   (a) Statistical analysis: There are significant differences in the three assessment indicators before and after therapy ($p < 0.05$). There are nine patients with zero myodynamia of triceps muscle of arm in all the patients. After training, myodynamia is recovered to 2.08 grades. Autonomous joint motion is recovered.
   (b) Security of equipment: There is no injury in all the patients during the training. Equipment design is rational, safe and reliable. The operation of the equipment is easy and flexible.
4. Discussion: The characteristics of upper limbs are flexibility, coordination, elaboration and skillful movements. The number of motor neurons in the cortex motor area that control upper limbs is bigger than that of motor neurons that control lower limbs. The relationship between them is complicated. Therefore, the functional compensation not only takes a long time, but also is complicated, which is the main reason for bad and slow functional recovery of upper limbs. Some researchers think that more intensified training is required to promote the functional recovery of upper limbs.

Although central nervous cells are lack of regeneration capacity, motor neuros are different from other tissue cells. Their number is big and they are the material basis of central nervous tissue potential. After partial motor neurons damages, cells around the injured area are trained to replace the functions of the injured cells, which is functional reorganization. However, cells around the injured area cannot obtain the functions like that of the injured cells unless they are received special repeated training.

At present, in clinic, the method used for functional recovery of upper limbs mainly is occupational therapy, which includes the training of passive, active and daily life ability. These methods are lack of enhancement degree and there is no training method for the upper limbs without autonomous movement. There is also no significant effect. Upper limbs in uninjured side are bind and upper limbs in injured side are forced to move. The therapy has a certain therapeutic effect. However, some kind of whole movement requires the patients' autonomous movements to complete. Meanwhile during the process of completing the movements, the patients merely try to do it no matter it is completed or not. Therefore,

Table 3.4 Functional assessment comparison table of triceps muscle of arm in paralyzed side before and after training ($\bar{x} \pm s$)

Assessment items	Before training	After training	p
Myodynamia	1.32 ± 0.65	2.62 ± 1.21	<0.05
Electromyographic signal	26.18 ± 8.36	87.31 ± 23.66	<0.01
Range of joint motion	19° ± 2.36°	36° ± 7.68°	<0.05

exception for lack of sense of urgency, because of the fixation of upper limbs in injured side, it is possible to have an accident. In addition, for the patients without autonomous movements or with severe obstacle of upper limbs in autonomous movements, it is difficulty to do this training and the therapeutic effect is not ideal. That is why this technique cannot be widely applied in clinic.

Therefore, investigation of the method for development and utilization of brain potential plays a key role in functional recovery after central nervous system damages, which is urgently necessary for clinical rehabilitation.

There are many examples that people can conquer difficulties and hardships using willpower and in dangerous condition people can burst into superman condition and tide over difficulties, which indicated that the human potential can be better developed in dangerous condition or with target and willpower. However, if the patients are diagnosed with hemiplegia or cerebral palsy, they may be with some severe protopathies such as hypertension, diabetes and heart disease. In dangerous condition, the training may exacerbate the disease state. Obviously, in dangerous condition, potential development training cannot be used for rehabilitation of this kind of patients.

Potential development training equipment can provide safe and reliable protection for upper limbs training with the help of bearing frame and hammock and can make the training from easy to difficulty and step by step through changing the quantity of weight loss. On the basis of that, Daoyin technique in traditional Chinese medicine is used to guide the patients to complete the movements through regulation of mind, breathing and movement. During the process of completing the movements, the therapists should use the words "hold up, or you will fall" "push up, or you will bump" combined with protective effect to create "safe" dangerous condition that is to the benefit of brain potential development. The functional reorganization of central nervous cells that control the movement of upper limbs is promoted to recover motor function. During this process, Daoyin technique in traditional Chinese medicine plays a leading role and the equipment has a supportive therapeutic effect.

In the potential development training of upper limbs, when the patients want to complete some kind of movement and cannot complete it because of limited capacity, the therapists should help them to complete it. Because of the help from the therapists, the movement becomes passive. On the contrary, in the process that the therapists help the patients to complete the movement passively, the therapists guide the patients to complete the movement actively and make the movement active. However, the ultimate goal of training is to complete the entire movement in order to develop brain potential that control injured limbs and promote brain function reorganization.

Clinical rehabilitation equipment cannot have an effect unless they conform to the rehabilitation method. The equipment cannot be applied unless they conform to the mechanism of human functional recovery. Some automatic, complicated and large-size equipment that are not based on rehabilitation theory and method ignore the process that people can do active movement by themselves because of the strong replacement, which affect clinical effects. People do active movement, which is good for human potential development. Some rehabilitation medical engineering specialists believe mistakenly that the patients can be recovered if the equipment is developed. If an athlete wants to improve his performance, he can achieve it through hardworking, scientific and persisted training. Athletes use equipment to increase the amount of exercise, not to replace themselves. If the equipment replace athletes themselves, the equipment are trained, but not the athletes. Therefore, how to improve the performance of the athletes?

3.4.2 The Development and Clinical Application of Potential Development Training Equipments of Lower Limbs

Because of the regeneration capacity of central nervous cells, functional recovery after damages is dependent on that normal cells around the injured area replace the injured cells to play a function, which is potential development. Potential is the ability that is hidden in the human body and cannot be showed. Everyone has great potential and its basis is tissues. The key point is how to develop potential maximally in order to compensate functional defect after CNS damages. The author designed potential development training equipment of lower limbs in order to develop potential of cortex motor center and promote motor function recovery of lower limbs.

3.4.2.1 Materials and Methods

1. The components of potential development training equipment of lower limbs: Potential development training equipment of lower limbs is composed of bearing frame, pedestal, weight loss sandbag and protection system. Bearing supporting system is made of hot drawing welded steel tube whose diameter is 36 mm and thickness is 4 mm. The bend frame (150 cm × 200 cm) is connected to pedestal. The pedestal is made of the same tube, which is dual-tier framework (180 cm × 150 cm × 20 cm) and covered by aluminium alloy plate in surface. In the middle of the top of braced frame, one corner and side wall, pulley is welding fixed. Steel wire whose diameter is 3 mm is used to connect hammock in frame and handle or weight loss sandbag hook in side wall. Hammock is fixed to the chest and abdomen of the patients. When the quantity of weight loss is big, the hammock can be connected to huckle part in order to prevent the shift of hammock and compression to chest and abdomen. The weight of weight loss sandbag includes 5, 10 and 20 kg. The quantity of weight loss can be regulated through changing the number and kind of sandbag. Scaleplate is made of transparent soft plastic plate (30 mm × 50 mm, rectangle). There are three different maps of sole of the foot in facies medialis. The inner loop is the actual size of the foot, named 100 score, the middle loop is two times of the actual size of the foot, named 80 score, and the outer loop is the three times of the actual size of the foot, named 60 score. The higher the foot score is, the more difficulty the training is.
2. Training method
   (a) Preparation before training: The patients dress hammock. The therapists stand one side of or in front or behind the patients. According to sandbag in exercise prescription, the therapists can grip the handle during training and regulate the quantity of weight loss through assisted force.
   (b) There are two kinds of training such as standing up and sitting down. Standing-up training is defined as that the patients are on kneeling-squatting position and the patients move their body center to paralyzed side. The patients are guided to take a deep breathing, breathe out slowly, concentrate on deep inspiration and hold the breathing, and then concentrate on quadriceps femoris in paralyzed side. During the slow standing-up process, the patients should feel the contraction of quadriceps femoris. When the patients cannot stand up by themselves, the therapists should help them. When the extension angle of knee joint is more than 90°, the therapists reduce assisted force suitably according to the condition and use the words "push up, or you will fall; hold on, or you will bump" to create dangerous atmosphere. The therapist should encourage the patients to stand up by themselves. Sitting-down training is defined as that the patients move their body center to paralyzed side. The patients are guided to take a deep breathing, breathe out and sit down slowly. During the slow sitting-down process, the patients should feel the contraction of quadriceps femoris. When the patients cannot sit down by themselves, the therapists should help them. When the extension angle of knee joint is less than 90°, the therapists increase assisted force suitably according to the condition and use the words "push up, po you will fall; hold on, or you will bump" to create dangerous atmosphere. The therapist should encourage the patients to hold on in this position for 3–5 s.

(c) Limbs control ability training: In the weight loss and safe protection condition, the patients' two feet are on the inner loop of the scaleplate and the center of body weight moves to uninjured side. The therapists guide the patients to bends coxa, bend knees, lift injured limbs and then put injured feet back to the inner loop. The patients should shorten the completed time gradually.

Training time is 30 min every time and one time a day. One course of therapy includes 30 times. After one course of therapy, the therapist should assess the therapy effect and decide whether to do the next course of therapy or not.

3. Clinical indications, contraindications and cautions
   (a) Indications: It is appropriate for the acute or chronic lower limbs dysfunctions training and movement coordinated ability training in the patients in stable condition with such as hemiplegia, cerebral palsy, child cerebral palsy, incomplete paraplegia, peripheral nerve injury, bones and joint muscles dysfunction after CNS, bone joint and muscle damages. It is also appropriate for the patients whose lower limbs functions cannot be improved in traditional rehabilitation therapy.
   (b) Contraindications: Contraindications of potential development include the patients in acute stage with unstable condition, the patients in uncontrolled condition with severe hypertension and diabetes, the patients with severe heart disease, pulmonary dysfunction and low cardiovascular response capacity, the patients with obvious dizziness and drop of blood pressure when standing up.
   (c) Cautions: For the patients with infirmity or long-term bedridden patients, the patients should do standing bed training before this type of the training in order to increase the stress capability of the patients' angiocarpy. When the patients stand erectly for 30 min and blood pressure, pulse and electrocardiogram are stable, this type of the training should be done. The training should be step by step. The therapists regulate the training through changing the weight and training time. High training intensity should be avoided. During training, the enthusiasm of the patients and the training atmosphere should be fully activated. The therapists should use encouraging words and scolding and critical words should be avoided.
4. Clinical application: From April 2006 to September 2007, potential development training equipment was used to treat 67 patients with upper limbs motor dysfunction who are all the inpatients and outpatients in neurological rehabilitation training center in Beijing Tongren Hospital affiliated to Beijing's Capital Medical University. There are 42 males and 25 females. The age is from 34 to 76 years old. The average age is 54.3 years old. The shortest medical history lasts 15 months and the longest lasts 62 months. The average is 27 months. There are 39 patients with hemiplegia after cerebral infarction and 28 patients with hemiplegia after cerebral hemorrhage. There are 36 patients with right hemiplegia and 31 patients with left hemiplegia.

   At the beginning of the training and the end of the therapy, the therapists assess myodynamia of quadriceps femoris and autonomous range of joint motion. SPSS12.0 statistical software is used for T test analysis.

3.4.2.2 Results

1. Statistical analysis of data: There are significant differences in the three assessment indicators before and after therapy ($p < 0.05$). There are six patients with zero myodynamia of quadriceps femoris in all the patients. After training, myodynamia is recovered to 2.68 grades. Autonomous joint motion is recovered. The detailed clinical effects control study refers to another paper. The results refer to Table 3.5.
2. Security of equipment: There is no injury in all the patients during the training. Equipment design is rational, safe and reliable. The operation of the equipment is easy and flexible.

Table 3.5 Functional assessment comparison table of quadriceps femoris in paralyzed side before and after training

Assessment items	Before training	After training	*P* value
Myodynamia	1.45 ± 0.87	3.62 ± 1.33	<0.01
Range of joint motion	16° ± 3.23°	45° ± 8.37°	<0.01
Limbs control ability	67.82 ± 28.73	89.64 ± 21.37	<0.01

3.4.2.3 Discussion

Many research indicated that there is reorganization ability of structure and function in CNS, which is plasticity. After damages, residual cells or normal cells around the injured area acquire the lost functions through functional reorganization in a new way. This process is the adaptive and compensatory process after neural tissue damages. The active effect is obvious in the acute stage of the damage and become weak after functional recovery. Concrete realization of plasticity may be the results of adaption of neural cells to environment. Its manifestations are readaption of synaptic connection, long-term potentiation, axonal extension and establishment of new synaptic connection, which are the theoretic basis to promote functional recovery through rehabilitation training after damages. The experimental study demonstrated that the plasticity of motor cortex function is one kind of "skill and dependence" mechanism, but not a simple "use and dependence" mechanism. Without new skillful movement, the plasticity change of motor cortex function cannot be induced, which is meaningful for the research and application of guiding rehabilitation training.

The plasticity, functional reorganization ability and tissue reserve of brain are the basis of brain potential. CNS has a large tissue reserve just as other organs. The research demonstrated that there are about 10^{11} motor neurons in brain and neurogliocytes that is ten times of motor neurons. Under noram circumstance, there are partial cells (6%) in using condition and most of them are under resting state. From this, we can conclude there are many motor neurons and the potential is great.

At present, the plasticity theory of brain is usually used to explain the mechanism of functional recovery after CNS damages, which is not appropriate for promoting brain plasticity and functional reorganization. Traditional rehabilitation techniques such as Bobath, Rood, Brunnstrom, PNF and electrical stimulation are mainly through passive movement, original reflex, anti-resistance training, daily life ability training and afferent stimulus. The effect of rehabilitation therapy is not satisfying, especially for the patients with chronic central nervous damages for more than half a year. Recently, some researchers started to try new rehabilitation methods include new therapy methods and employment of rehabilitation equipment. Some therapy methods such as motor relearning program and constraint-induced movement therapy have some effects, but these methods still are lack of the consciousness of brain potential development and targeted measures and the therapeutic effect is not ideal. Therefore, investigation of the method for development and utilization of brain potential is the key point of functional recovery after central nervous damages, which is required for clinical rehabilitation at present.

In real life, there are many examples about brain plasticity and functions reorganization. There are many examples that people can conquer difficulties and hardships using willpower and in dangerous condition people can burst into superman condition and tide over difficulties, which indicated that the human potential can be better developed in dangerous condition or with target and willpower. The ability in dangerous condition is not the result of immediate functional reorganization of brain, but the acquired function. The ability can be activated only in dangerous condition. However, target and willpower are achieved by functional reorganization of brain through repeated training. From this, repeated training in dangerous condition and repeated training with target and willpower can make the existed functions be used again in order to promote reorganization of brain function and generate new functions or functional compensation.

Daoyin technique in traditional Chinese medicine is capable of inspiring and motivating the individual's stamina, and is an important method to achieve functional rehabilitation by Creating a "critical state" of no danger with Daoyin speeches and skillful movement. It has a very long history, in terms of rehabilitation of stroke hemiplegia, the book of "the General Treatise on the Cause and Symptoms of Diseases" in Sui Dynasty in 610 A.D. Wind disease in the first chapter include "hemiplegia after stroke", "the patients cannot extend or flex the limbs because of stroke", "the hands and feet cannot move smoothly" and "phemilateral wind", which are related to sequelae after stroke. There are more than twenty kinds of Daoyin techniques. The technique included static exercise with the breathing controlled by OBEs and dynamic exercise with OBEs, breathing and movements (imitation of various kinds of animals). Through regulation of the mind, regulation of breathing and regulation of movements, Daoyin technique could circulate main and collateral channels, regulate qi and blood, harmonize viscera, strengthen the body resistance to eliminate pathogenic factors, strengthen homeostasis and have favorable influence on body metabolism to recover motor functions. Modern medicine research indicated that Daoyin technique has a good regulatory effect on cardiovascular diseases, respiratory diseases, nervous diseases, digestive diseases and rehabilitation effect.

Potential development training equipment can provide safe and reliable protection for lower limbs training with the help of bearing frame and hammock and can make the training from easy to difficulty and step by step through changing the quantity of weight loss. On the basis of that, Daoyin technique in traditional Chinese medicine is used to motivate the patients' willpower to create dangerous condition in order to achieve "safe" dangerous condition that is to the benefit of brain potential development and the functional reorganization of central nervous cells. It is possible to improve the special skills and war power of special troops in special hard condition scientific training.

References

1. Xiangyang M, Maoxiang C, Fang X. The effects of "sports imagine" therapy on upper limb functional recovery in patients with cerebral trauma. Chin J Prev Contr Chronic Dis. 2008;16(5):506.
2. Xiangdong Z, Hengfang L, Qingcheng Y, et al. Research on plasticity of motor function after cerebral infarction. Chin J Pract Nerv Dis. 2006;9:6):6–8.
3. Jing H, Yuanwu M, Tang T. The plasticity and rehabilitation of brain after stroke. Chin J Rehabil. 2004;19(1):50–2.
4. Dewald JP, Beer RF. Abnormal joint torque patterns in the paretic upper limb of subjects with hemiparesis. Muscle Nerve. 2001;24(2):273–83.
5. Rice MS, Newell KM. Upper-extremity interlimb coupling inpersons with left hemiplegia due to stroke. Arch Phys Med Rehabil. 2004;85(4):629–34.

4 Comprehensive Application of Rehabilitation Technique of Neurological Training

Comprehensive application of rehabilitation technique of neurological training includes three principal aspects such as neural potential development, motor program reestablishment and motor pattern remodeling and many other training methods. All these methods should be combined and applied reasonably in order to obtain desired training effects. If these methods are combined and applied unreasonably or single method is used, it is difficult to obtain ideal effect.

In that way, how we combine and apply these methods reasonably? Before we explain this question, we must know the ultimate goal of rehabilitation training, the effect of various methods and the mechanism of motor function recovery.

For the motor function of human body, ultimate goal of rehabilitation training is to recover the voluntary movement ability, and the motor function that is fast, flexible, with less energy consumption and with more benefit. In order to achieve this goal, it is far from enough to recover the contraction ability of the muscle and voluntary single joint motion. It is necessary to recover coordinated and orderly body movements, which means normal motor pattern. Only normal muscle contraction and voluntary movement of single joint cannot make motor pattern normal. However, abnormal motor pattern cannot have the best movement effect.

Motor pattern is existed in the movements of arms and legs, such as coordinated movements of upper limbs in walking, running and jumping and independent operation of upper limbs and hands. Generally, single joint motion is called movement and multi-joint motions are called exercise. Motor pattern means the simultaneous or orderly and coordinated associated movement of multi-joint or multi-limbs.

The quality of motor function is dependent on whether motor pattern is normal or not. It is widely believed that the motor pattern of normal people without malformation is not completely normal and there are many imperfections in motor pattern, such as pigeon toe, splayed feet, heel friction ground, ball of foot friction ground, lateral foot friction ground and medial foot friction ground. These manifestations can be concluded from the shoe sole and are induced by abnormal motor pattern. In addition, in the people with same gender and age, some one run faster and some one run slower. Someone can run for a longer time and some one cannot. The phenomenon is related to congenital factor, living environment and exercise methods. The normal motor pattern is somewhat irrelevant to this phenomenon. People with normal motor pattern can move faster, consume less and are more efficient. There people run faster and longer. People with abnormal motor pattern move slower, consume more and are less efficient when doing the same movement. Therefore, they run slower and shorter.

Therefore, revering normal motor pattern is the ultimate goal of rehabilitation training. Based

W. Zhao, *Rehabilitation Therapeutics of the Neurological Training*,
https://doi.org/10.1007/978-981-13-0812-3_4

on this, we can set out rehabilitation training scheme. We must use various kinds of rehabilitation therapy of neurological training methods properly. We should first introduce the formation and harm of abnormal motor pattern. On the basis of prevention and rectification of abnormal motor pattern, we investigate how to use various kinds of rehabilitation therapy of neurological training methods properly and how to reestablish the mechanism of normal motor pattern.

4.1 The Formation and Prevention Mechanism of Abnormal Motor Pattern

4.1.1 The Formation Mechanism of Abnormal Motor Pattern

Motor pattern is a special movement form with which people can complete daily life movement, productive labor movement or athlete movement in order to achieve movement goal. Motor pattern is completed with bone, joint and muscle, which is the result of orderly multi-joint movement. Motor pattern is controlled by motor program of brain. Motor program is the result of orderly and coordinated function of many cortex motor neurons, which is the same as the robot made from imitating human functions. Motor pattern of robot walking is completed by the body movement of robot driven by gearing. The orderly movement of joint is controlled by the software dominated by the Central Processing Unit in robot. The software is compiled by the technician, which is motor program of robot.

From this we can conclude that human motor pattern is dominated by motor program of cortex motor center. Motor program is the inner form of motor pattern, while motor pattern is the manifestation of motor program. A small part of the formation of motor program is inherited and increase with age, which can be completed through trainings such as walking, running, jumping and speech. Most of them are acquired such as motor programs of cycling, swimming, driving, somersaulting and wirewalking. The motor program is established and used, which can be consolidated through precise training and become practical motor function—motor pattern that is necessary for daily life and labor work.

Deliberate normal motor pattern training can establish motor program that can control the movement in cortex motor center. The motor program can be consolidated through long-term training and the program can be used unconsciously to control normal motor pattern of muscle gradually. Similarly, long-term movement in abnormal motor pattern can modify abnormal motor program and then induce the formation of abnormal motor program, which can further aggravate abnormal motor pattern and make it hard to treat. These are the practical problems to be noticed in rehabilitation training.

That whether motor pattern is normal or not and its quality can directly affect precision of movement, difficulty of completing the movement, movement duration, energy consumption and its manifestations. Before the formation of motor pattern, during the formation and after it, some joint or muscle involved in motor pattern are injured for some reason such as motor neuron necrosis in cortex motor center, neural conduction pathway damages, neural fiber damages, skeletal abnormality, dysarthrosis and muscle paralysis, which can induce abnormal motor pattern. Central nervous system that generate signal source, conduction system, peripheral nerve and muscle lesion of joint motion, can induce the contraction function lost and joint position abnormity (drop-foot and strephenopodia). In order to complete necessary movement, human body can use other muscles or change the posture to compensate the lost functions of the muscle. However, this compensation can induce abnormal motor pattern. Motor program destruction due to CNS damages is the important factor of establishing abnormal motor pattern. For example, when the motor programs that control wrist extension and wrist flexion are destroyed, the joint motion of wrist can be totally lost in severe cases and abnormal joint motion of wrist can be induced in slight cases. When the signal intensity of wrist extension is weaker than that of wrist flexion, abnormal motor pattern of wrist flexion during wrist extension can be induced.

Especially after CNS damages, muscles dominated by the injured area of CNS may be paralyzed. If the patients want to walk before the function of the paralyzed muscle is recovered, in order to complete the walking, the function of the paralyzed muscle should be compensated by normal muscle around the paralyzed muscle. This compensation can mislead joint motion and induce abnormal gesture. For example, the patients cannot complete hip flexion because of the paralysis of hip flexor when walking. Paralyzed side limbs must lie on uninjured side. Meanwhile, the joint swing outside or the patients abduce the lower limbs because of the contraction of hip abductors. And then the patients adduct lower limbs because of the weight of limbs when setting foot down. Finally, the circle movement locus is formed because the patients abduce lower limbs and then abduct lower limbs, which is called "circle" gait. Because the paralyzed muscles are different, the compensatory way in walking is different and the abnormal motor pattern is different too.

The malformation of bone, joint and spinal cord, abnormal body gesture can induce abnormal motor pattern. However, this kind of malformation should be rectified through operation. We don't discuss these cases in this chapter.

In short, when the motor program is destroyed, the muscle is paralyzed, the contraction ability is decreased or the joint position is abnormal, abnormal motor pattern is different form normal motor pattern and can be induced by body posture change or other muscles compensation in the process of completing movement. Therefore, recovery of normal motor pattern should be started from the above aspects.

4.1.2 The Effect of Abnormal Motor Pattern on Physical Function

Motor pattern is scientific voluntary movement ability through practical application and training after birth. Abnormal motor pattern is faster, flexible, more efficient and less energy consumption and don't do harm to body. Abnormal motor pattern (abnormal motor pattern, AMP) is different, which is slower, involuntary, unskillfully, not flexible and more energy consumption. In addition, movement with long-term abnormal motor pattern can induce abnormal body posture or malformation, which further can damage bone, joint and muscle. Even the malformation of spinal cord or thorax can affect viscera function and do harm to body health.

For upper limbs, the function of motor pattern is to complete the motor function that is required for daily life and technical ability. In the movement, upper limbs and lower limbs can coordinate, restrict and affect each other. When walking and running, coordinated pendulum motion of upper limbs can balance the human body. When walking and running, the started side upper limbs move backward and the contralateral upper limbs swing forward. The bigger the pace is when running, the bigger the amplitude of swing of upper limbs is. Meanwhile, because upper limbs sway forward, the trunk rotates slightly to the started side and elevates which alleviate the bear load of lower limbs and are beneficial for the increase of stride frequency and stride. All these can accelerate paces and can transfer the swaying power of upper limbs to lower limbs, which can make the backward pedal more powerful. Some studies indicated that if the power of upper and lower limbs cannot keep balanceable, the whole body cannot exert strength coordinatingly, which can affect the running speed.

Because of abnormal motor pattern of upper limbs, not only some movements cannot be completed, but also work and life quality can be affected to varying degrees such as embroidery, playing a ball game and computer, meal, toothbrush and dressing. The hemiplegic patients with one side upper limb paralysis lose the balance between upper limbs or upper and lower limbs, which can affect the ability of walking and running.

Abnormal motor pattern of lower limbs includes circle gait, drag gait, swaying gait, gluteus medius gait, which affect speed and quality of walking. Because of the different movement locus, it is easy to bump, sprain or fall down, meanwhile it is difficult to achieve the walking goal and the energy consumption is big. Motor function of lower limbs and life quality are affected severely. Walking with long-term abnormal motor pattern can modify motor program in the cortex motor center and turn it into abnormal motor program. The more the patients take movement with abnormal motor program, the stronger the excitability is. Finally, establishment is achieved. And abnormal motor pattern is more severe and is difficult to be rectified, even irreversible. We should pay high attention to it in rehabilitation therapy.

4.1.3 Common Classification of Abnormal Motor Pattern

The movements of arms and legs, which are controlled by motor program in cortex motor center, are associated movements completed with orderly multi-joint and practical significance. It is an integrated functional system. Anyone in this system is damaged such as nervous system impairment, deformity of bone and joint and muscle dysfunction, can induce abnormal motor pattern. Abnormal motor pattern induced by severe deformity of bone and joint can be recovered through rehabilitation training after operative correction, which is not discussed in this book.

This book mainly introduces abnormal motor pattern induced by neuromuscular disorders. When some area of nervous system is damaged, it can induce paralysis of corresponding muscle or abnormal muscular tension, coordination lost or disorder of muscle group. Normal movement locus is changed or synkinetic movement is generated and different kinds of abnormal motor patterns are formed. This is the formation process of abnormal motor pattern.

Abnormal motor pattern may be formed with damages of joint and muscle or anatomic abnormality, because joint motion is the basic composition of movements. Therefore, abnormal joint motion is the basis of forming abnormal motor pattern. Prevention of abnormal movements in joint motion is the fundamental measure to prevent and rectify abnormal motor pattern. Certainly, recovery of CNS function that induces abnormal joint motion is the first problem to be solved.

According to the part of abnormal motor pattern, it is divided into four kinks such as faciocervical part, upper limbs, lower limbs and trunk. Abnormal motor pattern is normally observed in lower limbs, which can considerably affect daily life and work of the patients.

4.1.3.1 Abnormal Motor Pattern of Head, Face and Neck

- Head synkinetic movement: It is observed in hemiplegic patient. The head turns to injured side and the face turns to uninjured side.
- Musculus facialis synkinetic movement: It is usually observed in the patients with facial paralysis who is difficult to speak. Palpebral fissure becomes large in uninjured side. There is blepharoptosis in injured side. There is distortion of commissure in uninjured side in synkinetic movement.
- Twisted neck synkinetic movement: It is usually observed in the patients with athetosis child cerebral palsy and mixed type child cerebral palsy, especially the patients with dysphasia. When the patients use words to explain the event, they become nervous because of dysphasia. And then they wave their upper limbs, turn their face to the listeners, twist musculi colli and are usually with distortion of commissure.

4.1.3.2 Abnormal Motor Pattern of Upper Limbs

- Slow movement of upper limbs: It is usually observed in the patients with extrapyramidal damages who wave upper limbs involuntarily and objectlessly, especially the patients with difficulty in fine movement.
- Uncoordinated wave of both upper limbs: It is usually observed in hemiplegic patients with upper limbs dysfunction and flexor spasticity. During walking, the patients' upper limbs cannot wave coordinately and the walking speed and body balance are affected (Fig. 4.1).
- Synkinetic movement of upper limbs flexor: When the patients want to lift upper limbs in injured side, it is difficult to lift it because of lack of extensor strength. In order to complete movement, the patients' trunk inclines to the uninjured side, the patients shrug their shoul-

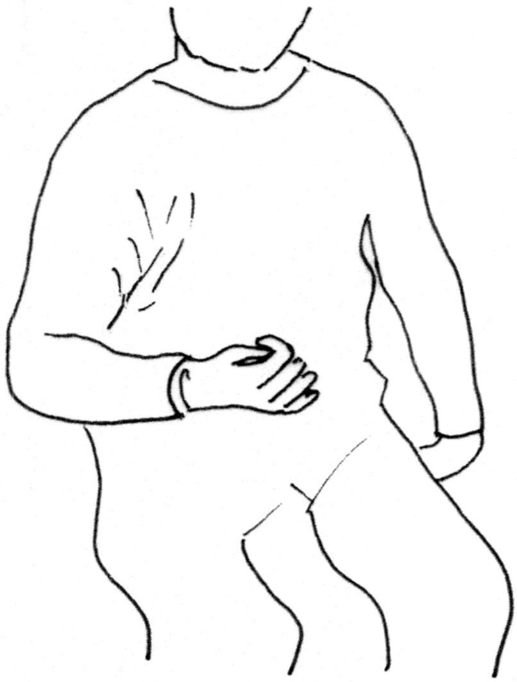

Fig. 4.1 Uncoordinated wave of both upper limbs

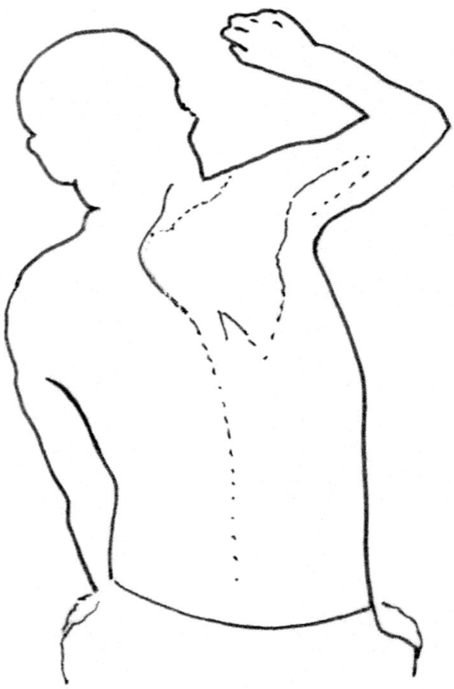

Fig. 4.2 Synkinetic movement of upper limbs flexor

ders and the patients lift their shoulder blade. Meanwhile, the patients are with flexion of elbow joint and pronation or supination of the forearm (Fig. 4.2).

- Synkinetic movement of extensor of upper limbs: It is observed in the patients who try to extend elbow joint hemiplegic side with internal rotation and adduction of shoulder joint, extend elbow joint and pronate, extend wrist joint slightly, in synkinetic movement of extensor of upper limbs with flexion of interphalangeal joint (Fig. 4.3).

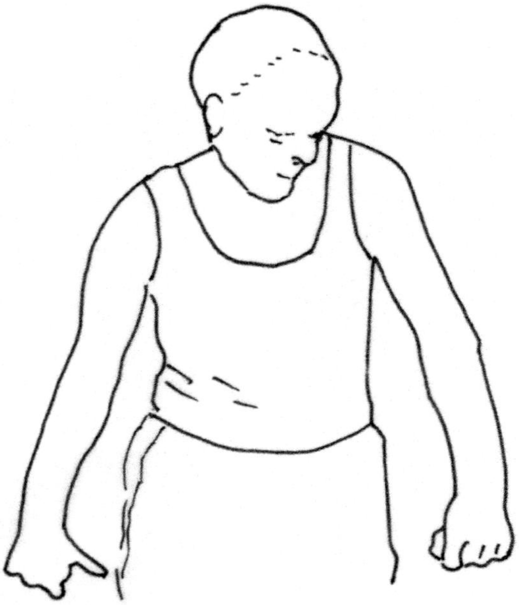

Fig. 4.3 Synkinetic movement of extensor of upper limbs

4.1.3.3 Abnormal Motor Pattern of Lower Limbs

The characteristic of abnormal motor pattern in lower limbs is abnormal gait. Its manifestation of it is abnormal posture in walking. There are many kinds of abnormal motor patterns in lower limbs due to different causes, which affect human functions greatly. Common abnormal motor pattern in lower limbs are as follows:

- Synkinetic movement of flexor of lower limbs: The patients try to flex hip, lift pelvis, abduce and abduct hip joint, flex knee joint, flex ankle joint plantarly and invert it. It is usually observed in the patients' hemiplegic limbs with foot drop and strephenopodia, which is called circle gait (Fig. 4.4).
- Synkinetic movement of extensor of lower limbs: The patients extend and abduce hip joint, unbend or extend knee joint, flex ankle joint plantarly and invert it, flex interphalangeal joint plantarly and abduce it (Fig. 4.5). There are hyperextension of knee joint, foot drop, strephenopodia, stiffness of lower limbs in injured side, walking difficulty, much energy consumption and joint injury in the patients with high muscular tension in hemiplegic side.
- Spastic paraplegia gait: It is usually observed in the patients with adductor muscles spasm in lower limbs after high level nerve injury, which induce myodynamia imbalance of adductor and abductor. When walking, the patients lift the leg and step forward, spasmodic adductor pull legs to adduct it, both legs cross inwards like the state that scissor is used to cut off the cloth, which is called scissors gait. It is usually observed in the patients with cerebral palsy such as child cerebral palsy.
- Sensory ataxia gait: It is observed in the patients with deep sensory disfunction such as the damages of fasciculus gracilis and fasciculus cuneatus of funiculus posterior medullae spinalis that transmit deep sensation. Its characteristic is big stride in walking, wide space between legs and high foot lifting. The patients can walk stably when they watch two feet and walk unstably when closing their eyes, even cannot walk.
- Festinating gait: It is slow to start walking. When the patients begin walking, the pace is small and random little step is shown up. The feet rub the ground, both upper limbs don't

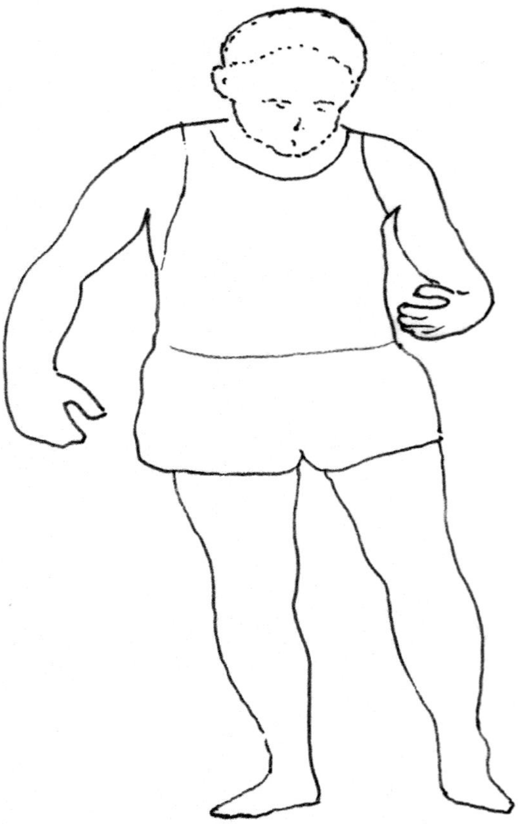

Fig. 4.5 Synkinetic movement of extensor of lower limbs (genu recurvatum)

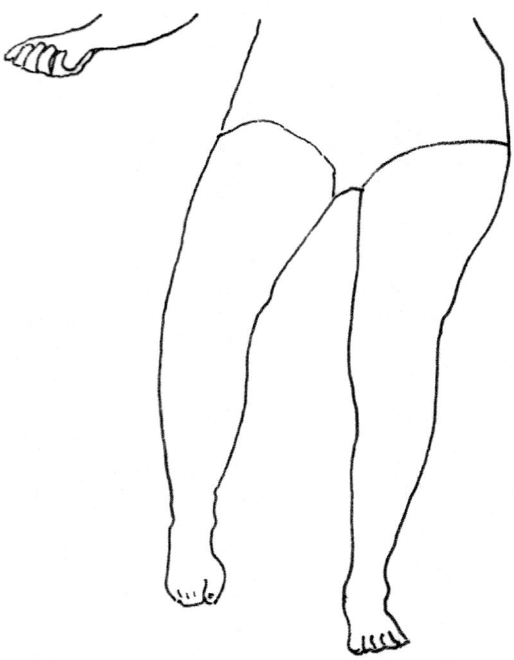

Fig. 4.4 Synkinetic movement of flexor of lower limbs (circle gait)

swing, the trunk forerake and center of body gravity move forward. Therefore, the patients use small paces to rush forward in order to balance the center of body gravity and cannot stop the paces, which is like a flustered man's gait and called chasing center of body gravity gait or propulsion gait. It is observed in the patients with shaking palsy and the diseases that can induce shaking palsy syndrome. There is high muscular tension in the whole body of the patients with these diseases.

- Steppage gait: It is usually observed in the patients with foot drop when they are walking. The patients have to lift the injured limbs higher in order to let the toe of foot drop off the ground. The posture is like leg lifting when crossing the threshold, which is called steppage gait. It is observed in the patients with tibialis anterior muscle paralysis induced by paralysis of common peroneal nerve.
- Dancing gait: When walking, the body is in involuntary movement state. The pace is big and irregular, which make the walking unstable, like salutatory gait or dancing gait. It is usually observed in the patients with neostriatum lesion.
- Swaying gait: Because of inability of pelvic girdle muscle and psoas and amyotrophy of lower limbs and pelvic muscle, spinal cord is in a lordosis state in order to keep balance of the body gravity. When walking, because the pelvis cannot be fixed, hip swings to the left and right like duck, which is called duck walking gait. It is usually observed in the patients with progressive muscular dystrophy.
- Drunkard gait: When walking, the body gravity cannot be controlled and the patients cannot stand steadily, the space between the legs becomes big, the body swing to two sides after leg lifting, both upper limbs usually shake in horizontal direction or back and forth, the patients cannot walk along straight line, which is like a drunken man's gait and is called drunkard gait. Because the patients shake back and forth and cannot walk forward, the gait is called staggering gait. It is usually observed in the patients with nervous system diseases, especially epencephalon or vestibular system lesion such as rickets, Kaschin-Beck disease, progressive muscular dystrophy or bilateral congenital dislocation of hip joint.
- Spinal muscular intermittent claudication: When walking after a certain time (1–5 min), there are inability, numb or pain in lower limbs in one side or two sides. Lower limbs cannot bear weight or load, the body inclines to injured side, weight bearing time of lower limbs is short in injured side and the patients limp. However, the right walking can be recovered after rest. It is usually observed in the patients with endarteritis of spinal cord, abnormal spinal cord development and spinal canal stenosis.
- Gluteus medius paralysis gait: Because of dysfunction of gluteus medius and decrease of myodynamia, when walking, hip joint cannot fixed in bearing load side and trunk bend to injured side and vacillate to the left and to the right. It is usually observed in the patients with progressive muscular dystrophy, polymyositis of gluteus medius and child cerebral palsy.
- Congenital myotonia: There is tetanic spasm of skeletal muscle when putting forth someone's strength. Therefore, when walking or running, if the patients want to stop walking or running, they may fall down because the muscle cannot relax immediately.
- Hysteric gait: There are many types in hysteric gait such as squatting gait and dragging gait. This kind of patients usually is accompanied with other functional disease.
- Star trail gait: When the patients close their eyes, move forward and move backward to injured side or to negative direction, after repeated moving, the gait is like star. It is usually observed in the patients with vestibular labyrinth lesion.

4.1.3.4 Abnormal Motor Pattern of Trunk

Abnormal motor pattern of trunk is usually due to spine malformation such as abnormal pattern of stoop and walking induced by young type kyphosis, motor pattern of trunk rigidity induced by ankylosing spondylitis (AS) and abnormal motor pattern induced by scoliosis. When the patients are not severe, orthotics is used to prevent the development of malformation or the malformation can be partially rectified. When the patients are severe, it is necessary to be treated through operation or there is no effective treatment method. Rehabilitation training can also alleviate the development of the diseases.

4.1.4 The Mechanism of Prevention and Rectification of Abnormal Motor Pattern

4.1.4.1 Prevention of Abnormal Motor Pattern

All aspects of the formation of motor pattern are damaged and lose functions because of some reason, which induce the loss of motor function, but abnormal motor pattern are still not formed. During the process that original functions are recovered through all kinds of methods such as rehabilitation or before it, the method is used to prevent the formation of abnormal motor pattern.

According to the fact that the formation of abnormal motor pattern is usually after muscle disability, before trying to complete original movement, the lost functions can be compensated by other muscles or body posture. The mechanism of the formation of abnormal motor mode means that the formation of abnormal motor pattern can be prevented through avoiding body movement before autonomous innervation and certain myodynamia (three-level) of paralyzed muscle are recovered. With the measures that prevent abnormal joint motion effectively (training equipment for motor pattern modelling) and lose weight, the training of motor pattern remodeling can be done.

4.1.4.2 The Mechanism of Rectification of Abnormal Motor Pattern

1. According to the mechanism of "target and motivation", active anti-resistance joint motion induced by six-step Daoyin technique in traditional Chinese medicine is the basic method to develop neural potential and promote CNS plasticity and functional reorganization.

Fundamental measure to rectify abnormal motor pattern is to reestablish normal motor pattern in cortex motor center, which include motor program in cortex motor center IV area that dominates single joint and motor program in cortex motor center IV area that dominates associated movement. Motor program of single joint is the basis of dominating muscle contraction to complete joint motion. Motor program of associated movement is to dominate muscles to complete multi-joint motion orderly and coordinately.

However, the basis of forming motor program is numerous motor neurons, destruction of motor program and the formation of abnormal motor program. Except abnormal motor pattern induced by functional defect of bone, joint and muscle and abnormal motor program induced by long-term abnormal motor pattern, abnormal motor program is due to damages of CNS cells and conduction system for various reasons. Therefore, one of the significant mechanisms is reestablishing motor program. The significant measure and mechanism of reestablishing motor program primarily is that reserved CNS cells and conduction system around injured area are trained to replace the functions of injured CNS cells and conduction system. Single joint motion is the movement without any practical function such as drinking, combing, jumping and running. One single joint motion cannot be used to complete the movement mentioned above. However, functional recovery of CNS cells to complete single joint motion should be firstly achieved, because single joint motion is the basis of multi-joint associated movement. Where there is multi-joint associated movement, there is single joint motion. Cortical motor area VI can give out signal to motivate every single joint involved in movement orderly to form meaningful and functional movement such as drinking with teacup and dressing. Certainly, because cells and conduction pathway cortical motor area VI are damaged, reserved cells and conduction pathway around injured area are also required to recover coordinated and orderly associated motor function.

All these above are the process of neural potential development. According to the mechanism of "target and motivation", active anti-resistance joint motion induced by six-step Daoyin technique in traditional Chinese medicine is the basic method to develop neural potential and promote CNS plasticity and functional reorganization.

2. According to the mechanism of "target and motivation", active joint motion induced by six-step Daoyin feedback technique in traditional Chinese medicine is the effective method to coordinate new activated CNS cells and reestablish motor program.

Through training, CNS cells around injured area replace injured nervous tissue, which means an army recruit young soldiers and the young soldiers improves their constitution and master operation knowledge of firearms through drills and learning, but this is not the case that young soldiers improve their actual combat skills. On the basis of theoretical learning, the soldiers must combat actually in order to turn previous drill achievement into actual combat skills. New activated CNS cells are like this and can possess coordinated ability to dominate joint motion through further drill.

A joint motion requires many pieces of or many groups of muscle such as agonistic muscle, antagonistic muscle, coordinated muscle and neutral muscle. Moreover, coordinated and orderly contraction and relaxation of the involved muscle are required to complete the movement. For example, during elbow extension, the contractility of triceps muscle of arm must be strong and the contractility of bicipital muscle of arm must be weak, which means that the elbow extension can be completed with strong contractility of agonistic muscle and weak contractility of antagonistic muscle. Meanwhile, neutral muscle plays neutralization role and coordinated muscle plays coordinated role to make elbow extension flexible and smoothly. Multi-joint body movement requires sequential joint motion and joint motion with specific pattern. However, limbs movement of joint motion and multi-joint movement can be completed through muscle contraction and relaxation. Muscle contraction signal is from CNS cells. These sequential and different proportional electrical signals are called motor program, which is the result of coordinated and orderly cooperation of many central motor neurons.

Because of the degree of injury and different injured area, CNS does not certainly be damaged. Therefore, some area can perform the functions, but others cannot or seldom perform functions. At this moment, CNS would have lost normal coordinated work ability, but still with partial function, which can usually cause abnormal work program and abnormal motor program is formed.

Whether motor program is completely lost or normal motor program is established on the basis of abnormal program, we should know motor program that the cells in cortex motor center dominate muscles to complete joint motion so that we can judge the actual state of abnormal motor program in order to reestablish normal motor program training through rectifying abnormal motor program.

Electrical signal and pressure sensing device are used to display the tension change of agonistic muscle and antagonistic muscle and the signal intensity of agonistic muscle and antagonistic muscle from CNS real-timely during joint motion with the form of curve or sound. Transverse line is used to mark the intensity of surpassing and the degree of decreasing. Six-step Daoyin technique in traditional Chinese medicine is used to surpass the original target until normal motor program is established and consolidated.

In the process of establishing motor program, many patients don't understand the repeated and the same training even are fed up with it. And then they refuse to receive regulation training under the detection of motor program. Rehabilitation doctors and therapists should educate the patients patiently and can use the example of archery or shooting to explain how to do long-term training with display of motor program signal in order to make the patients understand why they should receive the training of reestablishing motor program. For example, if Chinese Olympic shooting champion Hai-Feng Xu shoot to the sky without target, does he can improve shooting accuracy? Why does he shoot to the target for months and years? And then the doctors should discuss with the patients and explain the mechanism to the patients. The purpose is to use practical example and common phenomenon in daily life to make the patients truly understand the mechanism of important role and repeated training of rehabilitation methods of neurological training. And then the patients can truly understand, actively participate, positively cooperate the training and become one of the members in the therapy but not the simple training receiver, which can improve training effect.

3. Practical usage training induced by six-step Daoyin technique in traditional Chinese medicine and applied by abnormal joint motion limiter is the essential procedure of remodeling abnormal motor pattern.

The author use recruiting soldiers, training them, making them do actual combat and forming fighting capacity to explain procedure and mechanism of rehabilitation therapy of neurological training. After recruiting soldiers, through drill and learning, soldiers master all kinds of skills including various firearms operation, military strategy of soldier formation and physical ability improvement. However, this is not equal to actual combat ability. The soldiers can turn knowledge and skills into actual combat ability through actual combat. The grow-up process of a Gong Fu master with actual combat ability and military accomplishments is also the case. After the drill of basic skills such as standing exercise and beating, the master does a series of skills and trick in wushu and combat method such as shaolin quan, wudang quan and military strategy of soldier formation. The master can turn previous drill result into practical combat skill through fighting hand to hand or fighting with each other.

On the basis of the mechanism mentioned above, the process of rehabilitation therapy of neurological training is developed according to the mechanism of autonomous movement of body dominated by CNS. It is far from enough that potential development training activates CNS cells around injured area to perform functions and motor program training makes new activated cells work coordinately and orderly. Practical function required for real life or work requirements is not necessary to be turned into practical motor function through practical applied training, which means that training method of remodeling motor pattern can turn reestablishment of motor program and development of CNS potential into useful practical motor function.

On the basis of preventing or rectifying abnormal motor pattern, through practical usage and motor pattern remodeling, normal motor pattern can be established. However, in the process of establishment, how to prevent abnormal motor pattern effective and how to guarantee the normal of reestablished motor pattern? These are practical problem needed to be solved in the process of rehabilitation.

Through clinical research and verification for more than 10 years, in the motor pattern remodeling of lower limbs, the author experienced simple restricted walking, abnormal gait rectification weight support treadmill with elastic band and motor pattern remodeling trainer. The author realized the meaning of rectifying abnormal motor pattern and remodeling normal motor pattern. Independent developed abnormal gait rectification weight support treadmill training equipment and motor pattern remodeling trainer can make the patients walk in the early stage and assure the patients can receive walking training under normal motor pattern on the premise of effectively restricting joint motion. This method not only improves the training effect of motor pattern remodeling, and also turns developed potential and reestablished motor program into actual motor ability to shorten therapy course obviously. Developed domestic motor pattern remodeling trainer is portable and can assure the self-training of the patients is correct so that recurrence is prevented effectively. Therefore, abnormal gait rectification weight support trainer and motor pattern remodeling trainer play an essential role in normal motor pattern remodeling training.

4.1.5 Rehabilitation Method Used for Rectifying Abnormal Motor Pattern at Home and Abroad at Present

From the mechanism of motor pattern remodeling mentioned above, we measure rehabilitation method used for rectifying abnormal motor pattern at home and abroad at present such as good limbs position placing in early stage, restricted off-bed walking, talipes varus and valgus orthotic board, standing training, wearing orthotics, Bobath technique, body weight-supported treadmill training (BWSTT) and gait training guided by the speeches of the therapists. These methods have a certain improving effect on recovering walking ability and gait symmetry of the patients with abnormal gait. However, because these methods cannot effectively restrict unnecessary joint motion in body movement, they have no correction effect on abnormal gait and there is no specific clinical indication. Moreover, they cannot restrict the exercise after training. Most of the patients walk with abnormal motor pattern when they are out of training room or hall, which go against reducing the excitability of abnormal motor center and make it difficult to rectify abnormal motor pattern. For example, a person with a craving for tobacco wants to quit smoking. In the smoking cessation room, some methods are used to explain the harm of smoking in order to alleviate the tobacco craving, but the patients still smoke when they out of smoking cessation room so that it is difficult to quit smoking.

In addition, these methods are usually in exclusive use and there is no training basis for pathogenesis of inducing abnormal motor pattern such as the training without neural potential development and motor program reestablishment. Gait training is directly done before reestablishing motor program. Like a new recruited army without operation knowledge of firearms and combat skills, it is impossible to obtain fighting capacity through immediate military exercise.

In addition, rehabilitation training at home and abroad at present is lack of dedicated device to cooperate gait training. Some researcher think that gait analysis system is the ideal gait assessment and training method, but is only used in detecting the gait condition in order to provide the basis for clinical diagnosis and therapeutic schedule, which is the assessment indicator of gait training effect. There is no report about application of gait detection device. Body weight-supported treadmill training is the expedite edition of walking training in natural state. It not only can decrease the field required for walking training, but also can regulate the walking speed. However, it still cannot restrict unnecessary joint motion in body movement effectively. Robot of rehabilitation training is the robot that helps the patients to do exercise. The exercise object may be the robot, but not human, which has no effect on rehabilitation.

There are defects in training methods of preventing and rectifying abnormal gait at home and abroad at present:

- There is no systematic rehabilitation training method of preventing and rectifying abnormal gait.
- Gait training is usually guided by the oral instruction, which cannot restrict the unnecessary joint motion in movement and go against the reestablishment of normal motor pattern.
- Training method of abnormal motor pattern at present is lack of definite indications and contradictions.
- There is no training equipment of rectifying abnormal motor pattern and reestablishing normal motor pattern.
- Most of the patients walk with abnormal motor pattern when they are out of training room or hall, which go against reducing the excitability of abnormal motor center and make it difficult to establish normal motor pattern.

These defects severely affect the training effects of prevention and rectification of abnormal motor pattern and reestablishment of normal motor pattern.

4.2 Three Stages of Rehabilitation Training Method in Neurological Training

4.2.1 The Division, Principal Method and Mechanism of Three Stages in Neurological Training

According to rehabilitation techniques of neurological training, three stages are divided in the whole training process from development of neural potential to recovery of normal motor function. After exploration and clinical verifications for many years, the author summarized a comprehensive rehabilitation training method through repeated adjustment and improvement. It is the high generalization and quintessence of rehabilitation methods of neurological training and has a good clinical training effect.

4.2.1.1 First Stage: The Stage of Neural Potential Development

For dyskinesia induced by CNS damages, the key point of therapy is to recover the functions of CNS cells at first, but the regeneration capacity of CNS cells is weak and they play limited role in or has no effect on recovering lost motor function. Therefore, it is necessary for normal cells around injured area to perform functions and for reserved conduction pathway to replace the injured pathway, which means that the lost functions can be compensated through CNS plasticity and functional reorganization. The plasticity and functional reorganization are in accordance with the principle "skillful use and dependence". CNS plasticity can be promoted through active movement. A number of reserved CNS cells and conduction pathways are the basis of CNS plasticity. Reserved cells are trained to perform functions and reserved conduction pathways are activated, which are the basis of promoting CNS function reorganization. The training method is the process of CNS potential development. Therefore, CNS potential development is the principal training target of this stage.

Main therapeutic method: from neural potential development, in the early phase of recovery of CNS damages, the key point of therapy includes two aspects:

- The first is to enhance muscle tension, prevent joint adhesion and occurrence of bad position, increase response ability of angiocarpy and improve internal environment. The methods include good limb position placing, electrical stimulation, active and passive joint motion, massage, blood circulation drive, standing bed training, regulation of disordered water, electrode and acid-base equilibrium, therapy of dizziness and arthralgia and maintenance of vital signs such as blood pressure and breathing.
- The second is the CNS potential development training. Active movement with target, willpower and "safe" dangerous condition is an effective principal method to develop potential. Six-step Daoyin technique in traditional Chinese medicine is mainly used for motor program signal enhancement training, a physical exercise therapy of neurological training and potential development training of upper limbs, lower limbs and trunk. This stage emphasizes on the enhancement of agonistic muscle signal, but not decrease of antagonistic muscle signal, which means the coordinated training of motor program proportion is not emphasized in case that it alleviates the function of CNS potential development due to motor program proportion. However, "goal and motive" mechanism is the method that we should pay attention to constantly, especially for the training induced by motor program signal to the muscle with zero myodynamia.

Some researches show that the sensitivity of receiving equipment of motor program signal (electromyographic signal) is about 360 times of that of MMT. Moreover, the recovery of motor program signal is earlier than that of myodynamia. Therefore, zero myodynamia is not equal to zero signals. The author tested 343 muscles with zero myodynamia of 77 patients with paraplegia and found that there are 11 muscles with zero myodynamia and the coincidence rate is only 0.3%, which demonstrate that the sensitivity of MMT is far below motor program the sensitivity of receiving equipment of motor program signal. Clinical observation found that if autonomous motor program signal of the muscle can be received, the functions of the muscle can be recovered to varying degrees through rehabilitation therapy of neurological training.

Autonomous contraction of muscle with zero myodynamia cannot be observed with eyes. During training, the patients try many times but they fail to see the effects and progresses. And then they will lose confidence. The therapists feel absent, feel difficult to continue the training and even give up therapy.

How to make the patients to see the progress of therapy? Except the specific training, it is useful for motivating the desire and confidence of the patients for rehabilitation. Six-step Daoyin technique with motor program signal reception and real-time display can induce motor program from CNS to muscle. Although the patients cannot see muscle contraction, the signal can be received from the skin surface. After amplification, the signal can be displayed on the screen in a curve form real-timely, which make the patients and the therapists see the effect and progress of training. In addition, the goal for the patients is like the cross bar in jumping, which is an objective indicator to reach or surpass. The patients must try their best to develop more potential in order to promote the intensity of this signal. Through the training of surpassing the peak of the last, neural potential is constantly developed and the lost motor function is finally recovered, which help the patients and their family to enhance confidence of rehabilitation. Through this method, after training, the functions of 343 muscles with zero myodynamia are recovered to varying degrees.

For the patients with abnormal motor pattern in the recovery stage and late recovery stage, the key points of therapy are as follows:

- Reduction of myospasm and relaxation of adhesion include standing bed, varus-valgus standing plate training, passive joint motion after thermal therapy and restraining force orthotics.
- Neural potential development includes upper limbs, lower limbs, tibialis anterior muscle, hamstring muscles and trunk potential development training and physical therapy of neurological training.
- Reestablishment training of motor program: After CNS damages, destruction of motor program induces abnormal motor pattern and long-term movement with abnormal motor pattern promotes excitability of abnormal motor program. And then the vicious cycle is formed. Ultimately, abnormal motor program is consolidated and is difficult to be rectified. Therefore, therapy in this stage is to decrease the excitability of abnormal motor center and reestablish motor program training. However, it is not all right to overemphasize the proportion of motor program because excessive motor restriction can affect training effects of neural potential development.

In this stage, the exercise (multi-joint coordinated exercise) of the patients are prohibited in case that abnormal motor pattern is formed or deepened because the function of paralyzed muscles is compensated by other muscles. For the patients with abnormal motor pattern, the exercise is prohibited to decrease the excitability of abnormal motor program, which can make the patients forget motor pattern under abnormal motor pattern in order to reestablish normal motor program. Therefore, that the exercise is prohibited is the fundamental therapeutic measure in this stage. However, for the patients with good motor function, they can do motor pattern remodeling training under the protection of motor pattern remodeling training equipment.

4.2.1.2 Second Stage: Reestablishment of Motor Program

The second stage is the process that new activated cells perform functions coordinately and orderly.

Through the previous potential development training, autonomic nerve innervation of paralyzed muscles is recovered to varying degrees, because the function of undead CNS cells is recovered through training to activate normal cells around injured area and reserved conduction pathway. Although there is new connection pathway between these cells and the dominant muscles, it is necessary to establish work coordination. Only if coordinated operational capability of CNS cells that dominate joint motion is established, it is possible to recover autonomous and coordinated motor function. This process is the process of reestablishing motor program, which is the basis of establishing and recovering normal motor pattern.

Reestablishment of motor program includes reestablishment of motor program of single joint and multi-joint coordinated exercise, which means that cortex motor center IV area and VI area are recovered separately. In the early stage of reestablishing motor program, the function of cortical motor area IV area should be recovered firstly, which means reestablishing motor program of single joint. Meanwhile, reestablishment of motor program of multi-joint associated movement should be considered. In the middle and later periods of reestablishing motor program, the training of reestablishing motor program of associated movement should be emphasized, which means recovering the function of cortical motor area VI area.

Rehabilitation techniques of neurological training are adopted in the training. On the basis of real-time display of motor program signal induced by six-step Daoyin technique, the patients are instructed to increase the signal intensity of agonistic muscle and decrease the signal intensity of antagonistic muscle gradually until the proportion of the motor program signals between them are returned to normal. Through repeated training, the proportion can be consolidated. In the training of physical therapy of neurological training, the patients are instructed to promote myodynamia of agonistic muscle and relax antagonistic muscle, because the actual state of motor program signal and its proportion cannot be observed in physical therapy of neurological training.

When the joints involved in associated movement are possessed with active joint motion, the therapists can start the training of reestablishing motor program of associated movement. Before therapy, the pattern of associated movement should be designed such as using teacup to drink water of upper limbs, stepping forward for walking of lower limbs and speech therapy for stammer.

In this stage, the training of remodeling motor pattern under the detection of motor program signal is mainly used such as walking training that is divided into two-step method, three-step method or four-step method in order to achieve the rehabilitation training principle of step by step and from easy to difficulty.

1. Operation process of two-step method of gait training only emphasize on the training of hip joint and ankle joint involved in gait motion (Fig. 4.6).
   - Hip flexion movement: The signal is induced from CNS to hip flexor to lift the legs and step forward.
   - Dorsiflexion of foot: The signal of tibialis anterior muscle is induced secondly to assure the degree of dorsiflexion of foot, make toe not rub the floor, make the heel touch the ground first and prevent varus.
2. Operation process of three-step method of gait training only emphasize on the training of hip joint, knee joint and ankle joint involved in gait motion (Fig. 4.7).
   - Hip flexion movement: The signal is induced from CNS to hip flexor to life the legs and step forward.
   - Flexion of knee: The signal of hamstring muscles is induced secondly to help flex knee joint in order to assure stride with certain length and height.
   - Eversion of dorsiflexion of foot: The signals of tibialis anterior muscle, peroneus longus and peroneus brevis are induced finally to assure adequate dorsiflexion of foot and strephexopodia degree.
3. Operation process of four-step method of gait training only emphasize on the training of hip joint, knee joint and ankle joint and four kinds of exercise involved in gait motion (Fig. 4.8).
   - Plantar flexion: The signal is induced from CNS to musculus gastrocnemius to induce

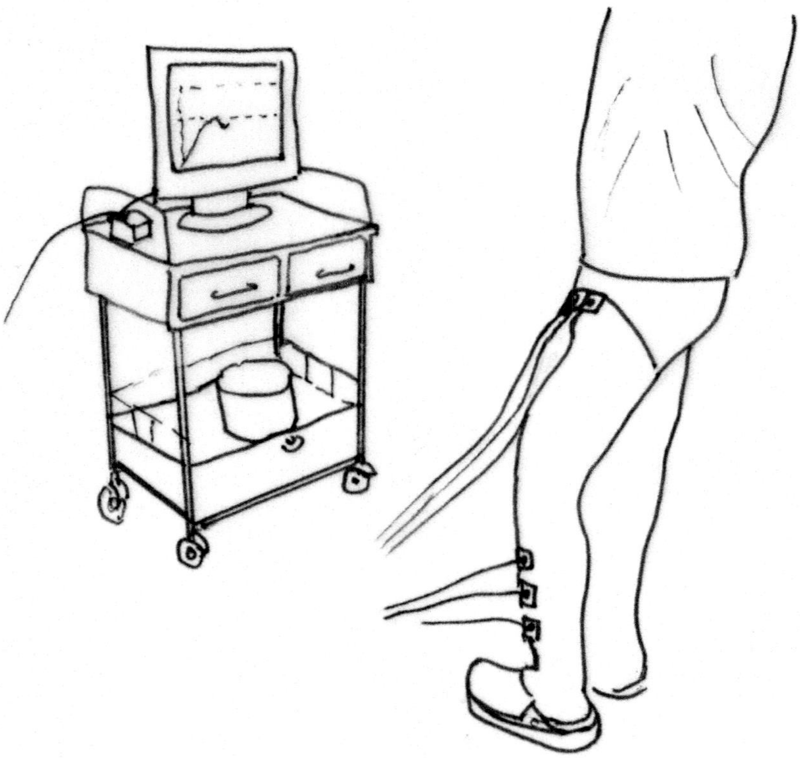

Fig. 4.6 Operation process of two-step method of gait training

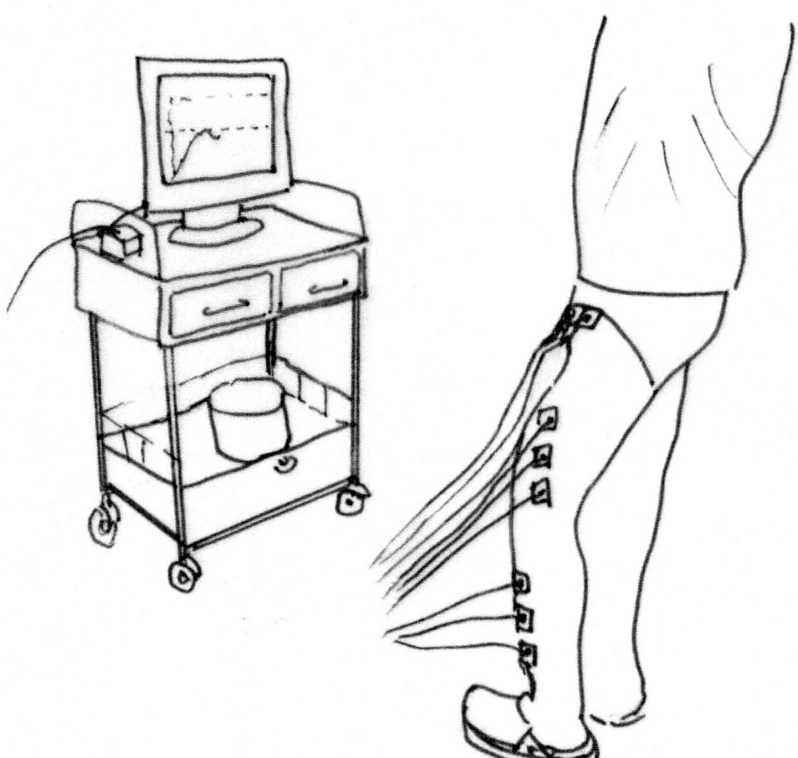

Fig. 4.7 Operation process of three-step method of gait training

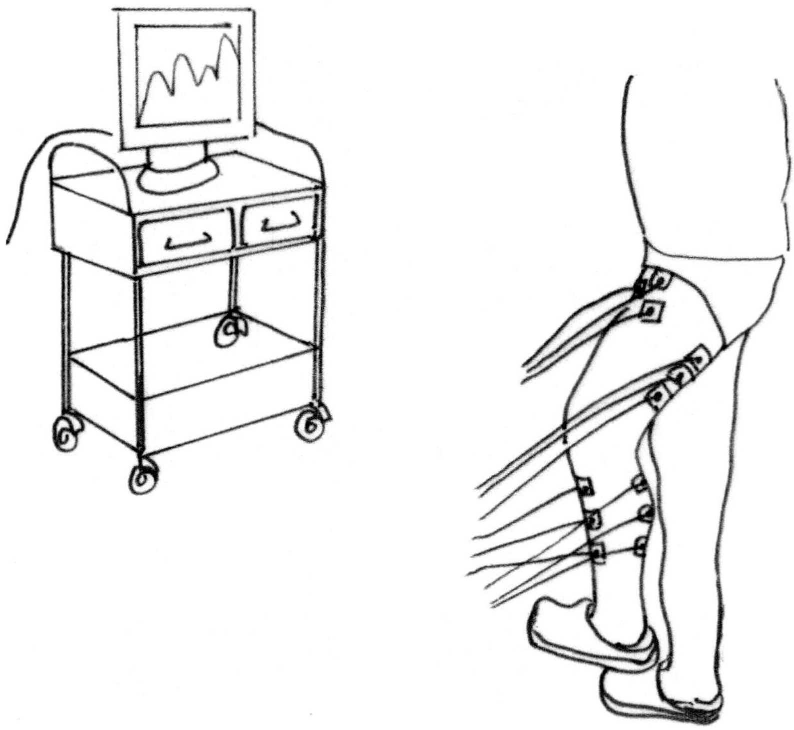

Fig. 4.8 Operation process of four-step method of gait training

plantar flexion of ankle joint so that heel is full of the strength of back step to make the body step forward.

– Hip flexion movement: The signal is induced from CNS to hip flexor to lift the legs and step forward.
– Flexion of knee: The signal of hamstring muscles is induced to help flex knee joint in order to assure stride with certain length and height.
– Eversion of dorsiflexion of foot: The signals of tibialis anterior muscle, peroneus longus and peroneus brevis are induced finally to assure adequate dorsiflexion of foot and strephexopodia degree, make toe not rub the floor, make the heel touch the ground first and prevent varus.

Associated motor pattern training can be arranged with real life demand according to actual state of functional recovery in the patients such as using teacup to drink water (Fig. 4.9), dressing and walking. Generally, too many and fine steps can make the patients difficult to distinguish them and induce disorder. Therefore, the training procedure should be as easy as possible on the premise of satisfying training demands. The principle of from easy to difficult and step by step should be abided by. When doing the multi-joint associated movement training, the therapists should avoid very difficult training. The patients are often pessimistic because they cannot meet the requirements, which can affect training effect.

In this stage, the patients are required to decrease the whole movement. The patients with good motor function can use motor pattern remodeling trainer and abnormal gait rectification weight loss walking device to do movement training. Combined with the training of reestablishing motor program, they can be seen as the early training of the third stage (remodeling stage of motor pattern).

4.2.1.3 The Third Stage: Remodeling Stage of Motor Pattern

Just as the items mentioned above, the motor programs of single joint and multi-joint associated movement are merely established, which is not

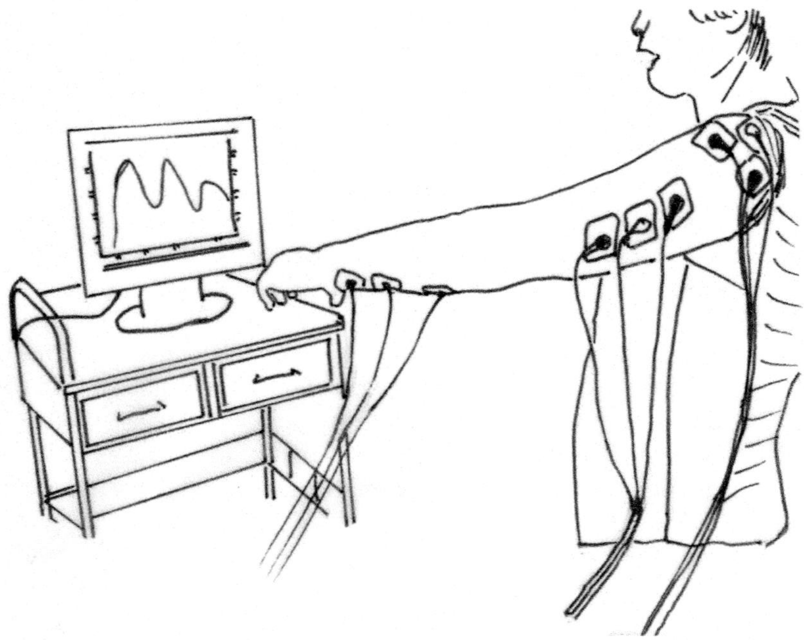

Fig. 4.9 Operation process of three-step method of grasping

equal to actual motor function. The established motor program can be turned into actual motor ability in daily life through actual practical training, which is a process of motor pattern remodeling. For example, in the walking motor pattern training, when the patients are capable to stand up with balance, flex hip and ankle joint of injured side actively, they can do gait remodeling training, shifting of weight, stride gait training, walking marked by gait and training with walking device marked by gait assisted by weight loss device. Along with the increase of the patients' walking ability, the weight of weight loss is decreased gradually, and then the training is turned into walking without weight, training with motor pattern remodeling trainer under protection in lower limbs and independent ambulation under protection. The patients' normal walking ability is increased gradually until they can walk without help.

In this stage, the patients are encouraged to do training of motor pattern remodeling step by step with guidance and protection, which can prevent abnormal joint motion of motor pattern remodeling trainer of upper limbs, lower limbs and trunk. It plays an important role in rectifying and remodeling motor pattern of upper limbs, lower limbs and trunk. Variable motor pattern remodeling trainer is complicated and heavy, which is inconvenient to put on or put off. It is appropriate for the patients with serious illness to do training in rehabilitation hall of hospital. According to individual demand, portable motor pattern remodeling trainer is light and easy to put on or put off, which can be used for the self-exercise of the patients out of hospital. The device can assure the correctness of motor pattern in self-exercise so that recurrence of abnormal motor pattern can be prevented effectively.

The first and second stage of the therapy is basic training. Its purpose is to recover autonomic nerve innervation of the muscle and reestablish motor program. The patients are required to avoid associated movement in abnormal motor pattern. Its purpose is to decrease or eliminate abnormal motor pattern effectively. The excitability of abnormal motor program in cortex motor center is in favor of reestablishment of normal motor program. In the third stage, training results of the first and second stage are turned into actual functional movement in daily life and labor work through motor pattern remodeling. Three stages supplement one another. According to the actual condition of the patients, they can be used flexible.

4.2.2 Basic Methods and Clinical Indications in All Stages of Neurological Training

4.2.2.1 The First Stage: Neural Potential Development Stage

1. Basic training method is the training method that is appropriate for neurological training to promote CNS plasticity and functional reorganization.
   - Potential development training: With the help of human potential development training device, the therapists can help the patients to regulate weight loss until the patients can stand up with lower limbs, hold up with upper limbs and stick out with waist. The weight is about one-third to one-fifth of the patients' weight. Six-step Daoyin technique in traditional Chinese medicine is used to guide the patients to do training of different parts on the basis of regulation of mind, breathing and movement such as standing up, squatting and control ability training of lower limbs and upper limbs.
   - Neurological training: Daoyin feedback technique in traditional Chinese medicine is used. The motor program signal induced by six-step Daoyin technique is displayed real-timely. Agonistic muscle signal is promoted through biological feedback. Meanwhile, it is time to attenuate the signal intensity of antagonistic muscle. In this stage, the proportion of motor program signals between agonistic muscle and antagonistic muscle cannot be emphasized. If we overemphasize the proportion of motor program signals, it is easy for the patients to affect the intensity of agonistic muscle signal because of worrying about excessive antagonistic muscle signal, which makes it difficult to promote CNS plasticity, especially the training induced by autonomic signal of weak myodynamia or zero myodynamia.
   - Physical therapy of neurological training: Six-step Daoyin technique in traditional Chinese medicine is used to guide the patients to do active joint motion. During the process of joint motion, the therapists use manipulation to exert resistance in the orientation of joint motion and use Daoyin technique to guide the patients to do anti-resistance training such as hip flexion, knee extension, dorsiflexion of foot, strephexopodia of lower limbs and shoulder abduction, elbow extension and flexion, wrist extension and flexion, finger extension and flexion of upper limbs. In the interval of training, the therapists can do passive joint motion for the patients in order to loose joint and soft tissue adhesion.
   - Standing bed or standing board training: For the patients in the early stage of recovery with poor cardiovascular stress response ability or foot drop and foot varus-valgus, the patients can do standing bed training or dorsiflexion of foot training, foot varus-valgus training in order to promote cardiovascular stress response ability of the patients, alleviate contracture and adhesion of soft tissue and provide condition for active movement training.
   - According to the specific condition of the patients, adjuvant therapy methods such as acupuncture, massage, thermal therapy and electrical stimulation are used to promote therapeutic effect.

   In this stage, the patients are allowed to do single joint motion exclusively and are prohibited to do associated movement of multi-joint motion.
2. Clinical indications
   - The patients in the early stage of the disease with dyskinesia who don't walk out of the bed.
   - The myodynamia of paralyzed muscle is less than or equal to level 2. The intensity of motor program signal is less than or equal to 80 μv.
   - The patients with potential development training who can stand erectly for 30 min and the vital signs are stable.
   - The patients with abnormal motor pattern of upper limbs, lower limbs, trunk or face such as circle gait, dragging gait and hemiplegic gait of lower limbs and the patients with uncoordinated swing of upper limbs and

posture malformation in trunk movement in recovery stage. The state of the illness is slight and the motor function can be recovered through three-stage method training.

3. Clinical contraindications
   - The patients with severe diseases and unstable vital signs
   - The patients with poor cardiovascular stress response ability who cannot stand erectly for 30 min
   - The patients with severe hypertension and diabetes who cannot keep state stable after corresponding medicine therapy.
   - It is used with caution in the patients with fractures of rib, spinal cord, pelvis and lower limbs and uncompleted healed after damages of joint and muscle.

4.2.2.2 The Second Stage: Reestablishment of Motor Program

1. Basic training method: It is appropriate for the training of coordinated work ability between CNS cells, which includes the training of single joint motion and reestablishment of motor program of associated movement. However, in this stage, we should consider the slow of CNS functional recover. The patients still do potential development training, but the training time is less than that of training of reestablishing motor program.
   - Neurological training: The proportion of motor program signal of agonistic muscle and antagonistic muscle that control joint motion is emphasized. Meanwhile, the training of enhancing agonistic muscle signal is continued, such as the proportion of motor program signal of single joint such as hip flexion, knee extension, dorsiflexion of foot and strephexopodia of lower limbs and shoulder abduction, elbow extension, elbow flexion, wrist extension and wrist flexion of upper limbs. Reestablishing motor program of multi-joint associated movement is continued too.
   - Potential development training: The trainings of standing up and squatting with lower limbs and body control ability are continued. Potential development trainings of upper limbs and trunk are continued too.
   - Basic training of reestablishing normal motor pattern: The first is stride gait training and shifting of weight training. Weight loss, stride gait and shifting of weight device are used for training. Regulation of weight loss can make the patients stand up and the weight loss is one-third to one-fifth of the patients' body weight. According to the length of stride, the training device is divided into five kinds. The training is from the primary to normal stride. The second is remodeling training of abnormal gait rectification and weight loss gait. Abnormal gait rectification and weight loss gait training device are used. The training is done in the training footpath marked with gait. Adjustment strength of lower limbs adduction and foot drop elastic orthotics band of this device can make the patients to prevent lower limbs adduction and foot drop when stepping forward. The third is flexibility training of segment of motor program in lower limbs, upper limbs and trunk.

   In this stage, the patients are still required to do the training mainly with single joint motion. If the restriction is not available, the training of associated movement of multi-joint motion can be started.
2. Clinical indications
   - The patients with stable blood pressure and without dizziness and nausea who can sit or stand with balance
   - The myodynamia of paralyzed muscle is recovered to level 2 to level 3.
   - The patients can partly complete active joint motion such as hip flexion, knee flexion, dorsiflexion of foot, strephexopodia, shoulder abduction, elbow extension and elbow flexion.
   - The signal intensity of motor program (sEMG) is from 80 μv to 150 μv.
3. Clinical contraindications
   - The myodynamia is less than level 2 and sEMG is less than 80 μv. The patients cannot do active joint motion.

- It is used with caution in the patients with fracture of rib, spinal cord, pelvis and lower limbs and uncompleted healed after damages of joint and muscle.

4.2.2.3 The Third Stage: Training Stage of Remodeling Motor Pattern

The purpose of the third stage is to turn the previous training results into daily life and work ability step by step through actual practical training of restricting effectively unnecessary movement in body exercise. However, reestablishment technique of motor program can be used to establish and consolidate motor program of associated movement.

1. Basic training method
   - Neurological training: The training of reestablishing motor program of multi-joint associated movement is emphasized such as reestablishing motor program of dorsiflexion of foot and strephexopodia in walking, two-step method, three-step method and four-step method gait training.
   - Motor pattern remodeling training: Motor pattern remodeling trainer is used. The patients with poor motor function such as unstable gait with lower limbs, can do the training with the help of abnormal gait rectification and weight support treadmill training device. The weight depends on the specific condition of the patients and is about one-fifth to one eighth of the body weight. The device can be also used for preventing the patients from falling down without weight loss function. During gait training, the patients should be walk on the footpath marked with gait. This footpath requires the patients to achieve clear objectives of the stride and stride width.
   - Gait training of weight loss: Weight loss walking trainer is used and the weight is about one-fifth to one eighth of the body weight. Track rotation speed of walking machine is started from 0.22 m/s and the speed is increased with the increase of walking ability. The patients are instructed to do the training on the track of the walking machine marked with gait (Fig. 4.10).

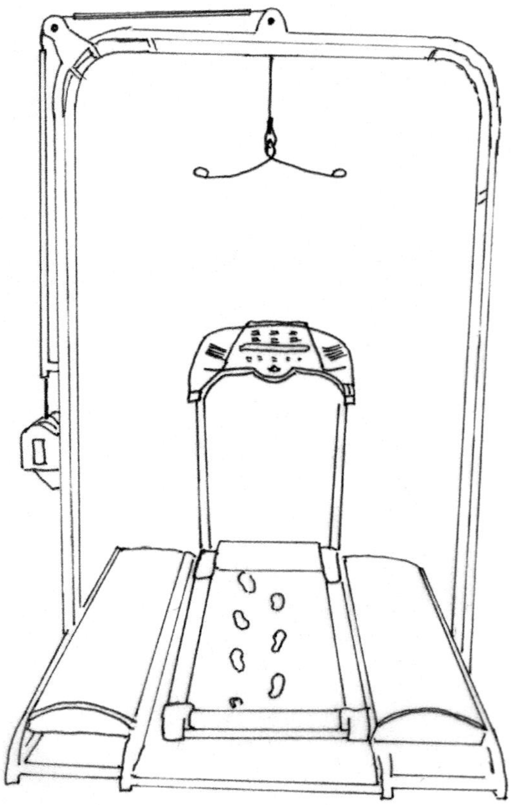

Fig. 4.10 Gait on the track of walking machine

   - Comprehensive walking trainings include walking training with balance bar or walking aid marked with gait, ascending and descending the stairs training and independent walking training marked with gait.

In this stage, the patients are required to try their best to do actual movement training without assistive device. For example, the patients try not to use wheelchair, walking stick and walking aid to do walking training in the remodeling of lower limbs. The actual practical training can be done such as combing and dressing of upper limbs without help.

2. Clinical indications
   - The patients without complaints in dependent ambulation.
   - The myodynamia of muscles of paralyzed side include deltoid, triceps muscle of arm, bicipital muscle of arm, extensor carpi and flexor muscle of wrist of upper limbs, hip

flexor, quadriceps femoris, tibialis anterior muscle, peroneus longus and peroneus brevis of lower limbs and lumbodorsal muscles is more than or equal to level 3.
  - The patients who can complete active joint motion.
  - The signal intensity of motor program of agonistic muscle is more than or equal to160 μv.
3. Clinical contraindications
  - The myodynamia is less than level 3 and sEMG is less than 160 μv.
  - The patients who cannot actively complete multi-joint associated movement.
  - It is used with caution in the patients with fracture of rib, spinal cord, pelvis and lower limbs and uncompleted healed after damages of joint and muscle.

4.2.3 The Training Time and Therapy Course of Three-Stage of Neurological Training Therapy

- The schedule of daily therapeutic programs: There are 4–6 therapy programs every day and the therapy time is 30–50 min. The interval time is about 5–10 min for the patients to have a rest.
- The schedule of therapy time: According to the particularity of CNS system development, reestablishing functions in the injured brain takes a long time, because human take 1 year to learn walking after birth. According to the patients, the patients' family, hospital beds, therapeutic effect and costs, long hospital days is bad for various aspects. After clinical exploration for many years, it is proved primarily that 3 months of one therapy course that includes three stages (1 month per stage) is appropriate for most patients' training. This scheme can achieve the expected therapeutic effect and the hospital time is short. The hospital time can be prolonged in special condition or the second therapy course is continued. After that, the patients can go home and do self-exercise. After six to twelve months, the patients can go to hospital for rehabilitation training as needed.

The training process of CNS potential development is like an army that needs to have a rest after long-term combat in order to fill soldiers, ammunition and living supplement and then can throw them into new combat. After a period of time, the potential ability of CNS is partially developed and the potential resources are consumed for a certain amount. Therefore, the patients feel fatigue and need to take a break to supplement nutrition. After that, they continue training to get better therapeutic effect.

4.2.4 Flexible Use of Three-Stage Neurological Training Therapy

In clinic, we found that three-stage therapy is appropriate for most patients. The therapy time (one month per stage) is enough to achieve the therapeutic effect but is not appropriate for the rehabilitation training of every patient. Therefore the therapists should use it flexibly in clinic.

4.2.4.1 In Each Stage of the Therapy, We Take One Therapy Goal as the Principal Thing and Take Other Methods as the Subsidiary Thing

Training time and content from three stages cannot completely satisfy the demands of CNS functional recovery, even draw a clear distinction. Neural potential development, reestablishment of motor program and remodeling of motor pattern all require long-term training. Rehabilitation training in hospital doesn't allow us to do the training according to neurodevelopment mechanism. The training time can only be short. However, in the therapy of every stage, we take one kind of therapy goal as the principal thing and take other methods as the subsidiary thing. They can make up with each other through cross-over application. For example, in the therapy of the first stage, we take neural potential development training as the principal thing and take reestablishment of motor program as the subsidiary thing. We cannot overemphasize the proportion of motor program, or it can affect the effect of potential development. Similarly, in the therapy of the third stage, we take remodeling of motor pattern as the principal thing.

The signal intensity of motor program and myodynamia of the patients cannot meet the requirements so that the training of neural potential development and reestablishment of motor program is still continued. The time spent on remodeling training of motor pattern is more than the time spent on the training of potential development and motor program reestablishment.

4.2.4.2 In Every Stage, the Therapists Can Adjust Indications Properly According to the Specific Condition of the Patients

During therapy, the therapists should analyze the specific condition of the patient comprehensively and ascertain the corresponding method to obtain better training effect. For example, the patients with higher myodynamia (it is more than or equal to level 3) can do the training of the second stage. For the patients with severe disease and slow recovery of autonomous motor functions, the therapy of the first stage should be prolonged.

4.2.4.3 The Idea of Accepting or Rejecting Should Be Established and the Severe Patients Can Do the Training of the Third Stage Directly

For the severe patients with long disease course (more than half a year) and without autonomous movement can do usability training in the motor pattern of weight loss during the training of potential development and motor program reestablishment. These patients can also do motor pattern remodeling training directly. If the patients still do the training according to three-stage method, the functions may be not recovered finally. For the patients with severe disease, "To accept the lesser of two evils" idea should be established in designing therapeutic principle, which means that the patients try to make the paralyzed limbs move and then let them move normally. Walking under abnormal motor pattern is better than lying on the bed. The author established the rehabilitation principle "standing on the early stage and walking for recovery". Satisfying clinical effect can be obtained after the training with specific principle.

4.2.5 Clinical Verifications of Three-Stage Neurological Training Therapy

4.2.5.1 General Data

From June 2006 to May 2008, there are 60 patients with hemiplegia who are all the inpatients in neurological rehabilitation training center in Beijing Tongren Hospital affiliated to Beijing's Capital Medical University. There are 52 males and 8 females. The age is form 15–69 years old. The average age is 48.2 years old. There are 29 patients with hemiplegia after cerebral infarction, 18 patients with hemiplegia after cerebral hemorrhage, 13 patients with hemiplegia after brain damage. There are 28 patients with left hemiplegia and 32 patients with right hemiplegia. The patients are divided into two groups include prevention group and rectification group and there are 30 patients in each group. Prevention group includes the patients who cannot walk off the bed. There are 25 males and 5 females. The average age is 48.1 years old. Therapy group includes the patients who can walk but with abnormal gait. The disease history is form 1 month to 5 years. There are 27 males and 3 females. The average age is 48.3 years old. The inclusion and exclusion criteria are as follows:

- The inclusion criteria: According to the diagnostic criteria of national cerebrovascular disease conference in 1995, the hemiplegic patients are diagnosed with cerebral infarction or cerebral hemorrhage and by CT or MRI; the patients without obvious dysgnosia (MMSE score is more than or equal to 20); There is no serious contracture of the knee joint or ankle joint and passive movement range is normal.
- The exclusion criteria: The patients with severe organ dysfunction such as heart and lung, severe infectious disease, bone fracture, dyscrasia and so on cannot do rehabilitation training; The patients with severe cognitive disorder or long-term drug use such as sedatives, antidepressants and diazepam cannot cooperate with therapy; the patients with fre-

quent epileptic attack; the patients with diseases such as various myopathy, bone and joint diseases and peripheral neuropathy that can affect movement; the patients stop therapy for any reason or cannot persist in the therapy for 90 times.

4.2.5.2 Therapy Method Includes Division of the Three Stages, Indications and Training Methods

- The first stage is neural potential development. Adopted rehabilitation training methods are as follows:
  - Standing bed or board training: For the patient with poor cardiovascular stress response, foot drop or varus and valgus in the early stage of recovery can use standing bed, dorsiflexion of foot standing board or varus and valgus standing board to do the training in order to enhance cardiovascular response ability and alleviate contracture of Achilles tendon and adhesion of musculus gastrocnemius (30 min per time).
  - Neurological training therapy: According to therapeutic schedule, six-step Daoyin technique in traditional Chinese medicine is used to do the training of hip flexion, hip abduction, knee extension, dorsiflexion of foot and strephexopodia. The training time is 10 min for one joint and the total time is 40 min.
  - Potential development training of lower limbs: Potential development training equipment of lower limbs is used and the regulation of weight loss can make the patients stand. The weight is about one-third to one-fifth of the body weight. Six-step Daoyin technique in traditional Chinese medicine is used to guide the patients to stand up, squat and do limbs control training. There are ten times per group and the training time is 30 min.
  - Neurological training: Daoyin feedback technique in traditional Chinese medicine is used to display motor program signal induced by six-step Daoyin technique in traditional Chinese medicine that is from cortex motor center to agonistic muscle and antagonistic muscle. Through biofeedback mechanism, agonistic muscle signal enhancement training of hip flexion, knee extension, dorsiflexion of foot and strephexopodia is done. In this stage, it is not appropriate to emphasize the proportion of motor program signal of agonistic muscle and antagonistic muscle. The training time is 10 min for one joint and the total is 50 min.
  - The above therapy is once a day and 30 time totally.
  - In this stage, the patients are required to sit on the wheelchair and is prohibited to walk.
  - Clinical indications of the first stage: the hemiplegic patients who cannot yet walk off the bed in the early stage of recovery; the patients with circle gait or dragging gait in the recovery stage; The myodynamia of hip flexion, quadriceps femoris, tibialis anterior muscle, peroneus longus and peroneus brevis is less than or equal to level 2; The signal intensity of hip flexion, quadriceps femoris, tibialis anterior muscle, peroneus longus and peroneus brevis is less than or equal to 80 μv.
- The second stage is the reestablishment of motor program. The adopted training methods are as follows:
  - Potential development training of lower limbs: The training of standing up, squatting and limbs control ability are continued and the training time is 30 min.
  - Neurological training: The proportion reestablishment training of motor program signals of agonistic muscle and antagonistic muscle of hip flexion, knee extension, dorsiflexion of foot and strephexopodia is emphasized. The training is 10 min for one joint and the total time is 50 min.
  - The training of stride, gait and shifting of weight: The training device of weight loss, stride, gait and shifting of weight is used. The regulation of weight loss can make the

patients to stand up. The weight is about one-fourth to one-sixth of the body weight. The length of stride is increased gradually. The training time is 30 min per time.
 - The above therapy is once a day and 30 times totally.
 - In this stage, the patients are required to sit on the wheelchair and is prohibited to walk, but they can walk with help from wheelchair to bed or from wheelchair to pedestal pan.
 - Clinical indications of the second stage:
 - The patients with stable blood pressure and without dizziness or nausea who is recovered to sit or stand with balance.
 - The myodynamia of hip flexor, quadriceps femoris, tibialis anterior muscle, peroneus longus and peroneus brevis in paralyzed side is from level 2 to level 3.
 - The patients who can actively complete the joint motions such as hip flexion, knee flexion, dorsiflexion of foot and strephexopodia.
 - The signal intensity of hip flexor, quadriceps femoris, tibialis anterior muscle, peroneus longus and peroneus brevis is from 80 to 150 μv.
- The third stage is the remodeling of motor pattern. The adopted training methods are as follows:
 - Neurological training: when the patients do the signal intensity enhancement training of agonistic muscles in hip flexion, knee extension, dorsiflexion of foot and strephexopodia, the proportion reestablishment of motor program signal of agonistic muscle and antagonistic muscle motor program is emphasized. The training time is 10 min for one joint and the total time is 50 min. The training time is 2–3 a week.
 - Remodeling training of Abnormal gait weight loss rectification: the weight is about one-fifth to one eighth of the patients' body weight. On the walkpath marked with gait, the patients dress motor pattern remodeling to do walking training. According to foot drop and elastic band of lower limbs adduction, the training is 30 min every time.
 - Weight loss gait training: the patients dress motor pattern remodeling trainer and do the training with weight loss gait training device. The weight is one-fifth to one-eighth of the patients' body weight. Rotational speed of walking machine is started from 0.22 m/s. The speed is increased with the enhancement of walking ability. The patients are guided to do the training according to the marked gait on the walking machine track. The training time is 30 min every time.
 - Comprehensive walking training includes walking training of balance bar or walking aid marked with gait, ascending and descending the stairs training and walkpath marked with gait training. The training time is 10 min for each item and the total time is 30 min. In the beginning stage, the patients dress motor pattern remodeling trainer to do training, and then they can walk without motor pattern remodeling trainer.
 - The therapy time is one time a day and the total number is 30.
 - In this stage, the patients are required to abandon the wheelchair. The patients are helped or guided to do walking training.
 - Clinical indications of the third stage:
 - The patients with no complaints who are recovered to sit or stand with balance.
 - The myodynamia of hip flexor, quadriceps femoris, tibialis anterior muscle, peroneus longus and peroneus brevis in paralyzed side is more than or equal to level 3.
 - The patients can actively complete joint motions of hip flexion, knee flexion, dorsiflexion of foot and strephexopodia.
 - The signal intensity of hip flexor, quadriceps femoris, tibialis anterior muscle, peroneus longus and peroneus brevis is more than or equal to 160 μv.

4.2.5.3 Observation Indicators

International functional assessment methods are used for evaluation, which include Fugl-

Meyer motor function of lower limbs, Lovett manual muscle test, the intensity and proportion of signal, stride, bearing time of injured limbs, range of joint motion in hip flexion, hip abduction, dorsiflexion of foot and strephexopodia. The assessment should be done and the data should be collected in the beginning of the therapy and at the end of the therapy. SPSS12.0 statistical software is used for statistical analysis.

4.2.5.4 Results

There are 30 patients in prevention group. There are 26 patients without abnormal gait and with normal walking pattern. There are four patients with unrecovered functions of peroneus longus and peroneus brevis. The patients with slight strephenopodia, walk with slight circle gait and can be rectified with foot aid. There are 30 patients in rectification group and the gait is obviously rectified, but there are two patients with foot aid. After therapy, there are significant difference in Fugl-Meyer motor function of lower limbs, Lovett manual muscle test, the intensity and proportion of signal, stride, bearing time of injured limbs, range of joint motion in hip flexion, hip abduction, dorsiflexion of foot and strephexopodia between before therapy and after therapy ($P < 0.01$) the results are referred to Tables 4.1 and 4.2.

4.2.5.5 Conclusion

Three-stage therapy of neurological training is the effective method of preventing and rectifying hemiplegic patients with abnormal motor pattern of lower limbs. The index of clinical indications is appropriate for every stage.

This paper is published on Chinese chemist and druggist 2011, 6(5): 621–623.

Table 4.1 Prevention of abnormal gait before therapy and after therapy ($\bar{x} \pm s$)

Assessment items	Before therapy	After therapy	t Value
FMA score of lower limbs	9.27 ± 5.06	27.47 ± 5.12	−21.44*
Stride (cm)	4.87 ± 7.08	23.36 ± 7.75	−10.87*
Bearing time (s)	0.15 ± 0.36	3.29 ± 1.12	−15.52*
sEMG (μV)			
Hip flexor	17.90 ± 13.06	57.27 ± 26.74	−11.81*
Quadriceps femoris	37.00 ± 27.23	101.67 ± 42.92	−14.28*
Tibialis anterior muscle	32.00 ± 25.23	97.26 ± 39.02	−9.23*
Peroneus longus and peroneus brevis	11.00 ± 12.04	50.30 ± 37.29	−7.51*
sEMG (μV)			
Hip flexor/gluteus	18.12 ± 9.64	67.33 ± 23.46	−10.56*
Quadriceps femoris/hamstring muscles	26.07 ± 22.97	86.10 ± 38.37	−13.94*
Tibialis anterior muscle/musculus gastrocnemius	14.12 ± 5.23	58.28 ± 19.36	−9.86*
Peroneus/tibialis posterior	6.63 ± 8.71	41.70 ± 32.30	−7.17*
MMT (level)			
Hip flexor	0.5 ± 0.50	3.5 ± 2.50	−5.67*
Quadriceps femoris	1.5 ± 0.50	4.5 ± 1.50	−8.32*
Tibialis anterior muscle	1.0 ± 1.0	3.5 ± 2.50	−6.54*
Peroneus longus and peroneus brevis	0.5 ± 0.50	3.0 ± 1.50	−7.82*
ROM (°)			
Hip flexion	6° ± 2.5°	52° ± 13.6°	−12.56*
Hip abduction	3° ± 2.5°	22° ± 10.14°	−11.47*
Dorsiflexion of foot	9° ± 5.8°	24° ± 12.7°	−9.32*
Strephexopodia	1.3° ± 0.4°	12° ± 6.4°	−8.97*

*$p < 0.001$

Table 4.2 Rectification of abnormal gait before and after therapy ($\bar{x} \pm s$)

Assessment items	Before therapy	After therapy	t Value
FMA score of lower limbs	18.10 ± 6.16	29.71 ± 3.36	−15.19*
Stride (cm)	14.77 ± 7.21	30.23 ± 4.94	−14.76*
Bearing time (s)	1.28 ± 0.75	5.93 ± 1.78	−17.83*
sEMG (μV)			
Hip flexor	22.03 ± 8.87	59.23 ± 20.53	−12.01*
Quadriceps femoris	35.84 ± 17.43	112.13 ± 36.60	−11.93*
Tibialis anterior muscle	14.12 ± 5.23	58.28 ± 19.36	−9.86*
Peroneus	12.52 ± 9.14	58.16 ± 29.43	−9.93*
sEMG (μV)			
Hip flexion/gluteus	46.33 ± 18.57	112.47 ± 44.22	−10.25*
Quadriceps femoris/hamstring muscles	27.94 ± 17.26	98.10 ± 34.33	−11.71*
Tibialis anterior muscle/musculus gastrocnemius	65.32 ± 31.66	−9.46*	9.61 ± 5.98
Peroneus/tibialis posterior	7.61 ± 8.67	45.42 ± 26.86	−8.46*
MMT (level)			
Hip flexor	1.5 ± 1.50	3.5 ± 1.50	−8.32*
Quadriceps femoris	3.5 ± 2.50	4.5 ± 1.50	−7.67*
Tibialis anterior muscle	2.5 ± 1.50	4.0 ± 1.50	−6.45*
Peroneus longus and peroneus brevis	1.0 ± 1.50	3.5 ± 1.50	−9.38*
ROM (°)			
Hip flexion	12° ± 7.6°	78° ± 16.8°	−11.45*
Hip abduction	16° ± 12.5°	42° ± 23.7°	−7.65*
Dorsiflexion of foot	12° ± 10.2°	43° ± 15.8°	−6.71*
Strephexopodia	3° ± 1.6°	19° ± 8.4°	−9.89*

*$p < 0.01$

4.2.6 Clinical Application Experiences in Three-Stage Rehabilitation Method of Neurological Training: A Philosophical Method with Dialectics and Natural Law

4.2.6.1 Three-Stage Rehabilitation Method of Neurological Training Is a Philosophical Method with Dialectics and Natural Law

Philosophy is the hypostasis and wisdom that can guide people's life and work. "Theory of use and disused" in Darwinian evolution and "sparks of fire, set the prairie ablaze" are the concepts that can make people reborn, which are the hypostasis that can guide human life.

In the three-stage rehabilitation method of neurological training and long-term development of methods, people don't realize that the methods are guided by philosophy to develop gradually. According to the requirements of functional recovery, the methods are added gradually. According to the methods, the equipment is developed. After development, people can analyze the condition and realize that the methods are guided by philosophy to develop gradually. In the three-stage rehabilitation method of neurological training, people found that the methods are guided by philosophy. Main representations are as follows:

- "Theory of use and disused": in the three-stage methods, the therapists should seek the method that active movements of limbs are dominated to recover brain function as soon as possible, which is in accordance with "theory of use and disused" in Darwinian evolution. Moreover, the patients are guided to do active movements of limbs are dominated by brain and the therapeutic effects are better.

- "Transcendence goals and motive force source": Goals are widely used in daily life such as "five-year plan". "The whole day's work depends on a good start in the morning and the whole year's work depends on a good start in spring.", which demonstrated that where there is no goal, there is no motive. In the three-stage rehabilitation method of neurological training, it is established on the basis of transcendence goal. Six-step Daoyin technique in traditional Chinese medicine of guiding collaterals through meridians is used to induce and encourage the patients to surpass the increasing goal to develop potential, reestablish program and remodel motor pattern. Therefore, rehabilitation methods of neurological training are not simple active movement training, but the training guided by Daoyin technique. Through creating safe state of emergency, speech encourage and inspiration, resistance of enhancing active movement to surpass goal, it is easy to develop and utilize neural potential.
- "There's no making without breaking" principle: If the original pattern or habits not removed, it is difficult to establish new pattern. If an old habit is not corrected, there is no way to establish a good one. During the process of rectifying abnormal motor pattern, on the basis of prohibiting and restricting the walking of the patients and eliminating old pattern, neural potential development and reestablishment of motor program are continued. And then the remodeling of motor pattern is started. With the help of effectively restricting abnormal joint motion of body movement device, normal gait remodeling training can be done, which is transited into independent walking. On the moment of "breakthrough", new normal gait training should be established form basis. And then the better clinical effects are achieved.
- "Yin and Yang in equilibrium and harmony is most precious" principle: In traditional Chinese medicine, unity and opposites of Yin and Yang are used to emphasize balance and coordination of functional movement in various organs and tissues, which summarize the rule of various vital movement. Explanation of "Yin and Yang in equilibrium, regulation of mind, Yin-Yang dissociation, exhaustion of vital essence" is meaningful for maintaining normal vital essence.

After CNS damages, the original steady state is destroyed and there are a series of dyskinesia. Six-step Daoyin technique in traditional Chinese medicine of guiding collaterals through meridians is used to clear and activate the channels and collaterals, regulate of Qi and blood, develop neural potential and recover equilibrium between Yin and Yang. Some researchers think that the role of rehabilitation methods of neurological training is related to homeostasis that is recovered by increased negative entropy in vivo after the training of clearing and activating the channels and collaterals and developing neural potential.

4.2.6.2 The Three-Stage Method Is in Accordance with Law of Nature of Functional Shift of Subject, Knowledge Subject and Functional Subject

Law of nature, also named natural rule, is the law that exists in the inner of objective things in natural world, which is the inherent essential connection of natural phenomena that is independent of human willpower. If there is necessary condition, the law can play a role repeatedly.

Human is the subject of application method. People learn methods through study, but this is not equal to actual function. People can use method to figure out problem better through practical application. It is like the process that the Gongfu master learn wushu and apply it. Hundred thousand soldiers do physical training, learn gunnery and soldier's formation, but they still need practical training (military exercise) to turn learned knowledge into actual skill ability.

In this process, in accordance with functional shift of "subject, subject with methods and subject with practical application methods", none is dispensable, which is internal law of nature that can turn method into function.

Rehabilitation methods of neurological training are the process that the methods are turned into functions in vivo. The subject is brain cell and it is the primary target in the training of the first stage. Through potential development methods, new cells are activated and reserved conduction pathway is activated. These cells learn to how to dominate body movement, which is the second stage. Motor program reestablishment technique is used to combine new activated brain cells and undead brain cells closely. These cells perform functions coordinately and orderly. After that, through motor pattern remodeling training (actual practical training) of the third stage, previous training results are turned into actual ability to dominate body movement. In accordance with inherent law of three-element process "activate cells, learn method and apply practically", if the method is proper, indications is appropriate and training time meets the requirement, there will be better clinical effect.

In the other hand, although natural law is independent of man's willpower, human can use wisdom and method to induce, regulate and control real object, energy and information in natural world, make them change or make them become stable for human body. This is the subjective initiative on the basis of objective law. In the three-stage method of neurological training, for the severe patients with severe cognitive dysfunction and low conscious state, rehabilitation principle of "standing in early stage and walking recovery" should be established. Guided by this principle through potential development, standing and walking training, the severe patients can learn methods and develop potential. The patients who use normal methods cannot do active movement training to recover functions, can do the required training, which is in favor of functional recovery.

4.2.6.3 Dialectical Therapy and Formation of Individual Rehabilitation Principle of the Three-Stage Method

In order to improve clinical therapeutic effect of rehabilitation methods of neurological training, on the basis of three-stage method, the specific individual therapeutic principle and scheme are formed. Through detailed functional assessment, the therapists find out primary stagnation point (the reason of circle gait is denervation of peroneus longus and peroneus brevis), ascertain final rehabilitation goal, rehabilitation principle, therapeutic scheme and implementation process (doctors, the therapists, site and time). In rehabilitation principle, for the patients who cannot get off the bed after the disease or whose functions can be better recovered through rehabilitation techniques of neurological training, even abnormal motor pattern is formed, the patients can use typical three-stage rehabilitation principle and do the training strictly in accordance with requirements of every stage. For the patients with dysfunction of individual part and the patients' function can be recovered quickly through assessment, the patients can use atypical three-stage rehabilitation principle and enter into therapy of the third stage after solving the primary problem. For the patients with severe dysfunction, old and frail or obvious cognitive function, rehabilitation principle of standing in the early stage and walking recovery is used for therapy. For the patients with child cerebral palsy, rehabilitation principle of standing in the early stage and walking development is used for therapy. On the moment doing the training of lower limbs potential development, abnormal gait rectification body weight support treadmill trainer is used to support walking training in order to develop neural potential and recover autonomous movement dominated by brain.

In addition, for the elderly patients with severe disease, according to choose the less of two evils, the patients should abandon the therapy of the part whose function is difficult to be recovered. Therefore, functions that are important for daily life ability are recovered. Compared dysfunction of upper limb with dysfunction of lower limb, because the function of upper limb is difficult to be recovered, upper limb can be protected in the functional position. The patients can do rehabilitation training of lower limb first. Moreover, upper limb of one side whose function is normal can complete daily life movement. However, if only lower limb of one side is normal, daily life self-help ability can be affected severely. Compared functional recovery of lower limb in one side with functional recovery of strephexopodia, functional recovery of strephexopodia is relatively difficult. The patients can use foot aid to rectify strephexopodia, which cannot affect walking function recovery of lower limb.

Standing and walking of lower limbs are vital for improving the self-help ability of the patients.

4.2.6.4 The Equipment That Cooperates with Method Is an Effective Instrument to Assure Therapeutic Effect

The equipment is the effective instrument to guarantee standard application of method, broaden applied range of method, improve method effect and decrease labour intensity. At present, rehabilitation methods widely used at home and abroad and invented in last century include Bobath, Rood, Brunnstrom, PNF (Proprioceptive Neuromuscular Facilitation), MRP (Motor Relearning Program) and so on. The required equipment only includes PT bed, balance bar and Bobath ball, and the others are manual performance.

Most of clinical applied rehabilitation equipment aim at symptoms such as standing bed for foot drop, CPM device for muscle and joint adhesion, rehabilitation training robot of lower limbs of the patients without walking ability and so on. Obviously, this equipment plays a role in some respects, but cannot affect functional recovery of brain because it is not in accordance with promoting brain plasticity. However, it is a reserved training of recovering brain function after rehabilitation training.

In the rehabilitation therapy of neurological training equipment, whether potential development, reestablishment of motor program and motor pattern remodeling training equipment or rehabilitation therapy of neurological training robot of guiding collaterals through meridians and one-to-many automatic training system of guiding collaterals through meridians, all are clinical applied design that aim at methods such as potential development equipment. With the function of weight loss equipment and protection, the patients with big body weight, severe symptoms, cognitive dysfunction and low conscious state can do autonomic move movement and auxiliary movement training or are forced to do active movement training, which can obviously broaden applied range of methods, is in favor of standard application of methods and improvement of effects, alleviate labor intensity of the therapists effectively. Especially autonomous rehabilitation therapy of neurological training equipment has an advantage.

4.2.6.5 Rehabilitation Process of Recovering Motor Function After CNS Damages Is a System Process

Recovery of motor function after brain damages, is different from therapy process of damages and lesions in various body parts, because the therapy of lesions in various body parts is the process of repairing or replacement of individual part. For example, if the battery or tyre of a vehicle is broken, after the battery is replaced or the broken tyre is repaired, the vehicle can run on the road intact. For example, if the liver is ruptured, through surgical repair or partial hepaolithiasis, function can be recovered after heal and the patients can return to work. The cancer of kidney can be removed through surgical extraction. After wound healing, daily life ability can be recovered. If the bone is broken, reduction fixation can be done through surgery. After taking a rest, the fracture is healed and the original function can be recovered through exercise. The patients can use rehabilitation training in the early stage to prevent complications effectively, promote healing and shorten course of disease.

However, recovering the lost motor function after brain damages is different. Not only the injured brain should be repaired, but also function of trunk and organs dominated by brain should be recovered. Therefore, for functional recovery of organs and body parts, recovering the functions after brain damages is the relationship between use and disuse on the basis of self-functional recovery. Brain can dominate body parts and organs and body parts and organs are dominated by brain. In the process of recovering brain function, the function of brain and the function of body parts dominated by brain both are recovered. Therefore, the functional recovery of brain is a system process. Moreover, for the brain function, not only the function of individual cell should be recovered, but also coordinated work function of brain cells should be recovered. For example, the functional recovery of hemiplegic patients with cerebral infarction in one side, at first, the function of injured brain cells should be recovered or replaced by other brain tissues. And then the coordination function between new cells and old cells should be recovered. On the basis of that, the function of domination of limbs movement is recovered. In addition, the function of limbs is required to be recovered such as muscle and joint adhesion, deformity (such as foot drop and varus). Finally, the limbs are dominated by brain to complete the movement. Therefore, rehabilitation process of brain functions that rehabilitation methods and medical engineering technology are used to make the disabled recover to the person with independent daily life ability and work ability if surgery and drug have no effect on recovery. It is a cultivating project and medical subjects with high technology.

In short, three-stage rehabilitation method of neurological training is philosophical scientific method that is in accordance with natural law. It is the specific manifestation of chiastopic fusion and compound integration of various rehabilitation techniques of neurological training and traditional rehabilitation technique. The author thinks that it is ultimately improved and developed with increase of clinical application, further research, updated method, continuous innovation and improvement of equipment type and quality, which can promote the development of rehabilitation work.

4.3 Three-Stage Associated Equipment and Clinical Verification of Neurological Training

4.3.1 Abnormal Gait Rectification Weight Support Treadmill Training Device and Clinical Verification

4.3.1.1 Objectives

In higher CNS damages (such as child cerebral palsy, brain damages and so on), because inhibition of lower nerve center is lost, the excitability of lower nerve center is released to varying degrees, which lead to abnormal increase in the excitability of muscles dominated by lower nerve center. And then there are spasm and abnormal gesture. Severe patients usually lose standing and walking ability and it is difficult to be treated in clinic. At present, there is no specific equipment and method for these patients to do walking training. The author developed weight support treadmill training device of abnormal gait rectification. The purpose is to develop a rehabilitation therapy of neurological training device for the patients who cannot stand, walk and do normal weight support treadmill training with the help of weight loss, prevention of abnormal gait and safe protection. Walking training in the early stage can improve motor function of lower limbs and promote recovery of normal walking ability through promoting functional recovery of higher CNS. The therapists observe the effect and discuss clinical indications.

4.3.1.2 Basic Composition

Weight support treadmill training device of abnormal gait rectification is made of weight device, abnormal gait rectification system and footpath.

- Weight loss system is composed of loading frame, weight winch, pulley, handrail and weight loss hammock. The loading frame is made of double joint of hot drawing welded steel tubes. The diameter is 36 mm and the wall thickness is 4 mm. Two tubes are curved to rectangle frame (150 cm × 180 cm) with two layers and the space between them is 50 cm. double joint U-tubes in parallel are welded in the middle of the frame. In the middle of the top of U-tubes, fixed pulley and its guard board are welded. In one side of the corner in the top of U-tubes and in the middle of middle point in the wall, fixed pulley and winch are welded. Steel wires (the diameter is 3 mm) are used to link hammock connecting rod in the frame and weight loss winch in the side wall. In the front and back of underside of rectangle frame, four universal wheels are fixed separately. Handrail is fixed on the middle of the front and the height is adjustable. Disassembly protection bar is connected to the back. Weight loss band is divided into swimsuit type and waistcoat type. The stress point of swimsuit is located in inguinal region, chest and double oxters. Waistcoat type is connected to thigh of both side through hammock and the stress point is located in chest and hip. According to the specific condition of the patients, the equipment is comfortable to wear, there is no press of local soft tissue and the activities are not influenced.

- Abnormal gait rectification system: Elastic traction belt of lower limbs abduction and dorsiflexion of foot with different elastic force are made from elastic bandages of different width and thickness. The function of lower limbs abduction band is to prevent excessive abduction of lower limbs in walking. One end is linked to the superstratum steel tube of loading frame and the other end is fastened to the underneath of knee joint of the patients with nylon thread gluing. The function of dorsiflexion of foot elastic bandage is to prevent foot drop and strephenopodia in walking. One end is fixed to the top of loading frame and the other end is fastened to the front of feet. Tightness of traction belt can be adjusted in order not to affect walking with adduction of lower limbs and foot drop.
- Footpath is made from transparent and soft plastic plate with 2 cm thickness. The width is 30–50 mm and the length can be adjusted according to the rehabilitation hall. Footprint is drawn on the footpath according to different stride of children and adult.

4.3.1.3 Training Methods

1. Preparation before training: The patients can dress the hammock in standing or sitting position. Based on movement prescription, through regulating overhang traction system, the patients drag hammock to lose weight. According to the specific condition of the patients, therapists stand on one side, the front or the back of the patients. The patients grasp frontal handrail with two hands. According to the degree of lower limbs adduction and foot drop, the therapists can adjust the tightness of elastic bandage. With the help of elastic bandage, walking cannot be affected by lower limbs adduction and foot drop.
2. Training includes auxiliary power, autonomic power walking training and disassembled gait slow motion training of Daoyin technique.
   - Auxiliary power walking training: The therapists push the training instrument forward and the patients step forward with the instrument.
   - Autonomic power walking training: The patients push the training instrument forward and step forward with the instrument.
   - Disassembled gait slow motion training of Daoyin technique: Six-step Daoyin technique in traditional Chinese medicine are used to guide the patients do disassembled gait training on the basis of regulation of mind and breathing. The specific procedures are as follows: The patients are guided to regulate breathing, concentrate, put the center of body weight on one side slowly and try to flex hip joint to step forward. For example, in the associated movement with lower limbs adduction, the patients try to abduce lower limbs at the same time and pay attention to tibialis anterior muscle and peroneus longus and peroneus brevis to do dorsiflexion of foot and strephexopodia in case of foot drop and strephenopodia. After that, the patients bend forward to step forward. According to the footprint on the floor, the patients make the foot touch the ground first and then the entire foot is on the footprint. The center of the body shift to this side and offside disassembled stepping training is done with the same method repeatedly.
   - Body control ability training: In the weight loss and safe protection condition, the patients are guided to do hip flexion, dorsiflexion of foot and hip abduction training in plgenius. The specific procedures are as follows: the patients put the center of body weight on one side in standing or sitting position. The patients are guided to flex hip joint quickly on the basis of regulation of mind and breathing. In the movement of lower limbs adduction, the patients are

guided to abduce hip joint at the same time, dorsiflex ankle joint quickly, make the heel touch the ground first and put the entire foot in the footprint on footpath. The purpose of this training is to improve speed and flexibility of body limbs movement. The patients are required to relax as much as possible and not to exert too much in case of excessive united reflection. The patients can shorten the movement accomplishment time gradually. With the increase of myodynamia of lower limbs hip flexor, abductor, tibialis anterior muscle and peroneus longus and peroneus brevis, autonomic control ability, body control ability and walking ability, the quantity of weight loss and the pull strength of traction belt are gradually decreased. The patients can gradually walk independently without weight loss, traction and handrail.

The training is 30 min per time and 30 times per therapy course. After one therapy course, the therapists should assess the patients to decide whether do the next therapy course or not.

4.3.1.4 Clinical Indications and Contraindications

Indications

It is appropriate for the patients with severe lower limbs motor dysfunction who cannot do normal weight support treadmill training and is in stable condition with acute, chronic and obsolete hemiplegia, cerebral palsy, child cerebral palsy, incomplete paraplegia after CNS damages and the patients with lower limbs adduction or foot drop induced by muscle spasm or paralysis who feel difficult to do normal weight loss walking training.

Contraindications

Contraindications include the patients in acute stage with unstable condition, the patients in uncontrolled condition with severe hypertension and diabetes, the patients with severe heart disease, pulmonary dysfunction and low cardiovascular response capacity, the patients with dizziness and drop of blood pressure when standing up.

Cautions

- For the patients with long-term bed and infirmity, the adaptive training should be done before this type of the training in order to increase the stress capability of the patients' angiocarpy. When the patients stand erectly for 30 min and blood pressure, pulse and electrocardiogram are stable, this type of the training should be done.
- The training should be implemented step by step. The therapists regulate the training through adjusting the weight and training time. High training intensity should be avoided.

During training, the enthusiasm of the patients and the training atmosphere should be fully activated. The therapists should use encouraging words and scolding and critical words should be avoided.

4.3.1.5 Clinical Verification

Cases Selection

From October 2004 to June 2006, potential development training equipment was used to treat 52 patients with lower limbs motor dysfunction who are all the inpatients and outpatients in neurological rehabilitation training center in Beijing Tongren Hospital affiliated to Beijing's Capital Medical University. There are 31 males and 21 females. The age is form 23 to 76 years old. The average age is 44.33 years old. The shortest medical history lasts fifteen months and the longest lasts 62 months. The average is 38 months. There are 29 patients with hemiplegia after cerebral infarction, 18 patients with hemiplegia after cerebral hemorrhage, five patients with hemiplegia after child cerebral palsy.

Functional Assessment

In the beginning of the training and the end of the therapy course, the therapists do functional ambulation category (FAC).

Zero Grade: The patients cannot walk or can walk with the help of two people.

First Grade: The patients can walk with the help of one person to lose weight.

Second Grade: The patients can walk with the help of one person to support continuously of intermittently.

Third Grade: The patients can walk under supervision of others.

Fourth Grade: The patients can walk on the flat ground independently but hey need help when they walk upstairs and downstairs, up the slope and down the slope, on unstable ground.

Fifth Grade: The patients can walk everywhere independently.

Myodynamia of hip flexor, range of motion in hip joint flexion and Fugl-Meyer methods are used for lower limbs motor function assessment. SPSS 12.0 statistical software is used for analysis. The difference before therapy and after therapy is analyzed with T-test.

Results

There are significant differences in four assessment indicators before and after training ($p < 0.01$). In all the 52 patients, there are six patients with zero myodynamia of hip flexor and the myodynamia is recovered to 2.68 grade after training. Autonomous hip joint motion of all the patients is recovered. The results are referred to Table 4.3.

The safety of the equipment: There is no injury of all the patients during training. The training devices run without fault, they are easy to be operated, flexible and convenient, manual and reasonable designed, safe and reliable.

Discussion

For the patients with hemiplegia after brain infarction and spinal cord injury, there are a lot of reports about body weight support treadmill training, which is a safe and effective therapeutic measure.

Some research demonstrated that central pattern generator (CPG) located in spinal cord or brainstem can receive specific proprioception afferent information, integrate them and generate rhythmic electrical activity, and induce circulation gait motion. However, this is the results from cats' spinal cord. Faster exercise treadmill speed is adopted and stretching exercise of hip is maintained by therapists. Meanwhile, foot position helps the patients with complete spinal cord injury to reestablish passive physiological gait. However, on the same conditions, primates cannot do stepping movement, because the walking of the primates is more dependent on efferent stimulus of superior spinal cord. Reticulospinal movement pathway that is descendent along ventral spinal cord is closely related to stepping and walking. Therefore, for primates, functional recovery of cortex motor center and activation of reserved conduction pathway are critical for recovering walking ability of the patients.

Theoretical basis of functional recovery cortex motor center is CNS plasticity, which is the reorganization ability of structure and function on the basis of "skillful use and dependence" principle. Some research demonstrated that the training under "state of emergency" and repeated training with "goal and willpower" can better promote functional reorganization of central nerves. During the process of weight supported walking, the patients try their best to keep the pace of the treadmill machine in order to walk on the treadmill machine. Therefore, the autonomic uniform rotation of treadmill machine track can provide a kind of "state of emergency" for the patients. Through weight support walking, the repeated and specific training is also a kind of

Table 4.3 Functional assessment control table in paralyzed side before and after training ($\bar{x} \pm s$)

Assessment items	Before training	After training	P value
FAC	0.27 ± 0.87	3.67 ± 1.45	<0.01
MMT	1.45 ± 0.87	3.62 ± 1.33	<0.01
ROM	8° ± 3.23°	45° ± 8.37°	<0.01
Lower limbs FM	12.82 ± 4.71	23.41 ± 11.37	<0.05

forced movement, which is good for central nerves plasticity and functional reorganization. During this process, information feedback of load bearing receptor plays an important role in promoting the recovery of the patients' motor function.

The purpose of treadmill walking training is to make the patients without load bearing ability and balance keeping ability to do walking training erectly in order to use the early stage of recovering potential when the disease is stable. However, treadmill walking training can be done by the patients with certain ability. For example, the average myodynamia of lower limbs is equal to or more than level 2. Treadmill walking training can be done by the patients with the help of one or two therapists. However, for myodynamia, especially for obviously insufficient myodynamia of primary muscles (such as hip flexor, tibialis anterior muscle and quadriceps femoris), the patients with complete paralysis and zero myodynamia or the patients with severe foot drop, strephenopodia or lower limbs adduction deformity (scissors gait), it is difficult for them to do this training. In addition, in actual weight support treadmill training, the author found that there are some patients whose lower limbs myodynamia is equal to or more than level 2, but they are still worry about the danger of walking on the treadmill machine. It is easy for them to generate fear and they even refuse to do this training.

The purpose of developing weight support treadmill training device of abnormal gait rectification is to make the patients do treadmill training who cannot do body weight support treadmill training or the weight support treadmill training is not appropriate for the patients in order to recover walking ability on the basis of recovering the excitability of gait motor center. For the patients with child cerebral palsy, load bearing in standing position has a promoting effect on development of joint and bone.

Under the protection of the equipment, according to the specific condition of the patients, through the regulation of weight support, the patients can do the training with the principle "from easy to difficulty and step by step". Through regulation of the tightness of lower limbs abduction traction belt, the patients can adduce lower limbs in order not to affect the patients' walking. Through regulation of dorsiflexion of foot elastic traction belt, the patients can walk and keep the front of the foot out of the ground. During training, the patients or therapists push the training machine forward and the forward speed is the same as the walking speed of the patients. Without the feeling of tension induced by autonomic uniform rotation treadmill machine track, the patients can avoid ataxia induced by tension and the training is closer to actual walking (Fig. 4.11, 4.12, 4.13, and 4.14).

In the beginning of the training, the patients try to decrease the walking speed and the therapists guide the patients to lift toe to overcome foot drop by themselves. The patients try to abduce lower limbs to overcome adduction of lower limbs in walking. When the patients cannot overcome it by themselves, elastic traction bandage can play a role in the walking of the patients. During this process, every step of the patients is completed by agonistic muscle and antagonistic muscle dominated by cortex motor center to complete unaccomplished body movement

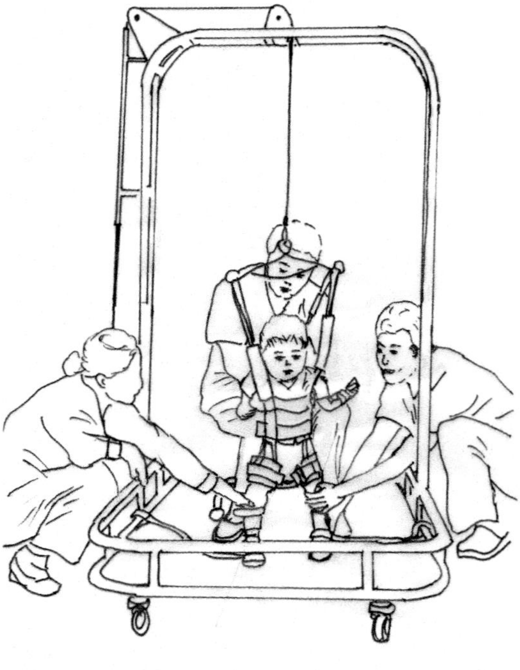

Fig. 4.11 Weight support treadmill training of abnormal gait rectification

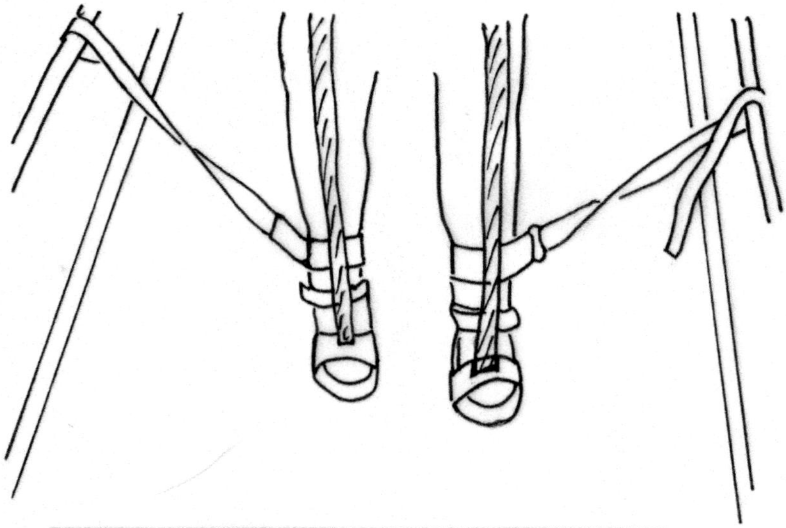

Fig. 4.12 Rectification elastic bandage to prevent foot drop and lower limbs adduction

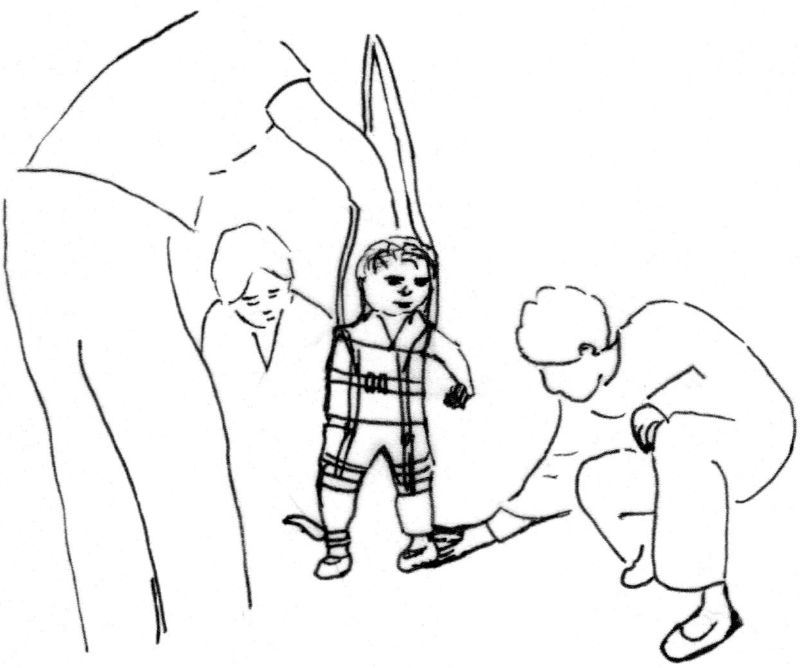

Fig. 4.13 The training for severe child cerebral palsy

before, which is good for neural potential development and functional reorganization. The function of footpath is to establish subjective indicators of stride and stride width for the patients. Stride can rectify the small stride of lower limbs in injured side and insufficiency of load bearing time. Stride width can induce the patients to rectify adduction of lower limbs, which is better for the training of hip flexor and hip abductor. Daoyin technique in traditional Chinese medicine is used to activate the willpower of the patients. The patients can complete walking and overcome the shortages in the walking by themselves. The comprehensive results are appropriate for "standing in the early stage and walking development" of the children or"standing in the early stage and walking recovery" of the adult, which is good for central nerves plasticity

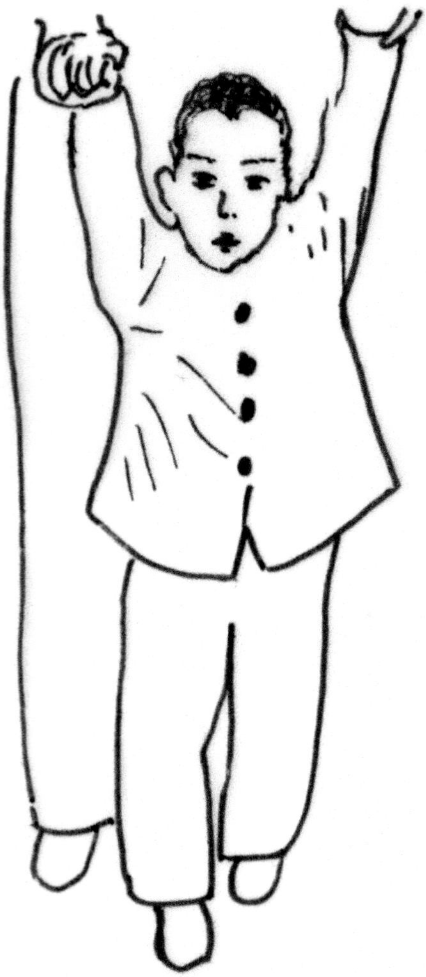

Fig. 4.14 Able to stand and walk after training

and functional reorganization and promote walking ability recovery finally.

This paper was published on Chinese Journal of Tissue Engineering Research 2009, 13(48):9455–9458.

4.3.2 Clinical Verification of Lower Limbs Motor Pattern Remodeling Trainer

Abnormal motor pattern of lower limbs is the common motor dysfunction after CNS damages, which is difficult to be treated in clinic. At present, in widely used rehabilitation methods at home and abroad, the training effect is greatly affected because there is no way to restrict the unnecessary movement in exercise. The author developed lower limbs motor pattern remodeling trainer and its purpose is to turn the training results of neural potential development and motor program reestablishment into normal walking ability and consolidate them in order to improve lower limbs motor function, enhance the patients' life quality and obtain good effect.

4.3.2.1 Purpose

It is necessary to develop a method to effectively restrict unnecessary joint motion in lower limbs movement, which assure the patients to walk with normal gait. On the basis of neural potential development and motor program reestablishment, normal motor patter of lower limbs is remodeled.

4.3.2.2 Basic Composition

Lower limbs motor pattern remodeling trainer is composed of waistline, assistive device joint prosthesis of hip, knee and ankle, aluminium alloy lattice framing, foot orthosis and fixed band. Joint prosthesis can confine range of activity and original angle (such as 15° flexed position) of hip, knee and ankle joint. The joint only allow the movement on the sagittal orientation (frontal axis). Joint prosthesis of hip, knee and ankle are connected with aluminium alloy lattice framings. The lattice framings between hip joint and knee joint or knee joint and ankle joint are double layers. There is a groove in the center and it can slide up and down. The length is adjustable and adjustable bolt can be used to fix it for the patients with different altitude to dress. The bottom of ankle joint prosthesis is connected to aluminium alloy foot orthosis (high temperature thermoplastic plate in domestic type). Bilateral hip joint is fixed on both side of waistline made of high temperature thermoplastic plate through rivet of lattice framing in order to support and restrict adduction and abduction of lower limbs. Foot orthosis is used to rectify abnormal joint position such as foot drop, strephenopodia and strephexopodia, which don't affect the ankle joint motion on the sagittal direction (frontal axis).

Lower limbs motor pattern remodeling trainer is divided into training type and maintenance type according to application. It is divided into double limbs type, single limb type, trunk double limbs type, trunk single limb type and local type according to different part. Training type can be adjusted according to limb length of the patients, which is appropriate for different individuals. It is used in rehabilitation hall of hospital. Maintenance type is made of lighter magnesium alloy according to different individuals, which is light and appropriate for the patients to do self-training when they leave hospital. It also can prevent relapse of abnormal motor pattern.

According to the specific condition of the patients, corresponding type is chosen to restrict abnormal joint motion effectively and make it comfortable to dress.

4.3.2.3 Clinical Verifications

Cases Selection

From October 2010 to June 2011, potential development training equipment was used to treat 30 patients with lower limbs motor dysfunction who are all the inpatients in neurological rehabilitation training center in Beijing Nanyang Hospital and Beijing Sun City Hospital. There are 21 males and 9 females. The age is from 38 to 65 years old. The average age is 48.3 ± 16.8 years old. The shortest medical history lasts 6 months and the longest lasts 78 months. The average is 33 months. There are 23 patients with hemiplegia after cerebral infarction, seven patients with hemiplegia after cerebral damages. There are 20 patients with circle gait and ten patients with dragging gait.

Training Methods

- Lower limbs potential development training: Wenru lower limbs potential development training device is used and six-step Daoyin technique in traditional Chinese medicine is used for lower limbs potential development training and lower limbs control ability training. The training time is 30 min every time and the frequency is one time a day. There are 90 times in one therapy course.
- Motor program reestablishment training: Neurological training instrument is used for motor program signal reestablishment training of agonistic muscle and antagonistic muscle in hip flexion, knee extension, dorsiflexion of foot and strephexopodia of lower limbs. During the process of enhancing the signal of agonistic muscle, the signal proportion training of agonistic muscle and antagonistic muscle is emphasized. The training time is 10 min for each joint and the total time is 50 min. The frequency is one time a day. There are 90 times in one therapy course.
- Motor pattern remodeling training:

Preparation before training: After the patients dress lower limbs motor pattern remodeling trainer, Wenru weight support treadmill training device of abnormal gait rectification produced by Beijing Xing Chen Wan You Science and Technology Ltd. and gait marked footpath are used for the patients to do the training. Based on movement prescription, weight support can be regulated. According to the specific condition of the patients, therapists stand on one side, the front or the back of the patients. The patients grasp frontal handrail with two hands or walk freely.

The training includes auxiliary power walking training and autonomic power walking training. Auxiliary power walking training: The therapists push the training instrument forward and the patients step forward with the instrument. Autonomic power walking training: The patients push the training instrument forward and step forward with the instrument. Disassembled gait slow motion training of Daoyin technique: Six-step Daoyin technique in traditional Chinese medicine are used to guide the patients to do disassembled gait training on the basis of regulation of mind and breathing. The specific procedures are as follows: The patients are guided to regulate breathing, concentrate, put the center of body weight on one side slowly and try to flex hip joint to step forward. According to the footprint on the floor, the patients make the foot touch the ground first and then the entire foot is on the footprint. The center of the body shift to this side and offside disassembled stepping training is done with the same method repeatedly.

Body control ability training: In the weight loss and safe protection condition, the patients are guided to do hip flexion, dorsiflexion of foot and hip abduction training in plgenius. The specific procedures are as follows: the patients put the center of body weight on one side in standing or sitting position. The patients are guided to flex hip joint quickly on the basis of regulation of mind and breathing. In the movement of lower limbs adduction, the patients are guided to abduce hip joint at the same time, dorsiflex ankle joint quickly, make the heel touch the ground first and put the entire foot in the footprint on footpath. The purpose of this training is to improve speed and flexibility of body limbs movement. The patients are required to relax as much as possible and not to exert too much in case of excessive united reflection. The patients can shorten the movement accomplishment time gradually. With the increase of myodynamia of lower limbs hip flexor, abductor, tibialis anterior muscle and peroneus longus and peroneus brevis, autonomic control ability, body control ability and walking ability, the quantity of weight loss is gradually decreased. The patients can gradually walk independently without weight loss, traction and handrail.

The training time is 30 min every time and the frequency is one time a day. There are 90 times in one therapy course.

Self-training at home: After abnormal motor pattern of lower limbs is rectified and normal motor pattern is formed, in order to shorten hospital stays, the patients dress domestic motor pattern remodeling trainer to do self-training at home, which require 6–12 months to maintain therapeutic effect. The normal motor pattern should be guaranteed to be consolidated.

Functional Assessment

In the beginning of the training and the end of the therapy course, the therapists do functional ambulation category (FAC). Range of motion of hip flexion, knee extension and dorsiflexion of foot, Fugl-Meyer lower limbs motor function assessment, signal intensity and proportion, and activity of daily living should be assessed. SPSS 12.0 statistical software is used for analysis. The difference before therapy and after therapy is analyzed with T-test.

Results

There are significant differences in six assessment indicators before and after training ($p < 0.01$). In all the 30 patients, there are six patients with zero myodynamia of hip flexor and the myodynamia is recovered to 3.25 grade after training. Autonomous hip joint motion of all the patients is recovered. The results are referred to Table 4.4. There is no patient with zero myodynamia of quadriceps femoris (more than level 2) and the myodynamia is recovered to level 4 after training. There are eight patients with zero myodynamia of tibialis anterior muscle and the myodynamia is recovered to 3.42 grade after training. There are 11 patients with zero myodynamia of peroneus longus and peroneus brevis. The myodynamia of three patients is recovered to level 3 after training, the myodynamia of five patients is recovered to level 2 and the myodynamia of four patients is not significantly changed. When walking, the patients need to wear foot aid to rectify strephenopodia. Average myodynamia is from 1.45 grade before training to 3.62 grade after training. Motor program proportion of knee extension is from 2.76 times before training to 6.34 times after training. Although there is difference between motor program proportion of knee extension and normal proportion (the proportion of agonistic muscle and antagonistic muscle is 10–1), there is significant difference before and after training.

The Safety of the Equipment

There is no injury of all the patients during training. The training devices run without fault, they are easy to be operated, flexible and convenient, manual and reasonable designed, safe and reliable.

However, during the follow-up, it was found that there were three cases of household-type broken due to the insufficient stiffness of the magnesium alloys stent. The bending strength of the magnesium alloys also need further improvement. At present, I adopt the aluminum alloys

Table 4.4 Functional assessment control table in paralyzed side before and after training ($\overline{\chi}$ ± s)

Items	Before training	After training	*t* Value	P value
FAC	0.27 ± 0.87	3.67 ± 1.45	7.01	<0.01
Hip flexion MMT	1.45 ± 0.87	3.62 ± 1.33	4.32	<0.01
ROM(0)				
Hip flexion	57.73° ± 34.55°	110.60° ± 17.91°	9.02	<0.01
Knee extension	110.68° ± 12.63°	160.86° ± 4.26°	10.11	<0.01
Dorsiflexion of foot	3.67° ± 6.49°	15.47° ± 7.10°	8.01	<0.01
FM	14.97 ± 25.01	29.60 ± 8.79	9.39	<0.01
sEMG (μV)				
Hip flexor intensity	23.70 ± 21.	60.97 ± 26.90	10.29	<0.01
Quadriceps femoris intensity	45.57 ± 33.69	103.73 ± 42.80	11.73	<0.01
Quadriceps femoris/hamstring muscles	2.75 ± 2.01	6.34 ± 2.33	10.54	<0.01
Tibialis anterior muscle intensity	15.77 ± 21.48	39.77 ± 28.04	6.39	<0.01
Tibialis anterior muscle/musculus gastrocnemius	1.47 ± 1.64	4.50 ± 2.37	9.43	<0.01
The intensity of peroneus longus and peroneus brevis	19.93 ± 24.90	41.47 ± 28.59	7.23	<0.01
ADL	55.83 ± 25.53	79.33 ± 11.72	7.02	<0.01

stent for children to produce motor pattern plastotype training devices. It both adds the rigidity of the stent and achieves the portable characteristic of household-type basically. Clinical application has got primary success.

Clinical Indications and Contraindications

- Indications: It is not only suitable for the training of the convalescence stage of obstacle of limbs movement accompanied with abnormal motor pattern, but in stable condition such as stroke and brain trauma, but also for the rehabilitation training of other lower limbs abnormal motor pattern patients whose rehabilitation methods training was ineffective.
- Contraindications: Patients with one of the following indications should be forbidden or careful to use motor pattern remodeling training device for training:

Hypertensive and diabetic patients whose condition has not been controlled effectively.

Patients after stroke whose condition is unstable.

Patients with lower limb fractures, articular cartilage and ligament injuries whose concrescence is not good.

Patients with pelvic fracture or injury of pelvic soft tissue.

Training Cautions

The training procedure should be step by step, and avoid by all means of blindly high-intensity training. Each training time should not be too long, generally 30 min. Patients who feel discomfort in training should stop training immediately and find out the reasons and then go back to training. It can also be regulated through reducing weight or shortening training time. It should be paid attention to use six-step Daoyin technique in traditional Chinese medicine correctly during training. The enthusiasm of the patients and training atmosphere should be fully activated, encouraging words can be used and rebuke and critical words should be avoided.

Discussion

At present, methods used to rectify abnormal gait in domestic and abroad are few. The most commonly used methods include good limb position in early stage, restriction walking off bed, varus-valgus rectification board standing, wearing orthotic devices, Bobath technique, body weight support treadmill training (BWSTT) and gait training under the verbal instruction of the therapists and so on. These methods have some certain effects on the aspect of recovering the walking ability of stroke patients and improving the gait symmetry and so on, especially like body weight support treadmill, which can be used to improve the adaptation of cardiovascular and walking ability. Some research reported that although Mobile Gait Monitoring System (MGMS) and lower limbs rehabilitation training robot have a better effect on improving the lower limbs motor function and the gait, both of them lack the correct effect on abnormal gait due to no restriction of unnecessary movement during exercise. Moreover, all of the training methods lack a valid movement constraint after training, so that most of the patients still walking according to the previous motor pattern once they left the training room. This is especially not good for the decrease of the abnormal motor center excitability, which make the abnormal motor pattern hard to be corrected and even easy to relapse.

There are many deficiencies of training methods at home and abroad that is used to rectify abnormal gait, which are as follows:

Most of gait trainings are mainly dependent on the verbal instructions of the therapists. There are no systematic rehabilitation methods to rectify abnormal gait. All of them cannot limit unnecessary joint motion, which is bad for the reestablishment of normal gait.

The gait training method at present is lack of definite indications and contraindications.

There is no training device that is used for rectifying abnormal gait and recovering normal gait again.

The patients still walk with original pattern, which make it impossible to decrease the excitability of the abnormal motor center effectively and is bad for the establishment and consolidation of normal motor pattern. Above-mentioned deficiencies affect the training results of the motor pattern remodeling.

Zhao Wenru and his colleague developed a therapy named three-stage therapy of neurological training, which includes neural potential development, reestablishment of motor program and motor pattern remodeling. The training time is two months for each stage. At the first two stages, the patients are prohibited to walk and are required to sit on wheelchairs. The purpose is to eliminate the excitability of the abnormal motor program in the cortex motor center in order to promote reestablishment of normal motor program. In the last stage, body weight support treadmill training device of abnormal motor pattern is used. Unnecessary joint motion is restricted in the lower limbs movement through an elastic band. Although there are some certain clinical effects, we found some shortage in clinical application:

In a long-term walking restriction, the patients cannot keep on it because it is difficult to accept.

Elastic band is used to limit abnormal joint motion, which is soft limitation. For the patients with severe abnormal joint motion, it is difficult to meet the requirements.

The time of motor pattern remodeling training only lasts one month. It is too short to be consolidated and it is easy to relapse.

The patients are required to do self-training for a long time aftercare. Although patients were told how to do the training when they left hospital, abnormal motor pattern often relapse because of wrong training, which affects remote therapeutic effect.

The mechanisms underlying remodeling motor pattern by lower limbs movement pattern remodeling training device. The motor program and the motor pattern interact with each other. The motor pattern is determined by the motor program and the long-term movement with the abnormal movement pattern can modify the motor program developed in the cortex motor center. On the contrary, in the normal motor pattern with limitation, due to the effective limitation of abnormal joint motion induced by abnormal muscle contraction, the myodynamia of this muscle gradually decrease. At the same time, it forced the muscle of this joint, which is produced normal activities, can be utilized. Therefore, the myodynamia gradually increase. For a long time, there can be a balance of the myodynamia that participate in the normal motion of this joint, which establish a normal motor program to dominate joint motion in the cortex motor center.

Lower limbs motor pattern remodeling device can rigidly limit the abnormal joint motion in lower limbs movement through the design of assistive device steel bar and the one-way joint motion, which assure the normal of the motor pattern. The muscles required to complete correct movement can be increasingly utilized, and the muscles formed abnormal joint motion is utilized on the decrease. Normal motor pattern is consolidated and then is gradually transited to normal walking without assistance.

As long as the patients can walk with weight loss or assistance, in the early stage, the motor pattern remodeling training can be done with potential development and motor program remodeling training. It can not only change the developed potential and reestablished motor program into motor function, but also satisfy the request of the patients who want to walk as soon as possible, improve the effect of rehabilitation training, shorten the time of training and inspire the patients' motivation for training. Moreover, the household-type guaranteed the correctness of self-training after the patients leaving hospital, which is good for the consolidation of the normal motor pattern.

The differences between the motor pattern remodeling device and the walking assistance device are as follows: There are significant differences in application and structure between the motor pattern remodeling device and the walking assistance device. Walking assistance device is mainly used for paraplegic patients, the function of which is to bear load and prevent joint motion. The joint is in a lock and fixed pattern condition when the patients are in passive standing and passive walking condition. While the motor pattern remodeling device is a proprietary training device that can change the established motor program into practical motor function. Every joint is activated when it is used. According to abnormal angle (like genu recurvatum) of the joint, the joint motion is restricted appropriately, the joint is only allowed to move in normal direction and movements to abnormal direction are restricted rigidly. The active training of motor pattern remodeling guided by the therapist can change the established motor program into exclusive training device of active movement with actual motor function.

There are many types of lower limbs motor pattern remodeling devices according to the differences of the body location and necessity of the training. It can be divided into training-type and household-type according to its usage.

The training-type device uses the double-layer assistive devices of aluminum alloy bar with strong capability of countering bending. There is a tank in its center and it is possible to slide up and down to adjust length. It is fixed by the adjustable bolts and can be used by the patients in different heights. This type of device is strong and durable, but the weight is big, which makes it relatively complicated when putting on and off. It is suitable for the recovery room of the hospital.

The household-type of lower limbs motor pattern remodeling device is a restrict device that is portable and used for maintaining the developed normal motor pattern. It is developed to protect the patients from the relapse of abnormal motor pattern due to the abnormal movement of the joint in the process of self-training. The device adopts magnesium alloy bar and usually use single bar. The waist and foot baseboards are made of thin layer of high-temperature thermoplasticized board. The characteristics of this type are as follows.

The unnecessary joint motion in the movement of lower limbs can be effectively restricted, while the joint motion to normal direction is not affected.

The abnormal location of the joint can be effectively corrected, such as foot drop, strephenopodia and strephexopodia, etc.

The weight of magnesium alloy is light, only a third of the weight of aluminum alloy.

It can be assembled as requirement and disassembled flexibly. It also can be dressed in a trouser. Therefore, it is convenient to wear and possible to wear in a long term, usually 6–12 months.

It is suitable for the patients whose normal motor pattern was basically set up after the motor pattern remodeling training. The weight of this kind of training device is light, but the bending strength is relatively poor so that it is suitable for the patients with self-training after leaving hospital, whose normal motor pattern was basically set up after the motor pattern remodeling training.

The differences between the training-type and household-type of movement pattern remodeling training devices are as follows: the training-type is used in the early-stage of the training and for the patients who just started to take the motor pattern remodeling training and whose abnormal motor pattern is relatively serious. High bending strength of double aluminum alloy bar is used. The whole structure is solid and the ability of supporting and restricting joint motion is strong so that it is suitable for recovery room of a hospital. It must be dressed outside the clothes. The household-type is a portable restriction device developed for maintaining the developed normal motor pattern and is suitable for the patients whose normal movement pattern is basically set up after motor pattern remodeling training. It also protects the patients from relapse in the process of self-training after leaving hospital. This type of training device use slightly poor bending strength of magnesium alloy bar whose weight is only a third of weight of the aluminum alloy bar. The whole weight is light, it can be dressed within the clothes and it is easy to wear. It also can be dressed for a long time, usually 6–12 months.

Besides, it can be divided into five types include double-limbs type, single-limb type, double-limbs of trunk, single-limb of trunk and local type according to the body part. It can be divided into children-type and adult-type according to the size. In order to lose weight and make it convenient to wear, the children-type is to the greatest extent made by magnesium alloy and thin layer of high-temperature thermoplasticized board.

The principles and structures of all kinds of types are basically the same, that is the abnormal angle and activities are restricted by the joint motion limiter and the restricting effects of the bars.

In brief, lower limbs motor pattern remodeling training device can effectively restrict the unnecessary joint motion in the lower limbs movement, it also can effectively remodel the normal motor pattern of the lower limbs training by this device on the basis of nervous potential development and movement procedure rebuilding training.

This paper is published on Chinese Medicine, 2013, 8(7):921–923.

4.3.3 The Design Principle and Clinical Verification of Limb Multifunctional Training Box

The training of limbs dyskinesia is lifelong. The functional training under the guidance of the therapist of the rehabilitation department in a hospital is relatively short. The more is self-training after leaving hospital. It requests not only a strong desire to rehabilitate and a strong willpower of the patients, but also require the correct training methods and the training devices. For this purpose, the author designed a training belt used for the training of every muscle and can be assembled into a box. It can be used to increase the muscle strength, maintain and increase the limbs function by combined the elastic force of the elastic belt with the application of Daoyin technique in traditional Chinese medicine. The training box is small and light and simple to use, makes it possible to use at any time in any place to achieve good effects.

4.3.3.1 Materials and Methods

Materials and Production

Six and eleven centimeter black or brown elastic belt sold in market is chosen and the tensile elongation elasticity is 2.4 times. The hip abduction resistance band is made of double layer and the others are all made of single layer. All of them are cut into elastic band that is 15 cm in length, and the two ends are linked by a black canvas whose width is the same as the elastic band. The nylon fastening tapes are fixed on the two ends of the canvas belt, respectively.

The training device for special parts and its production:

- Hip adductor training seat: an 11 cm depth stiff paper sponge can be chosen and is cut into a trapezoid block whose down base line is 22 cm, the top base line is 10 cm and the height is 18 cm. The two sides are cut into a concave shape, a corduroy soft cloth is enclosed.

- Wrist-hand training board: a wood board (30 cm × 15 cm × 1 cm) is chosen. The front of it is blunt and the shape is like a hand. Five set of rubber band that is linked with finger-stall is fixed on the front of edge after polished. A wrist flexion and extension training elastic belt is fixed on the location of metacarpophalangeal joints of the training board. A forearm fixing band is fixed on the location of wrist joint of the training board.
- Dorsiflexion of foot, strephexopodia training board: a wood board (30 cm × 25 cm × 2 cm) is chosen. A 10 cm groove is in the center of the front, clip the two sides of it and make them blunt and like shoe sole. Elastic belt is fixed on the two sides, 8 cm from the front edge, and the center groove after polished.

Shoulder abduction, elbow flection or extension, hip abduction, knee flection or extension, foot plantar flexion and special parts training board with operating instruction, video CD and guidance audio tape are packed for reservation.

Methods of Application

Choose the relevant training band according to the training parts and take training according to following steps after wear as required and fixation.

- Regulation of breathing: sit up and chest out, adjust your breath to stable.
- Regulation of the mind: relax your body and mind. In a state of tranquility, pay attention to the contralateral brain of the limbs which is going to be trained (pay attention to the left brain when training the right limbs and vice versa).
- Regulation of movement: The target point should be ascertained at first. For example, in the foot plantar flexion training, the target point of attention is anterior tibial muscle. Excitation pattern is adopted in order to take effort to contract anterior tibial muscle on the basis of regulation of breathing and mind to increase the angle of the foot plantar flexion as far as possible. Maintaining 6 s at the highest point you can reach, then breathe in deep and breathe out slowly, relax the mind to the greatest extent in order to relieve fatigue. The next training can be started after take a break and the same parts can be trained 6–8 times.

The training can be taken under the guidance of video or audio tape, and also can be taken with the help of families or caregiver.

The patients should take the training 30 min per time, two times per day, and should be kept on.

4.3.3.2 Indications, Contraindications and Cautions

Indications

The patients with limb dysfunction after CNS damages, such as the hemiplegic paralysis caused by cerebral hemorrhage, cerebral infarction, cerebral embolism and subarachnoid hemorrhage.

Incomplete paraplegia caused by spine injury.

The patients with decreased muscle strength and joint range of motion caused by osteoarticular muscle injury.

Children with cerebral palsy.

Muscle paralysis caused by peripheral nerve injury.

Contraindications

There are no obvious contraindications, but the patients with fracture and injuries of articular ligament, muscle tendon and muscle should take the training after the agreement of the in-charge physician.

Cautions

Before the self-training, the therapists should set an example to the patients on the basis of explanation of training mechanism and method of application to guarantee the correctness of the exercise. In addition, there are some cautions:

- The training should be done in a warm and quiet environment (indoor or outdoor) and the patients are required to concentrate.

- There are intervals for a certain time in the training. Increasing frequency too soon is not appropriate. Amount of training is enough when the patients sweat slightly and breathe smoothly. The patients can also do the training with the instruction of the video and audio tape.
- It is important to set a target point. During training, the patients try to pay attention to agonistic muscle of movable joint and feel the slight hotness of muscle contraction. Meanwhile, the patient should relax antagonistic muscle.

The training should be durable, but not intermittent.

4.3.3.3 Clinical Experiments

Materials and Methods

From June 2006 to February 2008, 52 patients with foot drop were all the inpatients in neurological rehabilitation training center in Beijing Tongren Hospital affiliated to Beijing's Capital Medical University. After 3 months' therapy, they left hospital. We chose 60 patients randomly. There were 30 patients using multi-functional training box in training group and there were 30 patients using self-training in control group. There were 21 males and 9 females in the training group. The age was 36–77 years old. The average age was 49.3 years old. The shortest medical history lasted 19 months and the longest lasted 59 months. The average was 40 months. There were 16 patients with hemiplegia after cerebral infarction, nine patients with hemiplegia after cerebral damages, two patients with hemiplegia after child cerebral palsy and three patients with foot drop after lumbar spine surgery. There were 19 males and 11 females in the control group. The age was 33–72 years old. The average age was 47.8 years old. The shortest medical history lasted 12 months and the longest lasted 60 months. The average was 42 months. There were 18 patients with hemiplegia after cerebral infarction, five patients with hemiplegia after cerebral damages and seven patients with foot drop after lumbar spine surgery.

Functional Assessment

Tibialis anterior muscle, Lovett MMT, range of motion of ankle joint, Fugl-Meyer of dorsiflexion of foot were used to assess the functions.

0: The patients cannot do dorsiflexion actively.

1: The patients can do dorsiflexion partially.

2: The patients can do dorsiflexion fully.

This criterion was used for functional assessment. T-test was used to analyze the data of functional assessment in hospital and out of hospital.

Results

Statistical analysis of three assessment indicators of training group demonstrated that there is no significant difference of Fugl-Meyer between discharge and three months later ($P > 0.05$) and there are significant differences of the other indicators between discharge and three months later ($P < 0.05$). There is no significant difference of all indicators between discharge and three months later ($P > 0.05$) in control group (Table 4.5). The results demonstrated that the patients in training group not only maintain function level 3 months later, but also improve it slightly. The function level of the patients in control group is decreased compared with that at the time of discharge.

Table 4.5 Functional assessment comparison table of training group and control group at the time of discharge and three months later $\bar{x} \pm s$

Assessment items	Group	Discharge	Three months later	p Value
Myodynamia	Training group	3.34 ± 0.65	4.06 ± 1.21	<0.05
	Control group	3.31 ± 0.47	3.36 ± 101	>0.05
Range of motion	Training group	18.23° ± 2.36°	19.43° ± 2.68°	<0.05
	Control group	16.12° ± 2.36°	16.47° ± 4.36°	>0.05
Fugl-Meyer	Training group	1.71 ± 0.50	1.82 ± 0.47	>0.05
	Control group	1.62 ± 0.50	1.70 ± 0.47	>0.05

Discussion

After CNS damages, rehabilitation of body limbs motor dysfunction takes a long time and most is the self-training post-discharge. Therefore, that how to use and exert the function of self-training play an important role in maintaining or promoting the effect of rehabilitation therapy, reducing family financial burden and improving daily life ability of the patients. However, family self-training is affected by many factors such as living space, training appliance, lack of instructions and improper methods so that it is difficult to do the training well. Family self-training mainly is simple walking, which is difficult to meet requirements and decreases functions. The foot drop of hemiplegic patients is one of the main obstacles that influence the patients' lower limbs motor function, which can lead to abnormal motor pattern of lower limbs. The patients in control group use voluntary walking as the main training pattern post-discharge. If the entire coordinated movement ability of lower limbs is not improved, there is foot drop to varying degrees in walking, which can affect normal gait.

Household equipment should be small, portable, easy to be operated, inexpensive and with good effect. Therefore, problems needed to be resolved that how to make the patients do correct self-rehabilitation training anytime and anywhere and how to improve enjoyment and effect.

Necrocytosis of axoneuron and destruction of conduction pathway are the root that can lead to dyskinesia of limbs after CNS damages. The key point of treatment is the functional recovery of axoneuron and conduction pathway. Because the axoneuron is unable to regenerate itself, the lost functions after central damages should be compensated by the normal cells around the injured area. The standby conduction pathway is activated to replace the functions (development and utilization of neural potentials) of injured cells, which is called neural potential development. Although the cells around injured area are the same as the injured cells, in normal condition, they cannot be used for life long. Only in special conditions, these cells can be used and exerted through special training. Therefore, there is potential ability of the neural tissues for injured CNS functions. The CNS contains great potentials that originate from numerous cells and synapses and is the basis of recovery of limbs motor functions through training after central damages. Therefore, development of neural potentials is the key of recovery of motor functions after central damages.

CNS potentials are the results of CNS plasticity and functional reorganization. However, the plasticity of nervous system is based on the "skillful use and dependence" principle, which means only active limbs movements can induce plasticity of motor cortex function and then improve the motor functions of limbs.

The question is that which kind of methods can quickly induce the potential of human body to compensate the lost functions. In normal life, people can overcome difficulties and hardships using willpower. In dangerous condition, people can get through the difficulties through bursting into extraordinary ability. In specified conditions, tough training can lead a person to be a superman, such as the training of special troops of liberation army. These examples showed that human potentials can be induced through dangerous conditions such as willpower, goal, stimulus, misfortune, disaster and accident. These factors can promote the development of human potentials. The human potentials mainly are CNS potentials, because all the muscles are dominated by CNS. However, patients with hemiplegia and brain paralysis always have serious protopathy, such as hypertension, diabetes and heart disease. Therefore, under imminent danger, train may worsen the condition. Obviously, under imminent danger, the potentials development training cannot simply be employed in the rehabilitation of patients with central lesion.

Regulation of movements based on regulation of mind and regulation of breathing is the basic technique of Daoyin technique in traditional Chinese medicine. The speech in Daoyin technique is able to enlighten and motivate human willpower commendably, which construct a safe "imminent danger" condition for functional rehabilitation. In modern opinion, the patients are instructed to concentrate to complete a designed movement and during this the therapists use

Daoyin speech to create a condition of imminent danger, such as "Stand up, or you will fall down", "Hold up your body or you will crash" and so on.

Daoyin technique in ancient traditional Chinese medicine has a long history. According to *Mister Lv's Spring and Autumn Annals,* in ancients time, people used dancing to prevent diseases and keep fit. Until 610 B.C., Chao Yuanfang in Sui Dynasty compiled *General Treatise on the Cause and Symptoms of Diseases* and systematically listed about 300 kinds of Daoyin techniques. There are 20 kinds of them that are used to treat hemiplegia. In 1973, in Changsha City of Hunan Province painting on silk Daoyin pictures from Mawangdui tomb 3 draw 44 Daoyin pictures with color, which reflect the diversity of Daoyin technique. From the origination, Chinese medicine rehabilitation therapy has close connection with Chinese traditional culture. Especially in the inheritance, the various factions summarized, replenished and developed it. The theory is extensive and profound, but inescapably mysterious, which is lack of definite concept. The principles are subjective abstract. Therefore, the application of Chinese medicine rehabilitation therapy is under restrictions. In addition, there is no objective indicator in the therapy and it is difficulty to be proved in basic research for application. Therefore, it is hard to be promoted in clinical rehabilitation. Modernization of Daoyin technique can promote renaissance of this technique. Six-step improvement Daoyin technique in traditional Chinese medicine is an attempt in this way.

Rehabilitation training is like other physical training. Definite quantitative index is very important for improving training effect. For example, a high jumper practices high jump without cross-bar elevation. It is hard for him to increase the altitude of the jump. The cross-bar is the indicator of new jump altitude on the basis of training achievement in last jump. In order to jump over the new altitude, the high jumper needs to adjust mood, run-up speed, take-off distance, ground force and throw-over gesture to develop jump potential adequately. Then the jump altitude will be increased gradually.

Elastic recoil of elastic bandage of multi-functional training box is exerted on the movement orientation of agonistic muscle that induce joint motion, which make the agonistic muscle to find the orientation easily. Therefore, it is easy for the induction of spontaneous movement of agonistic muscle under the action of Daoyin technique in traditional Chinese medicine. Elastic recoil of elastic bandage is directly proportion to stretched length (from zero to infinity), so that it can be used for most patients. Elastic recoil of elastic bandage in training methods keep on the point of maximal force for six seconds, which is the quantitative index of time and is good for neural nerve potential development. And then through promoting central nerves plasticity, functional reorganization can be achieved and motor function is recovered finally. For example, training plate of dorsiflexion of foot is used to do dorsiflexion of foot training. Through anti-resistance of elastic force on the orientation of dorsiflexion of foot, myodynamia of tibialis anterior muscle and autonomous movement degree can be increased, which is good for promoting the entire motor function of lower limbs.

Multi-functional training box of body limbs can be fully used by the patients in their spare time in or out of the hospital to help them recover. It is easy to be operated and portable. The patients can do specific training with the instruction of video with light music and audio tape, which can provide a good training condition and atmosphere. Persevering correct training can maintain and improve rehabilitation training effect.

4.3.4 Development and Clinical Verifications of Controlled-Release Force Ankle-Foot Orthosis

We usually see foot drop in clinic, which is an important factor to form abnormal motor pattern of lower limbs and affects the lower limbs function of the patients greatly.

Foot drop is usually induced by innervation of tibialis anterior muscle after coma, central nerve injury and peripheral nerve injury. If it is handled improperly, for a long time, spasm of musculus gastrocnemius and Achilles's tendon and fibrous adhesion of ankle joint affect the body limbs function and rehabilitation training of the patients. Surgical Correction can be given to severe patients. For the patients with conscious dysfunction, the surgery is doubted and then abandoned. Severe foot drop make it difficult for rehabilitation training and cause severe complications, even lead to life danger. The patients can lose hope for functional recovery. It is a problem in clinic need to be solved. According to the principle "small and sustained traction", developed controlled-release orthotics can help to solve the problem.

4.3.4.1 Materials and Manufacture Method

Materials

Macromolecule fibrous material and high temperature thermoplastic plate produced by Nanjing Shuang Wei Biomedicine Science and Technology Ltd. are used. The characteristics of macromolecule fibrous material are that before solidification it is as soft as mud, can adapt to the model and is easy to forming. After solidification it is air permeable, light, strong but pliable in texture, which doesn't affect X-ray examination and is comfortable to dress.

Manufacture of Controlled-Release Orthotics

For semi-finished product of macromolecule fibrous material modeling, ankle functional position orthotics materials are used. We open the packaging bag, take macromolecule fibrous material plate out, put it into room temperature water for six seconds, flatten it, cover it on ankle and shank of the patients, wrap it with pressure and fix it for 6 min. When macromolecule fibrous material is modelled, the therapists take it down, cut the edge, make the altitude of the edge of the shank is equal to that of vertical plane projection of tibia crista. The therapists cut a wedge-shape part in the rotation center of ankle joint in both sides, use it as axis and make it mobile like hinge. The outside of foot is tipped for 2 cm and the inside of the foot encases longitudinal arch. And then it is polished. The therapists punch a hole in the shank and ankle, use hollow rivet to fix fixing band and paste lamella artificial limb sponge slice onto the inner face of the modeled brace. During fitting, the technicians select proper elastic traction band. One end of the band is fixed on the toe part of the brace and the other is linked to upper end of shank through the front of tibia. The length of elastic band is adjustable. The traction of elastic band can increase the angle of dorsiflexion of foot gradually.

Structure and Function

Controlled-release force ankle-foot orthosis includes two parts. The main part is mobile ankle-foot orthosis of ankle joint according to foot and shank shape of the patients. Its function is to fix shank and pelma and generate dorsiflexion of ankle joint through exogenous process at the same time. The other is controlled-release force traction part, which means that elastic band is used to link toe to tibialis anterior. Small and sustained traction is produced by retractive force of elastic band to stretch contracture tendon and muscle in order to relax adhesive joint.

4.3.4.2 Clinical Verifications

Clinical Data

From July 2004 to February 2007, we produced 22 controlled-release force ankle-foot orthosis. The users are all the inpatients with foot drop. There are 18 males and four females. There are 13 patients with low conscious state and nine patients with spinal cord injury. Passive movement of ankle joint is restricted ($3.54° \pm 1.63°$). The average fixed angle of plantar flexion (minimum plantar flexion angle of passive movement of ankle joint) is $44.91° \pm 5.35°$. the patients cannot do the training in standing position.

Results

Controlled-release force ankle-foot orthosis is used to treat the patients for four weeks. The average range of passive movement of ankle joint is $28.09° \pm 9.26°$. There are 16 patients

Table 4.6 Data comparison of fixed angle of plantar flexion and range of passive movement of ankle joint before and after rectification ($\bar{X} \pm S$)

Items	Case number	Before rectification	After rectification
Fixed angle of plantar flexion	22	44.91° ± 5.35°	17.59° ± 10.04°*
Range of passive movement of ankle joint	22	3.54° ± 1.63°	28.09 ± 9.26°*

*$P < 0.05$

whose range of passive movement of ankle joint is equal to or more than 32.5°. The average fixed angle of plantar flexion is recovered to 17.59° ± 10.04°. There are four patients with 25° plantar flexion and foot drop, but they can do standing bed training. There is no improvement in two patients with severe tendon spasm and ankle joint adhesion.

T-test of SPSS12.0 software package is used to analyze data of fixed angle of plantar flexion and range of passive movement of ankle joint before and after rectification. There is significant difference in data comparison ($P < 0.05$), which can be referred to Table 4.6. The results demonstrated that Controlled-release force ankle-foot orthosis has an rectification effect on foot drop with spasm of musculus gastrocnemius and tendon and fibrous adhesion of ankle joint.

Controlled-release force ankle-foot orthosis made of macromolecule fibrous material has good air permeability and better adaptation for body limbs, which is easy to dress. There is no bruising in all patients. Small and sustained traction is produced by retractive force of elastic band to stretch contracture tendon and muscle in order to relax adhesive joint.

Clinical Indications, Contraindications and Cautions

- Indications: It is appropriate for the patients with foot drop induced by various reasons, especially with spasm of musculus gastrocnemius and tendon and fibrous adhesion of ankle joint.
- Contraindications:

  The patients with foot drop induced by scar contracture after deep burn of shank, foot and ankle.

  The patients with severe spasm of musculus gastrocnemius and tendon and no movement in passive movement of ankle joint.

  The ankle joints with fibrous ankyloses or bony ankyloses.

  The patients with ulcer of foot and ankle, lower limbs phlebothrombosis and severe varicosity
- Cautions: Partial bruising should be avoided in the training. Because body feeling of the patients is not good or is none, the condition should be observed carefully. In the first 3 days, every 2 h the therapists undress the orthotics to check if there is red and swollen and bruising. If there is no bruising, the orthotics can be dressed day and night.

Discussion

Foot drop is the common cause to induce abnormal motor pattern of lower limbs, which is usually in the patients with coma, low conscious state, central nerve injury, peripheral nerve injury. Because of innervation of tibialis anterior muscle and spasm of musculus gastrocnemius, plantar flexion of ankle joint lead to foot drop. In clinic, if there is no rehabilitation consciousness and no good limb position and passive joint motion, spasm of musculus gastrocnemius and tendon and fibrous adhesion of ankle joint can be induced after a long time. Therefore, unrectified foot drop is closely related to braking and apraxia of body limbs [1]. In the early stage of foot drop formation, through passive joint motion, spasm of musculus gastrocnemius and tendon can be stretched and adhesive ankle joint can be relaxed. And then orthotics is kept on the functional position. If the rectification opportunity in the early stage is lost, foot drop that can be alleviated can be turned into an implacable disease gradually, which bring about difficulty to rehabilitation therapy and affect the patients' standing, gait and walking ability training greatly [2, 3].

For foot drop with severe spasm of musculus gastrocnemius and tendon, fibrous and bony ankyloses, it is correct to be treated with surgery. For foot drop with passive joint motion, it is careful to be treated with surgery. For the foot drop in the patients with coma and low conscious state, it is inappropriate to be treated with surgery because there are no indications. However, because of extreme plantar flexion of ankle joint, the patients cannot do standing training and are forced to lie in bed for a long time, which can easily induce severe complications of respiratory, urinary, cardiovascular, digestive system, even death. At present, there is no rectification therapy report about this kind of foot drop. Although there are many kinds of ankle-foot orthosis at home and abroad, there is no report about controlled-release force ankle-foot orthosis [4, 5].

The author found that during the process of pulling rubber band, the stretched length in slow traction is more than the stretched length in quick traction. This phenomenon enlightened the author. Large traction of foot drop can induce bruising and make it difficult to relax spasm of musculus gastrocnemius and tendon. Retractive force of elastic band of controlled-release force ankle-foot orthosis and hinge in ankle-foot joint are used. Elastic band pull the pelma of orthosis and increase dorsiflexion angle of ankle joint gradually. Through small and sustained traction, spasm of musculus gastrocnemius and tendon and fibrous adhesive ankle joint can be stretched progressively, range of activity of ankle joint is increased, foot drop is rectified under micro damage condition without muscle spasm response, which create conditions for decreasing complications, promoting functional recovery such as rehabilitation training in standing position and rectification of abnormal motor pattern.

In a similar way, this kind of orthotics can also be used for rectification of other joints such as controlled-release force orthosis of knee joint, shoulder joint, elbow joint and wrist joint, which obtain good effect.

Controlled-release force ankle-foot orthosis can also be made of high temperature thermoplastic plate. The characteristic of high temperature thermoplastic plate can become soft under the temperature of 180 °C. After modeling, it is surface smoothing, good toughness, high strength and can be repeatedly heated to modify. However, the process is complicated with high temperature thermoplastic plate. At first, gypsum model is prepared, which requires plate heater. Because of the material without breathability, punch a hole for breathability is necessary. It is heavy and is uncomfortable to wear. Medium high temperature thermoplastic plate is selected and heated (180 °C) in plate heater for 10 min. After the plate is soft, it is pasted on the gypsum model and the space is drained to vacuum so that it is pasted to gypsum model completely. After solidification, take it down. The rest procedures are the same as the manufacture method of using macromolecule fibrous materials.

References

1. Tong W, Yong Z, Tao L, et al. An analysis of the effect of ankle foot orthosis on the function of lower extremity of foot. Theory Pract Chin Rehabil. 2004;19(1):30–1.
2. Hongtu W, Dongfeng H, Peng L, et al. AFO early intervention for cerebral apoplexy patients daily life activities ability and the quality of survival. Chin J Phys Med Rehabil. 2007;29(1):41–4.
3. Nan Y, Shui W, Ling L, et al. The production and application of dynamic ankle orthotics in adult hemiplegia patients. J Chin Phys Med Rehabil. 2002;24(4):232–4.
4. Lin S, Shumei Z, Jiading Z, et al. Improvement and application of ankle foot orthotics. Chin Rehabil Magazine. 2005;20(1):64–5.
5. Dawei Z, Jiankun Y. Effect of fixed ankle foot orthotics on lower limbs. Chin J Rehabil Med. 2006;21(9):829–31.

5 Training Method and Equipment of Virtual Neurological Training

5.1 The Mechanism and Significance of Virtual Training Methods

5.1.1 The Generation of Ideas of Virtual Neurological Training

The training methods of rehabilitation technique of neurological training mainly include neural potential development, motor program reestablishment and motor pattern remodeling, which can promote CNS plasticity and functional reorganization. These methods can recover motor function after CNS damages through clinical verification.

However, the training effect of rehabilitation methods of neurological training not only is related to the correctness of diagnosis and therapy scheme, but also is closely related to many factors.

1. It is related to degree of accuracy of the proficiency and implementation method of the therapists to this technique. The therapist should know the mechanism of recovering motor function after CNS damages well. The therapist must accept the important role and mechanism of neural potential development, motor program reestablishment and motor pattern remodeling, as well as the correct application of these methods. Because only actual therapists can really know the mechanism of these methods and remind of the concept of motor program usually. Daoyin technique in traditional Chinese medicine is used to guide the patients to try to complete designed movement and exert the role of these methods fully.
2. It is related to degree of encourage and correct instruction of the therapists. In the process of regulation of mind and breathing, the patients are required to enter into meditation “concentration without distracting thoughts”, which is called immersion. The patients can totally immerse in the surrounding and the method plays a role of clearing and activating the channels and collaterals. In the fourth step (stimulation) and fifth step (insistence) of six-step Daoyin technique, the therapists are required to increase tone and intensity and create a safe state of emergency by speech. In these processes, the therapists should be full of passion and encourage the patients to achieve the anticipated goal constantly. To some extent, the higher the therapists’ passion is, the bigger the activated willpower of the patients to overcome difficulties is, the better the training effect is. The passion is proportion to effect.
3. It is related to degree of understanding of the patients to rehabilitation methods of neurological training. Daoyin technique is the technique to guide the patients to play a role

W. Zhao, *Rehabilitation Therapeutics of the Neurological Training*,
https://doi.org/10.1007/978-981-13-0812-3_5

by themselves. In order to achieve this goal, the patients must know the mechanism of this method thoroughly. The therapists are required not only to understand and know the mechanism of the method correctly, and also use comprehensible and popular words to explain to the patients repeatedly. Therefore, there are cognitive disorder and recession of comprehensive ability and memory ability to varying degrees in many patients. In every therapy, the therapists are required to explain the training mechanism to the patients clearly and concisely in order to make the patients understand the mechanism thoroughly and obtain better training effect.

4. It is related to the progress of training effect. Because of the influence of the degree of species evolution, recovering motor function after CNS damages takes a long time, which is a long-term slow rehabilitation process. Therefore, the premise of training effect is long-term rehabilitation training. The premise of long-term rehabilitation training is the confidence of the patients and their families on rehabilitation method. The confidence come from the expectation of functional recovery and the effect of actual rehabilitation training, especially for the obsolete cases that the functions cannot be improved by rehabilitation training. The therapists should make the patients and their families to see the effect of rehabilitation training as soon as possible in order to increase the confidence of the patients and their families on rehabilitation method training, which is the most direct and credible measure to improve the effect of rehabilitation training. Therefore, before rehabilitation training, through detailed functional assessments, the therapist can find out the main obstacle that restrict the function and do interest training, which can make quick progress and is good for the confidence, understanding of rehabilitation method and the confidence for continued rehabilitation.

In the realistic clinical rehabilitation training, the author found that it is difficult to achieve the requirements mentioned above. The common influence factors are as follows:

1. The therapists cannot implement rehabilitation training method correctly because of fatigue. Labour intensity of rehabilitation training is big, especially rehabilitation training of neurological training, because the training is all active movement. At the moment of exerting proper resistance, the patients are guided to do a series of training for development of neural potential through anti-resistance joint motion. Especially the potential development training of upper limbs, lower limbs and trunk, the training should be done when the patients have no autonomic movement. Although the patients can lose weight through weight support equipment, auxiliary force of the therapists is 30–60 kg when they do compulsive and auxiliary active movement for the patients. One therapist treats 6–8 patients every day. They word 22–24 days for 1 month. In the weekend, they should guide the patients to do the training. They are very tired and the fatigue can influence the implementation of rehabilitation method.
2. Repeated explanation of the methods and the encouraging words of the therapists cannot be persisted. Explanation of the methods and the encouraging words can be achieved through speeches, which requires a therapist who trains several patients to keep high passion and explain to the patients tirelessly. It is difficult to achieve this. Because of fatigue, the therapist cannot guide the patients with passion or explain the mechanism to the patients clearly and the training effect is influenced.
3. Limited to the individual level of the therapists, it is hard to implement Daoyin technique correctly. Daoyin technique, especially six-step Daoyin technique of guiding the collaterals through meridians, the implementation should be in accordance with main and collateral channels, which brings about some difficulties to the training. There are two reasons. The first is that the rehabilitation doctor and the therapists graduated from western

medicine who are not familiar with main and collateral channels. The second is that disciplinary patients even don't know main and collateral channels, which brings about great difficulties to six-step Daoyin technique of guiding the collaterals through meridians. The patients think guiding the collaterals through meridians is entirely imaginary and unrealistic. Therefore, it is difficult to be implemented correctly, even the patients object to or refuse to do the training.

4. It is difficult to improve the therapy day by day and is easy to affect the therapy effect through influencing the patients' emotion. The improve of neural function is very slow, which is in accordance with the "all or none" law. When the training reach a certain level, corresponding function movement appear. If the function movement is not recovered, there is no obvious manifestation in motor function, which is called plateau period. However, if the patients continue training in this period, the accumulation of minor functions can lead to visible function movement. If the therapy is stopped, all their previous efforts are wasted. Neurological training equipment is an equipment that can receive motor program signal and display it real-timely. Its characteristic is to know real-time change of motor program signal, provide scientific basis for the establishment of the therapy schedule and set a surpassing goal for the patients. However, on the other hand, in the plateau period, there is no change of motor program signal for a longer time and the patients usually think that the training effect is halted and they may easily lose confidence to rehabilitation training because the patients can see the actual data.
5. The sensitivity of bio-electricity signal detecting system is strong and it is easy to be influenced by the environment. Another question of reality is that the signal should be amplified through amplification system after signal filtration and can be displayed in a smooth curve because the signal form CNS to muscle is very weak. Therefore, the sensitivity of signal reception equipment is high, which is easily disturbed by the surrounding and condition. These require medical ground electrode deeply buried under ground and copper wire mesh shield. Even so, the signal can still be affected by other signal source such as passing vehicle, strong phone signal and shake of signal conductor, even the position of the host machine in the training room, conductivity of skin electrode and scurf on skin surface. In many cases, because of the instability of signal baseline, it is hard to continue the training.

In order to solve the problems mentioned above, the therapists should study a method not only to implement rehabilitation methods of neurological training correctly in order to reflect the mechanism of rehabilitation methods of neurological training thoroughly, but also to alleviate labor intensity of the therapists. The patients can see the progress of the therapy and keep confidence of rehabilitation. Not only the patients can do rehabilitation training with a purpose, but also the patients can master the method and do the training with encouragement form the therapists. Not only it is good for the correct implementation of Daoyin technique, but also the patients can feel Qi in the main and collateral channels.

Therefore, the idea of investigating training system of virtual reality of neurological training is created. Through modern computer technology, virtuality, simulation, animation explanation, six-step Daoyin technique record guide and actual development method of neural potential, the actual problems of rehabilitation training can be solved in order to improve the effect of rehabilitation therapy and increase the understanding of the patients to the mechanism of the method, which can also alleviate labor intensity of the therapists.

5.1.2 Background of Related Techniques: Virtual Reality

5.1.2.1 Introduction to Virtual Reality

Virtual reality [1] (VR) is developed in 1960s. it is a virtual environment that imitate real object with computer and through multiple sensors, the users are put into this virtual environment to realize the natural interaction between users and virtual environment. The characteristics of VR technique are immersion, interaction and imagination. Immersion is the ability that VR system can see, hear, smell, touch, taste and so on, which can make users break away from external environment and immerse into virtual environment created by computer. Interaction is that users interact with various objects in virtual environment to make users immersive. Therefore, interaction is the key factor of man-machine harmony. Imagination is that through imagination virtual movement can generate real effect. For example, when VR technique is used to do surgery and the skin or muscle tissues are cut off by virtual scalpel, the manipulator can have the real feeling of tissue response.

General virtual reality system is composed of professional graphic processing computer, application software system, input equipment and display equipment. Through the information channel such as vision, audio, and touch, people can feel the senior user interface of designer' idea. The assisted hardware includes sensors such as helmet mounted display, data glove, three-dimensional eYes, data clothes. The feedback channel can be established through mouse and keyboard. At present, the most widely used is Helmet mounted Display. VR systems software is the key to realize VR technique. The application of VR technique in rehabilitation medicine is introduced in this chapter.

5.1.2.2 Current Situation of Rehabilitation Therapy at Home and Abroad

At present, rehabilitation therapy at home and abroad is mainly the therapists' manipulation, or manipulation assisted by some simple equipment. Through passive movement, auxiliary movement, active movement and anti-resistance movement, the motor function of muscle is recovered. Because of boundedness of existing rehabilitation instruments, it is unable to combine functional assessment, exercise therapy and psychotherapy together organically. Especially, the psychotherapy cannot run through rehabilitation therapy from beginning to end. In the traditional exercise therapy, the patients are in a passive position. The repeated and boring manipulations in the training can induce boredom of the patients, which is bad for the continue and in-depth of the therapy and affect training effect greatly.

However, virtual reality technique can figure out the problems mentioned above in rehabilitation therapy. Through virtual reality technique, functional assessments, specific therapy and mental regulation in rehabilitation therapy are closely combined together. Music, picture and voice prompt are used to increase training pleasure and improve therapeutic effect.

5.1.2.3 The Application of VR Technique in Limbs Motor Function Rehabilitation

VR technique provides a carefree environment associated with real life for the patients with stroke to promote the therapeutic interest of the patients in order to improve training effect. For example, the training of hand function, in the virtual environment, the patients can move, grab, grasp or put virtual object, take part in the environment, interact with computer actively, and receive the feedback information of vision, audio, touch and smell in their own operation real-timely. The patients can regulate themselves according to the feedback information to enhance the flexibility of finger movement in order to promote the generation of separation movement. VR technique is applied for gait training and balance function training. At present, researchers form Israeli developed a set of "computer-assisted rehabilitation environment system". Through simulation of boating, playing balls, jogging and so on can help the patients to improve balance capacity and recover body motor function. Novel training mode with abundant videos can make the training of the patients become easy like a game and motivate the enthusiasm of the patients fully.

5.1.2.4 The Application of VR Technique in Cognitive Training

With the development of computer technology, computer is combined with cognitive rehabilitation from theoretical research to development and application of products, especially the appearance of virtual reality. The higher combination of computer technology and cognitive science is promoted. Virtual reality technique is used to study rehabilitation medicine for many years in America. In the cognitive rehabilitation, they accumulate rich experience and develop various special VR techniques for different kinds of cognitive disorder (memory dysfunction, spatial cognitive disorder, disturbance of thought and so on).

The advantages of VR rehabilitation technique compared with traditional training method:

1. Various kinds and safe training: It can provide various virtual therapy scenes for the patients to do rehabilitation training in a safe environment.
2. Specific designed training items: According to the practical situation of the patients, VR system can design specific therapy process with the same scene and mission.
3. Feedback function: Through sensing equipment of various mode, VR system can master the state and effect of the patients for information feedback and data storage. The physician can master the illness of the patients.
4. Training with a purpose: The training can be done with a purpose. The training is scientific and interesting and the training time is short with more obvious training effect. There is superiority for rehabilitation of group disability induced by war, severe disabled accident and natural disaster.

5.1.2.5 The Application of VR Technique in Psychological Rehabilitation

It is generally acknowledged the application of virtual reality in psychological rehabilitation is started from 1993. At present, this technique is used for anxiety disorder, posttraumatic stress disorder, eating disorder and relieving pain. Virtual reality technique is used to treat anxiety disorder at the earliest, especially for acrophobia, aerodromophobia and agoraphobia. In 1995, Rothbaum treated 20 patients with acrophobia for 7 weeks. Our results demonstrated that compared with control group, the anxiety, avoidance, depression and other symptoms of virtual reality group are obviously alleviated. The view to altitude is more positive. This experiment demonstrated for the first time that virtual reality therapy can change human behavior in real world. After America's 911, the therapy of posttraumatic stress disorder attracted a wide spread attention. Difede and Hoffman used virtual reality technique to recreate the explode scene of World Trade Center Building. They let a patient who the traditional exposure therapy has no effect on enter into virtual explode scene again with vivid sound, the people from building to the street, collapsed building and towering smoke. Finally, the patient is cured.

Through virtual reality technique, the training is done and psychotherapy is developed and promoted. Because the therapy of the patients is controlled by the computer, the training to varying degrees can be done through different pathways. At the moment of treatment, all kinds of parameters such as physiological signal of the patients are collected constantly. Through analysis and regulation, VR system can make a decision according to the specific situation of individuals and provide different feedback information automatically such as encourage, implication and suggestion. Through these feedback information, the therapists can help the patients to adjust therapy mode timely. According to different scenery pictures and music generated from these signals, the patients do the training in a carefree environment to relax anxious mood and increase training interest and therapeutic effect.

5.1.2.6 Virtual Training Machine

There are many VR training systems of this kind, which is widely used in rehabilitation medicine. At present, the relatively mature is used for rehabilitation training of bone surgery and orthopedic surgery. Although the principle is based on traditional rehabilitation theory, it is totally different from traditional training pattern. Virtual training machine is intelligent, scientific and interesting. The patients can receive therapy and rehabilitation in an environment close to nature. Virtual reality exercise bicycle developed in Tsinghua University for rehabilitation and posture balance control training system made in Korea belong to this kind of virtual training machine.

5.1.2.7 Prospect

VR technique is already used in rehabilitation training and the development prospect is better. However, the application of this technique in rehabilitation medicine is in the primary stage. There are some problems need to be solved. For example, the display equipment cannot receive high-quality and verisimilar medical image splendidly. In complicated environment, the real-time performance and generating velocity need to be improved. Importantly, the rehabilitation method is in accordance with the principle of recovering motor function or not, especially the mechanism of recovering lost motor function after CNS damages. With the development of computer, multimedia technology, sensor technology and communication technology, this technique may be modified, improved and developed, which may be widely used in rehabilitation medicine.

5.1.2.8 The Assessment of VR Technique

Although there is certain therapeutic effect in rehabilitation training with VR technique in some reports, this technique is the real reflection of actual movement. For example, video equipment is used to record some joint motion or limbs movement and these movements can be displayed in the computer screen in synchrony so that the patients can see their own movement. The main function of this method is to increase the feeling of freshness of the patients, because they seldom see their own movement from the screen. The patients feel curious and the fun of the training is increased. However, the function of this method is the same as that the patients see joint motion directly. If the joint can be moved, VR technique can be used to see joint motion displayed in screen. If the joint cannot be moved, VR technique can be used to see that there is no joint motion displayed in screen. However, the current situation is that the patients need rehabilitation training, especially for the patients with motor dysfunction after CNS damages who has no obvious joint motion or has abnormal motor pattern. For these patients, a series of methods are required to recover the joint motion of the patients, while only VR technique cannot solve the problem. Scenario simulation is added to display the actual joint movement in VR technique, which is lack of the training effect guided by training method. It is different from psychotherapy and it can simulate the scene of America's 911 through virtual reality technique. People with anxiety duo to America's 911 can place themselves into the virtual explode scene again to alleviate anxiety through repeated emergence.

This is why there is a notion in rehabilitation medicine engineering that the patients can be recovered after development of rehabilitation equipment. Actually, rehabilitation equipment can assure the correct implementation of rehabilitation method to make full use of the method. The rehabilitation is from rehabilitation theory, but it is the method of research and development of equipment that is based on theory and its purpose is method implementation, which cannot achieve good effect usually. Only the combining rehabilitation medicine engineering and clinical rehabilitation medicine, rehabilitation equipment is the correct research and development way and is with actual therapy value, according to clinical actual demand.

5.1.3 Research Purpose and Meaning of Virtual Neurological Training System

1. Purpose: Modern virtual and simulation technique are used to develop a kind of mechanism and method that is in accordance with neural potential development and motor program reestablishment, which can provide virtual reality motor dysfunction and simulation motor program feedback signal. The machine can explain mechanism and methods and guide the patients with Daoyin speech. It also can simulate main and collateral channels in human body, promote the understanding of the patients to therapy method, alleviate labor intensity of the therapists, and reduce the instrument interference and environment restriction. The standardization of rehabilitation training of neurological training can improve training effect and make use of the widely used rehabilitation methods of

neurological training and the replacement training system of the equipment.

2. Meaning: According to rehabilitation training method of neurological training, virtual reality training system of neurological training use virtual reality motor dysfunction, simulation of motor program feedback signal, automatic Daoyin technique speech guidance and mechanism explanation to give the patients actual anti-resistance training. The training system is synthesized from the anti-resistance of the therapists. The development of this system is to overcome many defects in rehabilitation training of neurological training such as incorrect application of methods, inability of passional guidance and encourage of the therapists, lost enthusiasm of the patients due to misunderstanding of the mechanism of the method and the interference of signal detection equipment. Meanwhile, because the computer software can produce many kinds of motor program signals with music, the training is enriched and the boring training is avoided. Especially, the computer software is used to establish animation light spot automatic tracking display system of main and collateral channels pathway to make patients do the training correctly according to main and collateral channels pathway and promote the process of standardization of neurological training. It is the precedent of computerization of rehabilitation training of neurological training, which is meaningful for training effect, popularization and application of this technique.

5.2 Composition and Training Method of Virtual Neurological Training System

5.2.1 The Composition of Virtual Neurological Training System

5.2.1.1 The Composition of Virtual Neurological Training System

1. Virtual animation and dubbing: animation dubbing technique is used to explain the mechanism of motor dysfunction after CNS damages recovery of motor function.
   (a) Anatomy and basic functions of CNS: What is motor program signal and how to dominate and control general movement?
   (b) CNS cells are lack of regeneration ability, but through neural potential development is reserved cells and conduction pathways are activated to replace injured cells and conduction pathways. Through reestablishment training of motor program, the lost motor function can be recovered.
   (c) Active movement, willpower and state of emergency are the condition to develop neural potential. Six-step Daoyin technique in traditional Chinese medicine can guide the patients through creating safe state of emergency and active movement, which is a better method to develop neural potential.
   (d) The archers practice archery only toward bull's eye, which can improve the degree of accuracy. Through simulation of different intensity and proportional motor program signal curve in various joint motion, the training can be used to develop neural potential and reestablish motor program.
   (e) Human body animation imitates main and collateral channels pathway. Six step of guiding collaterals through meridians is used for speech guidance. Animation light spot flicker guides Qi to acupoint, main and collateral channels, which covers twelve main and collateral channels and all joint motion.
2. Simulation parts of motor program signal: it is necessary to know definite movement defects and imitate normal movement goal.
   (a) The therapists use video to know actual motor dysfunction. According to the fact that people are not familiar with their own voice and motor pattern, through camera, the joint motion of the patients with motor dysfunction is displayed on fluorescent screen.
   (b) Simulation of normal joint motion and establishment of therapy task and goal: The patients are guided to do the same movement in the same joint of the unjured

side to find movement difference in injure side and establish training goal and specific mission.

(c) Video simulation and virtual animation are used to explain the task, goal and mechanism of this therapy. Through simulation video of normal motor pattern in the same joint with explanation record, the therapists explain training mission and goal to the patients clearly. Through simulation animation, the therapist explain the mechanism of neural potential development, motor program reestablishment training and recovery of joint motor function.

(d) Simulation of motor program signal and setting of an surpassing goal: Animation technology is applied to imitate motor program of joint motion, which includes single line and double line. From zero to 640 μV, there 6–8 levels to be completed. If there are eight levels, they are 0, 10, 20, 40, 100, 200, 400 and 640 μV. After the 10 μV training is completed, pink line that stand for 10 μV is displayed in the screen of 20 μV and the patients are required to use this as the virtual goal. The patients try to make virtual blue line surpass the altitude of pink line. The rest can be done in the same manner and CNS potential is developed and utilized in this process constantly.

3. Active movement and anti-resistance training with actual guidance: according to animation light spot automatic tracking display system of main and collateral channels pathway, dubbing of six-step Daoyin technique, joint motions such as elbow extension or flexion, actual movement ability, the therapists select corresponding intensity virtual motor program signal. After starting animation video, according to dubbing tempo, when it reaches the summit of analog signal curve, the therapists exert resistance in the orientation of joint motion to make the patients find the way of the signal easily. Through anti-resistance training, neural potential development is further promoted. Background music can be selected according to the patients' affection. Slow, relaxed or passion music is used to activate therapy atmosphere and encourage the patients' passion to take part in the training actively.

4. Software operation interface of virtual neurological training system is as follows:

(a) Icon: Virtual reality training system of neurological training on the computer screen is opened and the icon is Wenru brand (square, colour). Clicking this icon, entering into the home page and then virtual reality training system of neurological training is displayed in the screen.

(b) Items selection: The therapists operate in this page. Clicking home page and enter into the page of items selection, which is the operation page of the therapists. In the double-screen display computer, the page is existing from beginning to end. The therapists fill the therapy items and press "Enter". The screen will show the selected therapy contents. In single screen display computer, the therapists select the item and press "Enter". The screen will show the selected therapy contents. The detailed information in this page are as follows:

The patients: ____ Age: ____ Gender: ____ Admission number: ____
Diagnosis: ____ Onset date of illness: ____ Year ____ Month ____ Day ____
Therapy date: ____ Year ____ Month ____ Day ____
Background music: Yes ____ No (click Yes and there are many kinds of musics, select one and press "Enter")
Mechanism demonstration: Yes ____ No ____ Therapy items: (kinds in appendix)
Selection of therapy state: sound ____ silence
Signal prediction: Yes ____ No (Through pressure sensor, the patients can feel real flection of their own movement)
Therapy demonstration: Yes ____ No (click Yes and then enter into therapy items filling page and fill the animation demonstration type; Click No and then enter into data selection)
Therapy data selection (μV)
Agonistic muscle ____ Antagonistic muscle ____
Processing of results: ____ Save ____ Pass ____ Quit

Instructions: Mechanism demonstration—click Yes, the screen will show the mechanism demonstration animation. If the therapists don't click Yes, the page will go to therapy items selection. Click Yes, the screen will show the mechanism demonstration animation. If the therapists don't click Yes, the page will pass.

Video accompanying sound selection: Click sound and there is accompanying sound instruction. Click silence ans there is no accompanying sound instruction.

Therapy items selection: the therapists establish database of various parts such as face, upper limbs, trunk and lower limbs, various joint motions such as elbow extension, wrist flexion and dorsiflexion of foot and mechanism demonstration and store them separately. Vista software management platform is used and according to therapeutic requirements, the therapists can select it in items selection page and activate it autonomically.

Therapy items column: click therapy items or fill it directly and then enter into items selection page: Face, trunk, shoulders, upper limbs and lower limbs, swallowing, diaphragm, sphincter, gait, coordinated movement. Click the facial appearance: the frontal muscle, the risorius, bite quadratus, round eYes, round mouth suck up muscles. Click the trunk: neck stretched out, hold out a bosom, stretching. Click the shoulder: shoulder shrug before outreach, shoulder, shoulder after the reach, shoulder rotation. Click the upper limb: the extension, flexion, wrist, wrist flexion, feet wide, radial deviation, and refers to, be, thumb outreach, thumb on the palm. Click the lower limbs: spin, hip, hip flexion outreach, hip adduction, knees, bend your knees, foot, foot dorsiflexion bends, strephexopodia, strephenopodia, extensor, toe. Click swallow: enter into therapy data selection directly. Click diaphram: enter into therapy data selection directly. Click sphincter: enter into therapy data selection directly. Click gait: enter into therapy data selection and time selection directly. Click center of body weight shift: enter into therapy data selection directly. Click coordinated movement: drinking, combing, leg stretching and steps.

Every item above is selected, press "confirmation" and enter into therapy data selection column.

In the data selection state, fill 0, 10, 20, 40, 80, 100, 120, 140, 160, 180, 200, 240, 280, 320, 360, 400, 480, 560, 600 and so on. After completion the numbers, click "Enter" and the virtual motor program curve image can be operated. The therapy is started.

Storage and analysis: after one training, training items, training degrees and training progress of the patients can be stored. Because virtual training is not real, it is only used for reference of the patients' training. It is not used for data analysis of training effect.

5. Hardware part: The softwares mentioned above should be installed on the central processing unit of the computer and training screen is used to display mechanism demonstration, animation and training curve. Operation screen is used by the therapists to select items, which include single screen and double screen. The single screen is portable, which is applied for bedside training and self-training of the patients post-discharge. Double screen is suitable for the training in rehabilitation hall of the hospital. The outline of the machine refers to Fig. 5.1.

5.2.1.2 Operation Process

Start the computer, click brand and enter into the page of virtual reality training system of neurological training. Click the page and enter into operation page of the therapists. After filling basic items, select mechanism demonstration and the computer will play mechanism demonstration animation. If the therapists don't click, the page goes to therapy items. Select sound button and animation video will be played with voice. Select No button and silent video will be played. Click therapy items and enter into pandect page of therapy items. Click therapy item and press "Enter". Select agonistic muscle in the therapy data (μV), press "Enter", 0 μV data video will be played in the patients' screen. Combined with video, the therapists guide the patients to do

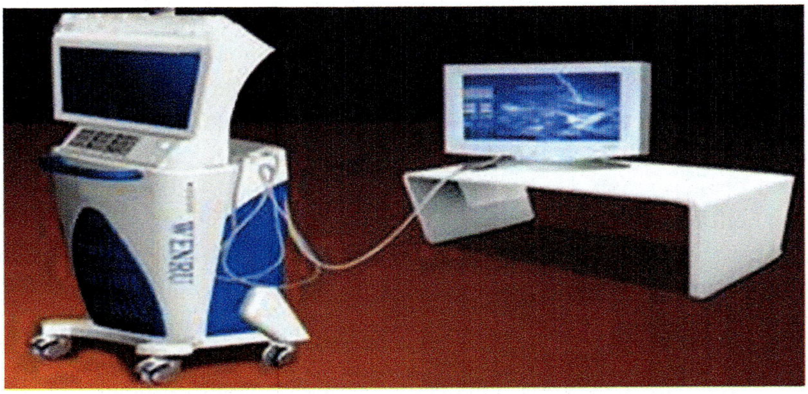

Fig. 5.1 Wenru brand training system of neurological training virtual reality

actual training. After one therapy, if the patients need to do the same items therapy, the therapists select other data in the therapy data and press "Enter". The patients can do the same item therapy with different data. The patients can do it repeatedly until selecting other therapy item.

The therapy process of other items are similar. During the therapy process, the therapists can save the data at any time, store therapy content, click quit button and log out. All kinds of animations and videos are stored in database.

5.2.2 Training Method of Virtual Neurological Training System

5.2.2.1 Voice Instruction of Daoyin Technique

Voice instruction of six-step Daoyin technique of guiding collaterals through meridians and animation light spot automatic tracking display is used. The example is the training of elbow extension. The description is accompanied with voice instruction of six-step Daoyin technique of guiding collaterals through meridians and animation light spot automatic tracking display.

Now we start to do the training of elbow extension, which belong to the Tri-energizer Meridian of Hand-Shaoyang. Please concentrate and take a deep breath. Concentrate again (low voice) and your mind originate form the tail end of the third finge, guide Qi to run along main and collateral channels indicatrix and run again. Okay, concentrate on outside of the upper arm and prepare for elbow extension. Take a deep breath, are you ready? Prepare for it, get up higher and higher (strong mood and long time). get up higher. One, two, three, higher, four, five. Great, relax, relax, guide Qi to run along main and collateral channels and disperse in pericardium slowly, great! You did great! (Fig. 5.2).

The second time: You did great just now. This time we use transverse line to mark the effect of last time. We try to make the signal intensity surpass the transverse line together. Okay, prepare for it. Take a deep breath, concentrate and your mind originate form the tail end of the third finger, guide Qi to run along main and collateral channels indicatrix and run again. Okay, concentrate on outside of the upper arm and prepare for elbow extension. Take a deep breath, are you ready? Prepare for it, get up higher and higher. Great, hold on and on. Good, relax, relax, and then relax. Guide Qi to run along main and collateral channels and disperse in pericardium slowly, great! You improve a lot.

The third time: We will do it again and let the signal line surpass the transverse line (Fig. 5.3). Take a deep breath, concentrate and your mind originate form the tail end of index finger, guide Qi to run along main and collateral channels indicatrix and run again. Okay, concentrate on outside of the upper arm and prepare for elbow extension. Prepare for it, get up higher. One, two, three, higher, four, five. Great, relax, relax, guide Qi to run along main and collateral channels and disperse in pericardium slowly, great!

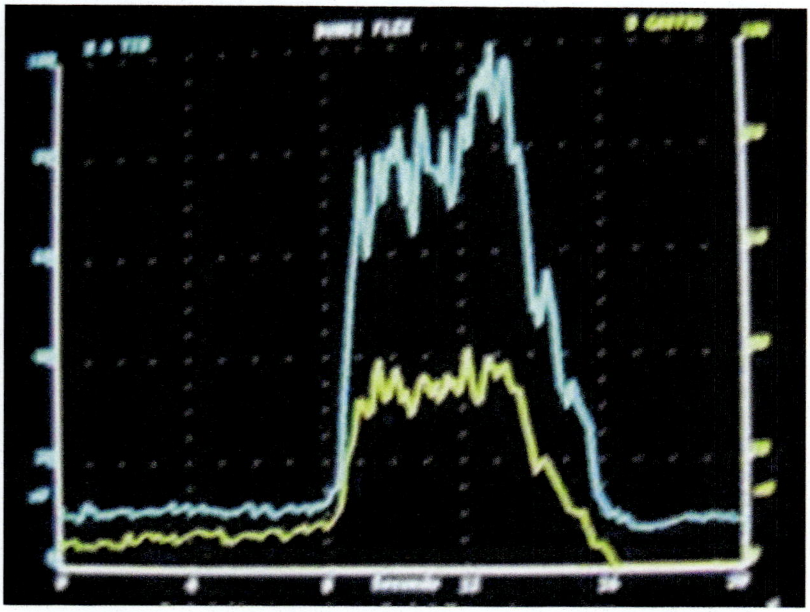

Fig. 5.2 Abnormal motor program of elbow extension on right side (blue signal line stands for signal intensity form CNS to musculus triceps brachii and yellow signal line stands for signal intensity form CNS to musculus biceps brachii. Imbalance of the proportion induce dysfunction of elbow extension)

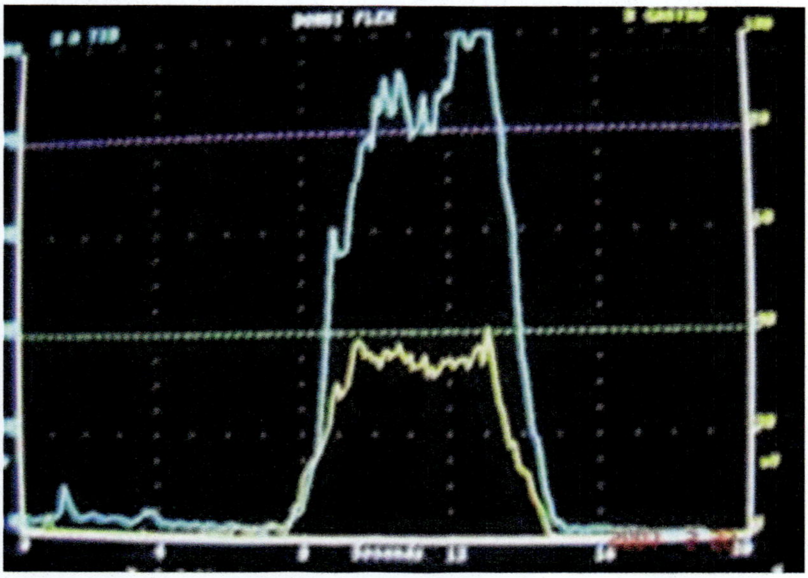

Fig. 5.3 The therapists guide the patients to promote the signal intensity of blue signal line. If the blue signal is too strong, the signal intensity of yellow signal is decreased. Pink line is the altitude of blue signal line of last time and is the target for the patients to surpass

The fourth time: Take a deep breath and relax, look out and let the signal line surpass the transverse line. Concentrate and your mind originate form the tail end of the third finger, guide Qi to run along main and collateral channels indicatrix and run again. Okay, concentrate on outside of the upper arm. Prepare for it, get up higher. One, two, three, higher, four, five. Great, relax, relax, guide Qi to run along main and collateral channels and disperse in pericardium slowly, great!

The fifth time: We will do it again and let the signal line surpass the transverse line. Take a deep breath, concentrate and your mind originate form the tail end of the third finger, guide Qi to run along main and collateral channels indicatrix and run again. Okay, concentrate on outside of the upper arm. Prepare for it, get up higher. One, two, three, higher, four, five. Great, relax, relax, guide Qi to run along main and collateral channels and disperse in pericardium slowly, great! What a quick pregress!

The sixth time: We will do it for the last time and let the signal line surpass the transverse line. Take a deep breath, concentrate and your mind originate form the tail end of the third finger, guide Qi to run along main and collateral channels indicatrix and run again. Okay, concentrate on outside of the upper arm. Prepare for it, get up higher. One, two, three, higher, four, five. Great, relax, relax, guide Qi to run along main and collateral channels and disperse in pericardium slowly, great! (Fig. 5.4).

The rest can be done in the same manner.

5.2.2.2 Clinical Indications and Contraindications of Virtual Neurological Training Method

Except for equipment, there is no difference of training method between neurological training virtual reality training method and rehabilitation methods of neurological training. Therefore, indications and contradictions of this therapy are the same as clinical indications and contradictions of three-stage of neurological training therapy.

5.2.2.3 Cautions of Clinical Application

In actual clinical application, several aspects that are paid attention to are as follows:

Immersion: Adopted virtual elevation and simulation of motor program signal are designed by human and they are not real elevation and motor program signal. The patients are need to be guided in the virtual environment. Through the surpassing training of virtual goal and simulation of motor program signal, neural potential is developed and motor program is reestablished. The therapists are required to guide the patients to immerse into therapy environment. The patients should be made to believe the virtual goal and simulation of motor program signal are real. Ang then there will be good training effect. Therefore, the therapists use the equiepement to explain the mechanism and make the patients to immerse into the training environment as much and deep as possible through regulation of mind and breath. If the patients can regard virtual elevation as real elevation and simulation signal as their own signal, which demonstrated that the therapy is in a deep state and there will be good training effect.

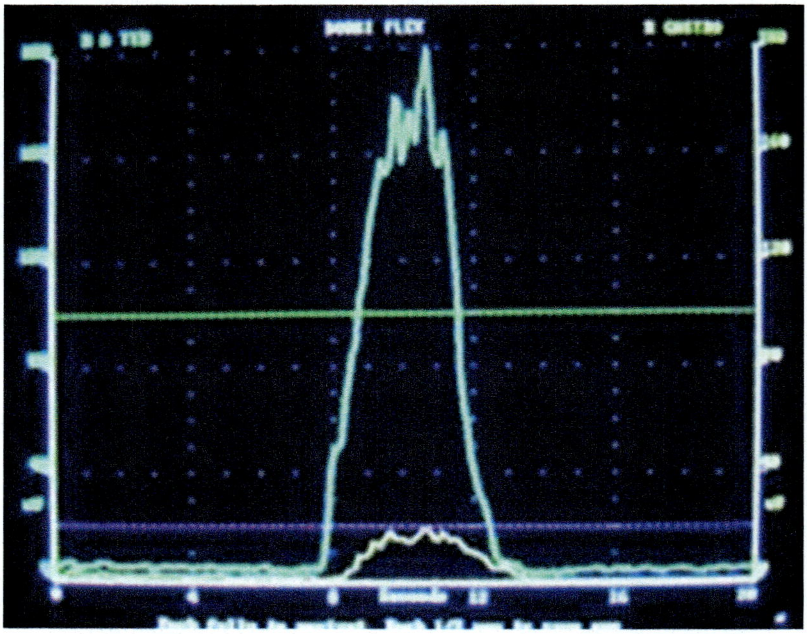

Fig. 5.4 Through training, blue signal line is increased obviously and yellow signal line is decreased obviously. Abnormal motor program can be rectified and be consolidated after repeated training. The function of elbow extension can be improved obviously

Actual anti-resistance process should be keep pace with the processing speed of simulation of motor program signal. In the actual clinical training, the patients should try to make the time of anti-resistance joint motion keep pace with the time and time frame (from the beginning to the end of motor program signal) of simulation of motor program signal in the screenrogram. The patients should try to make the beginning of anti-resistance joint motion keep pace with the beginning of motor program signal increase and the time of anti-resistance joint motion keep pace with the time of motor program signal processing. The system voice tells the patients to relax. When the motor program is zero, joint motion of anti-resistance must be stopped. Otherwise, there will be joint but not motor program signal and there will be motor program signal but not joint motion at the same time, which can make the patients think that the training is virtual and the effect is not real. Finally, the training effect will be influenced.

It is necessary to be combine with actual motor program signal detection. In order to increase the patients' reality to simulation of motor program signal. Virtual reality training method is combined with training with actual motor program signal detection, which can achieve good effect. Generally, in the first trainings of the patients in hospital, the training should be done in the actual motor program signal detection to know practical situation of motor program signal, which is good for the design of therapy method and is the reference index of therapy effect. In addition, because actual motor program signal keeps pace with joint motion dominated by brain, the patients can feel the relationship of brain and movement and the existence of t motor program signal he patients. Consequently, the patients can establish the concept and impression of joint motion dominated by motor program. After that, the virtual reality training system is applied for training and the patients are easy to enter into immersion state. Afterwards, every once in a while, such as 1 week, the training can be done in actual motor program signal detection to observe therapy effect and to deepen the impression of the patients to motor program signal further. In this aspect, the author insist to use one neurological training instrument with 3–5 virtual reality training system to do the training, which can overcome the defects of the training in actual motor program signal detection, know the benefits of that the actual motor program is good for diagnosis and achieve better clinical training effect.

5.3 The Mechanism and Function of Virtual Neurological Training System

5.3.1 The Mechanism of Virtual Neurological Training System

5.3.1.1 The Training System of Virtual Reality of Neurological Training Is Actual Training Underlying the Mechanism of "Goal and Motive"

The mechanism of "goal and motive" is an effective mechanism to develop neural potential and recover lost motor function after CNS damages. On the basis of animation simulation of motor program signal with surpassing goal, through actual anti-resistance done by the patients' manipulation, Virtual reality training system guides the patients to try to surpass the elevation constantly and promote neural potential in order to develop it further. During this process, these two factors play an important role.

1. Virtual motor program signal elevation and proportion: The elevation and proportion has no therapeutic effect, but they are essential. The elevation and motor program proportion are like the target of the archery, which is the definite orientation and surpassing goal for the patients. Just as the jumper without transverse bar are asked to jump and the archers are ask to shoot without target. No matter how to do the training, there is no improvement of the performance (Fig. 5.5).
2. Actual anti-resistance training: With the elevation but without body active movement

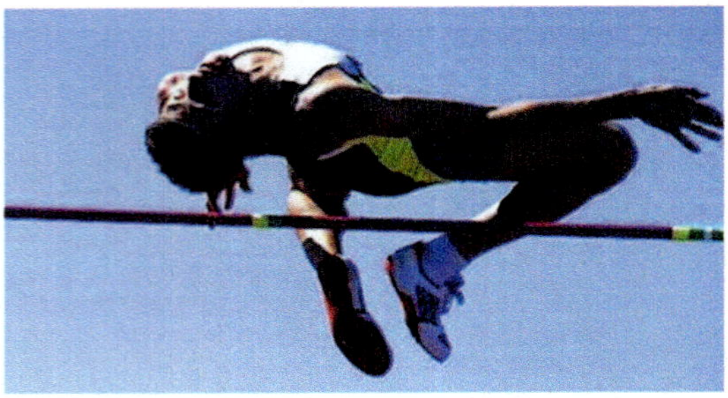

Fig. 5.5 Transverse bar is essential for improving the jump performance

dominated by brain, there is no effect. Only with definite surpassing goal, through genuine own efforts, the patients can complete designed mission or surpass designed goal in order to increase the ability. In the actual training, the therapists exert resistance in the orientation of the patients' joint motion and guide the patients to try to achieve or surpass the goal with the instruction of Daoyin technique speech together. It is a procee that the patients try to achieve the goal by. themselves and is the most important segment that can affect the results.

5.3.1.2 Speech Instruction, Mechanism Explanation and Function Display of Animation Light Spot Automatic Tracking Guarantee the Correctness of Qi Guided in the Main and Collateral Channels

The system provides automatic speech explanation for mechanism with the accompany of animation notice and use comprehensive public language to explain the following aspects: How does the brain dominate body movement? What is motor program? Why there is motor dysfunction after CNS damages? Why the function is improved through the therapy? These question can make the patients understand the pathogenesis and therapy mechanism and increase the enthusiasm of the patients to take part in the training actively. The adequate understanding from the patients is the spring of motivation. The patients with brain infarction and damages are usually accompanied with cognitive disorder. It is necessary to explain it to the patients repeatedly and the system can explain it at any time without resting.

Automatic speech instruction of six-step Daoyin technique in the system can keep the enthusiasm of the patients through increasing the volume of voice amplification system. In addition system can provide the pathway of main and collateral channels and animation light spot automatic tracking display to guarantee the correctness of regulation of mind in the pathway of main and collateral channels and increase the function of clearing and activating the channels and collaterals, which is the basis for implementing method and promoting effect.

5.3.2 The Function of Virtual Neurological Training System

Virtual reality training system of neurological trainin can satisfy the requirements of the theory and method of neurological training. Through motor program signal and elevation of various animations generated by software, the system can provide all kinds of feedback and surpassing goal for Daoyin technique and use automatic speech instruction and animation light spot automatic tracking indication technique of main and collateral channels pathway to increase the function of clearing and activating the channels and collaterals. The system overcomes the shortcoming of high enthusiasm and labor intensity, can relieve labor intensity of the therapists electively and can provide safe "state of emergency" created by speech that is good for potential development, which provide a good condition for development of CNS potential, reestablishment of motor program and improvement of motor function through Daoyin technique.

The comprehensive results of this system make the patients know their own dysfunction and the mechanism of recovering function, which is good for increasing active cooperation and emphasize on the consciousness of recovering CNS function. Especially the patients can know their own motor dysfunction and the gap between dysfunction and normal motor pattern. The system increases the excitability of chasing goal and bridge the gap. Through excitatory competitive inhibition of cerebral nuclei, the system can provide the goal of attention diversion for the patients, which is good for decreasing pathological inhibition of brain nuclei. Automatic speech explanation, indication and six-step Daoyin technique training speech instruction provide advantage of self-training and quality guarantee of self-exercise for the patients. The theory of development of CNS potential, reestablishment of motor program and remodeling of motor pattern is new. The method of six-step Daoyin technique in traditional Chinese medicine of guiding collaterals through meridians is new. The equipment is simplified and the computer animation is at low cost. There are many functions that are rational and scientific such as automatic speech, mechanism explanation and many actual training unit. The therapeutic effect is high. The patients know what to do and how to do and the system can let the patients keep high enthusiasm, which is good for the improvement of training effect. The userage is comprehensive. It can be used in many training items such as motor center training, potential development training and physical exercise therapy of neurological training. The moment the effect is improved, the enjoyment is increased.

Developed types at present include immobile table type and portable type. There are many functions such as divi-screen display, speech indication, virtual simulation in immobile table type. This type should be kept away from sound and light. This type is mainly used for the severe patients in the rehabilitation hall of the hospital. There are many functions such as single screen display, speech indication, virtual simulation in portable type, which can be used in training hall and at home.

The core content of both types are motion simulation, virtual elevation, actual training, development of CNS potential, reestablishment of motor program and remodeling of motor pattern.

The training system not only can be used in large hospital, but also can be used in community and grass-roots clinics, which can prevent the defects of poor therapeutic effect induced by simple equipment in grass-roots clinics and shortage of doctors.

5.4 Clinical Experiment of Virtual Neurological Training System

5.4.1 Clinical Data

5.4.1.1 Sampling

From June 2007 to June 2009, there are 120 patients with hemiplegia who are all the inpatients in neurological rehabilitation training center in Beijing Tongren Hospital affiliated to Beijing's Capital Medical University and neurological training ward of Hengxing rehabilitation centre. There are 84 males and 36 females. The age is from 45 to 85 years old. The average age is 52.1 years old. There are 58 patients with hemiplegia after cerebral infarction, 36 patients with hemiplegia after cerebral hemorrhage, 26 patients with hemiplegia after brain damage. There are 56 patients with left hemiplegia and 64 patients with right hemiplegia. The patients are divided into two groups include virtual simulation group and neurological training group and there are 60 patients in each group. Virtual reality group includes 41 males and 19 females. The average age is 51.8 years old. Neurological training group includes 43 males and 17 females. The average age is 52.3 years old.

1. The inclusion criteria: According to the diagnostic criteria of national cerebrovascular disease conference in 1995, the hemiplegic patients are diagnosed with cerebral infarction or cerebral hemorrhage and by CT or MRI; the patients without obvious dysgnosia (MMSE score is more than or equal to 20); There is no serious contracture of the knee joint or ankle joint and passive movement range is normal.
2. The exclusion criteria: The patients with severe organ dysfunction such as heart and

lung, severe infectious disease, bone fracture, dyscrasia and so on cannot do rehabilitation training; the patients with severe cognitive disorder or long-term drug use such as sedatives, antidepressants and diazepam cannot cooperate with therapy; the patients with frequent epileptic attack; the patients with diseases such as various myopathy, bone and joint diseases and peripheral neuropathy that can affect movement; the patients stop therapy for any reason or cannot persist in the therapy for 90 times.

5.4.1.2 Training Method

The training is done in the two groups according to training method in three-stage of neurological training such as development of CNS potential, reestablishment of motor program and remodeling of motor pattern. Virtual simulation group uses virtual reality training system of neurological training to do actual training through animation mechanism display and virtual signal and elevation. Neurological training group uses real-time signal detection of neurological training instrument and the therapists explain to the patients and guide the patients to do the training. The other therapy methods are the same as the content such as the training of shoulder abduction, elbow extension, hip flexion, knee extension and dorsiflexion of foot.

1. Neurological training: Virtual simulation group use Daoyin feedback technique in traditional Chinese medicine. Under the instruction of virtual mechanism display and automatic speech of simulation motor program signal and elevation, the therapists use anti-resistance training method, six-step Daoyin technique in traditional Chinese medicine and biofeedback to do the training. The time for every joint is 10 min and the total time is 50 min.
2. Physical therapy of neurological training: The six-step method includes motor imagination and simulation, assembly of "energy", confirmation of target point, trigger, insistence and relax. Six-step Daoyin technique in traditional Chinese medicine is used for the training. The time for every joint is 10 min and the total time is 50 min.
3. Potential development training of upper and lower limbs: Wenru brand potential development training device of upper and lower limbs is produced by Beijing Xing Chen Wan You Science and Technology Ltd. Regulation of weight loss can make the patients' upper limbs to support the trunk and the lower limbs support the standing. The weight is usually one-third to one-fifth of the patients' body weight. Six-step Daoyin technique in traditional Chinese medicine is used to guide the patients to push up and down with upper limbs, stand up and squat with lower limbs and do body control ability training. Potential development training of upper and lower limbs should be done separately. The training time is 30 min per time.
4. Motor pattern remodeling training: The first is weight support treadmill training device of abnormal gait rectification. Wenru weight support treadmill training device of abnormal gait rectification produced by Beijing Xing Chen Wan You Science and Technology Ltd. and gait marked footpath are used for the patients to do the training. Regulation of hip flexion, lower limbs adduction and foot drop rectification elastic band can help the patients to complete hip flexion, dorsiflexion of foot and lower limbs adduction. The training time is 30 min per time. The second is weight support stride and gait shifting of weight training. Wenru brand weight support stride gait and shifting of weight training device produced by Beijing Xing Chen Wan You Science and Technology Ltd. The weight is one-fifth to one-eighth of the patients' body weight. The therapists guide the patients to do stride gait and shifting of weight training. The training time is 30 min per time. The third is weight support gait training. Wenru brand weight support gait training device is produced by Beijing Xing Chen Wan You Science and Technology Ltd. The weight is one-fifth to one-eighth of the patients' body weight. Track rotation speed of walking machine is started at 0.22 m/s.

With the improvement of walking ability, the speed is increased gradually. The patients are guided to do the training according to the gait mark on the track of walking machine. The training time is 30 min per time. The fourth is comprehensive walking training, which includes balance bar or walking aid gait mark walking training, ascending and descending the stairs training and independent walking training on gait mark way. The training time is 10 min per item and the total time is 30 min. The fifth is upper limbs and hand function training, which includes tightening the nut, picking up balls and fastening the button. The training time is 30 min per time.

The patients can do the training once every day and the are 30 time in each stage. The total times are 90. The therapy items are adopted alternatively according to the specific condition of the patients. For example, in the training of the third stage, for the patients with low myodynamia, the potential development training can be added properly. For the patients with uncoordinated movement, the reestablishment training can be done on the basis of rectification of abnormal motor program.

5.4.1.3 Methods of Functional Assessment

At the beginning of the therapy and at the end of the therapy, international general functional assessment methods are used, which include Fugl-Meyer, Lovett manual muscle testing (Lovett MMT), surface electromyogram signal (sEMG) strength and proportion, range of joint motion (ROM), and ability of daily life (ADL) assessment. The data is collected to establish database.

5.4.1.4 Statistical Analysis

The analysis results are showed as Mean ± SD ($\overline{X} \pm S$). SPSS12.0 statistical software is used for statistic analysis. At pretherapy and post-treatment, within group therapy and between group therapy, T-test is used to compare the mean of the two groups.

5.4.1.5 Results

There is significant difference of Fugl-Meyer, MMT, sEMG, ROM and ADL between pretherapy and post-treatment in virtual simulation group and neurological training group ($P < 0.001$). At post-treatment, There is no significant difference of Fugl-Meyer, MMT, sEMG, ROM and ADL between virtual simulation group and neurological training group ($P > 0.05$). The results are referred to Tables 5.1, 5.2, and 5.3.

5.4.1.6 Discussion

The key point of recovering motor dysfunction induced by CNS damages due to cardiac and cerebrovascular disease is to recover CNS functions, but CNS cells are lack of regeneration ability. The functional recovery requires the function of normal cells around injured area and activation of reserved conduction pathway. CNS plasticity and functional reorganization are promoted to compensate the lost functions. The plasticity and functional reorganization is in accordance with "skillful use and dependence" principle. Only active movement can promote CNS plasticity. A large number of reserved central neural cells and conduction pathways are the basis of CNS plasticity. The functions of reserved central neural cells and conduction pathways are the basis of functional reorganization. Training method is the process of CNS potential development.

There is great potential in CNS and other tissues of the body. These potentials can be activated and used in specific condition. Their basis or origin is come from the functional enhancement of tissues or organ cells. However, the number of involved cells is not decreased. On the other hand, the reason may be the increase of cell without functional enhancement of single cells. There are both at the same time. However, functional enhancement of single cell is limited. The increase of involved cell number can improve the entire function. Therefore, human potential is root in reserved body tissues and cells. For example, there are 140 billion brain cells, but only 6% is in use. There are 300 million alveoli in human lung and the area is 70 m^2.

Table 5.1 Functional assessment scontrol table pretherapy and post-treatment of virtual simulation group ($\bar{X} \pm S$)

Items		Before therapy	After therapy	t	P
MMT (grade)	Deltoideus triangularis	2.20 ± 1.20	3.57 ± 0.95	14.86	P < 0.01
	Musculus triceps brachii	1.97 ± 1.18	3.30 ± 1.18	16.42	P < 0.01
	Hip flexor	2.43 ± 1.05	3.83 ± 0.76	14.20	P < 0.01
	Quadriceps femoris	2.67 ± 1.05	4.18 ± 0.65	15.26	P < 0.01
	Tibialis anterior muscle	1.28 ± 1.19	2.45 ± 1.35	10.93	P < 0.01
sEMG (μV)	Deltoideus triangularis strength	34.17 ± 28.02	88.98 ± 42.88	13.87	P < 0.01
	Musculus triceps brachii strength	32.63 ± 32.69	88.88 ± 66.54	9.60	P < 0.01
	Musculus triceps brachii proportion	1.91 ± 1.58	5.29 ± 2.79	13.33	P < 0.01
	Hip flexorstrength	21.03 ± 19.51	63.48 ± 42.34	11.28	P < 0.01
	Quadriceps femoris strength	41.93 ± 30.24	106.88 ± 48.46	13.88	P < 0.01
	Quadriceps femoris proportion	2.49 ± 1.61	6.01 ± 2.10	15.87	P < 0.01
	Tibialis anterior muscle strength	15.05 ± 21.84	41.80 ± 35.26	9.33	P < 0.01
	Tibialis anterior muscle proportion	1.39 ± 1.32	4.21 ± 2.26	13.22	P < 0.01
ROM (degree)	Shoulder abduction	52.42° ± 47.61°	96.88° ± 48.03°	13.86	P < 0.01
	Elbow extension	99.25° ± 32.79°	127.33° ± 31.86°	17.01	P < 0.01
	Hip flexion	64.40° ± 32.18°	105.02° ± 22.86°	11.44	P < 0.01
	Knee extension	114.58° ± 13.63°	132.92° ± 4.35°	11.20	P < 0.01
	Dorflexison of foot	4.03° ± 8.19°	13.65° ± 11.03°	8.86	P < 0.01
FMA		34.10 ± 25.76	53.12 ± 22.31	13.43	P < 0.01
ADL		51.33 ± 25.28	77.33 ± 14.71	11.87	P < 0.01

Table 5.2 Functional assessment scontrol table pretherapy and post-treatment of neurological training group ($\bar{X} \pm S$)

Items		Pretherapy	Post-treatment	t	P
MMT (grade)	Deltoideus triangularis	1.92 ± 1.17	3.27 ± 0.84	14.75	P < 0.01
	Musculus triceps brachii	1.80 ± 1.33	3.63 ± 0.52	9.66	P < 0.01
	Hip flexor	1.92 ± 1.03	3.63 ± 0.52	13.88	P < 0.01
	Quadriceps femoris	2.32 ± 1.00	3.97 ± 0.55	12.50	P < 0.01
	Tibialis anterior muscle	1.23 ± 0.98	2.57 ± 1.13	9.39	P < 0.01
sEMG (μV)	Deltoideus triangularis strength	18.63 ± 19.42	74.08 ± 40.56	16.1	P < 0.01
	Musculus triceps brachii strength	30.38 ± 33.24	100.02 ± 64.37	11.93	P < 0.01
	Musculus triceps brachiiproportion	2.47 ± 1.52	6.28 ± 2.89	13.09	P < 0.01
	Hip flexor strength	27.27 ± 17.51	74.75 ± 29.48	16.47	P < 0.01
	Quadriceps femoris strength	46.52 ± 34.80	112.08 ± 42.15	18.06	P < 0.01
	Quadriceps femorisproportion	2.38 ± 1.83	5.66 ± 1.88	12.75	P < 0.01
	Tibialis anterior muscle strength	11.13 ± 9.49	41.38 ± 25.58	10.61	P < 0.01
	Tibialis anterior muscle proportion	2.41 ± 1.24	4.86 ± 2.04	12.08	P < 0.01
ROM (degree)	Shoulder abduction	47.93° ± 35.85°	96.10° ± 43.19	19.83	P < 0.01
	Elbow extension	101.75° ± 11.38°	130.75° ± 5.03	19.81	P < 0.01
	Hip flexion	51.25° ± 27.32°	100.58° ± 19.18°	18.57	P < 0.01
	Knee extension	112.67° ± 12.30°	134.08° ± 4.17°	13.17	P < 0.01
	Dorflexison of foot	3.07° ± 4.39°	10.53° ± 6.04°	12.03	P < 0.01
FMA		31.02 ± 17.64	60.55 ± 19.54	16.08	P < 0.01
ADL		35.75 ± 20.66	75.08 ± 15.00	19.45	P < 0.01

Table 5.3 Functional assessments control table post-treatment of virtual simulation group and neurological training group ($\bar{X} \pm \mathbf{S}$)

Items		Post-treatment of virtual simulation group	Post-treatment of neurological training group	t	P
MMT (grade)	Deltoideus triangularis	3.57 ± 0.95	3.27 ± 0.84	1.84	$P > 0.05$
	Musculus triceps brachii	3.30 ± 1.18	3.02 ± 1.00	1.42	$P > 0.05$
	Hip flexor	3.83 ± 0.76	3.63 ± 0.52	1.68	$P > 0.05$
	Quadriceps femoris	4.18 ± 0.65	3.97 ± 0.55	1.97	$P > 0.05$
	Tibialis anterior muscle	2.45 ± 1.35	2.57 ± 1.13	0.51	$P > 0.05$
sEMG (μV)	Deltoideus triangularis strength	88.98 ± 42.88	74.08 ± 40.56	1.96	$P > 0.05$
	Musculus triceps brachii strength	88.88 ± 66.54	100.02 ± 64.37	0.93	$P > 0.05$
	Musculus triceps brachiiproportion	5.29 ± 2.79	6.28 ± 2.89	1.91	$P > 0.05$
	Hip flexorstrength	63.48 ± 42.34	74.75 ± 29.48	1.69	$P > 0.05$
	Quadriceps femoris strength	106.88 ± 48.46	112.08 ± 42.15	0.63	$P > 0.05$
	Quadriceps femorisproportion	6.01 ± 2.10	5.66 ± 1.88	0.97	$P > 0.05$
	Tibialis anterior muscle strength	41.80 ± 35.26	41.38 ± 25.58	0.07	$P > 0.05$
	Tibialis anterior muscle proportion	4.21 ± 2.26	4.86 ± 2.04	1.67	$P > 0.05$
ROM (degree)	Shoulder abduction	96.88° ± 48.03°	96.10° ± 43.19°	0.09	$P > 0.05$
	Elbow extension	127.33° ± 31.86°	130.75° ± 5.03°	0.82	$P > 0.05$
	Hip flexion	105.02° ± 22.86°	100.58° ± 19.18°	1.15	$P > 0.05$
	Knee extension	132.92° ± 4.35°	134.08° ± 4.17°	1.50	$P > 0.05$
	Dorflexison of foot	13.65° ± 11.03°	10.53° ± 6.04°	1.92	$P > 0.05$
FMA		53.12 ± 22.31	60.55 ± 19.54	1.94	$P > 0.05$
ADL		77.33 ± 14.71	75.08 ± 15.00	0.83	$P > 0.05$

Generally, only 1.8 million cells and 40 m^2 area are in use. It is always the case in other tissues and organs such as reserved conduction pathway of nervous system, blood reserve and muscle tissue reserve. When needed, these reserve can play functions. Previous training and special education are the premise to develop human potential. For a bridle-wise person, in an emergency, strong will and great potential may be activated. On the contrary, for a person without training and mental preparation, in an emergency, not only the potential cannot be activated, but also the function of nervous system is paralyzed. Not only the ability of resisting and defending danger cannot be improved, but also the function is decreased. And then the patients are in a dangerous and passive situation.

Potential can be activated in special condition such as state of emergency and there is no potential ability in normal condition. The potential ability in state of emergency can be transferred to ability in normal condition through rehabilitation training, which is the important mechanism of motor function recovery after CNS damages. At present, rehabilitation methods such as Bobath, Rood, Brunnstrom and PNF developed in 1950s abroad have a weak effect on functional recovery of CNS, because they take primary reflexes such as myotatic reflex and tonic neck reflex, passive movement and efferent stimulus as the principal thing. The effect of rehabilitation therapy is dissatisfactory [2].

Zhao Wenru improves ancient Daoyin technique in traditional Chinese medicine to six step method that can be used for clinic. On the basis of that, neurological training rehabilitation therapy technique is developed. Bio-electricity signal reception device is used to receive motor program signal real-timely and display it in a curve form. Motor program signal is used as feedback signal and Daoyin technique is used repeatedly to do motor program training with a purpose. The effect of this method is related to the factors as follows.

- The patients' understanding of therapy mechanism
- Correctness and passion of the therapists use six-step Daoyin technique
- Real-time reception and display of motor program signal
- The scheme of rectification of disordered motor program and reestablishment of normal motor program and the setting of the goal

Neurological training rehabilitation method is a therapy of active movement, which requires the involvement of the patients actively. Therefore, the patients' understanding of the mechanisms of therapy method that includes the mechanism of recovery and formation of motor dysfunction is the important factor that can influence the therapy process and effect. Meanwhile, training effect is affected by comprehension and memory of the patients, comprehension and expression of the therapists to therapy method. Because the therapists cannot use the method correctly, the therapy goal cannot be achieved. Because the patients misunderstand the mechanism, the therapeutic effect is influenced.

In the process of six-step Daoyin technique in traditional Chinese medicine, the therapists use speech to guide the patients to regulate mind and breath and then regulate movement on the basis of regulation of mind and breath. Regulation of movement is completing active movement of some joint such as dorflexison of foot. In this process, the correctness, passion and encourage words of Daoyin methods and the encourage degree of the patients are directly related to therapeutic effect. Especially when the curve of agonistic muscle reaches the peak last time and the therapists ask the patients to try to surpass it, the therapists should raise the voice and encourage the patients with passion. One therapist do this job in a short time and treats several patients every day. They can keep high enthusiasm. If the therapist do this job for a long time and treats 8–10 patients every day, it is difficulty for him to keep high enthusiasm.

The sensitivity of human bioelectrical signal reception and display equipment is high and the equipment can receive interference signal of electrocardio on the skin surface of lower limbs muscle. The signal of vehicle and cellphone in the surroundings can affect the reception greatly. The equipment works in room A, but cannot work in romm B. The equipment works today, cannot work tomorrow. Therefore, the equipment should be installed in a good environment such as deep medical ground electrode and copper net shield. In spite of this, the therapy is usually disturbed. In addition, the signal detection equipment is expensive, which can increase the clinical cost and family burden. It is difficulty to popularize and apply, especially in grass roots, community hospital and health-center.

According to the requirements of neurological trainingrehabilitation therapy, the patients should fully understand therapy methods. The therapists should use six-step Daoyin technique correctly and encourage the patients with high passion. The defects of motor program signal detection equipment, the mechanism of "goal and motive" and the anti-resistance in the orientation of joint motion are basic requirements. The patients understand the basic procedures of therapy and the mechanism of functional recovery through virtual animation. Through simulation of motor program signal curve and elevation, the objective goal is provided for the patients to surpass. Through six-step Daoyin technique indication record, high passion and encourage can be maintained. In the orientation of joint motion, the therapists can exert proper resistance to develop neural potential.

Rehabilitation is the process of achieving goal through special training method. The main difference between virtual reality training system and virtual reality technique invented in 1960s is that VR is the virtual environment created by computo. Through immersion, interaction and imagination, the users can throw them into the virtual environment and the users can interact with virtual environment naturally. Some researchers found that VR has some therapeutic effects on hemiplegia [3], but this is because VR is used to ease the patients' mood with display of completed functional movement. The patients can observe their actual movement. When the patients cannot complete active movement with autonomic movement deficiency, virtual reality technique cannot affect it too. VR technique is lack of the actual rehabilitation training process such as neural potential development, motor program reestablishment and motor pattern remodeling, which can influence practical therapy value and meaning.

Virtual reality training system of neurological training is appropriate for the therapy of neural potential development and motor program reestablishment and is the rehabilitation training equipment with rational design. It is simple and at low cost. The patients can better understand the therapy mechanism and can be motivated to take part in the therapy with it, which can alleviate labor intensity of the therapists and improve therapeutic effect at the same time.

Reference

1. Burdea G, Patounakis G, Popescu V, et al. Virtual reality-based training for the diagnosis of prostate cancer. IEEE Trans Biomed Eng. 1999;46(10):1253–60.
2. Sik Lanyi C, Laky V, Tilinger A, et al. Developing multimedia software and virtual reality worlds and their use in rehabilitation and psychology. Stud Health Technol Inform. 2004;105:273–84.
3. You SH, Jang SH, Kim YH, et al. Virtual reality-induced cortical reorganization and associated locomotor recovery in chronic stroke: an experimenter-blind randomized study. Stroke. 2005;36(6):116–7.

6 Rehabilitation Methods of Neurological Training in Special Diseases

6.1 Rehabilitation Methods of Neurological Training of Recovering Motor Function in the Patients with Severe Unconsciousness

6.1.1 Theoretical Foundation of Motor Function Recovery Training in the Patients with Severe Unconsciousness

In this section, we introduce the knowledge of the patients with severe disturbance of consciousness that include vegetative state and minimum conscious state. Rehabilitation methods of neurological training and mechanism of motor function recovery is introduced. We don't discuss the pathogenesis of these diseases and associated progress of therapy. However, for understanding and clinical application, we should introduce diagnosis, cardinal syndromes, classification and main therapy method of disturbance of consciousness in this chapter. Associated functional assessment of conscience is not introduced in this book. Please refer to associated professional books about rehabilitation assessment.

The patients with severe disturbance of consciousness, especially the patients in vegetative state VS: Vegetative State [1] and minimum conscious state [2], totally lose cognitive ability and communicative competence. Therefore, they cannot cooperate with the therapists to do rehabilitation training that take active movement as the principal thing and can promote CNS plasticity. The doctors and the therapists feel confused on these patients. They have nothing to do but adopt some sustained rehabilitation measures with passive movement and afferent stimulus that is difficulty to achieve effect.

For the patients with severe disturbance of consciousness, do they do rehabilitation training of functional recovery? At first, we should ascertain and re-recognize the diagnosis and prognosis of various disturbance of consciousness.

A lot of people think that the wake up possibility of Vegetative state is low, but some paper demonstrated [3–5] that the recovery rate of VS induced by traumatic accident 1 year after the accident is about 50% and the recovery rate of VS without traumatic accident is 15%. In addition, there are some reports that family affection is used to wake up VS in life. All these demonstrated that the patients with disturbance of consciousness are able to recover conscience, which include the patients in vegetative state and minimum conscious state. In addition, we know little about human CNS and the mechanism of formation and recovery of disturbance of consciousness. Therefore, it is necessary to research and investigate further.

We can be enlightened by noctambulism. Sleepwalk is a variant conscious state and the incidence rate is 1–6%. The number of Children

W. Zhao, *Rehabilitation Therapeutics of the Neurological Training*,
https://doi.org/10.1007/978-981-13-0812-3_6

with sleep walk is more than that of adult with sleepwalk. There is usually a family history. When in sleepwalk, the patients can complete some kind of job, movement or complicated operation unconsciously and speak the language that cannot be understand. When the sleepwalk is ended, the patients know nothing about the sleepwalk experience. This seems that human motor function can be separated from conscious state of self- sobriety. This may be the factual basis for the patients with low conscious state to do motor function training.

In addition, in the clinical rehabilitation work, the author found that at present, myodynamia assessment criteria at home and abroad is Lovett MMT (manual muscle test). The therapists use hands to feel the muscle contraction or the ability of anti-resistance to judge the myodynamia. The myodynamia is zero in this test, which doesn't mean the muscle is paralyzed, because the human perception is limited. Three hundred and forty-three muscles are tested by Lovett MMT with zero myodynamia. Surface electromyogram signal equipment is used to test them again and the results show that there are only 11 muscles with zero myodymania, because the sensitivity of bioelectrical signal reception device is 300 times more than human perception. Moreover, precision of the equipment can be increased with the improvement of industrial level of electronic instrument. For example, if we use hour as measurement criteria for human running speed, we cannot tell the difference of running ability between man and man. If we use second as measurement criteria for human running speed, we can tell the difference of running ability between man and man. If we use millisecond as measurement criteria for human running speed, we can tell the minor difference of running ability between man and man.

Similarly, the diagnostic criteria of VS in "Nanjing Standard 2001" established in our country include lost cognitive function, unconscious activities and inability of executing instruction. All these measurement criteria are dependent on the subjective perception and experience. The measurement is broad and not precise. If we used more sensitive method to assess the VS, the diagnosis of VS can be decreased.

On November 10, 2011, there is a paper in *The Lancet* found that electroencephalogram (EEG) can test latent consciousness in the patient is with VS. Compared with functional magnetic resonance imaging (fMRI) that can test slight consciousness in the patients with VS, it is convenient and at low cost, which is not affected by metal implant.

In this study, the researchers examined 16 patients with VS due to brain damages (trauma and anoxia) and 12 healthy control. When they wear the electroencephalogram monitor, the therapist asked the patient to imagine they can move their own fingers or toes. The researchers found that just like healthy control, three patients with brain damages can generate two different kinds of motor pattern according to command. One of the patients did it for more than 200 times that is more than that of healthy control. The researchers deemed that a new classification system is required to reflect the actual condition of these patients more precisely. Although they are diagnosed with VS, some of them are actually not in VS. VS actually is a new definition of behavior energy syndrome.

From the discussion above, we can conclude the following points:

1. The patients with VS can change or wake up with the time or stimulated by some kind of factor. Some researchers found that 1 year after trauma, the recovery rate of consciousness is about 50%, but the recovery rate of consciousness in the patients without trauma is only 15%.
2. Human motor function can be separated from conscious state. This may be the factual basis for the patients in unconscious state to do motor function training.
3. Through the investigation of EEG and MRI, according to clinical diagnosis criteria at present, some of the patients with VS are proved to have conscious reaction and they are not actual in VS. The researchers think that the assessment method at present is not precise, which require more precise assessment criteria.

Some research found that even the patients have been injured for many years and had no response ability. It is necessary to re-assess the condition. Especially there is some improvement noticed by the family or other people.

In a word, whether from the fact that the patients with VS are possible to wake up with time, or from the fact that some patients can wake up because of incorrect diagnosis, it is the truth that some patients with VS can wake up. Form the rehabilitation medicine, we don't think that rehabilitation training of the patients with VS is not valuable and merely do sustained training. We should improve the training method constantly in order to be adaptable to the recovery training of consciousness and motor function of the patients with VS and low conscious state.

6.1.2 The Introduction of Severe Unconsciousness

6.1.2.1 Classification of Severe Unconsciousness

Severe unconsciousness includes brain death, coma, VS, minimum conscious state and locked-in syndrome. All kinds of diagnostic characteristics referred to Table 6.1.

The definition and connotation of consciousness: Consciousness is the perception and comprehensive function of human body to themselves or outside world, which include the level, the range, the content. The maintenance of normal sober conscious state is dependent on the ascending reticular activating system of brain stem, relay integration of thalamus and cortex function.

1. Coma: coma is a severe pathological disturbance of consciousness. There is close binoculus, no spontaneous opening eyes and no sleep-wake circle, which are different from the syndromes of VS. Severe patients can lose any cognitive function and motor function. The vital signs cannot be maintained. Life support system such as breathing machine and medicine are used to keep them alive.
2. Locked-in syndrome: this syndrome is usually in the condition that both side of corticobulbar tract and corticospinal tract are damaged. The patients to almost completely lose motor function. There is only opening eyes, closing eyes or slight eyeball movement in the patients with complete perception and cognitive function. In clinic, the patients can response to the command through opening and closing eyes.
3. Minimum conscious state (MCS): this belongs to severe disordered conscious state. The patients can have cognitive function to themselves or outside world, spontaneous opening eyes and sleep-wake circle.
4. The part of vegetative state includes the definition, clinical manifestation and diagnosis criteria of vegetative state (Table 6.1).
   (a) The definition of vegetative state: the brain is damaged due to some kind of reason. The patients lost the cognitive function to themselves and outside world, but they can open eyes and have sleep-wake circle. The function of hypothalamus and brain stem is maintained.
   (b) Clinical manifestations of vegetative state: the clinical manifestations of the patients with VS are diverse, but the basic characteristic is no perception function to

Table 6.1 Clinical diagnostic characteristics of disturbance of consciousness

Classification	Cognitive function	Sleep-wake circle	Brain stem function	EEG
Coma	Lost	None	Stable or change	Severe abnormal
Locked-in syndrome	Definitely exist	Yes	Complete	Normal
Minimum conscious state	Limited but definitely exist	Yes	Basic complete	Severe abnormal
Vegetative state	Lost	Yes	Basic complete	Severe abnormal
Brain death	Lost	No	No	Mostly electrocerebral silence

outside world or themselves such as sense and perception, memory, thinking, emotion and willpower. The patients can open eyes, but there is no spontaneous speech. They cannot understand others' words. There is entire or partial sleep-wake circle. There is unconscious movement in the body and there is no response to pain. There is entire or partial brainstem reflexes such as pupillary light reflex, corneal reflection and eyelash reflex, cough reflex, swallowing reflex and sucking reflex. The vital signs are stable.

(c) Diagnosis criteria of vegetative state: The cognitive function is lost. There is no conscious movement and the patients cannot execute instruction. The patients can open eyes autonomously or under stimulus. There is sleep-wake circle. There is eyeball tracking movement without purpose. The patients cannot speak and understand the words. They can keep autonomous respiration and blood pressure. The function of hypothalamus and brainstem is normal.

(d) Diagnosis criteria of permanent vegetative state: traumatic VS lasts more than 12 months and non-traumatic VS lasts more than three months, which can be diagnosed with permanent vegetative state.

(e) Brain death: Whole brain functions including brainstem are damaged and lost irreversibly. There are no brainstem reflexes and autonomous respiration. Life support system must be used to keep them alive such as breathing machine.

6.1.2.2 Current Situation of Therapy Methods of Severe Unconsciousness

At present, there is no definite and effective measures in the therapy of severe disturbance of consciousness. Except for etiotropic therapy, there are many comprehensive measures such as nursing, nutritional support, medicine, traditional Chinese medicine, hyperbaric oxygen, electric stimulation and rehabilitation.

1. Traditional Chinese medicine: In traditional Chinese medicine, severe disturbance of consciousness belongs to neurological disease of heart and brain, which is induced by invasion of evil into heart and brain or blockage of heart and brain by exhaustion of qi and blood. The common therapy methods include acupuncture and moxibustion, massage and Chinese medicine, which can dredge brain, dredge main and collateral channels and clearing away the heart-fire, especially the injection made from prescription in ancient time through modern purification technology such as restoring consciousness jing. They are widely used in clinic and play an important role in treating the patients with disturbance of consciousness.
2. Hyperbaric oxygen therapy: Hyperbaric oxygen therapy is the essential method to treat the patients with CNS damages and low conscious state, which is recognized domestic and overseas [6, 7]. Some reports think that the quicker hyperbaric oxygen therapy starts, the longer the therapy course takes, the better the therapeutic effect is. The principal mechanism is to improve the oxygen supply of brain cells and the function of the cells in reversible state can be recovered, which can promote neural function recovery. Some papers found that the recommend oxygen pressure is 1.5 ATA. The therapy time is 1–2 times every day and 5 time for a week. The therapy course includes 30–40 days. The severe patients can receive 200 times.
3. Neural electric stimulation therapy includes electrical stimulus of peripheral nerve, high cervical spinal cord and deep brain.
   (a) Peripheral neural electric stimulation: it belongs to low-frequency electrical stimulation. Bilateral nervus peronaeus or nervus medianus are stimulated constantly, which have an effect on activating electroencephalogram to promote wake-up of brain, but it is not widely used in clinic at present.
   (b) High cervical spinal cord electric stimulation: Because the electrode of cervical spinal cord should be implanted through

surgery, the required condition is high and it is difficulty to be kept for a long time, it is unable to be used.

At present, the most widely used is high cervical spinal cord electric stimulation. In general anesthesia, the electrodes are placed in the middle part outside of dura mater from the second spine to the fourth spine. Electric intensity is from 2 to 5 V/0.1–0.5 ms. The frequency is 100 times/s. It is amplified to 15–25%. The stimulation time is 6–12 a day. If the electrodes are placed subdural, electric intensity can be decreased 50%. The mechanism is that electricity go up through cervical cord to brainstem and finally reach cerebral cortex through ascending reticular activating system and activation system of hypothalamus. Animals experiment found that electric stimulation can increase the acetyl choline in brain, improve brain electrical activity, increase α wave and decrease slow wave. For the patients with severe disturbance of consciousness induced by head damages, anoxic encephalopathy and cerebrovascular disease, there are some certain effect.

(c) Deep brain electric stimulation includes electric stimulation of thalamus, brainstem, midbrain and epencephalon.

Deep brain electric stimulation can increase the excitability of reticular formation of brain stem, activate ascending reticular system and wake up cerebral cortex. This operation can be done through stereotactic operation and the stimulation electrodes are placed into cuneiform nucleus of reticular formation of midbrain or non-specific nucleus of thalamus. The reception device is in subcutaneous of colpus. The stimulation time is more than 6 months. The electrode should be kept for 3–24 months. Some papers found that the therapeutic effect is definite. Some patients waked up from VS and the EEG showed that there was arousal reaction. The brain blood flow was improved.

(d) Neural stem cells transplantation is the hot spot in research at present, but it is not mature. The practicability and reliability remain further study and discussion.

(e) Rehabilitation methods: At present, the purpose of rehabilitation therapy for this kind of patients is maintenance therapy such as physical therapy, homework therapy, speech therapy and psychological therapy. The Rood method is the main method. Flapping quickly, squeezing and pressing, ice compress and hot water to stimulate the skin and sensitive part of the patients such as hand, foot and face to stimulate and induce autonomic movement of the patients. Neuromuscular proprioception promotion method is used to do passive movement. Through deep sensation of joint, central nerves can be connected and the training of maintaining and recovering joint motion can be done. And then the training is transmitted to standing balance and standing in cant board training. These training can improve the respiration, circulation, digestion and urinary system of the patients in VS. It is also important to enhancing the bearing ability of bone joint.

Various kinds of electro-optics stimulation such as ultrasound, frequency spectrum and infrared ray can improve brain blood flow and promote metabolism of neural cells. Electric stimulates peripheral nerves and muscles and photothermic effect improves body dysfunction. In speech therapy, there is entire or partial conduction pathway of audio, vision and touch in the patients without conscious activities. Visual and auditory stimuli are presented to the patients. Meanwhile, the vocal organ is stimulated such as stimulating oral cavity with ice swab and perioral muscles training.

6.1.3 Compulsive Active Movement Method of Neurological Training of Recovering Motor Function of the Patients with Severe Disturbance of Consciousness

According to the fact that consciousness can be separated from movement, at present, it is not precise to judge the level of unconsciousness and the factors such as safe state of emergency that is good for potential development. Except for maintained rehabilitation training and deep brain electric stimulation, the author studies the methods in allusion to recovering motor function and consciousness of the patients with severe unconsciousness. Compulsive active movements induced by positioning have achieved some certain effects in clinic.

6.1.3.1 The Mechanism of Compulsive Active Movements

Except for the patients with brain death and severe disturbance of consciousness, the patients can have some certain consciousness and the ability of responding to external stimulus. If there are some methods to amplify or enhance the consciousness and reaction ability, it is possible to promote consciousness recovery and functional recovery including movement controlled by consciousness. Under safe state of emergency, active movement can activate and amplify the existing consciousness and reaction. For example, human can be motivated to a superman in dangerous condition.

Compulsive active movement of neurological training is non-subjective consciousness movement using specific equipment and human assistance. Because of sudden change of assisted dynamics, the patients can be motivated to do resistivity active response movement that is instructed by deep consciousness and is good for eliminating danger. After repeated training of this kind of movement, the existing consciousness and reaction ability are amplified and enhanced, which can promote waking up and motor function recovery.

6.1.3.2 Training Equipment and Training Methods

Because the patients are in unconscious state, they cannot stand up and cooperate with movement. Therefore, developing the equipment that can make the patients to stand and move is key point of the training and is a tool to implement the method.

1. On the basis of training equipment of compulsive active movement in upper limbs and lower limbs, the author developed weight support and protect system of potential development training device in upper limbs and lower limbs to make the patients in low conscious state and the patients without standing ability to keep in standing position and not to fall down or bump in the training.

   Compulsive active movement in upper limbs and lower limbs lower limbs, it is easy to do compulsive active movement training in lower limbs and the effect is better. For the patients with severe dysfunction of conscious state, it is difficulty to do compulsive active movement training in upper limbs. Compared with compulsive active movement training in upper limbs, compulsive active movement training in lower limbs can enlarge or enhance the existing consciousness and reaction ability better.
2. Training Methods: Example of Compulsive Active Movement Training in Lower Limbs.

   In clinostatism, the patients wear weight support chest thigh band, with help of the therapists, the patients are in standing position and connect the hook of chest band to weight support hook of potential development training device in lower limbs. The therapists regulate the weight in order to make the patients keep in standing position with slight assistance. According to the specific condition of the patients such as body weight, lower limbs myodynamia and cardio-pulmonary function, the number of people that should take part in the training and the assistance can be ascertained. Generally, the training requires 2–3 people and they stand two side and behind the patients. People grasp the waist training band separately, one person commands the other people involved in the training and make the patients from standing position to kneeling-squatting position. The depth of squatting is progressive, from 15° flexion of hip and knee to 150°. And then, the therapists guide with speech or play Daoyin technique record to help the patients to stand up slowly and in a constant speed. Ascending every 5°, the three people should withdraw the force and grasp waist training band. When the patients fall down suddenly, they yell out "stand up, or you will fall down". Generally, the patient's body will react to the voice. Meanwhile, the therapists should help the patients back to the original position and help the patients to continue the training.

One training includes three groups and one group includes ten squatting training. The break between groups is 2 min. The training time is 30 min and one therapy course includes 30 times. After completion of one therapy course, the therapists do the assessment and decide to do the training of next therapy or not. The total training usually takes 3 months.

3. Cautions
   (a) Training of improving cardio-pulmonary function: before training, the training of standing bed should be done first to enhance cardiovascular response ability and bearing ability. When the patients can keep at 90° position for more than 30 min and the vital signs are stable, this training can be done.
   (b) Preparation of range of joint: there are adhesion of muscle and joint, even tendon contracture in the patients without rehabilitation therapy even joint motion for a long time. Therefore, before doing compulsive movement training in lower limbs, the training of range of joint should be done. Traction, physiotherapy and manipulation are used to relax the adhesion of joint and muscle. Meanwhile, constant passive movement equipment is used to achieve a better effect.
   (c) Prevention of accidental injury: because of long-term bed, this kind of patients have severe osteoporosis. Through standing bed training, the patients get better, but there is still osteoporosis. During training, the therapists should keep eyes on the force in case of bone fracture and soft tissue injury.
   (d) For very weak patients with long-term bed, the training should be done with electrocardiograph monitoring. Once there is abnormal situation, the training should be stopped in case of accident.
   (e) Application of sudden postural change: sudden postural change is the key point in the training. Because the therapists only use sudden postural change but not uniform and slow postural with proper Daoyin speech to create real state of emergency, which can motivate deep consciousness of the patients and amplify and recover consciousness.
   (f) The training of compulsive active walking in lower limbs: For the unconscious patients without standing and walking ability, the training can help them to stand and walk to recover the consciousness and walking ability of the patients. It is the training that can help the application of Daoyin technique.
      - The training mechanism of compulsive active walking in lower limbs: human walking center is located in sacral spinal cord. In the patients with in extremely low conscious state, because of long-term bed, the excitability of walking center is very low, even totally be lost. Therefore, recovering the excitability of walking center is the prerequisite to recover the walking ability of the patients. Assisted walking training in standing state is actual walking with bearing load of lower limbs and constant stimulation of deep sensation. Lower limbs walking support devices that are fixed on support frame are connected with bearing. Artificial hip and knee joint are bearings, which can increase the flexibility of joint motion in walking and make it suitable for the walking training of the patients in low conscious state. In addition, artificial hip and knee joint are equipped with rotation resistance regulation device that can increase the resistance and difficulty of lower limbs in the process of stepping forward and make it suitable for the walking training of the patients in consciousness recovery with bad walking ability in order to develop potential, increase the

excitability of walking motor center and actual walking ability.

- Walking training device or equipment for severe patients: training device is mechanical equipment without power-driven and feedback functions. Training equipment is modified from training device. Training equipment can detect and display motor program signal of quadriceps femoris in walking or resistance signal in walking, which is a biological feedback function and make the patients do the training with a purpose (Fig. 6.1).

  During training, the patients stand on the exoskeleton of lower limbs of gait training device and fix the fixing band. According to practical condition of the patients, weight support system is used to regulate weight to make the patients keep in standing position. The therapists stand on the pedal or both sides (when there is no pedal training device) of gait training device of lower limbs and the therapists regulate the resistance of artificial hip and knee joint resistance device of walking support device of lower limbs according to "step by step" principle to do the training with proper walking difficulty.

  Before the patients' consciousness is not recovered, because there is no walking ability, at the time of playing walking instruction record, the therapists pull the hauling cable of hip flexion fixed on knee joint to help the patients coordinate step movement synchronized with record. When the stepping leg is on the process of rising, the therapists suddenly loose the hauling cable of hip flexion and encourage the patients "raise up or you will fall down" and "pass over or you will bump". Meanwhile, the therapists try to lift the falling leg and motivate the consciousness recovery of the patients.

- Training time and therapy course: The training time is 30 min every time and there are 30 times in one therapy course. After one therapy course, the effect should be reevaluated and the

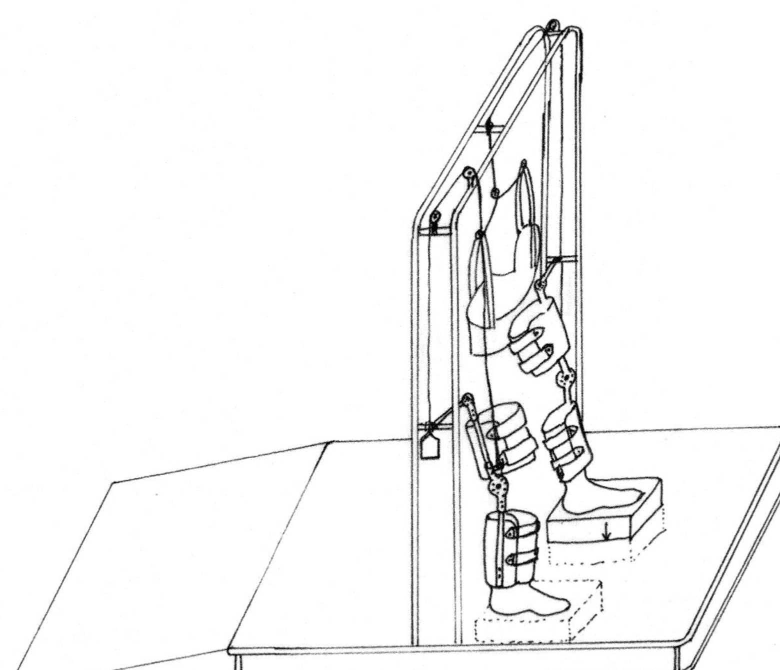

Fig. 6.1 Gait training equipment of severe patients

therapists decide to do the training of next therapy course or not. The training takes three months or longer time.

- Cautions: The cautions are the same as these in compulsive active movement training of lower limbs.

The therapy of severe disturbance of consciousness introduced in this chapter is one of the unsolved problems in clinic. Although there are many therapy methods, it is hard to ascertain which method is effective. The operating mechanism of CNS and therapy and rehabilitation training of nervous diseases require further investigation and study.

EEG has reference value for the prognosis of the patients with severe disturbance of consciousness. Normal EEG is composed of three waveforms and basic amplitude symmetry such as α, β, δ and two hemispheres asymmetry. The waveforms of coma are mainly flat wave and slow wave. If there is β wave, the patients may wake up. If the patients have sensitive reaction, the prognosis is good. Flat wave is the wave stand for brain cells death. Slow wave is the wave stand for brain cells apoptosis, which indicate that there are a few brain cells still alive. Apoptosis wave may recover to normal wave such as α and β waves.

6.2 Rehabilitation Methods of Neurological Training of Muscle with Zero Myodynamia

After central and peripheral nerve injury, there is disability phenomenon of the dominated muscle, unconscious muscle contraction. In clinic, manual muscle test is used to assess myodynamia in order to find the degree and the reason of low myodynamia, which is important for musculoskeletal and nervous system lesion, especially functional assessment of peripheral nerve lesion.

In this section, we mainly discuss the recovery training method of muscle with zero myodynamia tested by manual muscle test. Because the patients with zero myodynamia cannot do automatic muscle contraction and joint motion subjective consciously, the rehabilitation methods of this kind of muscle are only passive methods such as flapping, stretching, massage and electric stimulation, which can increase the excitability of the paralyzed muscle. Because these methods cannot promote SND plasticity and potential development, the therapeutic effect is not good. However, there is no better training method and there is no target for the training. Because the patients cannot see muscle contraction, joint motion and any training effect, they are easy to lose enthusiasm of the therapy, even give up.

6.2.1 The Mechanism of Rehabilitation Training of Neurological Training of Zero Myodynamia

Through the change of training mode and subjective indicator of myodynami, the training under "goal and motive" mechanism can induce active movement training. Muscles dominated by CNS are induced to complete joint motion, which can promote CNS plasticity and functional reorganization. Finally, the voluntary contraction of the muscle can be recovered and lost motor function can be recovered to varying degrees.

The change of training mode: Guided by six-step Daoyin technique, through change of body posture such as standing up and squatting, the purpose of compelling and helping active movement training can be achieved. Meanwhile, Daoyin speech with safe state of emergency can encourage the patients to try to complete intended goal with the help of the therapists. During this process, CNS potential can be developed and utilized to promote plasticity and functional reorganization.

The change of subjective indicators of myodynamia: according to the intensity of myodynamia, within limits, it is in direct proportion to drive signal from CNS to muscle and the signal recovery is quicker than myodynamia recovery. This signal can be measured by V, mV and μV, which makes very weak signal become visible indicator. During the process that Daoyin technique is used to guide the patients to use brain to control joint motion. Through bioelectrical signal reception device, motor program signal can be received real-timely from brain to muscle and be displayed in the fluorescent screen in a curve form, which is visible subjective indicator of muscle contraction. The patients can see their effort and enhance the confidence for rehabilitation training. In the premise that last signal intensity surpasses the goal of this training, because the patients have definite surpassing goal, anti-resistance method of six-step Daoyin technique is used in this training to encourage the patients to make the signal intensity surpass goal intensity. Through repeated training, CNS potential is developed and functional recovery is achieved. When the signal is strong enough, there are visible muscle contraction and joint motion.

Many people don't understand anti-resistance training in zero myodynamia. They think it is impossible to do anti-resistance training in zero myodynamia. However, it is proved to be practical in reality, because zero myodynamia is not equal to zero drive signal of muscle, even not equal to muscle without tension. The author detects 343 muscles with zero myodynamia and found that when the patients try to control muscle contraction, although there is no visible muscle contraction, almost all the muscle drive signals from CNS synchronized with muscle contraction can be received. There are only ten muscles without drive signal. The results demonstrated that most of muscles with zero myodynamia in clinical test still connect with CNS and are controlled by CNS, which also demonstrated that central nervous tissue still have some functions after damages.

Because muscles with zero myodynamia are relaxed, the patients try to complete joint motion through active contraction and cannot induce muscle contraction due to weak intensity of drive signal. There is no sensation of proprioception stimulation induced by muscle contraction and it is easier to make the patients lose the target of muscle drive signal and is harder to induce muscle contraction. At this time, in the fixed orientation of joint motion, the therapists exert resistance to increase muscle tension through stretching it and stimulate proprioception receptor in the muscle to some extent. Proprioception receptor is the target and destination of muscle drive signal from CNS. Neurological training equipment can detect very weak signal and display it in a curve form. The patients can see their own effort. The therapists use this signal intensity to make an elevation transverse line that is the surpassing goal of next training. With guidance, drive signals from CNS are promoted, which is good for promoting recovery of voluntary muscle contraction.

Whether the patients with zero myodynamia in the early stage of the disease, or the patients with zero myodynamia in the recovery period, they are all the indications for training methods mentioned above. In the early stage of injury, muscle with zero myodynamia partially due to temporal muscle contraction dysfunction induced by transient dysfunction (shock) after nervous damages. In acute period, the patients' myodynamia is possible to be recovered. Through training methods mentioned above, the functions of paralyzed muscle can be recovered quickly and the complications can be prevented. After acute period, for the patients with zero myodynamia, the muscle function is difficulty to be recovered because of organic pathologic changes of injured nerves. The training methods must be used to recover the lost functions.

6.2.2 Training Methods of Zero Myodynamia

6.2.2.1 Rehabilitation Training Method of Neurological Training

This method can real-timely display the effect of Daoyin technique on the moment normal or six-step Daoyin technique of guiding collaterals through meridians is used. Through establishing different surpassing goal and biofeedback, under the mechanism of "goal and motive", the patients are trained with a purpose to develop neural potential and promote CNS plasticity. Finally, functional reorganization is achieved and the lost motor function is recovered. The specific methods are as follows:

1. Neurological training equipment method: bioelectric reception device of neurological train-

ing equipment can receive electric signal guided by Daoyin technique from CNS to muscle and display it in fluorescent screen in a curve form. Through establishing surpassing goal, Daoyin technique is used constantly to guide the patients to do neural potential development, motor program reestablishment and motor pattern remodeling with a purpose. The signal intensity is measured by μV. The patients can see their own minor progress and enhance the confidence of rehabilitation training, which is good for the improvement of training effect.

2. Myodynamia Daoyin equipment method: myodynamia Daoyin equipment can receive tension force generated by muscle contraction through tension force receptor. Its sensitivity can be measured by mg or μg. Where there is muscle contraction, there is detection. Tension force can be transformed to visible curve in the fluorescent screen. The precision of this method is less than that of bioelectrical signal reception device, but it can display subjective indicator of Daoyin technique and make the patients do goal surpassing training with a purpose.
3. Muscular tension Daoyin equipment method: muscular tension Daoyin equipment receives the pressure of pressoreceptor on the skin surface of agonistic and antagonistci muscle induced by muscle tension when the patients are guided to do joint motion, turn it into curve form and display it on fluorescent. Therefore, the patients can do the training of potential development and motor program reestablishment with a purpose under the mechanism of "goal and motive". The sensitivity of this equipment can be measured by μg, so it can display muscle tension change in a curve form when muscle tension is changed slightly. The patients can see their own effort, enhance the confidence of training and improve training effect.
4. Virtual reality training method: Virtual reality training system of neurological training is used to do the training. This technique cannot detect or display the muscle drive signal and pressure really. Whereas, both virtual technique and Daoyin technique display simulative muscle drive signal and elevation. When Daoyin technique is used to guide the patients to do joint motion, the therapists exert resistance in the orientation of joint motion and ask the patients to do anti-resistance according to virtual signal intensity in order to develop neural potential constantly. The interference factor of this method is few and virtual signal designed by human can be increased. Artificial virtual signal is always increased. The patients should not misunderstand their trainings are not progressive and feel sad because of low intensity of actual detected signal. They should keep optimistic rehabilitation state that is good for progress of training. The key point of this method is to make the patients fit in training environment as much as possible through "immersion" technique. When the patients regard virtual signal as their own achievement, the therapeutic effect is better.

6.2.2.2 Assisted Active Movement Training Method Through Body Position Change

Upper limbs, lower limbs and trunk potential development training device are used for the training that is different from the training in the patients with severe disturbance of consciousness the patients. Most of the patients with zero myodynamia are conscious people who can cooperate with training and organically combine the guidance of the therapists and the patients' effort. Therefore, this training is not compulsive but assisted active movement training. The patients should bring their subjective initiative. Daoyin technique is used to guide the patients to try to complete designed movement. When the patients cannot complete the movement, the therapists help them to complete it.

In the example of active movement assisted with lower limbs, after the patients wear weight support chest thigh band, regulating weight make the patients keep in standing position. Normally, one therapist helps the patient and in in particular cases two therapists help the patient at the same time. The therapist help the patients from standing position to squatting position (the depth of squatting from hip and knee flexion 25–150°), and then the therapists use speech or play Daoyin technique record to encourage the patients to try to get up slowly by themselves. If there is difficulty in the getting up process, the therapist should yell out "stand up, or you will fall down". The patients try to get up by themselves. If the patients cannot get up, the therapists can help them to get up. When the patients are able to get up by themselves, the therapist can exert resistance on the injured shoulder in the orientation of standing up and encourage the patients to get up in order to develop more potential.

The training time is 30 min and one therapy course includes 30 times. After completion of one therapy course, the therapists do the assessment and decide to do the training of next therapy or not. The total training usually takes 3 months.

In clinic, the author found that if there are physiological reflexes such as patellar tendon reflex and achilles tendon reflex in the body with zero myodynamia and there is no pathological reflexes such as patellar clonus, ankle clonus and Babinski's sign. Whether the disease time is long or short, through the training mentioned above, most of the patients' voluntary autokinetic movement can be recovered.

6.2.2.3 Cautions

1. The training should be in accordance with the principle "step by step and from weak to strong". It is forbidden to increase training intensity, especially for the feeble patients. The training can be done with electrocardiograph monitoring. If there is any abnormity, the training should be halted in case of accident.
2. The therapist can increase resistance gradually: The muscle with zero myodynamia is accompanied with sensory deficiency. During the training of anti-resistance, the resistance should not be too strong in case of injury of muscle and tendon.
3. Preparation for range of joint: the patients don't do rehabilitation therapy and joint motion for a long time. There are muscle and joint adhesions, even tendon spasm in most patients. Therefore, before active movement training of upper and lower limbs, range of joint training should be done first and manipulation is used to relax adhesion of soft tissues such as muscle. After the training, continuous passive movement (CPM) can also be used to help joint motion.
4. Prevention of accidental injury: because of long-term bed, the patients are lack of standing and walking exercise. There will be rarefaction of bone to a certain extent even severe rarefaction. The bone is fragile and easy to be broken. During the training, the intensity should be paid attention to in case of bone fracture and soft tissue injury. It is better to do standing bed training in case of accident.

6.2.3 Clinical Research of Neurological Training Therapy of Zero Myodynamia

In order to verify the training effect of neurological training rehabilitation of the muscle with zero myodynamia, we do clinical experiment study of 343 upper limbs muscles with zero myodynamia of the patients with obsolete spinal cord injury and observe the relationship among training effect, myodynamia and electromyographic signal (motor program). We analyze the reason, investigate the mechanism and provide theory and clinical experiment basis for rehabilitation training of muscles with zero myodynamia.

6.2.3.1 Materials and Methods

1. Materials: there are 77 patients with spinal cord injury. There are 62 males and 15 females. The male female ratio is 4:1. The age range is from 11 to 64 years old. The average age is 31.7 years old. The injured spinal cord are from C1 to C5. There are 40 patients with C5 injury, which accounts for 51.9% of all the patients. There are 19 patients with C4 injury, which accounts for 24.7% of all the patients. The injury reason is mainly vehicle accidents (60 patients, 77.9%). There are eight patients with exercise injury, which accounts for 10.4% of all the patients. The disease history

is 0.5–20 years after injury. The average disease history is 4.2 years. All the patients are the people whose functions cannot be recovered through various kinds of routine rehabilitation method therapy for many times. The patients in this group complete one therapy course. The EMG biofeedback therapy time is 50 min per time and there are 15 times in each therapy course.

2. Equipment: Neuroeducator II with 3 M Ag-AgCl surface electrode produced by Therapeutic Alliances in America is used in this training. The function of Neuroeducator II is to analyze the EMG signal to provide EMG signal for feedback. Through root mean square of potential of EMG signal (less than 140 dB) whose noise level is less than 0.2 μV and bandwidth is from 10 to 1000 Hz, the signals are analyzed to get feedback signal. If the combination of EMG signal is more than 0.1 s, it can be standarded into μVs. The data of one-tenth second is displayed in the color screen in a continuous curve form. Scanning limit of every screen is 20 s and can be storaged in the soft disk for analysis.
3. Therapy methods: In a quiet and lucifuge therapy room, the patients sit in front of display. The therapists put two 3M surface electrodes on the skin surface of two ends of muscle belly and place ground electrode between the two electrodes. Surface electrodes are connected to corresponding leads of Neuroeducator II through wire. The therapists ask the patients to watch the EMG signal change on the display. Meanwhile, the therapists use Daoyin technique to guide the patients to do shoulder abduction, elbow flexion, elbow extension, wrist flexion, wrist extension, finger flexion and finger extension actively. The strongest EMG signal collected from this movement is the raw data for recording and is used to make a marked line. The therapists ask the patients to try to make the EMG signal intensity surpass the baseline level and let the patients not concentrate on joint motion and muscle contraction but watch the EMG signal curve on the display. If the EMG signal surpass baseline, the new summit is the new baseline. In the next joint motion guided by Daoyin technique, the patients should try to make new EMG signal surpass the baseline. The rest can be done in the same manner until EMG signal cannot surpass the baseline, which requires 6–8 movements. The therapy time is 50 min per time and there are 15 times in one therapy course.

6.2.3.2 Observational Indicators

International general assessment methods are used in the therapy. Pretherapy and post-treatment, the therapists do functional assessments.

1. Measurement of myodynamia: according to modified Lovett manual muscle test (MMT), pretherapy and post-treatment, the therapists measure myodynamia of each muscle and classify them.
2. EMG data collection: the raw strongest EMG data of each muscle before therapy and the strongest EMG data at the end of therapy are recorded separately, which are used for comparison and statistical analysis.

6.2.3.3 Results

There are 343 muscles with zero myodynamia in 77 patients. There are 16 middle deltoid, 21 musculus biceps brachii, 28 musculus triceps brachii, 31 extensor muscles of carpus, 61 musculusflexor carpi, 97 extensor digitorum muscle and 89 flexor of fingers. Pretherapy and post-treatment, electromyographic signal and statistical analysis results of myodynamia of each muscle refer to Table 6.2.

Pretherapy and post-treatment, the data of electromyographic signal and myodynamia of 343 muscles are used for statistical analysis. The analysis of electromyographic signal demonstrated that there is significant difference between pretherapy and post-treatment ($P < 0.001$).

There are only 11 muscles with myoelectric potential in 343 muscles with zero myodynamia. After one therapy course of 11 muscles with zero myodynamia, the myodynamia increases to 0.15 grades. Compared with pretherapy, there is no statistical significant difference ($P > 0.05$). The

Table 6.2 Statistical analysis results of raw and post-treatment EMG signal data

	Electromyographic signal (μV)				Myodynamia	
Name	Number*		Pretherapy	Post-treatment	Pretherapy	Post-treatment
Middle deltoid	16	$\overline{X}$	27.69	134.81*	0.00	0.67*
		SD	28.72	69.65	0.00	0.54
Bicipital muscle	21	$\overline{X}$	26.10	105.76*	0.00	0.74*
		SD	41.08	124.79	0.00	0.58
Triceps muscle	28	$\overline{X}$	21.39	165.21*	0.00	0.92*
		SD	33.14	188.18	0.00	0.84
Wrist extensor	31	$\overline{X}$	24.19	120.45*	0.00	0.46*
		SD	21.84	124.80	0.00	0.64
Wrist flexor	61	$\overline{X}$	34.59	95.69*	0.00	0.75*
		SD	137.73	153.97	0.00	0.81
Extensor digitorum	97	$\overline{X}$	16.89	78.96*	0.00	0.27*
		SD	32.89	97.65	0.00	0.46
Flexor of fingers	89	$\overline{X}$	24.75	70.04*	0.00	0.39*
		SD	44.92	95.51	0.00	0.82

*P < 0.01

average of myoelectric potential increases to 8.01 μV. Compared with pretherapy, there is statistical significant difference ($P < 0.05$). There are 121 muscles with myoelectric potential that is less than 10 μV in 343 muscles. After one therapy course, the myodynamia increases to 0.32 grades. Compared with pretherapy, there is statistical significant difference ($P < 0.01$). The average of myoelectric potential increases to 45.34 μV. compared with pretherapy, there is statistical significant difference ($P < 0.001$).

6.2.3.4 Discussion

According to the definition of manual muscle test, muscles with zero myodynamia mean that the therapists cannot feel muscle contraction on the skin surface of the muscle when the patients are guided to do muscle contraction, which demonstrates that the muscle is in denervated completely paralyzed state. Except that zero myodynamia of the patients' muscles due to spinal shock in acute period may be recovered, for the patients in chronic period, it is impossible to recover independent contractile activity of the muscle. Most of the patients abandon therapy and functional exercise, especially for the patients with zero myodynamia due to obsolete nerve injury for more than 1 year. If innervation of the muscle is impossible to be recovered, the patients lose the ability of functional recovery and improving life quality. The disease history of this group is 0.5–20 years and the average is 4.2 years. After therapy, there are statistical significant increases in electromyographic signal and myodynamia. The results may be related to the following factors:

1. The sensitivity of manual muscle test is low. Manual muscle test is the assessment method that is used for diagnosis, therapy program development and therapeutic effect assessment in clinic. This method can distinguish the grade of myodynamia well and assess it quantitatively. The comparability and repeatability are high. The method is easy to be mastered and memorized without the help of special equipment, which is widely used in clinic. MMT is one of the most credible and subjective methods for the assessment of motor dysfunction due to pain of lower limbs and waist. It is usually applied in rehabilitation domain. Bohannon thinks that MMT has

good coherence to range of joint in lower limbs myodynamia.

Some reports indicated that the sensitivity of MMT is less than that of sthenometer for assessing myodynamia that is less than grade IV. If the grade of myodynamia is equal to or more than IV, MMT is better than sthenometer. Compared with isokinetic myodynamia assessment method that is used for myodynamia assessment after spinal cord injury, we found that the sensitivity of MMT to myodynamia assessment is not enough. The sensitivity of MMT is less than that of isokinetic myodynamia assessment method. Through root mean square of potential of EMG signal (less than 140 dB) whose noise level is less than 0.2 μV and bandwidth is from 10 to 1000 Hz, the signals are analyzed to get feedback signal. It is very sensitive. There are 11 muscles with zero myoelectric potential in all 343 muscles with zero myodynamia and the coincidence rate 3/1000, which demonstrated that the sensitivity of MMT is far from that of myoelectricity biological feedback signal reception device. If the equipment can receive autonomic electromyographic signal, through therapy, the functions of the muscles can be recovered to varying degrees.

2. Weak electrical signal display provides effective surpassing target. The disabled patients are always pessimistic and are accompanied by severe mental disorders. Especially the patients' functions cannot be improved through rehabilitation therapy or the doctors tell them that it is impossible to recover the functions, the patients may be pessimistic. Therefore, the way to make the patients see their own progress is vital for motivating the rehabilitation desire and confidence further. The effective method to induce autonomic muscle contraction and joint motion is to induce the appearance or enhancement of autonomic nerve signal that dominate the muscle through active movement. The autonomic contraction and joint motion of muscles with zero myodynamia cannot be observed with eyes. The patients tried many times but lose confidence because of no progress. The therapists feel deeply out of their head. The therapy cannot be carried out and the patients give up the therapy. With the monitoring of electromyographic biofeedback equipment, when doing autonomic contraction and joint motion of muscles with zero myodynamia, the equipment can receive very weak electromyographic signal that can be amplified and processed by the computer to be displayed in the screen in a curve form. At this time, the therapists must explain the origin and meaning of the curve to the patients and guide the patients to watch the change of the curve and to increase the altitude of the curve. The patients should not pay attention to muscle contraction and joint motion and the autonomic nerve signal is easy to be induced. The patients and the therapists can see the therapy progress anytime to enhance the confidence of rehabilitation.

   Some researches found that the intensity of electromyographic signal is not in direct proportion to myodynamia. The received electromyographic signal is actually mixed signal that takes EEG as the principal signal, which means the curve stands for the functional level of muscles dominated by brain.

3. Daoyin feedback technique in traditional Chinese medicine provides surpassing objective target. Objective indicator is essential for learning and functional training. In daily life, there is a truth that archery athlete aims at arrow target to practice archery so that degree of accuracy in archery can be increased. Otherwise, the degree of accuracy in archery cannot be increased without target. This is because archery is a motor program that is constructed in cortex motor center. Through repeated practice, the archery skill will be promoted continuously. When archery athlete aims at arrow target to practice archery, the first arrow may be shoot in the above of the bull's-eye. The archery result is sent to the brain and the brain will analyze numerous factors (altitude of arrow target, distance, wind direction, bow weight, arrow weight, arm strength and emotion) comprehensively. After calculation, the gesture of the second arrow

can be decided such as lowering the arrowhead. The second arrow may be shoot in the below of the bull's-eye. The archery result is sent to the brain and the brain will know the arrowhead is too low. The gesture of the third arrow can be decided such as raising the arrowhead. The third arrow is shoot in the bull's-eye. After repeated training, the speed and accuracy of the movements are controlled precisely by the brain so that the speed and accuracy of the movements will be increased. Daoyin feedback technique in traditional Chinese medicine provides biological feedback signal that is equal to target. The results feedback to the patients; brain through vision. Brain can regulate the intensity and precision of the signals. It goes full circle and promote the functional recovery of brain cells, reestablishment or enhancement of nervous signal transduction pathway and finally improve the body functions.

4. There are residual nervous signal transduction pathways after spinal cord injury. Some reports deemed that the occurrence rate of spinal cord injury is low, which may be related to anatomical structure of spinal cord. Generally, after spinal cord injury, if there are one-third normal spinal cord, the functions remain normal. If original conduction pathway is destroyed, the latent conduction pathway can be activated, but this process requires proper training methods. For example, scientific training can improve the performance of the athletes. For muscles with zero myodynamia and without zero myoelectric potential, through active movement training, the electromyographic signal can be received and surpassing target can be established. During the process of surpassing the target, it is easy to activate the latent conduction pathway. For muscles with zero myodynamia and zero myoelectric potential, during the active movement training, the electromyographic signal cannot be received and surpassing target can be established, which demonstrates that there is severe damage of the diseased region and it is difficulty to activate the latent conduction pathway. At this time, the therapists must have confidence and encourage the patients to try their best to move the muscles through giving out signal from brain. The therapists can use assisted active movement method to induce autonomic signal. For example, bicipital muscle of arm can induce autonomic signal and activation of conduction pathway through assisted pull-up and quadriceps femoris can induce autonomic signal and activation of conduction pathway through assisted standing up from half kneeling-squatting position. The author found that if there is autonomic signal, it will be increased and never lose. Sometimes, the reflex signal form spinal cord can induce autonomic signal.

6.3 Beauty Method of Neurological Training

In daily life, there are some phenomena we can observe. For example, the actors' face is younger than their actual age. The face of the females who live in foggy and humid south is fine, smooth and roseate. People who are broad-minded and with good psychological quality live a long life and their face is younger than their actual age.

Why these factors include actors, moisture and psychological quality can influence beauty? We should analyze it from the actors. Actors major in performances. Before appearing on the stage, they should coat make-up preparations on face. Dose make-up preparations influence the beauty? Make-up preparations are chemical agent. Long time use not only cannot influence beauty, but also do harm to the skin. Obviously, the reason that the actors' face is younger than their actual age is not make-up preparations.

In that way, are the actors with good psychological quality and less sadness? It is known that the actual life of the actors is not as right as rain. They undergo great pressures such as ups and downs of career, love frustration and social disputes that can induce mawkishness and sadness. Obviously, psychological quality and mentality not always influence the beauty, but the person with peaceful mind without sadness can keep the endocrine system at a virtuous circle state, which is good for the normal functions of respiration, circulation, urinary, reproduction, digestion and endocrine system and can delay senescence.

The residual factor is the emotion of happy, anger, sorrow and delight expressed by facial mimetic muscle in the performance. Therefore, active contraction of facial mimetic muscle may be the key factor of good appearance, fine skin and gloss.

The beauty of active movement of mimetic muscle may be related to the following factors:

1. Active movements can increase blood circulation of face and promote metabolism. When the facial mimetic muscle is in active contraction, the partial blood circulation can be increased and the metabolism is promoted. On the moment of increasing myodynamia, the increase of muscle volume is promoted or the decrease is delayed. The facial shape cannot collapse or shrink with age.
2. Active movements can burn subcutaneous fat and prevent skin expansion. Muscle contraction requires a lot of energy and can burn more fat, which can prevent facial subcutaneous fat deposits in order to prevent facial skin expansion due to subcutaneous fat deposits. Eliminating the subcutaneous fat decrease due to age can finally lead to facial or cervical cutis laxa and shrinking.
3. Active movements can keep facial skin elasticity. Long-term repeated contraction of facial muscle can promote blood circulation and make the facial skin full of blood with vigorous metabolism. Repeated contraction and relaxation of skin can increase skin tension of the muscle and keep skin elasticity in order to delay facial senescence.
4. Active movements of facial muscle can promote discharge of metabolite. The contraction of facial muscle can promote partial blood circulation and enhance metabolism. It can keep the temperature in a high level. High skin temperature can open the trichopore and further promote vessels dilation and blood circulation. Sweats can promote discharge of metabolite so that acid metabolic waste cannot harm facial skin and the face is hard to age.

Therefore, usual active contraction of facial muscle can make facial skin keep elasticity and gloss, which is the key factor to delay senescence.

Moisture and warm weather can promote blood circulation and metabolism. Moisture can prevent facial dry skin and is good for sweat pore opening and metabolite discharge so that people can keep face gloss. However, the effect is very little.

In short, active movement of facial muscle is the important measure to delay senescence. According to this mechanism, active movement beauty training methods of neurological training is introduced as follows:

6.3.1 Active Movement of Facial Muscle Training Method of Neurological Training

In a warm and quiet room, on the moment six-step Daoyin technique is used, neurological training equipment is used to receive signal from CNS to facial muscle through single channel and display it in a curve form. The therapists used this baseline as the elevation. In the next training, through exerting resistance in the negative orientation of muscle contraction, the patients are guided to try to make the signal intensity surpass the elevation. The rest can be done in the same manner in active movement training of facial muscle. Through enhancement of motor program signal, the moment increasing the sensitivity of muscle contraction, myodynamia and muscle volume are increased constantly.

The training of frontal muscle and orbicularis oculi muscle, cheek muscles, musculus risorius, bite quadratus, orbicularisoris muscles, cervical anterior muscle and musculus nuchae are done separately and orderly. Every muscle is trained for 5 min (6–8 times). The total time is 50 min and there are 30 times in one therapy course. After one therapy course, the patients rest for 6 months and do the second therapy course. During the rest, according to self-exercise schedule, the patients do self-exercise every day.

6.3.2 Active Movement Training Method of Facial Muscle of Virtual Neurological Training

Training system of virtual neurological training is used to do the training. Six-step Daoyin technique record is used to do the training according to simulated signal curve and elevation. The patients try to do active contraction of facial muscle and the therapists exert resistance in the negative orientation of muscle contraction. The patients are guided to try to do active contraction of facial muscle with the increase of simulated signal curve. Before training, immersion technique is used to guide the patients to immerse into virtual environment as much as possible until the patients think the simulated signal curve is from their own body. Their own efforts show similar changes with the simulated signal curve and the training effect is better than that of signal detection of neurological training equipment. However, it is better to do actual signal detection training before this training to make the patients relate muscle contraction to motor program signal. It is easy to make the patients immerse into virtual and simulated environment.

The training of frontal muscle and orbicularis oculi muscle, cheek muscles, musculus risorius, bite quadratus, orbicularisoris muscles, cervical anterior muscle and musculus nuchae are done separately and orderly. Every muscle is trained for 5 min (6–8 times). The total time is 50 min and there are 30 times in one therapy course. After one therapy course, the patients rest for 6 months and do the second therapy course. During the interval of training, facial manual massage can be used.

6.3.3 Manual Active Movement Training Method of Facial Muscle of Neurological Training

Manual active movement training method of facial muscle of neurological training is a method that the therapists use six-step Daoyin technique in traditional Chinese medicine to guide the patients to do active contraction training of facial muscle and exert resistance in the negative orientation of muscle contraction. During this process, the therapists use Daoyin speech to create state of emergency and encourage the patients to promote the intensity of muscle contraction. During training interval, the therapists can do facial massage of the training muscle for the patients to increase blood circulation and skin elasticity.

The active contraction and anti-resistance training of frontal muscle and orbicularis oculi muscle, cheek muscles, musculus risorius, bite quadratus, orbicularisoris muscles, cervical anterior muscle and musculus nuchae are done separately and orderly with the same method.

Every muscle is trained for 5 min (6–8 times). The total time is 50 min and there are 30 times in one therapy course. After one therapy course, the patients rest for 6 months and do the second therapy course.

6.3.4 Self-Training Method of Facial Muscle of Neurological Training

In the therapy or after therapy, the patients go home and do self-exercise method of facial muscle. The training can be done in front of the mirror. According to training method of signal detection with neurological training equipment, the patients do active contraction exercise of facial muscle and use finger to exert resistance in the negative orientation of muscle contraction (The finger control point is on the outside and upward of orbital cavity in frontal muscle contraction) for 6 s. During exercise interval, the patients can do facial massage by themselves.

The active contraction and anti-resistance training of frontal muscle and orbicularis oculi muscle, cheek muscles, musculus risorius, bite quadratus, orbicularisoris muscles, cervical anterior muscle and musculus nuchae are done separately and orderly with the same method.

Every muscle is trained for 5 min (6–8 times). The total time is 50 min and there are 30 times in one therapy course. After one therapy course, the patients rest for 6 months and do the second therapy course.

6.3.5 Facial Physiotherapy

Far infrared mask (or helmet) is used to do the therapy. Far infrared mask is equipped with infrared light heating and atomization system automatically controlled by temperature and humidity. Its purpose is to increase facial blood circulation, wet facial skin, promote facial metabolism and discharge of metabolite, increase muscle nutrition and keep the elasticity and gloss of facial skin.

Therapy time and therapy course: the therapy time is 30 min per time and there is one therapy a day. There are 30 times in a therapy course. The therapy can be done in the interval of facial care.

6.4 Active Movement Conceptions and Methods of Aged Care: New Concept of Modern Aged Healthcare

Since the beginning of the reform and opening in 1978, our country has sustained economic development, the society is in a long-term secular stability, human life get better and better and average life of a nation increases greatly. On the other hand, the problem of aging in our country is bigger and bigger. According to statistics, in 2005, the number of the aged who are more than 60 years old is 145 million, which accounts for 11% of the gross population. The increase rate is 3.3% every year. According to the standard of the United Nations, if the proportion of the aged who are more than 60 years old is more than 10%, the society is aging society.

Moreover, the moment our country enters into aging society, the proportion of empty nest phenomenon is increased rapidly. Empty nest phenomenon means that there are only the old in the family because the children grow up and go out for a living. In addition, there is still imbalance phenomenon between urban and rural areas. With the increase of people's life standard, acceleration of rural urbanization, obvious improvement of medical sanitary condition and development of body-building, expectation of life will increase constantly and the degree of aging society will be aggravated. Empty nest phenomenon will be the main mode of aging population family in cities even in rural area in twenty-first century.

For the biggest developing country of the world, we encounter a series of challenges because of aging of the population. Therefore, we can accelerate the reform and development of old-age care, which is the important measure to solve the inconvenience and confusion induced by aging and empty nest phenomenon.

At present, the most popular ways of old-age care are home-based care for the aged, gerocomium-based care for the aged and apartment-based care for the aged. Regardless of what kind of way of old-age care, old-age care concept is to look after the old as best as we can, do what we can for the old, alleviate the burden of the old and satisfy the need of the old in daily life. Even there are some excessive cares. For example, some nursing institutions for the aged use good service as key propagandist point. The service staffs do many things for the old such as tooth brushing and face washing. The service staffs do the things that the old can do by themselves. For a long time, the motor function of the body can be decreased. The old cannot complete daily life activity with time. In addition, the functions of organ and tissue are decreased such as bones, muscles, joints, digestion, respiration, circulation, and urinary system. Therefore, excessive care and movement replacement actually promote functional decline and aging of the old.

Of course, this is not to say that it is not necessary to take care of the old. Especially for the completed disabled old man, they should be taken good care of. However, for the old with functions who can improve functions through training, we should discuss how to take care of the old and what we should do that is the best for improvement of life quality and physical and psychological health of the aged.

The first we should figure out is that what the happiness is for the old. The happiness is that they are taken good care of by others or by themselves.

In daily life, we can obtain happiness from doing many things such as taking a walk, traveling, riding a tricycle, fishing, exercise and eating by ourselves. In other words, we are able to do these things and obtain happiness through completing them. One person strives for experience and wealth for a lifetime. In the old age, it is time to enjoy them and to do something that they want to do but don't have time to do in childhood. If they cannot do these things due to their physical state, there is only regret and no happiness.

In addition, age is one of the symbols of experience, technique and knowledge. They went through a lot, received a lot of lessons and had much successful experience. Through life and work of a lifetime, they understand the life thoroughly. They can teach young people the experience and learning in order to contribute to the society. Therefore, we do not treat the old as the burden of the society. They are useful for the development of the society, because they are the initiator of human civilization, teacher of social experience, knowledge and skills, valuable wealth to promote the development of the society. On the other hand, imparting knowledge and experience require healthy body and vigor.

Therefore, to recover self-function of the aged and prevent the function reduction is not only the important goal to improve life quality of the aged, but also the requirements of promoting society development. Only in this way, the aged can be able to enjoy themselves and have stamina and vigor to impart their experience and learning to the descendant and the society.

According to the mechanism of promoting CNS plasticity and functional reorganization, recovering self-function and slowing down function reduction require not only increasing proper nutrition and abundant rest, but also functional training of active movement. Only active movement can develop neural potential. On the basis of that, body motor function, active old-age care concept and pattern can also develop neural potential.

Existing nursing institution for the aged, whether gerocomium or apartment for the elderly, take physical exercise as one part of old-age care. There is exercise room or hall that is equipped with treadmill, balance bar and dumbbell, even advanced fitness equipment. They organize the aged to travel, playing gate ball and dancing with music regularly or irregularly, these are appropriate for the aged with good condition to do self-exercise or do training with instruction and protection. Moreover, most of the aged are impatient and neglect of using fitness equipment to do training. The exercise room becomes the exhibition room of fitness equipment. For completed or partial disabled old man, they give up because it is difficult for them to do training with fitness equipment.

Therefore, developing method and equipment in allusion to improvement of motor function of the aged and delay aging process of the aged is essential to enhance the life quality of the aged and play roles of the aged.

According to the characteristic that active movement of neurological training can promote CNS plasticity and functional reorganization, mechanism of "goal and motive", safe state of emergency and other neural potential development concept and method, in allusion to the body characteristic of the old, different cognitive state and cooperative degree, we use different rehabilitation training method and equipment.

6.4.1 Active Movement

It is appropriate for the aged with stable fundamental state, clear consciousness and normal cognitive ability who can partially complete autonomic joint motion. With the cooperation of the old, whether the old can complete the designed movement or not, the therapists exert resistance in the orientation of joint motion and do anti-resistance training guided by Daoyin technique. The training is done on the basis of the original functions to increase the ability of active movement and delay exercise aging, which is called intensified active movement training. The specific methods are as follows:

1. Neurological physical therapy (NPT): The therapists use normal or guiding collaterals through meridians six-step Daoyin technique in traditional Chinese medicine to guide the patients to do designed active joint motion on the basis of regulation of breathing and mind.

When active joint motion is on the summit, the therapists exert resistance in the orientation of joint motion and use counting method to encourage the patients to insist for 6 s. During this process, Daoyin speech such as "life up, or you will bump!" and "higher, or you will fall down!" is used to create safe state of emergency to encourage the patients to try to achieve the goal.

2. Neurological occupational therapy (NOT) is appropriate for the fine movement training of upper limbs and hands. According to the requirements in daily life, we designed different training items such as combing, tooth brushing, face washing and dressing. Daoyin technique is used to encourage the patients to complete the designed movement and during this process Daoyin speech is used to encourage the old such as "hold on, or your comb will drop; try, you are great" and make the old feel joyful after the movement.
3. Neurological training: Normal or guiding collaterals through meridians six-step Daoyin technique is used and motor program signal from real-time detection of neurological training equipment is used as baseline that is marked as the elevation. Daoyin technique is used again to encourage the patients to try to make the signal intensity curve surpass the elevation and guide the old to insist for 6 s at the summit, which is good for CNS potential development. Afterwards, the new summit is regarded as the baseline for the elevation. The same method is used to guide the patients to try to make the curve surpass the elevation. The rest can be done in the same manner to develop potential constantly and improve motor function.
4. Myodynamia Daoyin method: Daoyin technique is used to guide the patients to use brain to dominate muscle contraction. During this process, myodynamia Daoyin equipment is used to receive the signal of muscle contraction and turn it into curve in order to display it in the fluorescent screen. Initial curve intensity is used for the elevation and Daoyin technique is used to encourage the patients to try to make intensity of myodynamia surpass the elevation and keep at the summit for 6 s to develop potential. Afterwards, the new summit is regarded as the baseline for the elevation. The same method is used to guide the patients to try to make the curve surpass the elevation. The rest can be done in the same manner to develop potential constantly and improve motor function.
5. Muscle tension Daoyin equipment method: Daoyin technique is used to guide the patients to use brain to dominate muscle contraction. During this process, muscle tension Daoyin equipment is used to receive the signal of tension change of agonistic muscle and antagonistic muscle and turn it into curve in order to display it in the fluorescent screen. Initial curve intensity is used for the elevation and Daoyin technique is used to encourage the patients to try to make intensity of myodynamia surpass the elevation and keep at the summit for 6 s to develop potential. Afterwards, the new summit is regarded as the baseline for the elevation. The same method is used to guide the patients to try to make the curve surpass the elevation. The rest can be done in the same manner to develop potential constantly and improve motor function.
6. Virtual reality training methods of neurological training: Virtual reality training methods of neurological training system is used to do the training. Guiding collaterals through meridians six-step Daoyin technique record is used to instruct the patients to do joint motion through regulation of mind and breathing. The therapists exert resistance in the orientation of joint motion and use record to encourage the patients to try to increase the virtual signal line. In the next training, there is virtual signal line elevation. At this time, the same method is used to encourage the patients to make signal line surpass simulated signal line elevation. The rest training is done as the same way. The advantage of this method is that the actual signal cannot decrease and the patients can keep the confidence of the therapy because the simulated signal intensity is increased constantly. In addition, six-step Daoyin technique record can make the patients maintain high

enthusiasm all the time and can relieve the labor intensity of the therapists, which is good for promoting the training effect of rehabilitation training.

6.4.2 Assisted Active Movement Training

It is appropriate for the weak aged with stable fundamental state, clear consciousness and normal cognitive ability who can have consciousness of active movement but cannot complete autonomic joint motion by themselves.

For this kind of old people, assisted active movement training of body position change is used, such as push up and down of upper limbs, standing up and squatting of lower limbs. During the process of assisted active movement training of lower limbs, lower limbs potential development training device is used. The patients wear chest hip band and connect weight support system hook. According to the specific condition of the patients, the weight is regulated to prevent falling down and bumping. The therapists stand one side of the patients and grasp the waist training belt. On the basis of regulation of mind and breathing guided by Daoyin technique, the patients are guided to squat slowly. In the squatting process, the therapists should suddenly reduce the support and use Daoyin speech to encourage the patients such as "stop, or you will squat!" and "get up, or you will fall down!" to prevent fall down (Fig. 6.2). Along with the increase of stamina of the patients, the therapist can reduce support gradually until they can complete the movement by themselves.

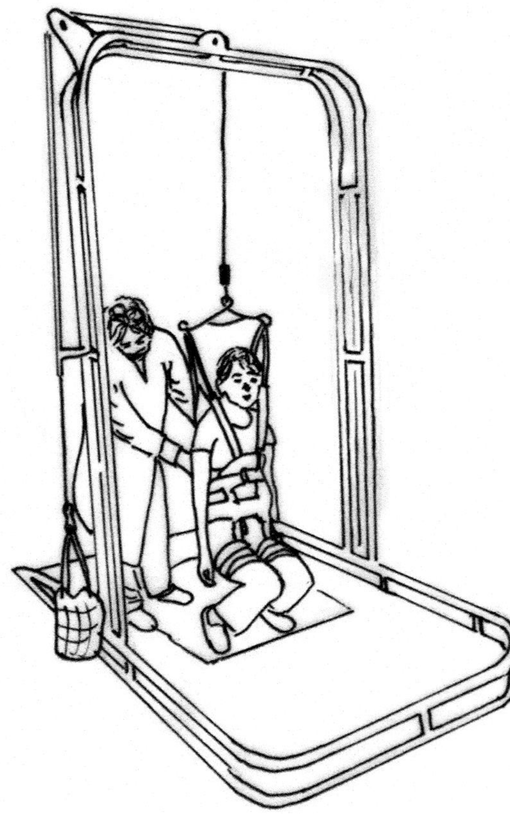

Fig. 6.2 Gait training equipment of severe patients

Meanwhile, the therapists should choose movement training of daily life such as assisted ascending and descending the stairs (Fig. 6.3) and assisted walking training (Fig. 6.4).

6.4.3 Passive Active Movement Training

It is appropriate for the aged with stable vital signs and clear consciousness who lost motor function of body limbs due to diseases. This kind of training usually requires two or more therapists. According to the specific condition of subject, the therapists choose proper training items. The patients can do the training with bare hands or use potential development training device of upper limbs, lower limbs and trunk.

1. Bare-handed passive active movement training method is the training without training equipment (Fig. 6.5). In the passive active movement training of lower limbs, the therapists dress the patients training waistband. Two trainers stand two sides of the patients. One is the main trainer and the other is the assisted trainer. The trainer make the patients stand up slowly. According to the principle "step by step", the patients squat to a certain extent. The therapists use Daoyin technique to guide the patients to regulate mind and breath-

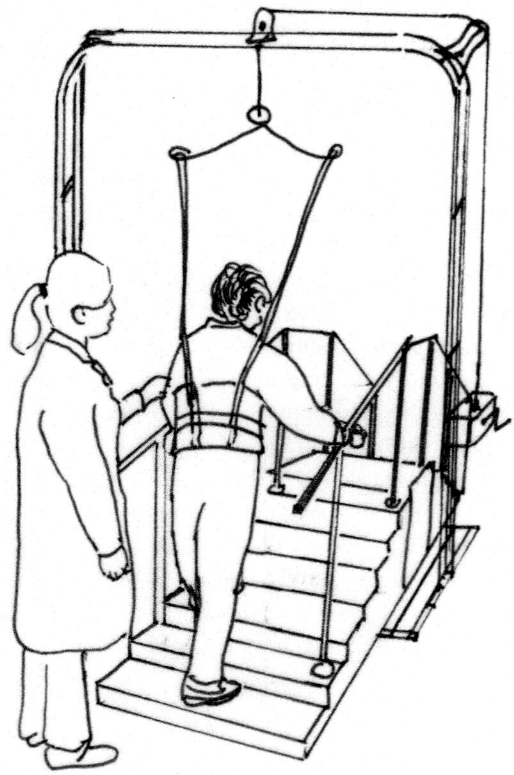

Fig. 6.3 Gait training equipment of severe patients

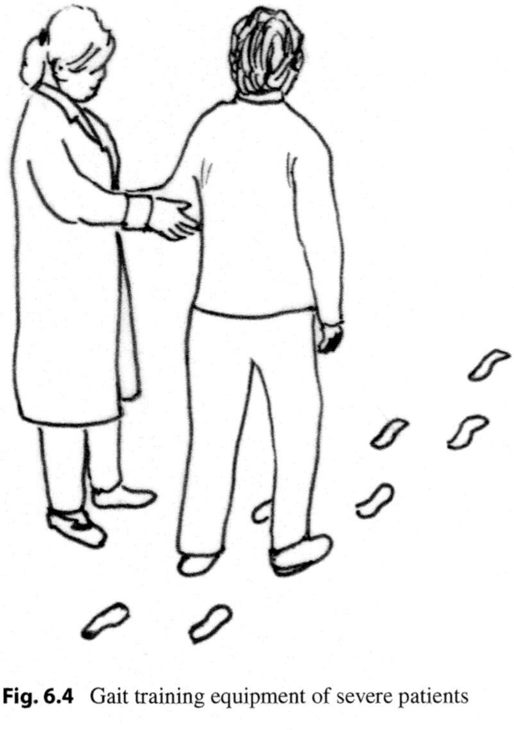

Fig. 6.4 Gait training equipment of severe patients

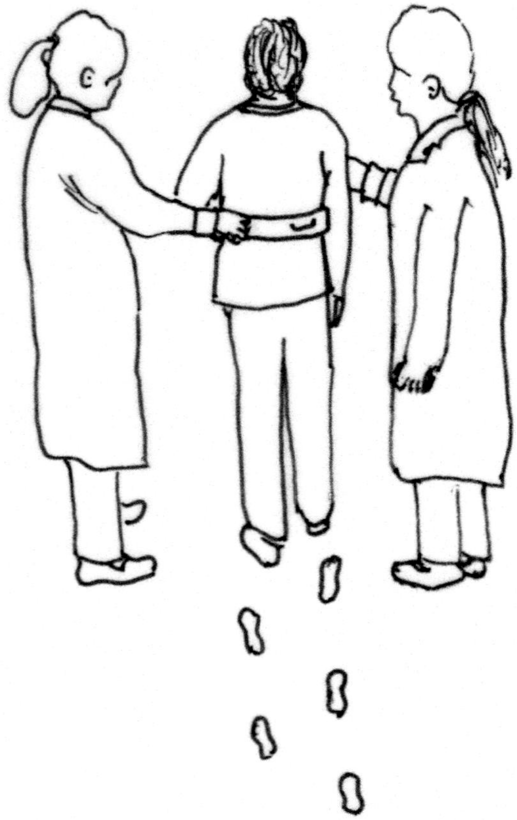

Fig. 6.5 Gait training equipment of severe patients

ing. They let the patients stand up slowly and use Daoyin speech to motivate the patients to get up by themselves. During the standing process, the therapists suddenly reduce support. During the process of falling down, the therapists use speech to motivate the patients such as "stand up, or you will fall down". The therapists help the patients to get up.

2. Passive active movement training with equipment: Corresponding training equipment is used to do the training of upper limbs, lower limbs, trunk, neck and ankle such as passive active movement training of upper limbs (Fig. 6.6). Upper limbs potential development training device is used. The patients wear shoulder chest training waistcoat, lie in a prone position on training mat of potential development training device of upper limbs.

The therapists connect straps of shoulder chest training waistcoat to weight support hook of the training device and suspend weight support sandbag on the other end. The weight can make the patients stretch upper limbs straightly with the help of the therapists. During training, the patients use hands to support their body on the training mat and are guided to regulate mind and breathing. The patients use upper limbs to push down their body and make the chest touch the training mat slowly. Meanwhile, the therapists strain weight support handle and let the patients flex elbow, which is called pushing down training. On the contrary, upper limbs of the patients are on a flexed position and the patients are guided to stretch upper limbs straightly slowly on the basis of regulation of mind and breathing. Meanwhile, the therapists strain weight support handle and control the elbow extension speed of the patients. During this process, the therapists can use Daoyin speech such as "push up, or you will bump head" to motivate the patients to develop potential in order to induce automatic movement.

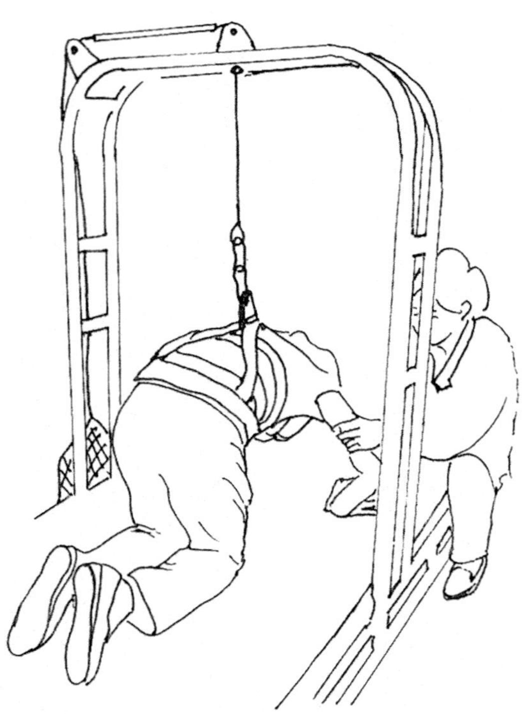

Fig. 6.6 Gait training equipment of severe patients

6.4.4 Compulsive Active Movement Training

It is appropriate for the aged with stable vital signs and unclear consciousness and is also appropriate for the old with clear consciousness and cognition impairment who don't cooperate with active movement training.

Before the training, the therapists should explain the goal and advantage of the training and its possible risks to the old. With the permission of the family, the training can be done, because the mentality and body function of the old may fluctuate during the training.

Compulsive active movement training includes standing up and squatting training (Fig. 6.7), which requires two or more therapists. The two therapists stand on two sides of the patients and use potential development training device of lower limbs to do the training. According to the

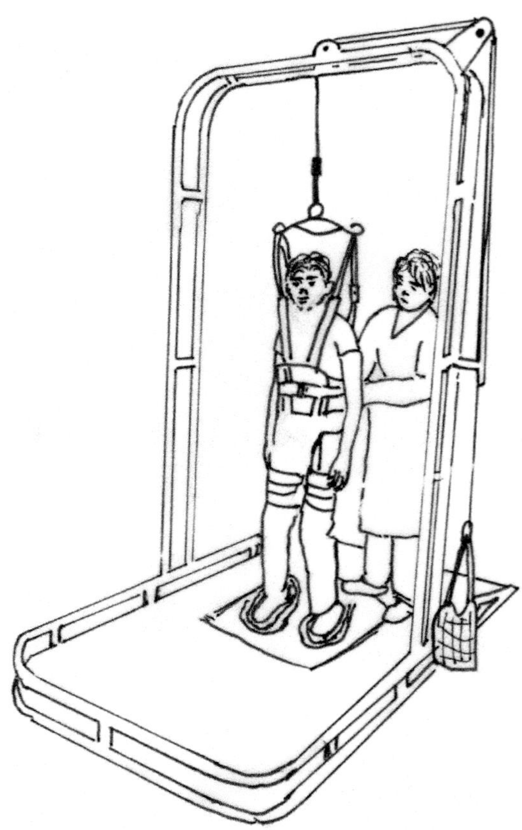

Fig. 6.7 Gait training equipment of severe patients

principle "step by step" and the specific condition of the subject, the therapists ascertain the training intensity. In the standing training, the therapists help the subject to squat at first and the depth is from 150° flexion of knee joint. According to the condition, the depth can be increased gradually. Daoyin speech is used to encourage the subject to stand up and the therapists suddenly reduce support in this process. At this time, the subjects fall down and the therapists use Daoyin speech to create state of emergency to encourage the patients to stand up again with the help of the therapists. Squatting training is from the standing position and the subjects is helped to squat slowly. During the squatting process, the therapists suddenly reduce support and encourage the subjects to maintain the body position in case of squatting.

Through repeated compulsive active movement training, movement response and autonomic motor function recovery of the patients are induced. During this process, for the old with clear consciousness and cognitive disorder, the therapists should be patient and guide the patients to adapt to the training and form habit. It is difficult to communicate with this kind of old people, so it is better to let them form the habit just like three meals in 1 day. For the old who are reluctant to do the training, it is hard to do the training. This kind of old people without cognitive disorder are reluctant to do the movement. The therapists should pay attention to the pattern and make the old realize the function of the training and cooperate with the training through increasing the training pleasure.

6.4.5 Self-Exercise Method of Neurological Training

It is appropriate for the old patients who can do self-exercise to recover consciousness and motor function to a certain extent through rehabilitation training of neurological training.

Portable virtual reality training system of neurological training and multiple functions band are used to do the training. Virtual reality training system of neurological training is equipped with explanation of training mechanism, Daoyin technique record and specific training video. Training content and method are chosen for the training such as elbow extension of six-step method of guiding collaterals through meridians. The trainer put the distal end of the elbow extension band on the dorsal part of the forearm on the upper end of wrist and put the other end on the back of forearm. After the training is activated, main and collateral channels of elbow extension appear. Daoyin technique record is used to guide Qi to go along with virtual main and collateral channels to triceps muscle of arm. Record can encourage the patients to initiate joint motion of elbow extension and make them to try to reach the altitude of simulated curve for 6 s. Afterwards, the patients relax, let Qi go along residual meridians (Fig. 6.8) and let it disperse in collaterals. The training of all joints and trunk can be done in the same manner.

The training frequency is one time a day and the time is 0.5–1 h every time. The patients should stick to the training.

6.4.6 Cautions

1. During training process, the therapists should increase the difficulty gradually and abide by the principle "step by step". The amount of training should be dependent on the ability of the subject. The patients should do the training according to one's abilities and don't push it too much in case of accident.
2. Pay attention to the selection of training pattern: The therapists can design training items with different pattern, difficulty and goal according to the specific condition of the aged. The therapists should increase the amusement and interest of the training.
3. The therapists should lay emphasis on basic training and do not do it with hesitation. Before training, especially the standing up and squatting training of lower limbs, the patients should do standing bed training at first. The patients can stand erectly for 30 min or more with stable vital signs and without discomfortableness.
4. At the beginning of the training, the therapist should pay attention to monitoring of

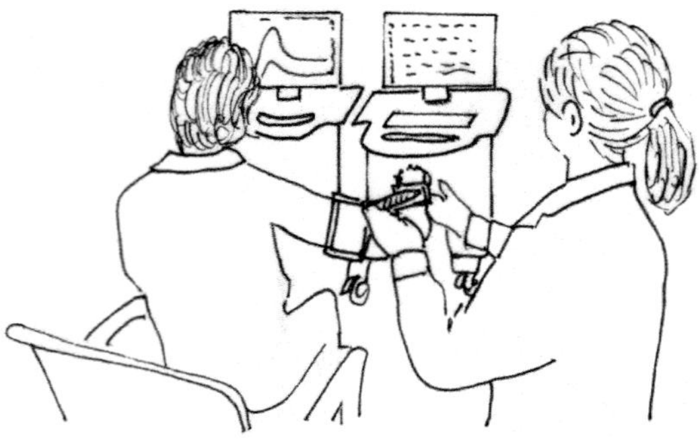

Fig. 6.8 Gait training equipment of severe patients

biological signs. At the beginning of the training, the training should be done with electrocardiogram monitoring in order to find the problem timely and in case of accident. After a period of time, the patients adapt to the training and can do the training without electrocardiogram monitoring.

5. In the training, the therapists should be patient and caring. The aged cannot cooperate with the training that is affected by stamina, understanding ability and memory ability. The therapists should be patient, confident and caring. They cannot give up and use scolding speech. They should use encouraging and complimentary words all the time to activate the enthusiasm of the patients.
6. The therapists should lay emphasis on training ingredient. The therapists should teach the patients how to do the training but not teach the patients to do what. In the training, some therapists just let the patients know how to do and to do what. The training should be concentrated on the lost functions of the patients. The therapists tell or ask the patients to do what, but the patients cannot do it without practical training. Therefore, the therapists should teach the patients by themselves and help the patients to complete the movements. Through repeated training, the patients are possible to recover the functions, which is the problem that the therapists should pay attention to in practical training.

Initiative way of old-age care not only can satisfy the health requirements of the old, but also increase the life quality of the aged to make them enjoy better happy life in old age.

Reference

1. Wade DT, Johnston C. The permanent vegetative state: pratical guidance on diagnosis and management. BMJ. 1999;319(7213):841–4.
2. Yuanxiang L, Ruxiang X. Minimally conscious state: definition, diagnostic criteria and clinical features of consciousness disorder. Chin J Neuromed. 2005;4(2):203–5.
3. Giacino J, Hins JJ, Mchado A, et al. Central thalamic deep brian stimulation to promote recovery from chronic posttraumatic minimally conscious state: challenges and opportunities. Neuromodulation. 2012;15(4):339–49.
4. Smith AC, Shah SA, Hudson AE, et al. A Bayesian statistical analysis of behavioral facilitation associated with deep brain stimulation. J Neurosci Methods. 2009;183(2):267–76.
5. Shah SA, Baker JL, Ryou JW, et al. Modulation of arousal regulation with central thalamic deep brain stimulation. Conf Proc IEEE Eng Med Biol Soc. 2009;2009:3314–7.
6. Zhongfu Z, Qingxi C, Jianli S. Effects of hyperbaric oxygen and acupuncture combined treatment in severe craniocerebral injury. J Chin Clin Rehabil. 2002;6(14):2106–8.
7. Yang R, Hong L, Ping P. The curative effect of hyperbaric neurosurgery and simple neurosurgery on patients with severe craniocerebral injury. Chin Clin Rehabil. 2002;6(14):2120.

7 Function Assessment and Therapeutic Schedule of Neurological Training Rehabilitation

Rehabilitation evaluation is the important measure [1] for rehabilitation therapy schedule and rehabilitation therapy effect assessment, which can guarantee the effect of rehabilitation training and is the crucial basis of verifying the effect of rehabilitation method. The application can affect the rehabilitation training effect and the assessment results of rehabilitation method directly.

Rehabilitation evaluation is similar with clinical diagnosis. Through objective and precise examination, the therapists judge the characteristic, part, range, degree and residual functions of dysfunction of the patients and estimate the development, outcome and prognosis of dysfunctions. It is good for the protocol of rehabilitation goal and rehabilitation therapy schedule. It is also a process that the therapeutic effect is judged and the patients can go on with the rehabilitation therapy or not.

There are many books about rehabilitation evaluation method, which account for a lot in rehabilitation books. However, most of them are used for evaluating the residual functions and abilities of the patients and the effect of rehabilitation training method. Although it is important for and handicapped degree of the patients the advantage and disadvantage of the rehabilitation methods, some assessment method have no effect on rehabilitation therapy schedule. In this chapter, we introduce functional assessment method that can influence neurological training rehabilitation training schedule. Activities of Daily Living (ADL), functional independence measure (FIM), movement assessment scale (MAS), and visceral function assessment are not introduced in our book.

7.1 The Main Methods of Rehabilitation Functional Assessment

7.1.1 The Principle of Neurological Training Rehabilitation Evaluation

In the clinical rehabilitation work for many years, the author thinks that international rehabilitation evaluation items are used for the assessment of rehabilitation training effect. The assessment should be done before rehabilitation training, in the midterm of rehabilitation training and at the end of rehabilitation training to accumulate data. Through statistical analysis of the data, the training effect of rehabilitation method is judged. Sometimes, these assessment items have no effect on rehabilitation training schedule. Because rehabilitation is a training that should be adjusted anytime, for therapy schedule, the principle of assessment method of application function are as follows:

W. Zhao, *Rehabilitation Therapeutics of the Neurological Training*,
https://doi.org/10.1007/978-981-13-0812-3_7

7.1.1.1 Selecting Simple Assessment Method to Reflect Dysfunction Part and Degree

1. Somatic movement function assessment: The therapists should select simple operative part that can be easily located such as one muscle or joint and degree such as the intensity of myodynamia to do functional assessment. Generally, muscular strength assessment, range of joint and muscle spasm degree are used for assessment.
2. Functional assessment of speech, cognition and swallowing function: Selective alogia assessment, dysarthria assessment, cognitive function assessment, swallowing function assessment and sensory function assessment are used for assessment.

7.1.1.2 Selecting Assessment Method That Can Reflect Partial or Entire Function Degree

Motor dysfunction induced by CNS damages varies in the degree and type of motor dysfunction due to different injured part and degree. The manifestation of brain stem damage is balance motor dysfunction. The manifestation of right cerebral hemisphere damage is motor dysfunction of upper and lower limbs in left side to varying degree. The manifestation of motor area IV of cerebral cortex damage is functional limitation of single joint motion. The manifestation of motor area IV of cerebral cortex damage is functional limitation of associated movement with multiple joint motion.

Partial function degree stands for the ability of contraction of one muscle and the function of motion of one joint, which is the basic requirements of single joint motion. Single joint motion is unable to complete functional movement needed for daily life. The entire function is the ability to complete functional movement required for daily life and work, which is composed of associated movement with multiple joints. In most cases, normal single joint motion is not equal to normal associated movement with multiple joint motion. Therefore, it requires further detailed assessment of partial and entire motor function.

1. Assessment of partial motor function: Motor program signal check of single joint motion, muscular strength assessment and range of joint motion are used for assessment. These assessment items can exactly reflect the contraction of every muscle, the intensity of myodynamia, motor program signal intensity and ratio between agonistic muscle and antagonistic muscle and ability of autonomic joint motion, which can provide reliable reference for analysis and judgement of single joint motion ability.
2. Assessment of entire motor function: the therapists can select assessment of coordinated and balanced function and gait analysis, motor program check of associated movement to know the functions of brain stem and motor area VI of cerebral cortex, which can reliable reference for rehabilitation therapy schedule.

7.1.1.3 Selecting Assessment Method That Can Be Used to Judge Main Dysfunction Point and Is Good for Training Schedule

The ultimate goal of recovering lost motor function is to recover functional movement that is meaningful for daily life and work, which means motor pattern and ability of associated movement. Abnormal motor pattern will influence associated movement to varying degrees. Abnormal motor pattern is composed of one or two obstacle points. For example, the circle gait is due to varus and hip flexor paralysis. Through detailed assessment, the therapist can find the principal obstacle point, which is good for formulating specific rehabilitation training schedule. It is the basic premise of obtaining good rehabilitation training effect.

1. Assessment of motor pattern includes functional assessment of upper limbs and lower limbs, gait analysis and balanced function assessment, which can be used to analyze functional ability of upper limbs, lower limbs and entire movement. According to the assessment results of motor pattern and myodynamia, the therapists can find out principal obstacle point of abnormal motor pattern.
2. Motor program examination of associated movement: The signal form cortex motor center

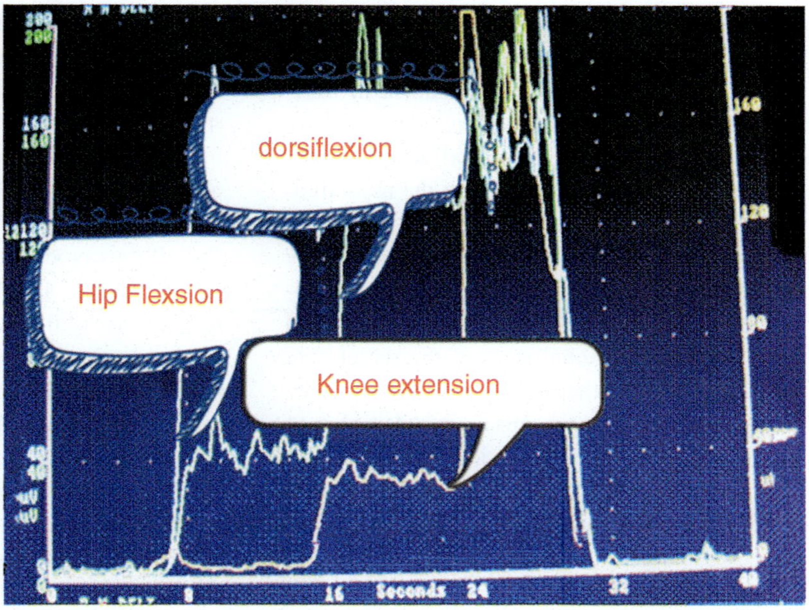

Fig. 7.1 Establishment training of walking motor pattern of lower limbs

to muscle of associated movement are examined and the therapists can observe the intensity of sequence of signals. The therapists can analyze the reason of abnormal motor program of associated motor pattern to provide reference for reestablishing normal motor program (Fig. 7.1).

7.1.2 The Main Content and Assessment Stages of Rehabilitation Evaluation

7.1.2.1 The Main Content of Assessment

1. Functional assessment of the trunk includes range of joint motion assessment, muscular strength assessment, functional assessment of upper limbs and lower limbs, gait analysis, nerve electrophysiology assessment, spasm assessment, sensory function assessment, coordinated and balanced function assessment.
2. Mental and psychological function assessment includes apraxia and agnosia assessment.
3. Linguistic function assessment includes alogia and dysarthria assessment.
4. Swallowing function assessment includes muscular strength assessment and electromyographic signal of swallowing muscle.

7.1.2.2 The Stages of Rehabilitation Evaluation

According to the process of rehabilitation training, from the beginning to the end, the purpose of rehabilitation evaluation is to observe the effect of the method and provide reference for therapy schedule [2].

1. Assessment in preliminary stage is the assessment of the patients in hospital before rehabilitation training. The purpose is to know the functional state, dysfunction degree, disability reason and prediction of rehabilitation prognosis, which is the important evidence of rehabilitation goal and therapy schedule and is the basic data of measuring effect of rehabilitation training method.
2. Assessment in midterm is the assessment that is done in stated midterm of rehabilitation time. Assessment in midterm should be done at least once a month. The purpose of it is to know the effect of rehabilitation method, find out shortcomings and defects and analyze the reason.

The therapists should know the functional state of the patients after a length of therapy, which can provide basis for the adjustment of rehabilitation training schedule.

3. Assessment in the late period is the assessment that is done in the end of the rehabilitation. The purpose is to assess the functional state of the patients after a length of therapy and to assess the effect of rehabilitation training. According to the cooperative situation and actual functional state of the patients in the therapy, the therapists can formulate self-exercise method and subsequent visit plan of the patients and suggest the patients to go home, go back to work or receive further rehabilitation therapy.

7.1.3 Assessment Method

7.1.3.1 Myodynamia Assessment

Manual muscle test and its classifications

1. The common method used for assessing myodynamia is manual muscle test [3] that was invented by K.W. Lovett in 1916. It was modified but the principle is not changed. In a certain position, standard test movements are used to observe the movement completion ability of the muscle. Although the classification method is rough and the assessment is related to subjective judgment ability, the method is simple and the indication is clear, which cannot be influenced by the difference of muscular strength between man and man and is the most valuable and the most common myodynamia assessment method in clinic.

   The myodynamia in every grade of this assessment method can be divided into two grades, which are manifested with "+" and "–". If the myodynamia is stronger than some grade, the "+" should be marked on the top right corner of the number that stands for this grade. On the contrary, if the myodynamia is weaker than this grade, the "–" should be marked on the top right corner of the number that stands for this grade.

   Generally, it is used for assessment of clinical therapy schedule six grades (include zero grades) myodynamia assessment can satisfy the requirements. For clinical effect research, twelve grades assessment method is more sensitive. The standard of myodynamia assessment classification refers to Table 7.1.

2. Muscular strength test with equipment: if the myodynamia is more than three grades and it is necessary to do further precise quantitative assessment, special equipment can be used to do muscular strength test. According to the muscle contraction type, the test types are various such as isometric muscle strength, isotonic muscle strength and isokinetic muscle strength test. In the general rehabilitation evaluation books, there are detailed descriptions of application methods and classifications. The readers can refer to these books if necessary. They are not introduced in this book.

Table 7.1 Lovett myodynamia classification standard

Grades	Name	Standard	Percent of normal myodynamia
0	Zero	Undetectable muscle contraction	0
1	Slight contraction	Slight contraction	
		But cannot induce joint motion	10
2	Bad	Can do entire range of joint motion	
		In weight support state	25
3	Can	Can do antigravity entire range joint motion	
		But cannot doanti-resistance joint motion	50
4	Fine	Can do antigravity and anti-resistance	
		Entire range joint motion	75
5	Normal	Can do antigravity and anti-resistance	
		Entire range joint motion fully	100

3. Cautions of muscle strength test: In order to guarantee the precision, better repeatability and comparability of the results, we should pay attention to the following aspects in the muscle strength test.
   (a) Correct test position: correct position can make the muscle give full play to contraction ability, which can prevent effectively supplement of other muscles and compensatory contraction.
   (b) Standardization of test method: The orientation of exerting force should be correct in order to make the muscle give full play to contraction.
   (c) Comparison test: in every examination, the comparison test of myodynamia of the same muscle in both sides. If the myodymania difference of the same muscle in both sides is more than 10%, there is clinical significance.
   (d) Proper assessment time: The subjects should be in proper excited state and cooperate with the test. Before examination, the subjects do warm-up exercise to warm up the muscle. It is forbidden to do this test after exercise, in fatigue state or when the subjects are full in case of affecting the accuracy of the results.
   (e) Contraindications: in the muscle strength test, especially isometric muscle strength test, constant isometric muscle contraction can increase the blood pressure of the patients significantly and possibly induce Valsalva effect. It should be used with caution in the patients with severe blood pressure and heart diseases.

7.1.3.2 Range of Joint Motion (ROM) Examination

1. The purpose of ROM examination includes the factors of hindering joint motion, degrees of joint movement disorder, the basis of formulating therapeutic schedule and the effect of assessing therapy method.
2. The type of ROM examination includes active and passive range of joint motion examination.
   (a) Active movement: the subjects should complete range of joint motion with their own ability, which belongs to active joint motion.
   (b) Passive movement: the subjects can move joint with outside force, which belongs to passive joint motion.
3. Basic position: all the joints should be placed in 0° of anatomical position. In the forearm movement, palm surface is in 0° vertical plane state. The concepts of axis and surface are the same as that in anatomy.
4. ROM measuring method: The therapists use protractor to do the test. Normal protractor is composed of two rulers and a semicircular protractor or whole circle protractor. Finger joint is measured with small semicircular protractor. In usage, the central point of protractor aims at the center of joint motion axis precisely. The distal end of two rulers is parallel to the long axis of the body. Along with the movement of distal limbs of joint, distal ruler moves. The therapists can read the number of degrees of range of joint motion in dial of protractor. The specific operation and normal motion range of every joint refer to Table 7.2.
5. The manifestation of ROM: The manifestations of ROM are various. One of them is in 0° of anatomical position in flexion or extension. When the extension of joint is limited, measure angle may be negative. The other is 0° in full extension in flexion movement and is 180° in full extension in extension movement. The therapist can choose any one and record the absolute value of range of joint motion, but not the negative value.
6. Cautions of ROM examination: In range of joint motion examination, except the normalized operation, there are many announcements: the subjects should fully expose joint. The therapists should prepare separate room for the female and the third person should be present when the opposite sex is tested. The patients should relax fully and the position should be correct. The position of limb immobilization should be at the proximal end or distal end of the joint but not on the joint. The axis of goniometer is in accordance with the axis of the joint, which cannot hinder the parallel translation of the axis. Before joint motion and

Table 7.2 Range of joint motion examination

Joint	Movement	Position	Protractor placement mark			0 Point	Normal value
			Center	Proximal end	Distal end		
Shoulder	Flexion and extension	Anatomic position, stand with the back on column	Acromion	Midaxilla (plumb line)	Lateral epicondyle of brachialis	Two rulers overlap totally	Flexion 180° Extension50°
	Abduction	ditto	Ditto	Ditto	Ditto	Ditto	180°
	Internal and external rotation	Lie on one's back, shoulder abduction, elbow flexion90°	Olecranon	Plumb line	Styloid process of ulna	Ditto	90°
Elbow	Flexion and extension	Anatomic position	Lateral epicondyle of brachialis	Bone peak	Styloid process of ulna	Two rulers are in alignment	Flexion 150° Extension0°
Wrist	Flexion and extension	Anatomic position	Processus styloideus radii	Vertical axis of forearm	The second head of metacarpal bone	Two rulers are in alignment	Flexion 90°
	Ulnar and radial flexion	Anatomic position	Midpoint of wrist joint	Ditto	The third head of metacarpal bone	Ditto	Radial flexion 25° Ulnar flexion 65°
hip	Flexion	Lie on one's back, hip hyperextension offside	Trochanter major	Horizontal line	Lateral femoral epicondyle	Two rulers are in alignment	125°
	Extension	Lie on one's back, hip flexion offside	Ditto	Ditto	Ditto	Ditto	15°
	Adduction, abduction	Lie on one's back in case of thigh rotation	Anterior superior spine	Anterior superior spine offside	The center of patella	Two rulers are at right angles	45°
	Internal and external rotation	Lie on one's back, lateral drop of two crus	Extremitas inferior of patella	Plumb line	Anterior border of tibia	Two rulers overlap totally	45°
Knee	Flexion and extension	Lie on one's back	Lateral malleolus of thighbone	Trochanter major	Lateral malleolus	Two rulers are in alignment	Flexion 150° Extension 0°
Ankle	Flexion and extension	Lie on one's back	Malleolus medialis	Malleolus medialis of thighbone	The first head of metatarsal bone	Two rulers are at right angles	Flexion 150° Extension 0°
	Varus and eversion	Lie prostrate	The midpoint of two ankles at the back of ankle	Vertical axis at the back of crus	The midpoint of heel	Two rulers are in alignment	Varus 35° Eversion25°

after joint motion, goniometer is used for measurement twice. Contrast measurement of the same joint in both sides is proceeded to guarantee the correctness of the results.

7.1.3.3 Gait Examination

Gait is the motor patter of associated movement with multiple joints in lower limbs, which is widely used in clinic.

1. Basic information of gait: From heel in one side touches the ground to the other heel touches the ground and then the heel touches the ground again, this is called gait cycle or stride. From heel in one side touches the ground to the other heel touches the ground, this is called step.

   In gait cycle, every foot should be through the stance phase and the swing phase.

   (a) Stance phase: there are five courses such as heel stride (HS), foot flat (FF), mid-stance (MST, the center of gravity is in the upward of ankle joint), heel off (HO, the body move forward until the heel off the ground) and toe-off (TO).

   In a gait cycle, two legs both are in stance phase, which is called double support (DS) and is the characteristic of walking. In a gait cycle, if there is no double support and there is soar of two feet, it is called running.

   (b) Swing phase: from the toe off the ground, through acceleration period, to vertical impaction of lower limbs, this is called mid-swing (MSW). After that, through deceleration period, the heel touches the ground.

   In a gait cycle, the time of stance phase is more than that of swing phase. The time of stance phase accounts for 60% of the entire cycle. The time of swing phase accounts for 40% of the entire cycle.

   Cadence stands for the walking times in every minute. The cadence of adult is 110-120 steps per minute. The fast cadence can reach 140 steps per minute. Step width (SW) stands for moving distance of one step, which is related to cadence and stature. The step width of the male is 70–75 cm.

During walking, the center of body weight moves forward like a complicated revolved curve. The projection in vertical plane or horizontal plane is sinusoid. The center of body weight moves forward in sequential acceleration and deceleration. In order to keep the smooth and steady of the movement of the center of gravity in axial view, the movement and acceleration of four orientations should be decreased. The subjects can not only decrease energy consumption, but also cooperate with the movement of hip joint, knee joint and ankle joint and the horizontal displacement and four orientations incline of pelvis.

During walking, normal variations of movements mentioned above are the characteristics of the diversification of gait. The variations go beyond a certain range due to pathological factors, which form abnormal gait. The inspectors are familiar with the configuration of normal gait and basic characteristics of common pathological gait. Through observation, the inspectors can do gait assessment and use multidimensional continuous camera, digital protractor and multiple-lead electromyogram to observe and acquire activity routines of muscle, joint or center of body weight in walking in order to compare with normal activity routines. Finally, they can judge the form and degree of abnormal gait.

Their efficiency of normal gait is very high, especially when they walk with the speed of 4.5-5 km per hour. The energy consumption in unit distance is low. At this time, the myoelectric activity is the least. The impetus of moving forward of body in walking is not totally provided by muscle contraction, but mainly is provided by gravity and inertia. In abnormal gait, the energy consumption is increased. When the patients with paraplegia wear assistive device or the patients with amputation wear artificial limbs in walking, the energy consumption is more prominent and the walking speed is limited. For example, the patients with paraplegia walk with crutch and the walking speed is confined to 1.6–2.4 km/h.

2. The common pathological gait: The classification is made according to pathology and pattern of abnormal gait.
   (a) Short leg gait: when the length of one leg is shorten 3.5 cm than that of the other leg, in the loading period of the injured leg, ipsilateral pelvis and shoulder submerges, which is called oblique shoulder step. When swinging the injured leg, there is compensatory foot drop.
   (b) Joint rigidity gait: when there are spasm and contracture of joint in lower limbs, the range of joint motion is limited and the gait is changed. Especially when the joint contracture is in the malformation position, the gait is changed more obviously. For example, flexion and contracture of hip joint can lead to compensatory anterior pelvic tilt, lumbar vertebra hyperextension and stride shortening. When the angle of flexion and contracture of knee is more than 30°, there is short leg gait. When knee is in extension contracture state, in swing phase, there are abduction of lower limbs or lifting of ipsilateral pelvis in case of toe mopping. When ankle is in plantar flexion contracture state, heel cannot touch the ground. The subjects compensate ankle through hyper flexion of hip and knee like hurdles, which is called hurdle step. In the stance phase of injured limbs, there is usually overexertion of knee and genu recurvatum.
   (c) Joint unsteady gait: The patients with congenital dislocation of the hip wag from side to side like a duck, which is called duck gait.
   (d) Pain gait: Limbs lesion due to various reasons can induce pain when the injured limbs are bearing load. In order to relieve pain, the patients shorten the weight bearing time of injured limb in stance phase as much as possible. Therefore, the patients use contralateral leg to move forward with small and saltatory stride, which is called briefness gait.
   (e) Muscle weakness gait: tibialis anterior muscle gait: Myasthenia of tibialis anterior muscle lead to foot drop. In swing phase, flexion degree of hip and knee is increased in case of toe mopping, which is hurdle gait. When the triceps surae is weak, in the late stance phase, the injured hip drops and the body moves forward slowly. Due to myasthenia of quadriceps femoris gait, injured limbs cannot maintain stable knee extension actively in stance phase. The patients can make the body incline forward to make line of gravity pass through the front of knee in order to extend the knee passively. Microbending of hip lead to tension increase of gluteus and hamstring muscle and backswing of distal femoral, which is good for passive knee extension. In the early stance phase, constant hyperextension of knee usually leads to genu recurvatum as one kind of compensatory stabilization. Accompanied with myasthenia of hip extensor, the patients should bend the body and press thigh with hands to make the knee extend straightly. Gluteus maximus gait: Due to myasthenia of gluteus maximus (hip extensor), the patients make the body tilt backward to make gravity line go through the back of hip joint in order to maintain passive hip extension and control inertia forward movement of the trunk, which forms the posture of chest up and entasis. Gluteus medius gait: Due to myasthenia of gluteus medius gait (hip abduction muscle), the patients cannot maintain lateral stability of hip. Therefore, in stance phase, the patients have to make the body incline to the injured side to make gravity line go through the lateral of hip joint in order to maintain the stability with adductor in case of drop of contralateral hip. Meanwhile, the patients can lift contralateral lower limbs and swing it. When hip abductor in both sides are damaged, the patients vacillate to the left and right like a duck, which is called duck gait.
   (f) Myospasm gait is due to muscle spasm. Hemiplegic gait: there are foot drop, strephenopodia, extorsion or intorsion of

lower limbs and inability of relaxation and flexion of knee. In case of foot mopping in walking, the patients can make the injured limbs convolute forward through arc line, which is called circle gait. At this time, the upper limbs are in a flexion and adduction state and the swing is stopped. Scissors gait is also called cross gait, which is seen in the patients with child cerebral palsy or incomplete high paraplegia. The reason is adductor spasm. During walking, two hips adduct and two legs cross over in the severe patients, which lead to unstable gait and walking.

(g) Other gait due to CNS damages: the patients with ataxia of epencephalon shamble like a drunken man, which is called drunkenness gait. In the patients with Parkinson's disease or other basal ganglia diseases, there are small stride, quick walking speed and paroxysmal acceleration. The patients cannot stop or turn around at will. The arm swing slightly or is stopped, which is called propulsion gait or festinating gait. Bizarre gait is that there is no certain powerless muscle and there is no explanations for abnormal gait except for hysterical gait whose characteristics are inconsistent gait (sometimes fast and sometimes slow) that is different form inconsistent myodynamia. In muscle tension examination there is gear-like reaction.

3. Gait examination: The therapists ask the patients to walk autonomously or with assistance and observe the body balance especially the balance of lower limbs include stride, cadence and shifting of weight. The gait and upper limbs swing are coordinated or not. Secondly, the therapists ask the patients to walk quickly or slowly. If necessary, the patients should relax or concentrate on walking and the therapists observe the movements separately. The patients can do the movements such as standing still, turning around, turning round, walking up and down stairs or slope, bypassing obstacle, going through door opening, sitting down and standing up, marching on the spot slowly or standing with one foot and standing with closed eyes. As the circumstances may require, the patients are asked to walk with closed eyes and the therapists observe the abnormal condition of gait.

   For the patients using crutch to walk, the therapists should examine the gait of the patients with crutch or without crutch, because crutch may cover the actual condition of abnormal gait.

   Gait examination and basic condition examination are used for analysis and the therapists can judge it with examinations such as physical examination of nervous system, myodynamia and muscle tension examination of various muscle groups, range of joint motion examination, the length test of lower limbs and morphological examination of spinal cord and pelvis, which are important for determining the reason, characteristic and rectification method of abnormal gait.

7.1.3.4 The Intensity and Proportion of Motor Program Signal

Motor program signal test is good method to ascertain the origin of abnormal motor pattern. Through this test, the therapists can find out specific muscle group or single muscle of abnormal motor pattern and provide basis for formulating rehabilitation therapy schedule.

Motor program signal intensity is in direct proportion to myodynamia with limits. The stronger the signal is, the stronger the myodynamia is. Signal intensity stands for the quantity and quality of central nervous cells that dominate muscle contraction. The proportion of muscle signal intensity between agonistic muscle and antagonistic is the specific manifestation of coordination of central nervous cells that dominate the joint motion.

Motor program of single joint located in motor area IV of cortex is tested to find out that there is mainly the signal that dominate agonistic muscle and antagonistic muscle and the other muscles that is involved in joint motion can be ignored such as neutralized muscle and congener muscle. Generally, the normal proportion of signal between agonistic muscle and antagonistic muscle is 10–1. When the signal of agonistic muscle can drive joint motion, if the signal of antagonistic muscle is too strong, there are difficult joint motion, inflexible activity, slow-movement, inability of movement and even the wrist flexion when the patients are asked to do wrist extension due to tension increase or spasm of the muscle.

There are many types of motor program of multiple joints associated movement located in motor area VI of cortex. According to the actual condition of abnormal motor pattern of the patients, if there is cycle gait in the walking of the patients, the therapists can test the signal intensity of hip flexor (hip flexion), hamstring muscles (knee flexion), tibialis anterior muscle (dorsiflexion of foot) and peroneus longus and brevis (strephexopodia). The reason of cycle gait is the weak signal of hip flexor, tibialis anterior muscle or peroneus longus and brevis. The measure goal of motor program of associated movement is not the proportion of muscle signal intensity between agonistic muscle and antagonistic, but the sequence and the intensity of signal of agonistic muscle of all joints involved in the movement. From this, the therapists can judge the program is normal or not and analyze the reason of abnormal motor pattern in program signal.

Rehabilitation therapy schedule of recovering motor function includes myodynamia measurement, balance ability measurement, muscle spasm degree measurement, motor program signal test and cognitive function assessment, which have essential significance.

7.2 The Formulation of Rehabilitation Therapy of Neurological Training Schedule

7.2.1 The Composition of Combination Therapy Group

Recovering lost motor function of the patients is very complicated, which involves not only rehabilitation medicine, but also neurology department, general medicine, neurosurgery, department of orthopaedics, spine surgery, vascular surgery and rehabilitation medicine. The group should include complete experts and skillful techniques for functional assessment, schedule formulation and specific therapy execution and instruction, which are the guarantee of precise functional assessment, correct schedule formulation, proper therapy method and expected therapy effect.

1. Manning: Combination therapy group is led by head of department or rehabilitation chief physician, which includes rehabilitation associate chief physician, visiting staff, bedside physician, group leader of therapists and orthotics therapists. According to the state of an illness of the patients, the group can invite experienced physicians of related departments.
2. Responsibility of combination therapy group: the main responsibility of combination therapy group the patients are functional assessment, therapy schedule formulation, therapy implement, supervision and inspection, instruction and adjustment of therapy schedule. The group is also responsible for organizing symposium of case report and therapy schedule formulation.
3. Organization and implementation of symposium: For the patients in hospital or in outpatient service, before symposium formulated in rehabilitation therapy schedule, combination therapy group should notice all the doctors and therapists ahead of time. Bedside physician should know functional assessment of the patients and record actual condition of functional examination. Other physicians can do essential examination in person. Symposium should include case report and video playing of the patients to increase third dimension and precision of schedule formulation. Generally, bedside physician should first put forward preliminary therapy schedule and explain the basis of therapy schedule.

Symposium usually is presided by head of department or rehabilitation chief physician. The doctors, therapists and other personnel can declare themselves or modify the schedule for preliminary therapy in allusion to specific dysfunction of the patients and explain the reason to the patients. Head of department discusses with the participants and get final determination. They can explain the mechanism of some common problems. In addition, on the basis of modification and supplement of original schedule, they can improve the level of rehabilitation therapy.

7.2.2 Basic Principle of Formulating Therapy Schedule

The illness of the patients that need rehabilitation therapy is complicated, always with various kinds of dysfunctions such as exercise, mentality, emotion, cognition, swallowing, sphincter incontinence, joint deformity, spasm and contracture dysfunctions. There are protopathies such as hypertension, diabetes mellitus, nervous lesion. Therefore, the rehabilitation of the patients is extremely complicated, which requires a lot of disciplinary knowledge and skills. Therefore, the requirements of rehabilitation chief physician and head of department are more restrict than other subjects. Because the rehabilitation therapy in our country is still in preliminary stage, we know little about the importance of rehabilitation and don't emphasize talent cultivation of rehabilitation. The society looks down on the rehabilitation personnel, which lead to small number of rehabilitation practitioner, especially top-level talents. Under this condition, current rehabilitation personnel should give play to rehabilitation function and regularize the flow and method of rehabilitation to let the society see and feel the importance of rehabilitation. For this reason, simple therapy mode is transformed to medical model of therapy and function, which is good for the disabled in our country.

In a broad sense, rehabilitation is that various kinds of measures such as medicine, surgery, functional training, physics, mentality and biomedical engineering are used to recover the original functions of the patients as much as possible, which is the problem that cannot be solved by single drug, surgery and any other subject technology.

Rehabilitation training method is used to promote rehabilitation of the patients, which is an engineering, especially for the patients with complicated condition. It is a mammoth project. Rehabilitation chief physician can command various rehabilitation medical staffs such as doctors, exercise therapists, profession trainer, speech therapists, cognitive therapists, psychological therapists, physical therapist, potential development trainers, motor program reestablishment and motor pattern remodeling trainer and orthotics maker. In different therapy stages, various measures are used to recover and apply the functions of the patients rationally. For example, a general command all arm of the services to win a tough war. In this process, the crucial factor is formulating rehabilitation therapy schedule. The correctness and implement of therapeutic schedule are related to therapeutic effect. The basis of schedule assessment are accurate functional assessment and abundant medical knowledge and experience of rehabilitation medical staff.

The specific principle and procedure of formulating rehabilitation therapy of neurological training schedule are as follows:

7.2.2.1 Careful Comprehensive Assessment, Video Playing, Formulation of Preliminary Schedule and Group Discussion and Decision

First diagnosis responsibility should be used for the patients in hospital or in outpatients. First diagnosis doctor is responsible for the patients, especially the patients in outpatients. If the doctor is not responsible for the patients, there will be careless omission. If the therapists cannot adjust therapeutic schedule timely, the therapeutic effect will be affected.

Supervisor physician should first do comprehensive functional assessments that include not only the assessments about rehabilitation such as myodynamia, spasm degree, range of joint motion, motor pattern, cognitive function, sensory function and osteoarticular deformit, but also the assessments of the entire condition such as vital signs, visceral functions, nutrition condition, psychological states, emotional state and therapy compliance. Specific to the main dysfunction and therapy point of the patients, the therapists record the functional assessment and dysfunction degree. According to the results of functional assessment, responsibility doctors discuss with related doctors and therapists and formulate preliminary therapeutic schedule. The therapists can try to do rehabilitation training if there are no contraindications.

Generally, head of department or rehabilitation chief physician organize symposium of all department and formulation of therapeutic schedule at least once a week. Responsibility doctors should first report the case and propose therapeutic schedule. During the process of playing the video of the patients, the therapists should explain the purpose and mechanism of therapeutic schedule. After that, participants have a discussion specific to therapeutic schedule and put forward their opinion and suggestion. Head of department or rehabilitation chief physician summarize it, put forward rectification opinion and explain the reason and mechanism of rectification schedule. All the doctors reach an agreement and ascertain therapeutic schedule of the patients.

7.2.2.2 According to Specific Condition of the Patients, Final Individualized Rehabilitation Goal Should Be Established

According to the individual condition of different patients, the therapists formulate the plan to achieve training effect through rehabilitation training, which is final individual rehabilitation goal. This goal is the ultimate goal that can be achieved through training. In order to obtain better effect, incentive method of rehabilitation group is designed and is carried out in inside of rehabilitation group. This is not the statutory mission and the therapists should explain it to the patients and their family or there is no need to tell the patients and their family.

The formulation of final rehabilitation goal and basic rehabilitation principle is achieved through comprehensively analyzing the patients' state of an illness, body condition, age, the part and degree of dysfunction, therapeutic enthusiasm and cooperation, family economic status. For example, if the rehabilitation condition of the patients is good but family economic status is in a poor state, it is difficult for rehabilitation training to be completed. If the goal is set too high, it is possible to draw a blank. The rules of application for reimbursement health insurance in all parts of the country are different. Reimbursement cannot be applied in some areas and reimbursement can be applied completely in some areas and in special crowd. In Beijing, affected by period of validity of western rehabilitation method, the deadline of application for reimbursement health insurance for motor dysfunction induced by CNS damages is in half a year after onset of the disease. The deadline of application for reimbursement health insurance for dysfunction induced by peripheral nerve injury is in 3 months after onset of the disease. If missing the deadline, the patients should pay all the costs. For some patients with craniocerebral injury and cerebral infarction, they pay a lot of hospitalization costs in first-aid stage. In rehabilitation stage, some families cannot afford long-term rehabilitation therapy costs. Therefore, in formulating therapeutic schedule principle, except the requirements of functional recovery, the therapists should consider the actual condition of the patients. For example, in the patients with hemiplegic circle gait, the main obstacles of abnormal gait are hip flexion and paralysis of peroneus longus and brevis. In order to rectify abnormal gait, the therapists should train two muscles to recover autonomous contraction ability at the same time. The therapist should adopt three-stage rehabilitation principle to do the training that takes about 3 months. However, family economic capability of the patients is limited and they cannot do 3 months' therapy. At this time, the therapists can abandon the training of tibialis anterior muscle and peroneus longus and brevis. The therapists use foot tray to keep the foot in 90° dorsiflexion position. The therapists can only do the training of hip flexor and gait. After 1 month, the patients can wear foot tray to walk.

1. The basis of formulating final rehabilitation goal: The setting of final rehabilitation goal originates from objective understanding and judgement of the state of illness of the patients,

the dysfunction degree of the patients, cognitive state and rehabilitation desire, applied rehabilitation method and effectiveness of other measures. In order to increase the effectiveness of the method, except for formulating specific therapeutic schedule, there are several principles that should be paid attention to in order to achieve anticipated rehabilitation goal.

(a) The principle of recovering the function that is good for promoting self-care life ability: Human functional rehabilitation includes movements, sense, cognition and speech, which is a chronic process. It is closely related to evolution extent of species. In this time consuming therapy, the patients and their family can abandon therapy because they cannot observe obvious rehabilitation therapeutic effect soon or over a period of time.

    Therefore, the therapists can select a part that is good for improving the daily life ability of the patients and is easy to achieve therapeutic effect in order to let the patients see the training progress as soon as possible, which can promote the confidence of the patients and their family to rehabilitation training.

    Compare with recovering functions of upper limbs, the reason to recover the function of lower limbs in priority is security objective. For rehabilitation training of the patients with hemiplegia, the first choice is to recover the function of lower limbs in hemiplegic side. Because the function of upper limbs in one side of the patients is normal, they can do the functions required for daily life such as face washing, tooth brushing, combing and clothing. Although the button is difficult to be fastened in dressing, we can change the dressing pattern to solve it. If the function of lower limbs cannot be improved such as severe strephenopodia or foot drop, they may have accidents due to ankle joint sprain or tumble in mobility limitation or walking.

(b) The training principle of recovering the function in the part that is easy to be recovered. In the formulation of rehabilitation training schedule, the therapists should first select the part is easy to be recovered for rehabilitation training. For example, if the function of head is normal, the therapists select trunk for training in order to recover the sitting by themselves and balance ability in sitting position as soon as possible. If the therapists select hand and wrist for functional training, because the fine movements of hand and wrist require a huge number of central nervous cells, it is difficult to develop so many cells to replace the functions of injured cells in a short time. Although the therapy time is long, the functions are not improved obviously, which affect the training of other parts.

    Generally, the complexity sequence of functional recovery of human is head and neck, trunk, lower limbs and upper limbs. From functional recovery of single limb, functional recovery of the proximal end is easier than that of the distal end. For example, the sequence of functional recovery of upper limbs is shrug, shoulder abduction and adduction, elbow extension, elbow flexion, wrist extension, wrist flexion and finger. The functional recovery of finger is difficult and takes a long time.

    The reason of recovering the functions of head and neck is that head and neck is the rudder of human movements that can regulate orientation, feel the surrounding and adjust body movement balance. If the functions of head and neck are not recovered, it is hard to recover motor functions of trunk and other parts.

(c) Functional training principle of choosing the less harmful one: the age and body limbs function of the patients are also the factor that should be considered in formulating training schedule. For rehabilitation training of children and adult, the main purpose is to recover daily life ability and work ability and go back to home, society and post of duty, which require long-term and comprehensive rehabilitation training schedule. This schedule can be completed in different stages, even beyond the year. For the old, the main training purpose is to recover basic self-help ability. In order to achieve this purpose, rehabilitation training schedule should be prominent but not comprehensive. For an old patient with hemiplegia whose age is 80 years old, the upper limb function in one side is good and the self-help ability required for basic daily life is completed. With the permission of the patient and his family, it is possible to abandon the functional training of upper limb in hemiplegic side and focus on rehabilitation training of lower limbs functions, which can increase the time of lower limbs training time and obtain better functional recovery. The old are able to walk independently or walk with crutch. They can take a walk and talk with their friends, which can increase their happiness index in old age.

For the patients with paralysis of lower limbs in one side and foot drop, strephenopodia and circle gait, they can do the training of tibialis anterior muscle and peroneus longus and brevis to recover independent contraction ability of peroneus longus and brevis, which is difficult and takes a long time. For the old patients or the patients with severe central nervous injury, they can abandon the therapy of foot drop and strephenopodia and use foot tray for therapy. The training point is the functional recovery of hip and knee joint and the remodeling of motor pattern, which is easy to recover the walking ability of the patients. They should do the training of tibialis anterior muscle and peroneus longus and brevis at regular intervals. With time, CNS can activate more cells to replace the injured cells in compensatory mechanism. In addition, the training can promote compensatory mechanism and functional recovery.

Omnibearing training can decrease the training time of the parts whose functions can be recovered, which lead to that the parts whose functions can be recovered are not recovered and the parts whose functions cannot be recovered are not improved. Because of long-term training, the patients are easy to lose confidence of further therapy and feel suspicious or dissatisfied with rehabilitation training method.

2. The types of individualized final rehabilitation goal: After understanding the state of illness of the patients comprehensively, according to the significant degree of rehabilitation principle, the therapists can anticipate the possible final results.
   (a) Motor function is close to the normal: the symptom is slight and protopathies such as hypertension and diabetes mellitus are controlled in a stable state with drugs. Through three-stage rehabilitation training method of neurological training, motor function and pattern can be recovered to the normal.
   (b) The patients can walk independently with simple assistance: These patients usually have entire abnormal motor pattern due to dysfunction of individual part, which decrease athletic ability. However, motor dysfunction cannot be recovered through rehabilitation training of neurological training. At this time, the patients can use assisted device to recover the function of obstacle part and then improve the entire function. The functions of the patients with circle gait due to strephenopodia cannot be recovered completely after training, but they can use foot tray to keep the foot in a 90° dorsiflexion position. Through the training of motor pattern remodeling, it is possible to recover the independent walking ability of the patients. After the second therapy course of rehabilitation training, the patients can walk without foot tray.
   (c) The ability of walking with crutch: The patients with severe CNS damages can recover most of the functions through the training. Through assisted device, the joint can be kept in a functional position. The patients' independent walking ability can be recovered with the help of axilla

crutch or elbow crutch, four legs cane or single leg cane.

(d) Assisted walking device is used to recover standing and walking ability: it is suitable for the patients with involuntary movements due to development of limbs and joints and incomplete spinal cord injury. The motor function of this kind of the patients is in a certain extent, but they cannot stand up or walk because of muscle spasm, joint deformity and involuntary movement. After rehabilitation training of neurological training, body motor function can be increased and the body limbs can be stretched to the functional position. After wearing walking assisted device or not using crutch, the standing and walking ability of the patients can be recovered.

(e) With the help of other methods, orthotics or assisted device are used to recover standing and walking ability, which is suitable for the severe patients with older child cerebral palsy, poliomyelitis, spinal damages and severe joint deformity. It is hard to recover involuntary motor function in this kind of patients, but after rehabilitation training, joint deformity can be rectified and the standing and walking ability can be recovered with the help of orthosis or walking assisted device. The patients can walk in the balance bar or weight support equipment.

Because of the different state of the patients, the formulations of rehabilitation goal are various, which requires comprehensive analysis and judgement of actual condition, however, the formulation of rehabilitation goal is not essential for rehabilitation training. The author deemed that the anticipation of rehabilitation goal can make the rehabilitation medical staff form clear rehabilitation idea and training process. Before rehabilitation training, the entire training plan is formulated to do the entire training with a purpose in order to obtain orderly rehabilitation training rational rehabilitation method, timely adjusted training schedule and functional recovery to a maximum extent. From this, the formulation of final rehabilitation goal is valuable in clinic.

7.2.2.3 Ascertaining Definite Principal Training Schedule of Achieving Rehabilitation Goal

Through functional assessment and actual condition of the patients, the principle of rehabilitation goal in this therapy course should be ascertained, which is important for the purpose of functional recovery of the patients. For example, the development of our country requires five-year plan. The whole day's work depends on a good start in the morning and the whole year's work depends on a good start in spring, which are required in the progress of enterprise and individual work. If we want to make a progress in the work, we should have a plan. Without requirements and goals, we cannot obtain good marks.

For the patients, according to actual condition of the patients and the function of various kinds of rehabilitation methods, anticipation goal should be set up for the patients in order to recover the function maximally. After that, we should ascertain the general guideline of rehabilitation method of actual goal. For example, for an old patient (80 years old) with stroke and hemiplegia who is with cognitive disorder and cannot stand up for 6 months, hypertension and diabetes mellitus can be kept in a normal level with drugs. Through examination of lower limbs in hemiplegic side, the myodynamia of hip flexor is grade III. The myodynamia of hip abductor and adductor are grade II. The myodynamia of quadriceps femoris is grade II. The myodynamia of tibialis anterior muscle and peroneus longus and brevis are zero. The understanding ability and memory of the patients are good with great rehabilitation desire. For an old weak patient with many diseases, except that the myodynamia of tibialis anterior muscle and peroneus longus and brevis are zero, the myodynamia of other muscles are more than grade II. The patient has greater rehabilitation desire and ability of understanding and memory. Through 3 months' rehabilitation training, the functions can be recovered to a certain extent, but the weak patient with many diseases cannot walk for a long time. Therefore, the training goal should not be too high. The functions can be recovered to the extent that the patients can take care of themselves with the help of walking aid or crutch.

The functions should be recovered as much as possible. Meanwhile, recovering normal motor pattern is ultimate rehabilitation goal. On the basis of this, according to different actual conditions and requirements of the patients, principal schedule of rehabilitation therapy of neurological training for achieving rehabilitation goal includes several kinds as follows. The specific therapeutic schedule is introduced in rehabilitation therapy of neurological training of various diseases.

1. Three-stage rehabilitation principle training schedule of neurological training: Three-stage rehabilitation training method is the comprehensive application pattern of rehabilitation technique of neurological training, which is suitable for the prevention and rectification of abnormal motor pattern.
   (a) Prevention of abnormal motor pattern: It is suitable for the patients in the early stage of the disease whose motor function cannot be recovered and who cannot do movements out of bed. Before the functions of the muscle are totally recovered, the patients cannot do movements out of bed. When the movements cannot be completed because of paralyzed muscle, other muscles or body gestures are used to compensate abnormal motor pattern. For this kind of patients, the training schedule is establishing the normal and preventing the abnormal. With the limitation of the patients' walking out of bed, on the basis of potential development, the patients can do the training of motor program reestablishment, which is the basis of establishing normal motor pattern.
   (b) Rectification of abnormal motor pattern: For the patients in recovery phase, with obsolete motor dysfunction or abnormal motor pattern, they can do movements out of bed or even walk independently. Because of the inappropriate walking time, abnormal motor pattern can be induced by the compensatory functions of the muscle. Long-term walking in this abnormal pattern, abnormal motor pattern can be consolidated in varying degrees. The patients and their family deemed that it is good to walk more, but they don't realize that under abnormal motor pattern, abnormal motor can be consolidated and it is hard to be rectified with more and more walking.

   Therefore, for rehabilitation training of this kind of patients, the training schedule of using stop as establishment and recovery step by step is proper. During the process of limitation of walking, on the basis of rectifying disordered motor program, through repeated training, the therapists should use normal motor program to do the training of motor pattern remodeling in order to recover normal motor pattern.

   All these principles should be achieved through three-stage rehabilitation method of neurological training, which includes neural potential development, motor program reestablishment and motor pattern remodeling. With the help of forbidden walking, limitation of walking and walking in motor pattern molding instrument, the patients can walk without assisted device. For prevention kind of patients, walking should be restricted in the first stage in order to prevent abnormal motor pattern. For rectification kind of patients, walking should be restricted in the first stage in order to make the patients forget abnormal motor pattern, which is good for the reestablishment of normal motor pattern.
2. Principal training schedule of motor coordination: in fact, uncoordinated movement is one kind of abnormal motor patterns. Although there is no obvious abnormal motor pattern, there is uncoordinated condition of body motor function in practical work and daily life such as fine movement of hand, uncoordinated swing of upper and lower limbs in walking, slight strephexopodia, strephenopodia or inflexible movement of lower limbs in walking. In addition, there is normal single joint motion, but it is difficult to do entire body movement (associated

movement of multiple joints). Motor pattern of limbs is normal, but it is hard to start the movement or the patients are slow-moving.

For this kind of patients, the principal training is motor program reestablishment of associated movement and movement starting speed (signal transduction) training but not potential development training, but the patients usually need long-term motor pattern remodeling training.

3. Principal training schedule for different symptoms: For the patients with facial paralysis, speech disorder, swallow disorder and gatism, according to the actual condition of the patients, the adopted methods and the doctors' experience, the main goal and therapeutic schedule can be ascertained. For the patients with facial paralysis, the method at home and abroad is normal therapeutic measure, which is short of functional training. Through functional training method, this kind of patients can obtain better therapeutic effect with other measures such as adhesion release, pulmonary functional training and clean catheterization. This kind of patients should use active functional training as the principal method and use other trainings as the subsidiary method. The rehabilitation goal cannot be set up too high, especially for the training effect of gatism. Through clinical practice, the therapeutic effect of the current method for gatism is not ideal, especially for the therapy of gatism due to spinal roots injury in sacrococcygeal region.

7.2.2.4 Principal Training Schedule of Assault Fortified Positions Specific to Main Functional Obstacle Point

In most cases, in recovery stage, the patients' motor dysfunction usually is induced by one or several paralyzed muscles. The circle gait of lower limbs in the patients with hemiplegia may be induced by paralyzed hip flexor. The patients cannot complete hip flexion with their myodynamia, and hip abductor and the trunk compensate to the uninjured side, which induce circle gait. Peroneus longus and brevis paralysis in injured side may lead to strephenopodia. During walking, the patients want to make the injured foot touch the ground and they have to move injured limb forward through hip abduction to make the outside of the foot touch the ground first. After that, lower limbs abduction can make the entire foot touch the ground and bear load. Under the circumstances, the patients lift injured limbs and move it forward, which indicated that the myodynamia of the patients' hip flexor is normal. The main obstacle of abnormal motor pattern may be paralysis of peroneus longus and brevis.

Therefore, through precise functional assessment, the therapists can find out the main obstacle point (paralyzed muscle) and formulate principal training schedule specific to the paralyzed muscle in order to employ the limited time on the training of the main obstacle part, which is good for shorting the therapeutic course and obtain better training effect. If the therapists don't find out the main obstacle point, it is forbidden to do a physical exercise therapy or professional training without a purpose, which may get half the result with twice the effort and affect training effect greatly.

7.2.3 The Implementation and Adjustment of Therapeutic Schedule

7.2.3.1 Implementation of Therapy Method

That whether therapeutic schedule can be implemented correctly or not is essential for the anticipated effect of the training. In principle, therapeutic schedule is one kind of medical prescriptions. The medical staffs must carry it out, but rehabilitation training should be completed by rehabilitation doctors, therapists and the patient. The training is completed with the detailed explanation and instruction of the doctors, guideline of therapists' enthusiasm and positive cooperation of the patients, which dependent on the correctness of manner of execution of the therapists, the quality of implementation method and the time of practical training. On the other hand, it depends on the understanding and cooperation of the patients. Because the neurological training is entire active movement, the patients are required to cooperate with the training actively and take part in the training, which is different from taking medicine in safe dosage according to medical prescriptions. Therefore, corresponding measures and regulations should be formulated to guarantee the effective implement of the method.

1. Therapeutic schedule and specific item therapy card system: In order to know the basic information of the patients, therapeutic principle and specific therapy method, regulation of therapy chest card can be used. General information, the main dysfunction point and rehabilitation therapy principle are written in one side of the card and specific therapy items, place, time and the therapist are written on the other side. The card should be written with a pencil so that it is easy to adjust the therapeutic schedule and therapist who is responsible for the patient.

The patients are required to put this card on bedside in ward and wear it in the chest in the rehabilitation training hall to make the patients, their family, caregivers, therapists and doctors know the therapeutic condition of the patients at any time, which is good for specific practical implement condition and adjustment of therapeutic schedule. Physical photo of therapy card refers to Figs. 7.2 and 7.3.

Fig. 7.2 The information side and rehabilitation principle side of the therapy card of the patients

Neurological training rehabilitation prescription

Name: Sex: Age: Bed number: Diagnosis:

	project	content	time	Therapist
Date of hospitalization:	NT			
Hospital number:	LIPD			
Rehabilitation objectives:	UIPD			
Principle: 1.Typical three stages;	VS			
2. Atypical Phase III; 3. Early standing and walking development;	SSGS			
4. Early standing and walking recovery	DGMP			
Main obstacles:	GR			
	SUBT			
	PT			
Particular considerations:				
Physician: Date:	other			

NT : Neurological training ; LIPD : Lower limb potential development

ULPD : Upper limb potentia ldevelopment ; VS : Virtual simulation

SSGO : Six-Step guidance operation ; GR : Gait remodeling

DGMP : Development of gastrocnemius muscle potential

SUBT : stand-upbed training ; PT : Physical therapy

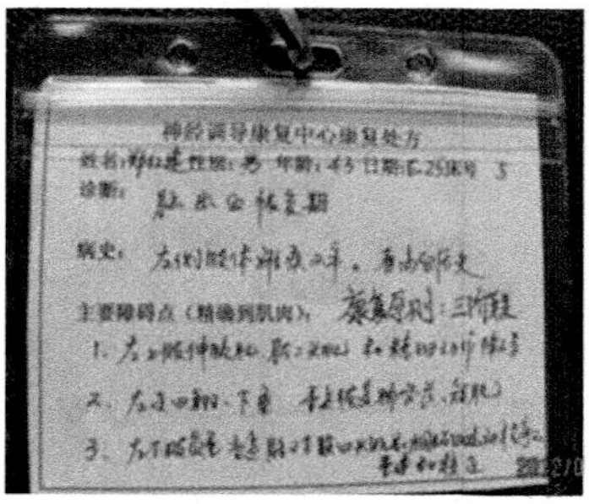

Rehabilitation Prescription

NAME: F/M AGE: DATE: BED NO:
Diagnose:

History:

Major disabilities:

Fig. 7.3 The specific therapeutic content side of the rehabilitation therapy card of the patients

2. Group leader responsibility system: There are many rehabilitation therapy staffs in the neurological training rehabilitation center of a big hospital. The therapists with professional technique and managerial experience can be selected to hold the post of group leader and belong to the key group of the department. They can help to manage the department and know the therapists and the difficulties in work. The specific tasks of the group leader are to assign therapeutic task, arrange therapy time, examine the implement of the schedule and instruct the technique. They organize morning conference of the therapists every day and hold vocational study conference of the therapists at regular intervals.

   Neurological training is a brand new technique. According to the therapy and method of rehabilitation technique of neurological training, they use special corollary equipment of neurological training for the rehabilitation of the patients, which is one of the primary conditions. The therapists are required to keep high enthusiasm to encourage the patients to gradually complete unaccomplished active joint motion before. The labor intensity is high. At present, western rehabilitation method takes passive movement as the principal thing and is widely used at home and abroad. When the therapists move the joint of the patients passively, they can keep in a position for a while and there is no speech encouragement, which can save labor. Therefore, the therapists prefer to move the joint of the patients passively, but it is not in accordance with the mechanism of the plasticity of central nerves. Form the view of motor functional recovery, there is no obvious training effect. Therefore, it is necessary to do technique instruction, inspection and supervision.
3. Physician-therapist pairing system: At present, in domestic rehabilitation medical establishment, the doctors receive the patients, write medical record, give the patients various examinations and prescribe medicine. The doctors only formulate the therapy principle generally, but they don't take part in the practical rehabilitation training and are not familiar with all kinds of rehabilitation therapy techniques. The responsibility of the doctors is equal to that of neurologists. There is severe gappy phenomenon between rehabilitation doctors and rehabilitation training. The author called it little neurologists, which is bad for the development of rehabilitation technique and improvement of rehabilitation therapeutic effect. Compared with rehabilitation therapists, rehabilitation doctors received comprehensive and long-term rehabilitation medical knowledge education and restrict training. The questions and solution abilities are better than the therapists. If they don't contact rehabilitation training and work on practical rehabilitation therapy, they cannot understand the mechanism and effect of various kinds of rehabilitation training. They are not familiar with the practical problem and unreasonable method of rehabilitation training. The new theory, method and equipment of rehabilitation cannot be accomplished.

   In order to solve this problem and eradicate rehabilitation doctors to become neurologists, rehabilitation doctors should take part in rehabilitation training and the pair regulation of rehabilitation doctors and therapists is necessary. Both head of rehabilitation department and rehabilitation resident doctor should take part in practical rehabilitation training. Head of department and chief physician mainly assess and treat new inpatients for the first time, explain the mechanism of neurological training rehabilitation, reassess the functions when leaving hospital and explain announcements of self-exercise out of hospital. Rehabilitation chief physician and resident doctor complete medical record and clinical therapy of the patients and select one or two difficult rehabilitation training or scientific research training items to do practical training. Treatment team is composed of one rehabilitation physician and 3–5 rehabilitation therapists. The doctors are responsible for holding a symposium every week and analyzing the effect of training schedule. If there is problem, they should propose solution and submit to superior physician. The combination of doctors and therapists is good for rehabilitation method and new problems, which provides opportunity for improvement and innovation of rehabilitation method.

4. First-diagnosis and last-diagnosis system of head of rehabilitation department or chief physician: Because head of department is in charge of the work of the entire department, especially clinic, outpatient service, budget, declaration and implement of scientific research task. The primary task of head of department is chief executive officer of the department. Therefore, First-diagnosis regulation can be established, which is helpful for head of department to know actual dysfunctions of the patients, instruction of therapeutic schedule and ultimate determination of therapeutic schedule. First-diagnosis can be done with motor program signal detector in neurological training room, which is good for the correctness of functional assessment and rehabilitation therapy of neurological training. It plays an important role in the understanding of the method and mechanism of rehabilitation therapy of neurological training and in activating the therapy enthusiasm of the patients. The head of the department and chief physician do functional assessment of the patients before leaving hospital and know the actual effect of the method, which is good for the improvement and development of the method.

7.2.3.2 Timely Adjustment of Therapeutic Schedule

For established therapeutic schedule specific to the patients' dysfunctions, it is not invariable. The schedule should be adjusted in time through assessment in order to obtain better training effect, especially three-stage rehabilitation training schedule of neurological training. The therapy time of every stage is not confined to 1 month. After 1 month's training, the condition of the patients should be assessed, reassessed, adjusted and re-adjusted in order to decide whether to do the training of the second stage or not. Generally, before every therapy, the therapists should assess the patients briefly and know the changes after last training and the actual condition of the patients' dysfunction at present. The therapists can judge the adaption and sensitivity of therapeutic schedule in solving the dysfunctions of the patients. If there is any problem, they should report to the doctors in charge, put forward individual opinion and apply for the adjustment of training schedule. Doctors in charge should take part in the training and know the actual condition of the training. The therapists should examine the patients in detail and adjust the therapeutic schedule in time according to the examination result. Head of department or chief physician make the rounds of the wards every week, examine the severe patients with difficult symptoms in detail and know the effect of original schedule, the therapy response of the patients and the condition of the disease, which is the basis of adjustment of therapeutic schedule.

The doctors are not responsible to give the tasks of therapeutic schedule to the therapists and let the therapists to do therapy with their personal experience and will. The therapists cannot complete therapeutic schedule. It is improper that the therapeutic schedule is not changed from admission to hospital to out of the hospital, which is irresponsible for the therapy of the patients.

7.2.4 The Role of the Patients and Their Family in Rehabilitation

Rehabilitation is a complicated project that takes time and labor and is related to the economic capability of the patients' family. Especially in most areas of our country, medical insurance reimbursement of rehabilitation is limited and the family should afford to all the costs. Financial burden can block the rehabilitation of the patients. In addition, the insistence of the patients is related to effectiveness of the rehabilitation method. There are three factors can affect rehabilitation effect and anticipated rehabilitation goal such as family affection, tenacity and rehabilitation method.

7.2.4.1 Family Affection

Because there is no regeneration ability of CNS, it is difficult and chronic to recover the dysfunctions of movements, cognition and speech due to damages. There are three stages in the emotion of the patients.

1. Deny and incomprehension: the patients cannot accept the fact that they are sick. They think they are healthy before and they don't understand why they fall ill suddenly. They will feel wronged and be down in spirits. They has lost all desire for food and drink and cannot fall asleep at night.
2. Sadness and hopeless: with the understanding of the disease, the patients find that they can fall ill just as other people. They will accept the fact. They don't know the severity of the disease, the recovery condition, the time of recovery, self-care condition, working ability, the pain of the disease, the financial burden and the burden of the family. The patients feel hopeless about the future. They usually feel upset and sorrowful. They don't cooperate with the therapy even give up the therapy or have other ideas.
3. Rise against the disease: With the time, the patients adapt to the disease and recognize that sadness has no effect on functional recovery. The only way is to rise against the disease. Therefore, they get up the courage and confidence to defeat the disease and start to cooperate with the therapy. In this stage, the disease is in the chronic phase. The family cost a lot of money in the acute phase of the disease and they will encounter economic problems.

In every stage, the patients can encounter different difficulty. Solving these problems is related to the care and devotion of the family members. Especially when these patients lose self-help ability, the destiny of the patients depends on their family. Therefore, the care and devotion of family member and the degree of the care and devotion are related to rehabilitation training and the degree of functional recovery of the patients.

There are significant differences in the care and devotion of the family member to the patients. Some families are not rich, but they can devote everything to the rehabilitation of the patients. Parents can do this for their children. Some families are rich, but they don't support the rehabilitation therapy of the patients. Furthermore, they ask the doctors to say to the patients that there is no therapy method for this disease. They are unwilling to devote to the patients. The reason why there is so big difference is related to the following factors:

Morality: happiness is due to love in the world and selfish help and devotion are the spring of happiness. Life is the most important in all the treasures.

Financial condition: with the limitation of the family financial condition, the family cannot afford to the therapy costs.

The recognition and importance of rehabilitation: the patients think that rehabilitation is dispensable and only surgery and medicines are effective. They don't realize that rehabilitation training is essential and irreplaceable in functional recovery. For example, the patients remain in bed with motor skill disorder and abnormal motor pattern a housing estate or village. They take medicines do self-exercise for years and the disease cannot be improved, but they cannot accept the rehabilitation training.

Therefore, rehabilitation medical staffs should understand rehabilitation deeply and explain it to the family of the patients ahead of schedule. The therapists should use effective method to make the patients and their families see the effect of rehabilitation training to increase the confidence of rehabilitation therapy, which provide precondition for the entire rehabilitation of the patients.

7.2.4.2 Toughness

Scientific training guided by the doctors, attic faith and remorseless toughness are the premise of functional recovery. In rehabilitation training, the power of determined will and toughness of the patients can make the patients obtain ideal rehabilitation training effect, which is related to the particularity of rehabilitation training.

1. It takes a long time to recover lost motor function after CNS damages, because the regeneration ability of central nervous cells is poor. Development, mature and repair after damages take a long time. Human take 1 year to learn how to walk after birth, while lower animal

such as sheep can learn to run a few hours after birth. Clinical practice indicate that functional recovery of paralyzed lower limbs takes 3 months, while functional recovery of upper limbs takes more than 6 months. Functional recovery needs long-term training, which is not a circumstance to taking medicine to bring down a fever. Therefore, rehabilitation training may make the patients think that there is no effect of the therapy. It is more difficult to recover the functions of injured brain tissues than to establish functions in neonatal brain.

2. It is hard to be rectified after abnormal motor pattern is formed. Every movement of human body is controlled and dominated by motor program in motor center of brain cortex. After brain cells damages, motor program can be destroyed in various degrees. Because of compensatory role of human tissues, the lost functions of some parts can be replaced by that of tissues of other parts. If there is no timely training to consolidate these compensatory functions, it will lead to disorder of associated movement and abnormal motor pattern. For example, the hemiplegic patients with foot drop cannot do dorsiflexion of foot and cannot lift the leg away from the ground. When hip flexor is paralyzed, the patients cannot incline to the uninjured side to make the foot away from the ground. They can only move the limbs forward through dragging, which induce drag gait. After a long time, disuse of hip abductor and tibialis anterior muscle can lead to weak myodynamia and the abnormal intensity of drag gait is more and more severe. Finally, abnormal motor program is formed in brain cortex and it is difficult to be rectified.
3. Self-training is lifelong after rehabilitation training. With limitation of regeneration ability of central nervous system, functional recovery after damages should be replaced by the normal cells in injured area and be compensated by reserved conduction pathway. Compared with original cells, the functions of reserved cells and conduction pathway are poor. The lost function cannot be recovered to the level before damages. It requires repeated self-exercise to consolidate the recovered functions.
4. The patients should take part in rehabilitation training actively. The patients should not take part in normal therapy such as medicine and surgery actively. The therapeutic effect depends on the effect of medicine and surgery. The patients accept the results passively. The purpose of rehabilitation is to recover the lost motor function of the patients. Through training process of motor relearning program, the anticipated goal can be achieved. All the measures and methods can play a role through the endeavor of the patients. Therefore, the patients must take part in it to achieve it. For example, in cycling and swimming, the learner can learn to cycle or swim only through practical self-training. The learner cannot learn to cycle or swim without practice even if the coaching technology is good.

Therefore, the cultivation and guidance of rehabilitation self-confidence of the patients should be emphasized. The preserved rehabilitation determination and strong willpower of the patients are established, which are the basis and important fundament of rehabilitation training.

7.2.4.3 Rehabilitation Method

The purpose of rehabilitation therapy is to recover self-help ability, improve life quality and return to society. Therefore, family affection and toughness are the premise and basis, but they are not enough. A good therapeutic effect of rehabilitation method can promote functional recovery of the patients and solve practical problems. Therefore, we should investigate and use rehabilitation training method to promote central neural plasticity and functional reorganization, which is essential for functional recovery. Rehabilitation medical staffs should focus on functional recovery of the patients and recognize the mechanism and effect of various kinds of rehabilitation method. The therapists should be practical and realistic, not worship things foreign and fawn on foreign countries and not follow suit. The therapists should investigate and explore new methods to increase the effect of rehabilitation therapy.

Functional recovery after CNS damages is peculiar, chronic, difficult. The patients should stick to it for a long time and take part in it actively. It requires the full recognition and definite confidence of rehabilitation medical staffs, the patients and their family who have fortitudinous willpower and prepare for protracted war, which can provide basis for realizing anticipated goal of rehabilitation. All rehabilitation medical staffs should pay attention the mechanism and effect of rehabilitation method and investigate new rehabilitation method that is in accordance with CNS plasticity to increase the effect of rehabilitation training and life quality of the disabled in order to bring benefit to all the disabled and contribute to the society.

References

1. Delisa JA, Gans BM. Rehabilitation medicine: principles and practice. 3rd ed. Philadelphia, PA: Lippincott-Raven Publishers; 1998.
2. Dengkun N, editor. Rehabilitation medicine. 2nd ed. Beijing: People's Health Press; 2001. p. 10.
3. Yulong W. Rehabilitation evaluation. Beijing: People's Health Publishing House; 2000. p. 88.

8 Integrated Method of "Physiotherapy-Physical Exercise and Self-Exercise"

The range of physiotherapy is extensive such as sound therapy, phototherapy, hydrotherapy, electrotherapy, cold therapy and thermal therapy, which is an inalienable part of rehabilitation medicine and plays an important role in modern and traditional medicine. It is used to treat many kinds of diseases in all disciplines. The methods and mechanisms of physiotherapy are introduced in *physiatry* that is chiefly compiled by Jiao Zhi-Heng and Fan Wei-Ming. It is published by Science and Technology Literature Press. We don't discuss these in our book.

Our book is mainly to the pathogenesis of common bony joint and muscle diseases. We discuss the reason why the disease is difficult to be cured and easy to relapse and propose specific integrated therapy method of "physiotherapy-physical exercise therapy and self-exercise.

8.1 The Reason Why Bony Joint and Muscular Painful Diseases Are Difficult to Be Cured and Easy to Relapse

8.1.1 Soft Tissue Adhesion After Damages Is Not Lessened Effectively

Bony joint, especially soft tissue around joint, includes muscle, ligament, tendon and joint capsule. Due to trauma, inflammation and tractive sprain, tear and muscle fiber necrosis and exudation are induced. The manifestations in acute stage are local swelling, pain and limitation of joint motion. According to the degree of damages, the clinical manifestation and disposition are different. The severe patients require decompression in closed operation, debridement or repair. In less serious cases, the patients require cold compress, immobilization, elimination of swelling and other physiotherapies [1].

Joint soft tissue injury can lead to pain. Meanwhile, joint motion can aggravate the pain, which is one kind of protection mechanism. Limitation of joint motion is to prevent the aggravation of tissue injury and to promote tissue healing. When the injure tissues are repaired or healed to a certain extent, there is no pain in joint motion, but soft tissue injury and exudation, inflammatory and joint limitation can lead to adhesion of muscle fiber, ligament, joint capsule and nervus vascularis and the adhesion between cartilages in articular surface, which affects the range of joint motion. According to the injured degree and the course of disease, if the patients don't receive timely and effective therapy, the adhesion may get worse and the tendon may contract and shorten. After that, severe tissue adhesion is induced such as articular fibrous ankyloses. Finally, with the deposition of calcium salt, incurable bony ankyloses of bony joint is formed [2].

W. Zhao, *Rehabilitation Therapeutics of the Neurological Training*,
https://doi.org/10.1007/978-981-13-0812-3_8

Some researches show that adhesion between soft tissues induced by shoulder joint with plaster immobilization of 1 day requires 7 days' joint motion to make the range of shoulder joint to be recovered to the original motion range. If the shoulder joint are immobilized for 3 weeks, the range of shoulder joint can be recovered to the original motion range through 300 days' joint motion. Therefore, joint immobilization is an important factor of soft tissue adhesion.

Different levels of adhesion of joint and soft tissue around joint can influence the range of joint motion to varying degree. During the process of joint motion, adhesion tissue can be stretched and nerve endings may be compressed or stimulated to induce different levels of pain. The pain can further affect joint motion. Limitation of range of joint motion can further aggravate adhesion between tissues, which forms a vicious circle.

The therapy methods used for osteoarthritis usually are medicine and physical methods, which emphasize the relief of pains such as thermal therapy, electrotherapy, acupuncture in traditional Chinese medicine, cupping and massage. It cannot lessen the tissue adhesion effectively. Therefore, after physiotherapy, during the process of joint motion, the patients' soft tissues are stretched so that it is easy to induce slight laceration and sensation of pain through stimulating neural ending. This is the reason why bony joint and soft tissue inflammation cannot be cured and are easy to relapse.

8.1.2 The Factors That Induce Soft Tissue Inflammation of Joint and Muscle Aren't Rectified

Osteoarthritis is one of the most common arthritis, which belongs to degenerative change, aging of joint. It often involves the mostly used and load bearing joints such as hand, knee and lumbar vertebra, which usually induces fibrosis, fracture, ulcer or loss of cartilago articularis. It is the main reason to cripple the elder.

There are many factors that can induce osteoarthritis such as age, obesity, inflammation, trauma and genetic factor. The factors are summarized as follows:

1. Age: The morbidity of osteoarthritis increases with age. In the middle age of human life, the functions of muscle and peripheral nerves decrease gradually, nervous reflex recede and the conduction time extend, which can lead to the incongruity between nerve and muscle and joint injury. In addition, the blood supply of bone and cartilago articularis decreases with age. Due to inanition, cartilago articularis becomes thin. Cartilage matrix decreases and it is easy to induce fibrosis. Inorganic substance of bone increases and the elasticity and tenacity, which make the cartilage easy to be damaged [3].
2. Obesity: Occurrence rate of knee osteoarthritis of the patients with obesity is high, because mechanical pressure of body weight to joint is high. The research indicated that the occurrence rate of knee osteoarthritis in the female with obesity is three times more than that in the female with normal body weight.
3. Overuse: Joint overuse and repeated injury can lead to osteoarthritis. Some occupational labor and strenuous exercise (weightlifting) can induce overloaded stress to joint and degenerative alterations of chondrocyte. Degenerative cells can decrease the synthesis of matrix and aggravate the destruction of chondrocyte. The vicious circle is formed and lead to osteoarthritis finally.
4. Repeated injury: Slight but repeated joint injury is the nosogenesis of osteoarthritis such as exercise without warm-up of joint and muscle and repeated and unexpected stepping empty, which can induce soft tissue injury of joint and around joint.
5. Climatic factor: The persons who usually live in humid and cold environment are easy to be diagnosed with osteoarthritis. For example, some young white-collar wear skirt and work in air conditioning environment for years. They are the high risk group of osteoarthritis. This is because that in cold environment they don't keep themselves warm and local blood circulation is affected. Inclement weather is the factor that induces or aggravates osteoarthritis. In cold environment, if the person cannot keep themselves warm, vasoconstriction can decrease tissue blood supply. In this case,

work, exercise or walking can easily lead to the injury of soft tissues of cartilago articularis and around cartilago articularis.

6. Special type of work and unhealthy life styles: A sedentary life and no exercise can induce arthritis. Cartilago articularis of miner, heavy worker, professional athletes or dancer receive high-intensitive stress wear for a long time and are easy to be injured. For example, the joint motion is decreased in the persons who bend over one's desk in work and there is adhesion of soft tissue easily. The joint capsule is easy to contract or compressed for a long time, which induces blood microcirculation disturbance and degenerative change of tendon, ligament and cartilago articularis.

In unhealthy life style, high-heeled shoes is related to the formation of arthritis, because walking with high-heeled shoes, the bearing pressure of knee increases and are easy to lead to damages of cartilago articularis, which is the biomechanics factor of osteoarthritis.

No matter what induce the disease, the result is injury of soft tissue of cartilago articularis and around joint without expectation. After tissue injury, self-repair mechanism can be activated. At ordinary times, most tissue cells are in dormant state when they are not injured. Once they are damaged, they can feel the environment change and there is plasma leakage in the injure vessels, which lead to the migration of fibroblast into injured tissue. When the fibroblast contact with the injured tissues, they form collagen to seal wound. Through regeneration type such as mitosis, new tissues are formed. The regeneration is limited. After minor injury, through regeneration, the original morphology and function can be recovered. After severe injury, the wound is recovered in scar and the original morphology and function are hard to be recovered such as elasticity of tissue. Repeated minor injuries, during the process of the tissue repair, fiber texture increases, blood supply decreases, tissue elasticity decreases and the tissue is in a sclerosis state. With time, there is calcinosis and ossification, which forms "bony spur". According to the position of bony spur, it can stimulate the peripheral soft tissue in joint motion. It can stimulate nerve or vessel and induce different symptoms such as pain, numb and insufficient blood supply such as dizziness, nausea and vomiting.

Except for cartilago articularis, bony spur usually occur in joint capsule and adhesion area between ligament and bone. For example, in spinal centrum, the position of bony spur is at the top and bottom edge of centrum. After the repeated injury of fibrous rings of intervertebral disc and ligament, during repeated repair of tissue, repair is overdone and calcification is formed.

Therefore, if the factors that include inflammation of soft tissue in cartilago articularis, muscle and ligament cannot be rectified effectively, the disease is possible to relapse although the symptoms are relieved or cured.

8.1.3 Single Therapeutic Method Without Comprehensive Therapeutic Method for Pathogenesis and Complication

In treatise and textbook of physiotherapy, there are many descriptions about the therapy of the disease such as physical agent intervention of relieving pain, massage of lessening adhesion, massage and joint mobilization, self-exercise method for preventing relapse. However, in practical therapy, the patients receive different therapies in different departments, but the therapy is not comprehensive. For example, some patients think that the effect of physiotherapy is better and they go to physiotherapy department for physiotherapy therapy such as ultrashort wave, far infrared and so on. Some patients trust traditional Chinese medicine and go to traditional Chinese medicine department. The doctors in traditional Chinese medicine department usually use massage, acupuncture, cupping and so on. All these therapies such as physical agent to relieve pain, simple acupuncture, moxa-moxibustion or massage are not comprehensive. These therapies cannot relieve pain effectively, lessen soft tissue adhesion and prevent relapse of adhesion at the same time.

Because adhesion of soft tissue is not lessened effectively and bad habit that induces osteoarthritis is not rectified, adhesion of the tissue can be stretched when the patients go home and try to move adhesive joint. Adhesive tissue can be stretched to compress neural ending. When the stretched strength is large, it can induce slight tear of soft tissue to a certain extent and damage neural ending directly. All these can induce pain, which can make the patients don't want to move joints. Immobility can aggravate the degree of adhesion and induce the pain of joint and limitation of range of joint motion. In addition, the patients work and live as usual and the pathogenic factors of arthritis are not eliminated. New arthritis is formed. The new symptoms cannot be relieved and the original symptoms are aggravated gradually.

8.2 Neurological Training Rehabilitation for Osteoarthritis

In the principle of dealing with injuries of soft tissue in cartilage of bony joint and around joint, therapies at different stages are as follows [4]:

8.2.1 Early Stage

Twenty-four to forty-eight hours after injury, tissue ischaemia induced by microvascular injury can lead to acute aseptic inflammation. A lot of tissue percolate lead to local tissue swelling. Principle of management in this stage is immobilization, hemostasis, detumescence, analgesia and alleviating inflammation. After injury, immobilization, cold compress, pressure dressing and injured limbs lifting should be done as soon as possible, but it is forbidden to do massage and thermal therapy in the injured area.

8.2.2 Middle Stage

After 24–48 h after injury, bleeding stops and acute inflammation starts to fade away. There is local extravasated blood and granulation tissue is formed. Tissue is to repair them. This stage lasts 1–2 weeks. Principle of management in this stage is improving local blood circulation and promoting metabolism and repair of tissue. Thermal therapy, massage, medicine and physiotherapy are used alternatively. Meanwhile, functional rehabilitation training with little amount of exercise can be done.

8.2.3 Late Stage

In this stage, local symptoms such as edema and pressing pain disappear. Injured tissue is repaired. However, intensity, elasticity and function of healed tissue are lower than that of normal tissue. Tissue adhesion still exists. Principle of management in this stage is lessening adhesion, recovering range of joint motion and enhancing myodynamia. Functional training is the main training with physiotherapy, massage and rehabilitation training.

Our book aims at the therapy of late stage or obsolete osteoarthritis induced by soft tissue injury. This kind of disease includes three aspects of symptoms:

1. Pain there are many reasons such as injury, osteoporosis, gout, periostitis, osteoarthritis, rheumatism and rheumatoid arthritis, arthromeningitis and meniscus injury, which can affect joint motion and induce pain in joint motion.
2. Soft tissue adhesion and contracture and ossification of joint capsule and ligament: The patients are afraid to move joints because of pain. Cellulose in inflammatory exudates can induce adhesion of soft tissue in articular surface and around joint. With time, adhesive tissue, joint capsule, ligament and tendon may contract and ossify, which can further affect range of joint motion and aggravate the pain in joint motion.
3. Limitation of joint motion: Both pain and adhesion can affect the range of joint motion, which can limit range of joint motion and immobilize the joint motion (fibrous ankyloses

or bony ankyloses of joint). It can affect the joint functions in varying degrees.

Three symptoms interact with one another and interact as both cause and effect. Pain can restrain joint motion. Limitation of joint motion can lead to adhesion of soft tissue. Severe adhesion further aggravates the degree of joint motion limitation. Limited joint can induce pain when joint motion causes tear of adhesive tissue. Therefore, therapy method for osteoarthritis should be give consideration to the three symptoms. If the therapy method only figures one of the symptoms, the therapeutic effect is affected inevitably. The effect cannot last long and the disease is easy to relapse.

The purpose of integrated therapeutic method in physiotherapy-physical exercise therapy and self-exercise of neurological training is to give consideration to three factors mentioned above in order to obtain stable therapeutic effect.

8.2.4 Physiotherapy

The purpose of physiotherapy is to relieve pain, increase blood circulation of injured part, alleviate swelling and promote heal of injured tissue. There are many physiotherapy methods. We only introduce the frequently-used methods in "physiotherapy-physical exercise therapy and self-exercise" in our book.

8.2.4.1 Far Infrared

Far infrared is the ray of light outside of red light. The wave length is 0.76–400 μm, which belongs to electromagnetic wave. It is a kind of radioactive ray with intense thermal effect that we cannot see with our eyes. According to the wave length of infrared, it is divided into near infrared, middle infrared and far infrared.

The thermal effect of infrared is the important part in therapeutic effect. The thermal effect is generated by the arrangement of dipole and free charge according to the orientation of electromagnetism in electromagnetic field. During this process, aggravated random motion of molecule and atom can generate heat. If the heat of the infrared exceed heat dissipation potential of living body, local temperature of the body increases, which is called thermal effect of infrared [5–7]. The therapeutic effect of thermal effect is related to biophysics mechanism of thermal effect.

1. Activation of bio macromolecule is good for the functional activities of bio macromolecule such as regulation of metabolism and immune, which can recover body function, prevent disease and cure disease.
2. Promotion and improvement of local and entire blood circulation: infrared acts on the skin and the energy is absorbed by the skin. The absorbed energy is transformed into heat and it can increase local skin temperature. Therefore, it can stimulate thermoreceptor in skin. It can relax vascular smooth muscle, dilate blood vessel and accelerate blood circulation through thalamus reflex. In addition, thermal effect can induce the release of vasoactive substance, lower angiotasis and dilate superficial arteriole, superficial capillary and superficial vein, which can promote local blood circulation.
3. Enhancement of metabolism: The thermal effect of infrared can enhance the vitality of cells and adjust neurohumour mechanism. It can also strengthen tissue metabolism and make the substance exchange in a stable state.
4. Increase of immune function: Infrared can increase the function of phagocytosis of macrophage and can promote the functions of human cells and humoral immunity.
5. Antiphlogosis and detumescence: Infrared can improve blood circulation, enhance tissue nutrition, activate tissue metabolism, boost cell regeneration ability, which is good for localization and control of inflammation and repair of nidus. In addition, thermal effect can enhance the stability of cell membrane, regulate ionic concentration, promote excretion of toxic substance and metabolite, accelerate absorption of exudate and promote control of inflammation and fade of edema.
6. Analgesia: The thermal effect of infrared can decrease excitability of neural ending and increase threshold of pain. With improvement of blood circulation and fade of edema, chemical

and mechanical stimulus of neural ending are relieved, which can alleviate pain.

8.2.4.2 Ultrashort Wave

1. The characteristic of ultrashort wave: The wave length of ultrashort wave is 1–10 m and the frequency is 30–300 Hz. The wave length of domestic therapeutic machine of ultrashort wave is 6, 7.2, 7.34 and 7.7 m. The frequency is about 50 MHz. Because the wave length of ultrashort wave is short and the frequency is high, electricity of ultrashort wave is easy to pass dielectric medium. Therefore, in the therapy the electrode does not directly touch the skin.

   Ultrashort wave act on human body and induce physiological reaction includes thermal effect and non-thermal effect. This is because the electricity of ultrashort wave is divided into continuous and impulse type. Current oscillation of continuous electrical curve continuously exists and there is a lot of thermal energy. On the basis of continuous ultrashort wave electricity, the electricity of impulse ultrashort wave is added with low frequency pulse modulation and amplification, which forms intermittent rectangle ultrashort wave electricity. There is no thermal inductance in therapy and its effect on human body comes from oscillation effect of pulse train.

   In the thermal effect of ultrashort wave, thermal energy is hard to spill out of the blood because there are few blood vessels in fat layer. Therefore, the temperature is higher than that of muscles with abundant blood supply. Some researches indicated that when the wave length of ultrashort wave is 7.34 m, the ratio between temperature rise of fat and temperature rise of muscle is 8–1. There still are some defects such as overheating of fat. The space between skin and polar plate is adjusted to increase deep tissue temperature and lower the temperature of subcutaneous fat. In practice, we should pay attention to the distance of the skin.

   Non-thermal effect is observed in ultrahigh frequency and low intensity ultrashort wave. Ultrahigh frequency electrical oscillatory wave can induce substance resonance in cells and change surface tension of liquid. Surface tension of some substance increases and surface tension of other substance decreases. Under the influence of high speed alternating high-frequency electromagnet wave, when the electric field intensity is maximal, cells stretch to electric field direction and become normal when the electric field intensity is minimum. Proper frequency electric field can make cells stretch out and draw back fully. It can produce special stimulus to cells and tissues and induce specific biological function.

   Although low-intensity ultrashort wave doesn't increase tissue temperature, its biological effect is still obvious. Under the same circumstance, exogenous heat has no such effect. Short time ultrashort wave without heat is used for therapy. The therapeutic effect for acute inflammation is more obvious than long-term warmth and can induce reaction of other tissues and organs, which is called non-thermal effect. Non-thermal effect is more obvious under the influence of low field intensity (lower than 40 mW/cm^2).
2. Physiological and therapeutic effects of ultrashort wave
   (a) Medium-small dosage of ultrashort wave has a sedative effect. Nervous system is very sensitive to ultrashort wave field, because nervous tissue is similar to dielectric medium, especially for brain cells, autonomic nerves and visceral peripheral nerves. Medium-small dosage of ultrashort wave acts on head, which can induce suppression phenomenon of central nervous system such as drowsiness except sense of warmth. It can lower tensity of sympathetic nerve, alleviate vasospasm, promote collateral circulation, improve histotrophic nutrition and increase functions.
   (b) Analgesia: Ultrashort wave has an inhibitory effect on sensory nerve and its analgesic effect is obvious. Moreover, small dosage of ultrashort wave can accelerate the regeneration of incomplete broken nerve fiber.
   (c) Improvement of microcirculation: In certain extent, increase of ultrashort wave

intensity can dilate blood capillary even blood vessel of deep viscera, increase vascular permeability, accelerate blood flow and improve blood circulation of tissue and organ.

(d) Sterilization: not only ultrashort wave can kill bacteria directly, but also little dosage ultrashort wave increase phagocytic ability of macrophage, which is good for sterilization.

(e) Promotion of wound healing: Clinical and experimental research indicated that ultrashort wave can accelerate the regeneration of connective tissue and growth of granulation tissue and promote division growth of vascular endothelial cell and phorocyte. Therefore, ultrashort wave can accelerate wound healing and promote escharosis. Large dosage ultrashort wave for a long time can dehydrate and age wound and connective tissue around it, which make the wound become hard and difficult to be cured.

(f) The influence on inflammation process: Ultrashort wave has a good therapeutic effect on inflammation, especially acute suppurative inflammation. In the therapy of acute inflammation, small dosage ultrashort wave has obvious antiinflammation. Large dosage can aggravate the state of disease. Small dosage ultrashort wave is suitable for the therapy of acute inflammation of superficial tissue. In the therapy of deep visceral infection, the dosage should be increased. This is related to the distribution and loss of ultrashort wave penetrating human electric field.

3. Therapeutic dose of ultrashort wave: In actual work, the dosage should be determined according to the feeling of the patients, luminance of neon lamp and meter reading (Table 8.1).

Grade 1 (8–10 min/time) or grade 2 (10–12 min/time) is used for the therapy of acute inflammation. Grade 3 (15–20 min/time) is used for the therapy of chronic inflammation or chronic disease. Grade 4 is used for the therapy of killing tumor cell, not for normal inflammation.

The frequency of 8–12 min/time is used for children. Course of treatment depends on the state of disease. The frequency of 6–8 min/time is used for acute inflammation. The frequency of 12–24 min/time is used for chronic inflammation.

4. Key points of operation include the patients' position, the place of electrode and the distance between electrode and skin.

(a) Position: The patients place themselves in a comfortable position and don't expose therapeutic area. Thickness of the clothes should be calculated.

(b) Electrode: The therapists should select proper electrode and aim at therapeutic area. The thickness of underbed should be determined according to the depth of lesion.

(c) The place of electrode capacitance electrode method is mainly used in ultrashort wave therapy. Its electric field distribution is closely related to the place method of electrode, pole plate and skin distance to make intensive power line get through the target. Two-pole method and body cavity method are usually used. Two-pole method is divided into contrapost and apposition. Contrapost is used for the therapy of the deep or visceral lesion and apposition is used for superficial lesion or extensive and superficial lesion. Body cavity method is a peculiar form of two-pole method. Tailor-made body cavity electrode (such as rectum and vagina) is placed in the

Table 8.1 Ultrashort wave dosage classifications and indications

	Classification quantity of heat	The patients' feeling	Luminance of neon lamp
1	None	No sense of warmth	Faint light of neon lamp
2	Slight	Slightly tepor	Full bright of neon lamp, dim light
3	Warm	Comfortable tepor	Brightness of neon lamp
4	Hot obvious hotness, but can tolerate	Brightness of neon lamp	

corresponding cavity. Another plate or band electrode can be placed in abdomen, lumbosacral spinal or around pelvis, but this electrode cannot be used in the therapy of osteoarthritis.

(d) The distance between electrode and skin is called air distance. The size of sir distance is related to therapeutic area and output power of the equipment. In the superficial lesion, the distance is small and the distance is big when the lesion is deep. If we used the therapy equipment with big power, the distance should be enlarged. On the contrary, the distance should be shrinking. In practice, we should consider the range of the lesion and the size of the electrode. When we used therapy equipment with small power and electrode, the distance is 0.5–1 cm. When we used therapy equipment with big power and electrode for deep lesion, the distance is 3–4 cm. In order to prevent uneven effect, the air distance should be small for uneven surface.

(e) Contraposition should be used with caution in children's head. The dosage shouldn't be too large for the therapy of human head. In apposition, the distance between two electrodes should not be shorter than the diameter of electrode or shorter than the radius of electrode.

5. Main indications and contraindications of ultrashort wave
   (a) Indications:
   - Various inflammation diseases including inflammation of soft tissue, joint, bone, the five sense organs, viscera in pleuroperitoneal cavity, nervous system and genitals. It has a good therapeutic effect on acute and sub-acute inflammation.
   - Painful diseases including neuralgia, causalgia, myalgia, acroaesthesia and the diseases of vasomotor nerve and some autonomic nervous dysfunction.
   - Traumatic wound and ulcer: Ultrashort wave can accelerate the fade of various traumatic reactions such as pain, edema, hematoma, hemarthrosis, hydrops articuli, bone fracture and swelling after replacement of dislocated joints. The ultrashort wave therapy should not be used for too many times. The frequency is less than 15 times in case of inducing tissue dehydration and aging of granulation tissue and new epithelial tissue.

   (b) Contraindications: The patients with bleeding tendency, hypotension, heart failure, active tuberculosis, cancer (except for killing tumor cells through high thermal energy), pacemaker or valvular replacement.

8.2.4.3 Medium Frequency Electrotherapy

1. The definition of medium frequency electrotherapy: Medium frequency electrotherapy is a method that pulse current with the application frequency (1000–100,000 Hz) is used for treating diseases. Interferential current therapy, modulated medium frequency electrotherapy, width sine intermediate frequency (voice frequency) and medium frequency electrotherapy controlled by computer are usually used in clinic.
2. The characteristics of medium frequency current
   (a) No electrolytic action: Medium frequency current is sine alternating current. There is no positive and negative electrode and no electrolytic action. Therefore, it is easy to be operated.
   (b) Reducing tissue impedance and increasing action depth: Medium frequency current can overcome tissue impedance and has a deep therapeutic effect.
   (c) Excitable effect on body tissue: After action potential of motor nerve, there is absolute refractory period and the duration is about 1 ms. If every stimulus can induce action potential, the frequency of medium frequency current should be less than 1000 Hz. Therefore, the current with the frequency that is less than 1000 Hz is called low frequency current. Medium frequency current with the frequency that is from 1 to 100 kHz cannot induce action potential every time, but combined action

of many stimuli can induce one action potential, which is called combined effect of medium frequency electrical stimulus.

(d) The characteristics of the stimulated effect of medium frequency current on neuromuscular stimulation: medium frequency current can stimulate the skin sensory nerve but cannot induce excitement of fiber of sensory pain. There is comfortable vibration sense but no pain. Therefore, current with strong intensity can induce intensive contraction of deep muscle, but cannot induce burn pricking of electrode. Medium frequency current with the frequency that is 6000–8000 Hz can induce divergence phenomenon between muscle contraction threshold and threshold of pain. In this frequency range, there is strong muscle contraction but no pain.

(e) Physiologic characteristic of medium frequency current with low frequency: Medium frequency current with constant range can be adapted for human body to decrease stimulation effectiveness. At present, medium frequency current modulated by low frequency current (0–150 Hz) is used in clinic to make range of medium frequency current change with the frequency of low frequency current. The current has the characteristics of low frequency current and medium frequency current. Moreover, human body is difficult to adapt to the change of wave form, wave amplitude, frequency and modulated amplitude. This kind of current includes interference current and modulated medium frequency current. Rectified pulse medium frequency current can be used for medicine-inductiveness therapy.

- Physiological effects of medium frequency current with constant amplitude and low frequency modulated medium frequency current are different because of different frequency of current. The main functions are as follows:
- The effect on motor nerve and muscle: The current with frequency that is 1–10 Hz can induce single contraction of muscle. The current with frequency that is 25–50 Hz can induce tetanic contraction of muscle. The current with frequency that is 100 Hz can weaken or diminish muscle contraction.
- The effect on sensory nerve: There is obvious vibratory sense in the frequency of 50 Hz and analgesic effect in the frequency of 100 Hz.
- The effect on blood vessel: The current with frequency that is 1–20 Hz can increase tension of blood vessel and the current with frequency that is 50–100 Hz can dilate blood vessel.
- The effect on autonomic nerve: The current with frequency that is 4–10 Hz can excite sympathetic nerve and the current with frequency that is 20–40 Hz can excite vagus. When the frequency is 100–150 Hz, the current can inhibit sympathetic nerve.

3. Physiological effect and therapeutic effect of medium frequency current: Medium frequency current can ease pain, promote blood circulation, diminish inflammation, lessen adhesion and prevent scar formation.

(a) Analgesic effect: Medium frequency electrotherapy can induce threshold of pain in local skin. In clinic, it has good analgesic effects, especially low frequency modulated medium frequency current. Analgesic effect includes immediate analgesia and follow-up analgesia.

Immediate analgesia is that pain can be relieved quickly after therapy. The mechanism of immediate analgesia may be masking effect theory, cortex interference theory and humoral mechanism. Medium frequency current can induce obvious vibratory sense. When an impulse goes into any node of pain stimulus afferent pathway, the conduction of pain stimulus can be blocked or covered so that the pain can be stopped or relieved. Cortex interference theory is that when electrical stimulus impulse and pain impulse go into cortical sensory area at the same time, they disturb each other in the cortex. According to excited competitive inhibition of cerebral nuclei, the sense of pain can be relieved or covered. Humoral mechanism of immediate analgesia is that endogenous morphine-like peptides (OLS) is secreted from brain, pituitary body and intestines. It has the effect of morphine and is one kind of natural neurotransmitter with analgesic effect. Endogenous morphine-like peptides include encephalin (short duration of analgesia) and endorphin (long duration of analgesia, 3–4 h). Medium frequency current can activate neurons of endogenous morphine-like peptides and they can release OLS with analgesic effect. The analgesic effect of OLS is 3–4 time of that of morphine and they have no side effects.

Follow-up analgesia: under the influence of medium frequency current, local blood circulation is changed to relieve edema between tissues and between nerve fibers, decrease tissue tension, alleviate muscle spasm induced by ischemia, improve anaerobic condition, promote elimination of pathological chemical substances such as potassium ion, plasmakinin and amines, which have indirect analgesic effect.

Promotion of blood circulation: Medium frequency current, especially low frequency (50-100 Hz) modulated medium frequency current can obviously promote local blood and lymphatic fluid circulation, increase skin temperature and dilate arteriole and capillary. The mechanisms are as follows:

(b) Axon reflex: Medium frequency current can stimulate skin receptor. Impulse go into the afferent neuron and can conduct to arterial wall another branch of the same axon retrograde, which induce dilation of local blood vessel.
 - The effect of vasoactive substance: medium frequency current can stimulate sensory nerve and make them release a little substance P and acetylcholine that can induce dilation of blood vessels.
 - The effect of metabolite muscle movement: Metabolites of muscle contraction have obvious dilation of blood vessels effect such as lactic acid.
 - The effect of autonomic nerve: medium frequency current can inhibit sympathetic nerve to promote local blood circulation.
 - Skeletal muscle exercise: Low frequency modulated medium frequency current can induce skeletal muscle contraction. It has little stimulation on skin sensory nerve ending and no electrolytic action. It can be used for a long time. Depth of current penetration is good for the therapy of deep lesion.

(c) Softening scars and lessening adhesion: medium frequency current with constant amplitude (sound frequency current) can soften scar and lessen adhesion, which is widely used in clinic. Its characteristics are as follows:

(d) Instant effect: there is quick therapeutic effect in the therapy of spasm induced by cerebral palsy. Muscle spasm is due to higher central nerve injury so that the therapeutic effect doesn't last long.
 - The therapeutic effect is fast: the therapeutic effect of cerebral palsy spasm is fast, but the therapeutic effect of muscle spasm due to higher central nerve damages cannot last a long time
 - Painless: There is on injury and pain in medium frequency electrotherapy and most of the patients can adapt to it quickly.
 - Fewer side effects: Medium frequency electrotherapy seldom induces discomfort or anaphylactic reaction.
 - Enduring therapeutic effect: the therapeutic effect of medium frequency current can last long. This may be because that there are additive effects after repeated therapies. Taking medicine, after several hours, the medicine lose efficacy and the symptoms reappear.
 - In addition to this, we can select and apply rehabilitation department existing physiotherapy equipment of rehabilitation department for therapy such as laser, kerotherapy, decimetric wave,

centimetre wave and millimeter wave. According to the different responses and requirements, the medicine can be added properly.

- Non steroid analgesic and anti-inflammation medicine can inhibit the synthesis of inflammatory substances, withstand inflammation reaction, relieve joint edema and pain, but they have no effect on the progress of osteoarthritis. We can use ibuprofen, rebellin, voltaren (diclofenac sodium) and celecoxib.
- Sodium hyaluronate is the main ingredient of articular cavity synovia, which can lubricate joint, decrease tissue attrition, enhance vicidity of synovial fluid and lubrication, protect cartilago articularis, promote the healing and regeneration of cartilago articularis, relieve pain and increase range of joint motion. This medicine can be used for intra-articular injection once a week for 5 weeks.
- Glucosamine is to promote the synthesis of protein polysaccharide with normal structure in chondrocyte. Caleineurin polysaccharide can protect cartilago articularis cells from damage in order to improve range of joint motion, relieve joint pain and delay the progress of osteoarthritis. The medicine should be taken orally 250–500 mg per time, three times a day with meal.

The medicine can be combined with acupuncture and stimulation of main and collateral channels in traditional Chinese medicine to obtain better therapeutic effect.

8.2.5 Method and Mechanism of Physical Exercise Therapy

Physical exercise therapy is physical therapy (PT). Somatic movement, massage, traction and training equipment are used for therapy and training to prevent and treat injuries and recover functions. The physical agents are applied include electricity, light, sound, magnet, cold and heat. The classification is over-general, which covers a lot and is easy to be confused. With the development and progress of rehabilitation medicine, the definition should be more precise and the classification is easy to understand and master. For example, the definition of physical exercise therapy is that manipulation and training skills are used to increase or recover the original functions of the patients. The most prominent thing is that the patients take part in the training process actively. The definition of physiotherapy is that natural physical agents such as electricity, light, sound, cold and heat are applied for prevention and therapy of the injuries. The important thing is that the patients passively receive the therapy and there is no training process. However, both physiotherapy and physical exercise therapy are all the inalienable important ingredients of rehabilitation medicine.

We mainly introduce the rehabilitation method of neurological training applied for injury of bony joint and soft tissue and degenerative inflammation.

8.2.5.1 Neurological Training Rehabilitation

Daoyin feedback technique in traditional Chinese medicine is used for the training to relieve pain and recover the range and function of joint motion.

1. Method and equipment Neurological training equipment and Daoyin equipment of muscular tension are applied for the training.

   The essence of neurological training is to combine six-step Daoyin technique of guiding collaterals through meridians and biological feedback technique. The record of six-step Daoyin technique of guiding collaterals through meridians or the oral dictation of the therapists are used to guide the patients to move agonistic muscle of joint dominated by brain. Meanwhile, electronic equipment is used to receive motor program signal form brain to agonistic muscle and antagonistic muscle or tension signal of muscle contraction and dilation and display it in the fluorescent screen with a curve form. Through establishing surpassing goal with different signal intensity, the patients are guided repeatedly to enhance signal intensity of agonistic muscle and decrease signal intensity of antagonistic muscle with anti-resistance training to develop brain potential. Through active joint motion, tissue adhesion can be lessened, myodynamia can be strengthened and the range of joint motion can be increased.

The theory of neurological training equipment is that it can receive the motor program signal form brain to agonistic muscle and antagonistic muscle that are involved in joint motion, which provide the therapists the training of motor program establishment with a purpose to guide the patients.

The theory of Daoyin equipment of muscular tension is the same as that of neurological training equipment. The difference is the tension change during the contraction of agonistic muscle and antagonistic muscle that are involved in joint motion, which is the pressure of muscular tension on reception electrode. It is another outward pattern of manifestation of motor program. This pressure signal can be showed in fluorescent screen with a curve form. Through establishing surpassing goal with different intensity of muscular tension signal, it can provide the therapists the training of motor program establishment with a purpose to guide the patients.

2. Training part and the placement of electrode: According to the affected parts, the training part can be ascertained all over the body.
   (a) Neurological training of scapulohumeral periarthritis can be divided into the training of shrug, shoulder protraction, rear protraction of shoulder, shoulder abduction and shoulder cyclovergence. Single lead electrode is used for shrug and electrode is pasted on skin surface above shoulder joint. Three-lead electrode is used for shoulder abduction and it is pasted on skin surface of anterior, middle and posterior bundle of deltoid muscle. It should be used for the training of shoulder abduction, protraction of shoulder, rear protraction of shoulder and shoulder cyclovergence.
   (b) The training of strain of lumbar muscles: Two-lead paralleling electrode (the left and the right) are used and they are pasted on skin surface of musculus sacrospinalis 2 cm outside of spinous process of lumbar vertebra. The training of waist anteflexion and rear protraction can be done separately. The training of muscle in L1, L3 and L5 of lumbar vertebra can be done.
   (c) The therapy of hip arthritis: The training of anteflexion, rear protraction, adduction, abduction and cyclovergence of hip joint are done separately. The electrodes of anteflexion and rear protraction of hip joint are pasted on skin surface of hip flexor and extensor separately. The electrodes of hip adduction and abduction can be pasted on skin surface of hip adductor and abductor. Four-lead electrode can be used for the training of hip cyclovergence. Four electrodes are pasted on skin surface of hip flexor, hip abductor, hip extensor and hip adductor. Through establishing different surpassing goal, Daoyin technique is used to guide the patients to surpass the goal through active anti-resistance training.
   (d) The training of knee arthritis the electrodes of knee extension and flexion are pasted on skin surface of quadriceps femoris and hamstring muscles.
   (e) The training of ankle arthritis: The training of foot dorsiflexion, plantar flexion, strephenopodia and strephexopodia. The electrodes of foot dorsiflexion and plantar flexion are pasted on skin surface of muscle belly of tibialis anterior muscle and musculus gastrocnemius separately. The electrodes of strephenopodia and strephexopodia are pasted on skin surface of muscle belly of peroneus longus and brevis and tibialis posterior.
   (f) The training of musculi colli: The training of neck extensor and flexor is the main training. Two-lead paralleling electrode (the right and the left) are used in this training. The back electrode is pasted on skin surface of musculi colli and 2 cm

outside of spinous process of cervical vertebra. The front electrode is pasted on skin surface of muscle belly of cleidomastoid. The trainings of cervical flexion, extension and cyclovergence are done separately.

Daoyin equipment of muscular tension is applied for the training. Through receiving the pressure of muscle contraction on reception electrode and using it as the feedback signal, the electrode is hard to be placed in some area and the sensitivity of the electrode is not more than that of neurological training equipment. We can choose the therapy equipment flexibly.

3. Training time and therapy course: The training is 30 min per time and 15 times per course. The therapy can be done continuously.
4. Neurological training used to treat osteoarthritis and its mechanism: Neurological training equipment is not physiotherapy equipment. During therapy process, there is no intervention of physical agent, but therapeutic effect of chronic bony joint disease is significant. Its mechanism is related to the following factors:
   (a) Autonomic joint motion training and consolidation of therapeutic effect: Six-step Daoyin technique of guiding collaterals through meridians is the Daoyin technique according to main and collateral channels. Is has a good clearing and activating the channels and collaterals effect. The current of main and collateral channels can alleviate pain. Especially, six-step Daoyin technique is used to guide the patients surpass specific goal and do anti-resistance autonomic range of joint motion training, which can improve range of joint motion. Moreover, the inspired autonomic joint motion training through reestablishing motor program belongs to methodology training. Once there is therapeutic effect, it can be consolidated and is hard to relapse. Just like a person has learned to ride a bicycle, after 1 year or more time, he still can ride a bike.
   (b) The important measure of painless joint motion is attention diversion. The reason why neurological training method can lead to painless joint motion without any intervention of physical agent is attention diversion. Through stimulant competitive inhibition of cerebral nuclei, attention diversion can be achieved. There is competitive inhibition in the excitability of central cerebral nuclei. For example, when a cerebral nucleus is excited, the excitability of another cerebral nucleus can be inhibited. This is because that human central nervous system can receive or perceive the information of the most excited cerebral nuclei and neglect information of other cerebral nuclei with low excitability. However, the excitability degree of one cerebral nucleus with strong excitability can be influenced by other nuclei. In fact, in actual life, there is such phenomenon. For example, in competitive sports of the 110-m hurdles, if the performance of Liu Xiang is better than others, the entire world focuses on him. When his performance is lower than any of the others, the concerned person is changed. The patients with multiple injuries perceive the most severe injured part or organ of the body. When the severe part is treated, they can perceive the injuries of other parts or organ. In clinic, the therapists may overlook the injured part and delay the therapy. Most of the patients feel less painful in daytime because of accompany of other people and feel more painful at quiet night.

   Neurological training method is that the patients are guided to do active joint motion, meanwhile the equipment receive the drive signal form central nerve to muscles of joint motion and displays it on the fluorescent screen in a curve from. There are three key points in the training:
   - Through immerse technique, the patients are immersed into therapeutic environment.
   - Through Daoyin technique of regulation of mind and breathing, the patients focus on concentration training.
   - During the process of regulation of movement, the patients are guided to

concentrate on surpassing the signal intensity of agonistic muscle and forget the joint motion training. The three key points can better diverse the patients' attention. When the patients move their joints, the sense of pain is greatly relieved or there is no sense of pain. After the therapy, the patients find that the range of their joint motion is increased and the sense of pain is relieved. Moreover, there is no pain in the therapy and the confidence of therapy is doubled.

- With the range of joint motion, adhesive joint capsule, ligament, tendon and muscle can be lessened to promote increase of range of joint motion and remission of the pain. This is why biological feedback technique can cure scapulohumeral periarthritis and pain of lower waist. It can lessen soft tissue adhesion without inducing pain.

(c) Promotion of blood circulation and elimination of metabolite: After diagnosed with osteoarthritis, because of pain during joint motion, the patients cannot move or do less exercise and the range of joint motion is decreased, which can affect blood circulation of soft tissue around joint to a certain extent and block the elimination of metabolite. Accumulation of local metabolite, especially lactate metabolite, can stimulate nerve ending of local soft tissue, which further induce pain and discomfort.

In addition, lymph backflow obstruction aggravates local heaviness. The training of automatic joint motion can promote the contraction and dilation of local blood vessels with the increase of the time of muscle contraction and relaxation in order to increase local blood circulation. With the increase of local metabolism, elimination of accumulative metabolite and smooth lymph backflow are good for elimination or alleviation of local pain, tingling, swelling and heaviness.

(d) Enhancement of myodynamia: anti-resistance training of neurological training can strengthen myodynamia to smooth joint motion and increase the range of joint motion. The enhancement of myodynamia requires more blood supply to promote local blood circulation. The increase of the range of joint motion is good for the loose of adhesion. It can turn joint motion into a virtuous cycle of functional recovery.

8.2.5.2 Physical Exercise Therapy of Neurological Training

Physical exercise therapy of neurological training is a training mode of six-step Daoyin technique of guiding collateral through meridians with bare hands. The training is done without neurological training equipment. Its basic procedures are the same with the process with neurological training equipment. They are all active joint motion training. According to specific conditions of the patients, anti-resistance training can be done properly with the help of passive joint motion and massage of muscle and soft tissue.

In physical exercise therapy of neurological training, the movements of muscle training include isometric exercise training and isotonic exercise training. Isometric exercise training is that muscular tension is changed with constant length of muscle, which is also called silent contraction training. It is suitable for the patients with arthritis. Except for acute and severe arthritis, the patients in any stage or any time can use this training method. Isotonic exercise training is that the muscle tension is changed slightly before and after exercises, but the muscle length and joint position are changed. It is suitable for anti-resistance training.

Training time and therapy course: Physical exercise therapy of neurological training can be used for treating osteoarthritis. The training time is 45 min per time. There are 15 times in one therapy course (once a day).

8.2.5.3 Manipulation of Lessening Joint Adhesion

It is a therapeutic method that manipulation is used to lessen tissue adhesion and to increase range of joint motion. The doctors or the therapists can exert force on the joints of the patients to improve range of joint motion, promote joint functions and relieve pain. Passive movements are mainly used to lessen joint, relieve and eliminate soft tissue adhesion in order to recover physiological movement and accessory movement of joint. The operation speed is slower than that of massage.

1. The classification of joint motion includes physiological movement and accessory movement.
   (a) Physiological movement of joint: The joint motion can be complete in physiological range, which is called physiological movement of joint. It can be completed passively or actively.
   (b) Accessory movement of joint: in the allowable range of joint and tissue around joint, the movements can be completed passively, which is called accessory movement.

   There is accessory movement in every joint. Accessory movement is one kind of indispensable motion form. This movement cannot be completed actively and it requires the help of others or offside limbs such as joint separation and lateral movement of patella.

   When the joint is restricted because of pain and stiffness, physiological and accessory movement can be confined. When physiological movement is recovered, there are still pain or stiffness in joint motion. This may be because that the accessory movement of joint is still not recovered completely.

   Before improving physiological movement of joint, we should improve accessory movement of joint. The improvement of accessory movement of joint can promote the improvement of physiological movement of joint.
2. Basic methods are named according to application mode of force of the joint and the mode of movable joint.
   (a) Swing: Swing is the lever-like movement of bone, which is physiological movement. During swing, the proximal of joint should be fixed and the distal of joint is made to swing in order to lessen adhesion.

   During joint swing, in order to prevent tissue tear or bone fracture, it is necessary to do the operation when the range of joint motion is more than 60% of normal range of joint motion. For example, during the swing training of anteflexion of shoulder, it should be applied when the anteflexion of shoulder is at 100%. Otherwise, manipulation of accessory movement should be used. Swing training can be used when the range of joint motion meets the requirements.
   (b) Roll: When one bone is rolling on the surface of the other, the touch point is changing because of the bones with different shapes. The movement is angulation movement. The rolling orientation is to the orientation of angulation, usually with slide and rotation of joint.
   (c) Slide: When one bone is sliding on the other, if it is simple slide, the surface shape of the two bones should be identical, plane or hook face (concave-convex degree of the two bone surface should be equal). During sliding, one touch point of bone surface can touch the touch point of offside bone surface. The slide orientation depends on concave-convex surface of bony joint. The bulge means the slide orientation is opposite to the angulation orientation. The hollow means the slide orientation is the same as the angulation orientation.

   There is more sliding in the smooth joint surface and there is more rolling in the unsmooth joint surface. In clinic, sliding can relieve pain. Combined with traction, sliding can lessen joint capsule, relax joint, and improve range of joint motion. Therefore, it can be applied in many spheres.
   (d) Rotation means the touch point can rotate around the rotation axis of static bone surface. During rotation, the same point does circular movement. Rotation usually is done with sliding and rolling. It is rarely done independently.

(e) Separation and traction: Separation and traction are both called traction. Separation is that the surfaces of two bone of the joint are separated in a right angle under external force, which is called separation or intra-articular traction. Traction is that the external force moves along the long axis of the bone to make the joint shift in a long distance, which is called traction of long axis.

The difference between separation and traction: During separation the external force is vertical to joint surface and the external force is strong. The force can separate two joints. During traction, the external force is parallel to long axis of the bone and the joint surfaces may not be separated.

3. Classification of manipulation and application selection: The classification of manipulation is according to range of joint motion.

(a) Matland classification:

Grade I: In the beginning of joint motion, joint can be lessened rhythmically in a small range. Grade II: Within the allowable scope of joint motion, joint can be lessened rhythmically, but not touch the beginning and the end of joint motion. Grade III: Within the allowable scope of joint motion, joint can be lessened rhythmically and the therapists can feel the tension of soft tissue around joint. Grade IV: The point of action is at the proximal of the joint. The joint can be lessened rhythmically in a small range. When touching the proximal of the joint every time, the therapists can feel the tension of soft tissue around joint.

(b) Application selection: The manipulation of Grade I and Grade II can be used for the therapy of pain. The manipulation of Grade III can be used for the therapy of pain and joint stiffness. The manipulation of Grade IV can be used for the therapy of contracture and adhesion. The manipulation of Grade I–IV can be used for accessory movement. The manipulation of Grade I–IV can be used for physiological movement when the range of joint motion reaches 60% of normal ROM. In clinic, The manipulation of Grade III–IV are usually used, while gradeI is seldom used.

4. The therapeutic effect of lessening adhesion through manipulation, the indications of clinical application and operational programs.

(a) Therapeutic effect: physiological effect includes mechanical and neurological effect. Mechanical effect can promote the flow of synovial fluid, increase the nutrition of cartilago articularis and cartilaginous operculum to relieve pain and prevent joint degeneration. Neurological effect can inhibit spinal cord and brain stem to release pain factor and increase pain threshold. Maintain of tissue tenacity: the manipulation of grade III and IV can be used directly for traction of soft tissue around joint to increase extensibility and tenacity in order to improve range of joint motion. The increase of noumenon feedback: with the increase of range of joint motion, the sensitivity of the joint to sensory information increases such as the information of joint immobilization, movement speed and change, movement orientation, muscle tension and change. Therefore, movement form and body position can be adjusted to complete coordinated movement.

(b) Manipulation application: The movement orientation of manipulation can be vertical or parallel to therapeutic plane (the plane of spin axis of the middle point of joint surface). In the separation manipulation, the movement orientation is vertical to therapeutic plane. In the manipulation of sliding and long axis traction, the movement orientation is parallel to therapeutic plane. The degree of manipulation: For the confined joint, movement range should reach the limit of joint motion. For the joint with pain, movement range should reach the pain point. With the alleviation of symptoms, the movement range can be beyond the pain point. The movement range of stiff joint should be beyond the stiffness point. During therapy, manipulation should be balanced. The force should be even and rhythmed. The manipulation should be kept on the action point for 30–60 s.

(c) Therapeutic reactions: After joint mobilization techniques, it is normal that there is normal reaction. If the pain cannot be relieved in 24 h after that, even aggravated, it demonstrates that therapeutic intensity is too strong or the therapeutic time is too long. The therapeutic schedule should be adjusted appropriately.

(d) Clinical indications include joint dysfunctions due to any non-neuronal mechanical factor, pain, muscle intense and spasm, reversible limitation of range of joint motion, progressive limitation of joint motion and functional joint immobilization.

(e) Clinical contraindications: The patients with acute arthritis, unstable joint or severe deformation, swelling, tumor or unhealed bone fracture.

(f) Operational procedure: The body position of the patients should be comfortable, relaxed and painless. The position of the therapists: the therapists should be close to the therapeutic joint. The therapists use one hand to fix the end of the joint and use the other hand to lessen the other end. Assessment before therapy: the therapist should find out the existing problems such as pain, stiffness and their degree, design corresponding therapeutic schedule and put into effect.

8.2.5.4 Continuous Traction

Traction is one kind of method in rehabilitation therapeutic method. External force is used to exert traction on some part or some joint of the body in order to separate them to a certain extent. It also can stretch soft tissue around joint to achieve therapeutic goal. For osteoarthritis, the traction can be divided into traction of spinal cord and traction of four limbs joint.

1. Therapeutic effect of traction: The main purpose of traction of bony joint is to lessen adhesion and relieve pain. The main effects are summarized as following:
   - Lessening the adhesion of soft tissue and stretching contracture joint capsule, ligament and muscle tissue
   - Improving local blood circulation, promoting elimination of inflammation and edema and benefiting tissue repair
   - Relieving muscle spasm, relaxing muscle and alleviating pain
   - Restoration of incarcerated synovium of joint or dislocation of zygapophyseal joint or recovering normal physiological curvature of spine
   - Increasing foramen intervertebrale and relieving stimulation and oppression of nerve root
   - Increasing intervertebral space, relieving pressure in intervertebral disc, benefiting return of protrusion of intervertebral disc and alleviating bending degree and oppression degree of vertebral artery
2. Traction mode: The classification should be done according to the duration and action point of traction
   (a) Continuous traction: Tractive force should be kept during the process of traction.
   (b) Intermittent traction: Tractive force can increase or decrease regularly during the process of traction.

   For lessening adhesion of soft tissue, skin traction is usually used with small and continuous traction. Intermittent traction has a massage effect, but the stimulation is strong. It is suitable for old patients or the patients with obsolete lesion or severe condition. Continuous traction is usually used at first. The therapists can switch to intermittent traction if the therapeutic effect of continuous traction is not good.
3. Common tractions for the therapy of bony joint diseases include tractions of lower limbs, upper limbs, cervical vertebra, lumbar vertebra and spine.
   (a) Skin traction of upper and lower limbs: With the help of traction bed, traction bracket (Browns or Thomas traction bracket) or bedside traction bracket, the traction can be done through skin

traction band such as traction band of bare foot, lower limbs, wrist, hands and upper limbs.

Traction weight is about 3–5 kg and the body should be elevated to prevent edema. During the process of traction, the therapists should observe the peripheral circulation of the body closely in case of blood circulation disorder of the body and bruised soft tissue.

(b) Traction of cervical vertebra: it is suitable for vertebral artery type of cervical spondylosis, nerve-root type cervical spondylosis, joint sprain of cervical vertebra, herniation of cervical disc, cervical spondylolisthesis, retrogression of cervical vertebra, cervical small joint dysfunction and cervical muscle strain.

Occipital-jaw traction band is usually used to do traction in sitting position or in clinostatism. Traction force can increase intervertebral space of cervical vertebra, but not induce injuries of muscle and joint. Traction weight is about 2–3 kg in sitting position and 10 kg in clinostatism. Generally, continuous traction time is 15–20 min per time. Long time traction can induce static injuries of muscle and ligament. The magnitude of intermittent traction force is according to 10–20% of the body weight of the patients. Traction time is 20–30 min per time. There are 15 times in one therapy course (once a day). The angle of cervical vertebra in traction: the angle of anteflexion of cervical vertebra is 10–30°. In vertebra artery type cervical vertebra traction, the angle of anteflexion of cervical vertebra is 5°. In nerve root type, the angle of anteflexion is 20–30°. In spinal cord type, the traction should be protracted backward slightly. It is needed to pay attention to that no matter what kind of the traction, the traction should be adjusted timely according to the response of the patients to the traction. Traction mode: Continuous traction is usually used. Intermittent traction is also used or the combination of the two can be used.

The body position of traction of cervical vertebra usually is sitting position, but in supine position, the back of intervertebral space in C4–C7 can be broadened and the angle is easy to adjust. In sitting position, the traction is easy to operate, but the position is unstable and the angle change is small.

Contraindications: Cervical vertebra tuberculosis, tumor, severe osteoporosis, the long-term use of hormone, vertebral artery sclerosis, cervical spine deformity, myocardial infarction, cerebral arteriosclerosis and chronic cervical trauma.

(c) Lumbar vertebra traction: it is suitable for lumbar vertebra osteoarthritis, oppression of ischiadic nerve by protrusion of intervertebral disc, tension of dorsal muscle, strain of lumbar muscles and fiber inflammation, stiffness of facet joint in lumbar vertebra, soft tissue spasm and adhesion.

The key points of lumbar vertebra traction:

- The patients lie on their back and bend hip and knee until the lumbar vertebra anteflect to decrease stress of spine as much as possible.
- Traction force should be started from 20 kg or one-fourth of the body weight that can overcome the friction between the body and the bed. The weight can be gradually increased to 30–40 kg. A moment later, according to the endurance of the patients, the weight can be increased to half of the body weight.
- Traction mode: Intermittent traction is mainly used. The break and traction time can be adjusted in 30 s. The traction usually is 7 s and the break is 15 s.
- Traction time: Traction time lasts 20–30 min per time. There are 15–20 times in a therapy course (1–2 times a day).
- Traction announcements: the therapists should observe the feeling and response of the patients in traction and adjust the traction according to practical conditions. For the elder, traction time should be short and traction force should be

weak. If there is discomfort or the symptom is aggravated in traction, the therapists should stop traction immediately, find out the reason and adjust it or stop the therapy.

Contraindications: blood circulatory disorder in spinal cord, osteomalacia of vertebra, cauda equina syndrome, spondylosis, spinal cord disease, lumbar vertebra tuberculosis, tumor, severe osteoporosis, long-term use of hormone, severe hypertension, heart diseases and hemorrhagic disorders.

8.2.5.5 Application of Continuous Passive Motion (CPM)

In the setting motion range, CPM can be done continuously in a setting time through mechanical drive equipment to drive the joint, which belongs to passive joint motion. CPM can prevent joint adhesion, promote wound healing, accelerate repair of cartilago articularis and injured soft tissue around it, relieve pain, improve range of joint motion and decrease postoperative complications of joint.

There is random control study about the influence of CPM on postoperative complications after fracture of lower limb. The therapy and nursing are given to control group routinely. The observation group are given CPM through CPM machine. The therapists observe the differences of joint pain, edema and range of motion after operation between the two groups. The results showed that there is significant difference of therapeutic effect between the two groups. The therapeutic effect of observation group is better than control group. CPM of lower limbs joint can promote blood circulation of joint, improve synovium nutrition, relieve joint edema, prevent joint stiffness and alleviate pain.

1. Clinical indications of CPM: it is suitable for osteoarthritis, joint spasm, intra-articular fracture, hemiplegia, paraplegia, limitation of joint motion ability and range of joint motion due to muscle dysfunction, and postoperation of joint.
2. Application method: according to the endurance of the patients, the period time is 1–2 min and the activity time is 1 h per time (1–3 times a day).

CPM can be used for injured limbs immediately after operation, even the patients are still in narcosis or there are too many surgical dressing in the first 3 days after operation to block passive motion in other ways. After operation, according to the condition, the patients can do movements at the range of 20–30°. The range of motion can be adjusted every day or every time according to the condition.

For the patients with knee joint surgery, in supine position, operation part of CPM can be fixed on the middle of thigh and the upside of shank. In the first day after surgery, knee joint can be moved at the range of 30°. The period is 2 min and the activity time is 1 h. After that, the motion angle can be increased gradually and the activity period can be accelerated.

8.2.6 The Method and Effect of Self-Exercise

After a period of time of the interventional therapy of physical agents, osteoarthritis can be eliminated gradually and the pain is relieved. Through rehabilitation training of active and passive joint motion and lessening adhesion through manipulation, the adhesion of cartilago articularis and soft tissue around joint is lessened gradually to relieve or eliminate pain. The range of joint motion can be recovered to the level before injury or the range of joint motion can be obviously increased compared with pre-treatment. However, if there is no proper method to prevent the adhesion of cartilago articularis and soft tissue around joint, it is possible to induce adhesion and the cartilago articularis may occur repeatedly or relapse. After therapy, micro damaged wound surface of the lessened soft tissue is still not healed. If there is no effective joint motion timely (enough range and times), the adhesion can occur again and the symptoms relapse.

However, the therapy time of the patients in hospital is limited, even in the therapy course, because the patients usually receive the therapy in outpatient service. Obviously, it is unrealistic to move the patients' joints by the doctors and the therapists. The best method is to teach the patients to do self-exercise of joint motion in order to prevent adhesion of soft tissue of joint.

In the past therapy, the patients' self-exercise of joint motion is taught by the doctors generally. The doctors say to the patients that they should do self-exercise of joint motion such as shoulder upthrow and cyclovergence movement of shoulder. There are two problems. The first is that there is no diagram to explain the detailed to the patients. The second is that the doctors don't master the correct exercise indeed. In addition, these methods cannot reach full range joint motion so that the effect of self-exercise is affected.

If the self-exercise becomes self-training, the effect of exercise can be increased obviously. Exercise normally is based on personal motor skills. Through repeated movements, it can forge or smelt the body, willpower and morality. It is one kind of personal movement, but it can increase efficiency. For example, through productive labor, social fighting and working practice, personal consciousness and working ability can be increased. Through various kinds of physical exercise, normal development of the body can be promoted to increase the functions many times.

The training should be done with the help of professional skilled personnel in a planned way step by step. Through study and practice, some kind of skill can be mastered. The trainers change qualities and abilities of the trainees consciously to make the trainees acquire one behavior pattern or one kind of skill.

Therefore, the training is more scientific than the application method of exercise and the effect is better too. In order to obtain better effect in self-exercise of the patients with osteoarthritis the patients, on the basis of physical training of neurological training, the author simplified the methods into a set of self-training method that can prevent soft tissue adhesion of joint.

8.2.6.1 Physiological Effect of Self-Training of Joint Motion

Improvement of neural function and increase of the entire functions: it is the same as the theory of rehabilitation of neurological training. Through normal movement pattern, self-training can improve and increase CNS function. Therefore, the body can endure intensive work and the balance, flexibility and stamina are increased.

1. The training can make brain switch between excitation and inhibition orderly. It can eliminate fatigue, clear mind, sharpen thought, prevent anxiety due to hypertension of nervous system. With improvement of nervous system function, control and regulation of organ systems, especially motor system, can be promoted and improved and the functions of the whole body can be increased.
2. Increase of blood circulation and promotion of metabolism: some research indicated that blood volume of brain cells in work are 10–20 times of blood volume of muscle cells, which accounts for 20–25% of oxygen consumption of the whole body. The training can increase blood supply of brain cells, increase myocardia function, promote blood circulation and metabolism of the whole body, make it in an aerobic exercise state, which are good for functional improvement.
3. Facilitating skeleton calcinosis and increasing bone functions: according to Wolff law, bone grow is stimulated by mechanical stimulation to change structure. The bone advance with use and move back with obsolescence. Continuous movement of specific part can induce hyperplasia and hypertrophy of local bone such as humerus of tennis player. Continuous fixation of specific part can make the local bone absorb hyperplasia and hypertrophy such as collum femoris after complete arthroplasty, which is the direct evidence of bone morphology adaptation induced by stress.

Through muscle movement, exercise can exert stress on bone and stimulate bone formation. Bone cortex becomes thick obviously, the diameter of bone increases, bone marrow cavity decreases, and bone mineral density increases, which can make the bone endure bigger load.

For the elder, especially postmenopausal women, osteoporosis and occurrence rate of fracture of the old can be prevented or decreased. Someone compared bone mineral density of lumbar vertebra of older athletes with that of age-matched older people and found that bone mineral density of lumbar vertebra of older athletes is apparently higher than that of age-matched older people.

It is noticeable that the patients in old age or with postmenopausal osteoporosis cannot increase bone mass through large amount of hard exercise because bone is not sensitive to mechanical signal. There is risk that bone trabecula may be broke off. Therefore, exercise only can prevent osteoporosis, but it is not therapeutic method for osteoporosis.

4. Increasing muscle strength and improving ligament flexibility: After therapy of osteoarthritis, the purpose of self-training is to move joint, lessen adhesion and prevent the relapse. During training, rapid metabolism increase blood supply of the muscle, thicken muscle fiber and enlarge muscle body. The change of muscle structure can enhance the activity of enzyme, promote function of nervous regulating system and improve muscle functions entirely. The manifestations include strong strength of muscle, fast startup, good elasticity and strong endurance.

   Joint motion with a purpose can stretch joint capsule, ligament, tendon and muscle effectively to improve extensibility of soft tissue around joint, which can further increase range of joint motion, joint soundness and suppleness of joint. All these are good for avoiding or decreasing various injuries and articular surface injury.
5. Correct self-training after therapy of osteoarthritis can lessen adhesion fully, prevent adhesion of joint and soft tissue around joint effectively. It can also move the joint as much as possible, even in the full range. Therefore, cartilago articularis, muscle, tendon, ligament, nerve and blood vessel, and joint capsule can all be stretched to lessen adhesion, prevent adhesion, consolidate therapeutic effect and prevent relapse.

8.2.6.2 Self-Training Method of Joint Motion

During the therapy or after the therapy, self-training method of joint motion of neurological training is that the patients do self-training without help of other people according to six-step Daoyin technique of neurological training, which can be cooperated with the record of six-step Daoyin technique and some simple training instruments. After the patients master the methods, the training can be done without the record and training instruments.

1. Self-training method of neck: The most common discomfort in neck are ache of the back of neck and numb of upper limbs, which is due to working at the desk for a long time or neck injury that can induce mircodamage of muscle of the back of neck and soft tissue, calcification of ligamentum nuchae, osteoproliferation of cervical vertebra, protrusion of intervertebral disc, calcification of posterior longitudinal ligament and spinal canal stenosis.

   After surgery or physiotherapy, the purpose of self-training is to keep the fitness of spinal canal and suppleness of paravertebral soft tissue and soft tissue of neck to increase range of joint motion of cervical vertebra, decrease the stimulation and oppression to nerve root and blood vessels, lessen and prevent tissue adhesion, and relieve symptoms.
   (a) The training of anteflexion, rear protraction and lateral bending of the neck: this method is mainly used to train muscles around the neck to increase local blood circulation and stability of cervical vertebra, lessen and prevent adhesion of soft tissue and move cervical joint.

      The patients sit down, keep the trunk up-right, concentrate their mind and make a shell-like thing from elastic band. The patients grasp the front end and put the rear end behind the head. In the training of rear protraction of the neck, two hands cross over and put them on occipital nodule to replace elastic band. On the contrary, in the training of anteflexion, the front end of elastic band is put on facies frontalis and the rear end of elastic band is fixed on the back of a chair or the wall. In the training of right bending of the neck, elastic band is put on the right of the head. In the training of left bending of the neck, elastic band is put on the left of the head.

After the elastic band is fixed, the patients take a deep breath and concentrate on the training part of the neck. For example, in the neck extension training, the patients should concentrate on the rear of the neck, feel the warmth of training part, and overcome the resistance from elastic band or upper limbs. When the movement of the neck reaches the maximum range, the patients speak silently "1, 2, 3, 4, 5 and 6" for 6 s. After training, the patients take a deep breath and exhale slowly. The ratio of inspiration and expiration is 1–2. The patients try to relax cervical muscle and soft tissue. The training sketch maps refer to 8-2-1–8-2-4. After that, the patients do next training and the training time is 6–8.

(b) Self-massage of the rear of the neck: in order to cooperate cervical self-training, the patients can use massage to further lessen soft tissue adhesion, which can help to relieve stiffness of ligamentum nuchae.

The patients sit down or lie on their back. The patients extend their heads to relax the tissue of the rear of neck and rub the two hands until they are warm. The patients put one hand on the rear of the neck and use rub, seize, clutch, malaxation and pinch to do a massage on the rear of the neck. The patients can use rub method to warm local tissue and then use malaxation method to move it laterally. For the patient with stiffness or calcification of ligamentum nuchae, the manipulation should be soft at the beginning and intensity is increased gradually. The patients use massage method to move the rear tissue of the neck laterally and feel the stiffness or calcification of ligament. After a period of self-massage, the tissue of the rear of the neck include stiff ligamentum nuchae can be relieved to varying degrees.

Self-massage of the rear of the neck can be used for health protection measures of the neck. The massage time is 15–20 min and there are 15 time in one therapy course (once a day) (Figs. 8.1, 8.2, 8.3, and 8.4).

(c) Cervical cyclovergence: the patients sit down or stand. In standing position, the two feet separate and the space between the two feet is the same as the shoulder. The patients draw in the chest slight and erect the back with arms akimbo. Cooperated with breathing, the patients regulate breath, look straight ahead,

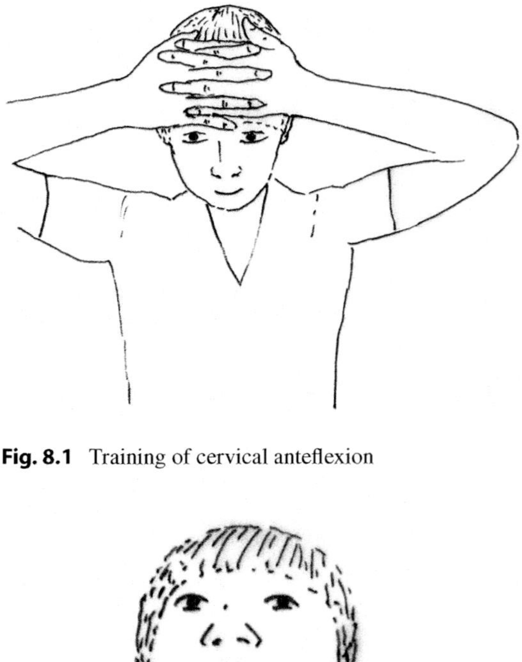

Fig. 8.1 Training of cervical anteflexion

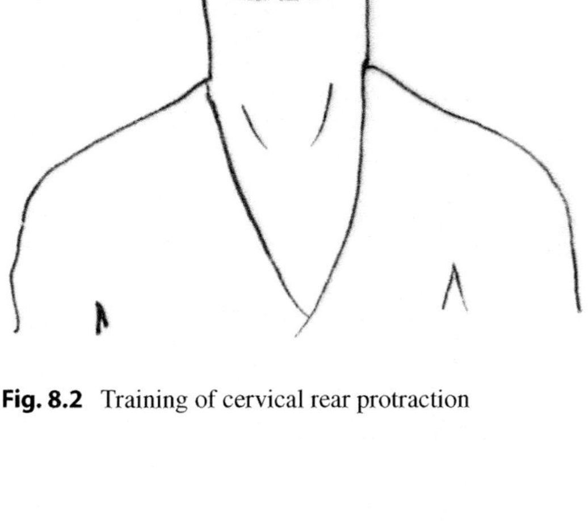

Fig. 8.2 Training of cervical rear protraction

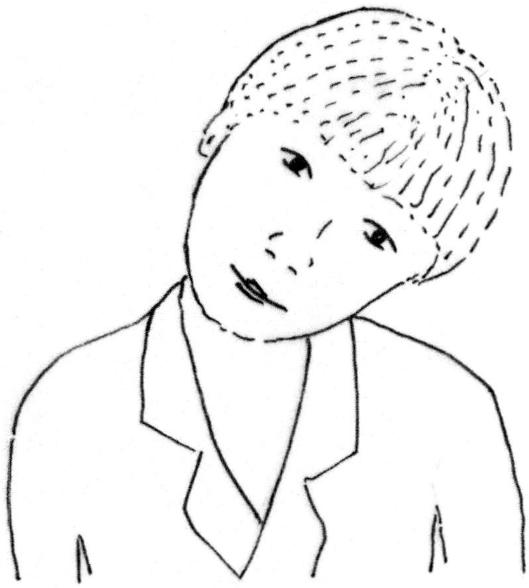

Fig. 8.3 Training of cervical left bending

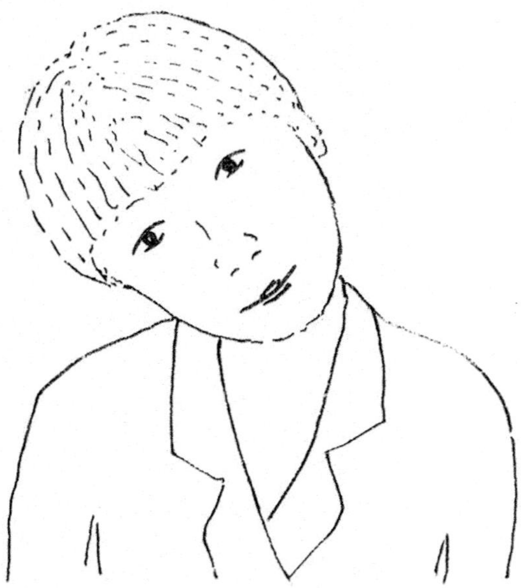

Fig. 8.4 Training of cervical right bending'

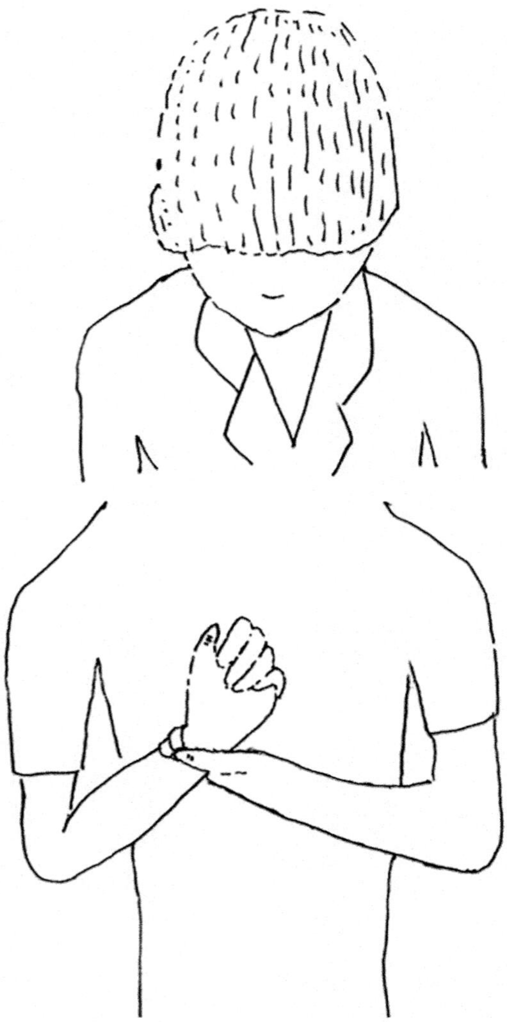

Fig. 8.5 Training of cervical cyclovergence

concentrate on the abdomen, rotate in clockwise direction of cervical flexion (lower their heads), left bending, cervical extension and right bending. The patients take a deep breath and exhale slowly. The patients concentrate on the abdomen and rotate in anti-clockwise direction (6–8 times). At the end, the patients do massage of the neck. In exercise, the patients cannot move the body (Fig. 8.5). The training time is 15–20 min. There are 15 time in a therapy course (once a day).

(d) Cervical cyclovergence and neck down: the patients take a deep breath, concentrate on the abdomen, lift two shoulders slowly, put down neck, rotate two shoulders downward and backward, lift the shoulder again, extend neck, exhale slowly and go back to neutral position (6–8 times). the patients take a deep

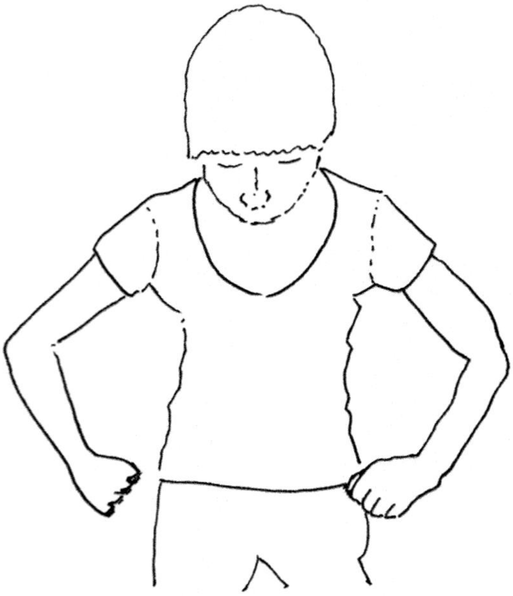

Fig. 8.6 Training of cervical cyclovergence and neck down

breath, concentrate on the abdomen, lift two shoulders slowly, put down neck, rotate two shoulders downward and backward, lift the shoulder again, extend neck, exhale slowly and go back to neutral position (6–8 times, Fig. 8.6). The training time is 15–20 min. There are 15 time in a therapy course (once a day).

(e) Bend forward and backward: when in inspiration, the neck should anteflect as much as possible to make the lower jaw be close to the edge of manubrium. In expiration, the head go back to neutral position. In the next expiration, the neck should protract backward as much as possible and in inspiration it goes back to beutral position with immobilization of waist and back (6–8 times). The training time is 15–20 min. There are 15 time in a therapy course (once a day).

(f) Do exercise of the neck in supine position: the patients are in supine position, remove the pillow, put the head on the center, face to the sky, put two hands beside the body and relax themselves. In inspiration, the head should anteflect and in expiration the head goes back. In inspiration again, the head protract backward and in expiration the head goes back. In the exercise, the movement should be done slowly and repeatedly. After that, the patients can do horizontal rotation. In inspiration, the head turn to the right and in expiration the head goes back to the center. In inspiration again, the head turn to the left and in expiration the head goes back to the center. The training time is 15–20 min. There are 15 time in a therapy course (once a day).

2. Self-training method of scapulohumeral periarthritis

Scapulohumeral periarthritis is chronic traumatic inflammatory inside and outside shoulder joint. It can aggravate or the disease phase prolongs if the therapy is not proper, even permanent dysfunction. Self-training after therapy has an effect on consolidation of therapeutic effect and preventing relapse.

(a) Katie·Chilly method: It is a therapeutic training method of shoulder joint developed for the therapists in England. It can be divided into primary, middle and advanced phase. The primary exercise is flexibility training of shoulder. The middle exercise is suppleness training. The advanced exercise is the training of intensity and stability. The patients can do one grade of exercise every time. If the patients don't complete the primary exercise, they cannot do the middle exercise.

From preventing soft tissue adhesion, auxiliary movement training of scapulohumeral periarthritis after therapy is suitable for primary exercise.

The movement of shoulder extension: the patients flex elbow, lift arm, extend forearm, anteflext shoulder joint, extort and intort shoulder joint.

Self-help movement of shoulder: this exercise can make upper limbs like pendulum. The shoulder swing naturally induced by their own weight in order to increase flexibility of shoulder gradually. Scapula control: the patients lean against the wall and the two feet keep away from the wall. The patients flex knee and the hip lean against the wall. Two upper arms relax and drop beside the body. The patients flex their elbows and two hands cross over before abdomen. The patients do abdominal curl and use scapula to push the wall. The patients insist and relax for many time. This method can increase strength of muscle around scapula. Shoulder extension: self-extension and self-flexion of shoulder.

Shoulder joint rotation: the patients flex elbow and the injured forearm is vertical to the ground. The patients put uninjured hands on the shoulder on the injured side. In order to feel the movement, the forearm rotate inside and outside.

Shoulder rotation: in sitting position, the patients sit upright. Two shoulders turn backward to form an arc. The patients stretch the muscle around scapula. When reach the maximum radian, the patients insist on for 10 s and relax for many times.

(b) Joint motion training of shoulder and chest: in sitting position, the patients draw in the chest slight, erect the back, flex elbow joints slightly, put upper limbs before abdomen. During exercise, accompanied with breathing, the patients look straight ahead, breathe to the pubic region, concentrate on medial margin of double scapula. The patients take a deep breath, lift two shoulders and make it be close to earlobe. The two shoulders intort forward slightly and stretch bilateral scapula for 6 s at the peak. The patients exhale slowly, lower shoulders and thrust the chest forward. The patients take a deep breath, lift shoulders and make it be close to earlobe. The shoulders extort backward slightly and squeeze the medial margin of bilateral scapula for 6 s at the peak. The patients exhale slowly, lower two shoulders and thrust the chest forward for 6–8 times (Fig. 8.7). The training time is 15–20 min. There are 15 time in a therapy course (once a day).

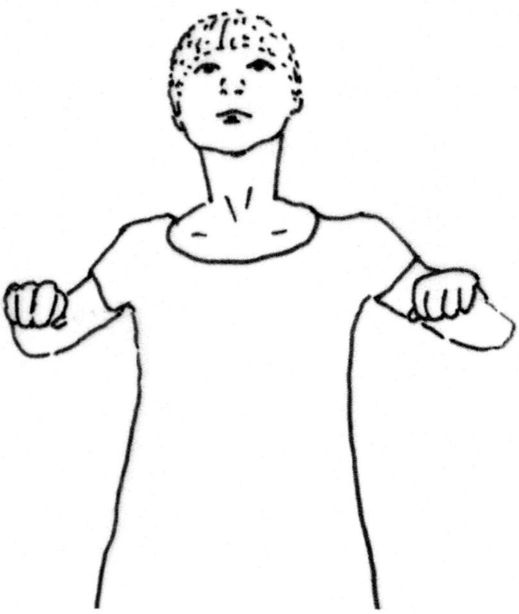

Fig. 8.7 Training of joint motion of shoulder and chest

(c) Range enlargement training of shoulder joint motion: With the help of offside upper limbs, the effect of this method can increase motion range of shoulder joint in the training side passively to lessen and prevent adhesion fully, enlarge the active motion range of joint, consolidate therapeutic effect in the early stage and prevent relapse.

Range enlargement training of standing on another's shoulders movement: in sitting position or standing position, the patients keep their heads up and thrust the chest forward. When the patients do joint motion of right shoulder, they use right hand to support the back of right elbow joint. When the patients do joint motion of left shoulder, they use left hand to support the back of right elbow joint. Upper limbs is at a 30–45° flexion position of elbow joint. The patients take a deep breath and lift upper limbs in the training side upward and inward. The patients use the hands of upper limbs in the training side to touch the offside shoulder until the shoulder joint in the training side reaches the maximum motion range. The patients fully relax upper limbs in the training side, use offside hand to support elbow joint, exert force inward and upward, stop when feeling the great resistance and hold on for 4–6 s at this point. The patients do support-relax and relax-support for three times and the intensity is increased gradually. After every trial, the patients exhale slowly, relax the whole body and prepare for the next time training. The same method is used for the training of offside shoulder joint (Fig. 8.8). The effect of this method is to fully stretch soft tissue of the back of shoulder, lessen joint capsule, ligament, tendon and muscular tissue of the back of shoulder to increase motion range of offside standing on another's shoulders.

Range enlargement training of upthrow movement: in sitting position or standing position, the patients keep their heads up and thrust the chest forward. When the patients do joint motion of right shoulder, they use left hand to grasp right wrist. When the patients do joint motion of left shoulder, they use right hand to grasp left wrist. The upper limb in the training side is at 120° elbow flexion position. The patients take a deep breath and lift upper limbs in the training side upward and inward beyond the head. The patients fully relax upper limbs in the training side, use offside hand, exert force inward and upward, stop when feeling the great resistance and hold on for 4–6 s at this point. The patients do support-relax and relax-support for three times and the intensity is increased gradually. After every trial, the patients exhale slowly, relax the whole body and prepare for the next time training. The same method is used for the training of offside shoulder joint (Fig. 8.9). The effect of this method is to fully stretch soft tissue of the inferoposterior part of shoulder, lessen joint capsule, ligament, tendon and

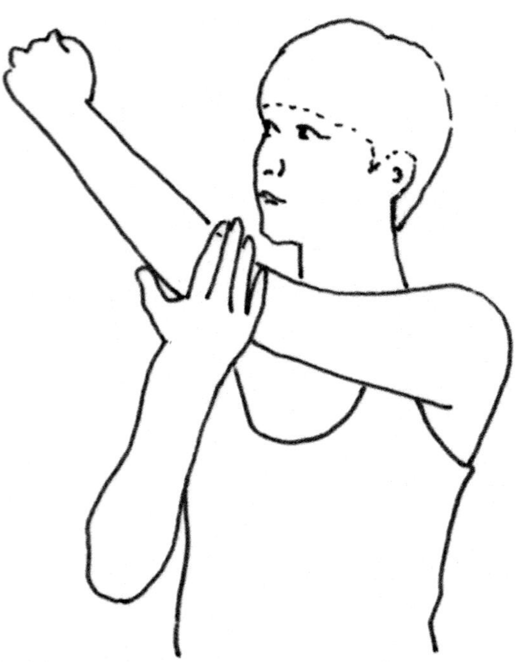

Fig. 8.8 Range enlargement training of stand on another's shoulders

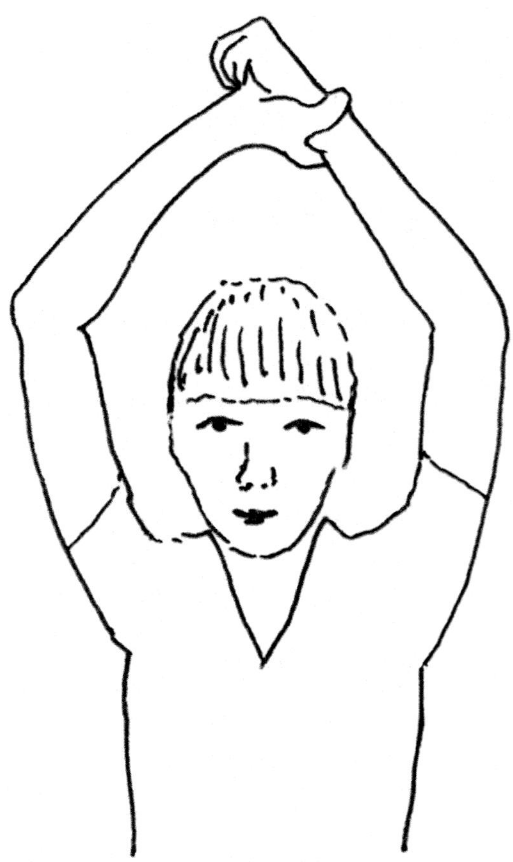

Fig. 8.9 Range enlargement training of upthrow movement

muscular tissue of the inferoposterior part of shoulder to increase motion range of lifting beyond the head of shoulder joint.

Range enlargement training of abduction movement: In sitting position or standing position, the patients keep their heads up and thrust the chest forward. When the patients do joint motion of right shoulder abduction, they use left palm to support the lower part of right elbow joint. When the patients do joint motion of left shoulder abduction, they use right palm to support the lower part of left elbow joint. The elbow joint is at a straight position. The patients take a deep breath and lift upper limbs in the training side upward and outward. The patients use offside hand to support elbow joint. The patients fully relax upper limbs in the training side, use offside hand to push upper limbs in the training side upward and outward, stop when feeling the great resistance and hold on for 4–6 s at this point. The patients do support-relax and relax-support for three times and the intensity is increased gradually. After every trial, the patients exhale slowly, relax the whole body and prepare for the next time training. The same method is used for the training of offside shoulder joint (Fig. 8.10). The effect of this method is to fully stretch soft tissue of the lower part of shoulder, lessen joint capsule, ligament, tendon and muscular tissue of the lower part of shoulder to increase motion range of shoulder joint abduction.

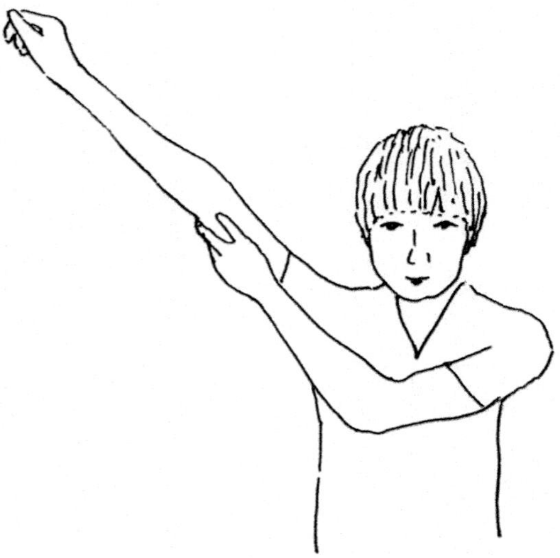

Fig. 8.10 Range enlargement training of abduction movement

Range enlargement training of front protraction movement: In sitting position or standing position, the patients keep their heads up and thrust the chest forward. When the patients do joint motion of right shoulder abduction, they use left palm to support the back of right elbow joint. When the patients do joint motion of left shoulder abduction, they use right palm to support the back of left elbow joint. The elbow joint is at a straight position or 90° flexion position. The patients take a deep breath and lift upper limbs in the training side upward and outward. The patients use offside hand to support elbow joint. The patients fully relax upper limbs in the training side, use offside hand to push upper limbs in the training side upward and outward, stop when feeling the great resistance and hold on for 4–6 s at this point. The patients do support-relax and relax-support for three times and the intensity is increased gradually. After every trial, the patients exhale slowly, relax the whole body and prepare for the next time training. The same method is used for the training of offside shoulder joint (Fig. 8.11). The effect of this method is to fully stretch soft tissue of the lower part of shoulder, lessen joint capsule, ligament, tendon and muscular tissue of the lower part of shoulder to increase motion range of shoulder joint extension.

Range enlargement training of standing on another's back movement: In sitting position or standing position, the patients keep their heads up and thrust the chest forward. When the patients do movement of standing on another's back of right shoulder joint, they use left hand to grasp wrist of right upper limb. When the patients do movement of standing on another's back of left shoulder joint, they use right hand to grasp wrist of left upper

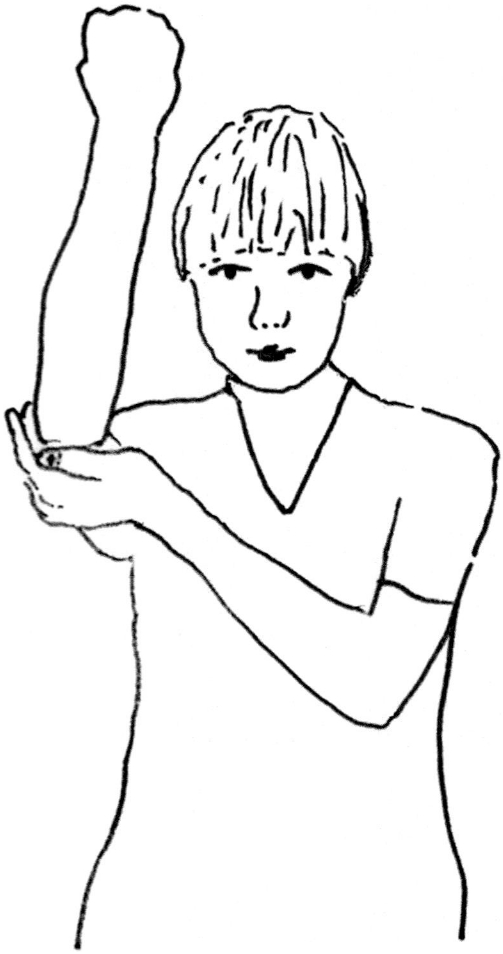

Fig. 8.11 Range enlargement training of shoulder front extension

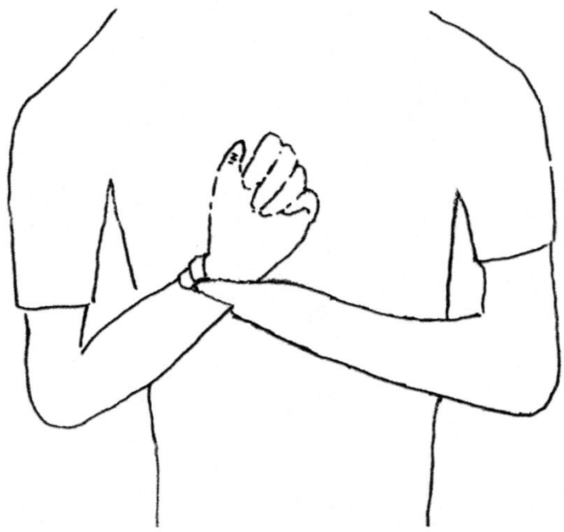

Fig. 8.12 Range enlargement training of stand on another's back

limb. The elbow joint is at a 45° flexion position of elbow joint. The patients take a deep breath and lift upper limbs in the training side backward, upward and inward. The patients use hand form the back to touch offside scapula until the shoulder joint in the training side reaches the maximum motion range. The patients fully relax upper limbs in the training side, grasp offside hand and pull upward, stop when feeling the great resistance and hold on for 4–6 s at this point. The patients do support-relax and relax-support for three times and the intensity is increased gradually. After every trial, the patients exhale slowly, relax the whole body and prepare for the next time training. The same method is used for the training of offside shoulder joint (Fig. 8.12). The effect of this method is to fully stretch soft tissue of the lower part of shoulder, lessen joint capsule, ligament, tendon and muscular tissue of the lower part of shoulder to increase motion range of offside standing on another's back of shoulder joint.

These methods can be used in turn for training. The training time is 15–20 min. There are 15 time in a therapy course (once a day).

(d) Self-anti-resistance training: The record of six-step Daoyin technique or self-regulation of mind and breath is used to do resistive joint motion with the help of elastic training band. Through anti-resistance training, it can increase local blood circulation, enhance myodynamia, further lessen and prevent adhesion in stronger muscle contraction and relaxation movement.

3. Self-training method of psoas: Pain in lower waist is usually seen in lumbar muscle strain, which accounts for the most part in chronic osphyalgia disease. The purpose of self-training of psoas is to further lessen and prevent soft tissue adhesion of waist, increase blood circulation of waist, promote metabolism, increase waist flexibility, which

are good for relieving the oppression of tissue in foramen intervertebrale, canalis spinalis and intraspinal on spinal cord or nerve root and relieve or prevent waist pain.

(a) Waist rotation exercise: In standing position, the space between two feet is as wide as the shoulder. Two hands cross over before the waist. The patients regulate breath, breathe to the pubic region and concentrate on lower waist. The patients protrude the abdomen slowly, rotate the waist in clockwise direction to the middle line of the trunk, bend waist to protrude the waist, rotate in clockwise direction to the middle line of right part of the trunk and protrude abdomen. After that, the patients exhale slowly and do the same training with the same method in anti-clockwise direction. A training includes two directions (Fig. 8.13). The training time is 15–20 min. There are 15 time in a therapy course (once a day).

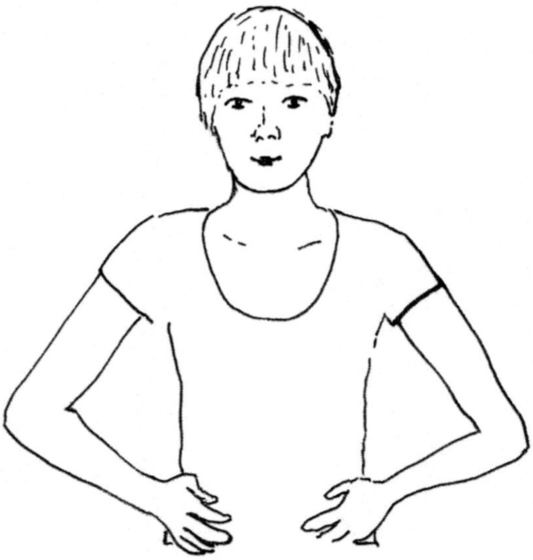

Fig. 8.13 Rotation training of waist

(b) The training of expanding chest and straightening waist: In standing position or sitting position, the patients regulate breath, breathe to the pubic region and concentrate on lower waist. The patients bend waist as much as possible, drop upper limbs naturally, expand chest and straighten waist slowly and hold on for 6 s at the peak (Fig. 8.14). The effect of expanding chest is to fully straighten waist in order to increase the intensity of psoas contraction. Deep bending waist is to fully stretch the tissue of waist and back. The training time is 15–20 min. There are 15 time in a therapy course (once a day).

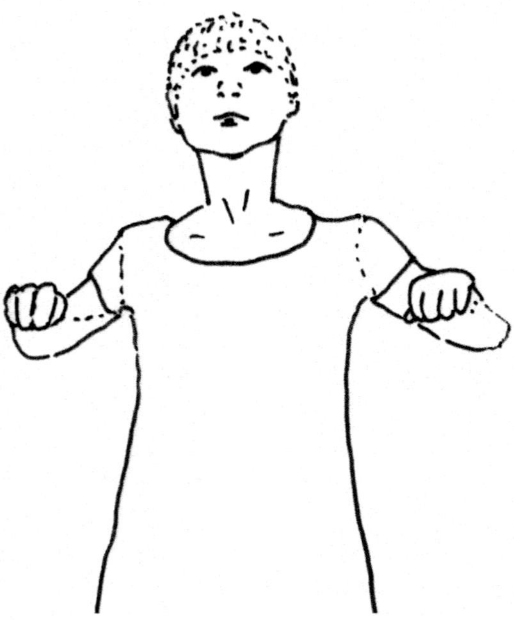

Fig. 8.14 The training of expanding chest and straightening waist

(c) The training of twisting hip and rotating waist: before this training, the patients should do warm-up exercise. In standing position, the space between two feet is as wide as the shoulder. The patients regulate breath, breathe to the pubic region and concentrate on lower waist. The left leg step forward and stand still. The right hip flex inside and forward. The upper part of the trunk and upper limbs rotate and swing to the right and backward. The right leg step forward and stand still. The right hip joint flex inside and forward. The upper part of the trunk and upper limbs rotate and swing to the left and backward (Fig. 8.15a, b). The training time is 15–20 min. There are 15 time in a therapy course (once a day).

(d) The training of bridging and swift flying: it is a combination of bridging and swift

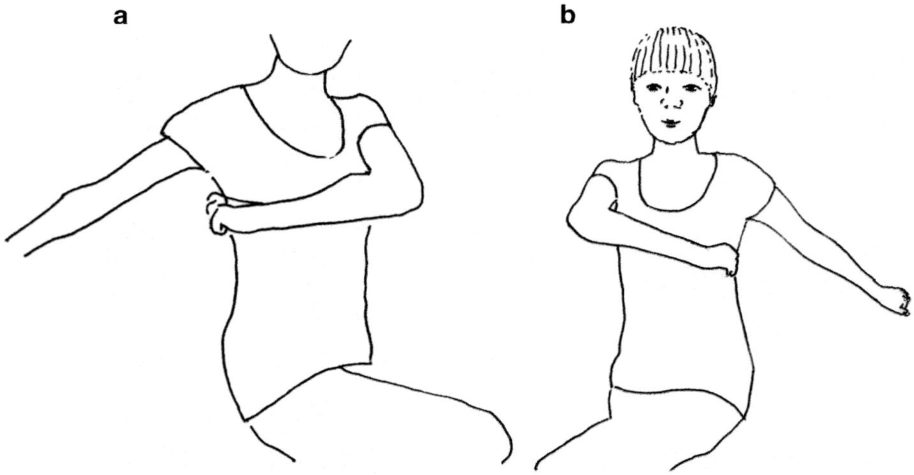

Fig. 8.15 (**a**) The training of twisting hip and rotate waist to the right. (**b**) The training of twisting hip and rotate waist to the left

flying. In the training of bridging, the patients lie on their back. In the training of swift flying, the patients are in ventral decubitus. The patients regulate breath, breathe to the pubic region and concentrate on lower waist. The patients use shoulder and two feet as the support point, protrude abdomen to support the trunk and waist, hold on for 6 s at the peak, relax and lie down on the bed. The patients inhale deeply and exhale slowly, and do the second training. The patients repeat the training for 6–8 times. In ventral decubitus, the patients regulate breath, breathe to the pubic region and concentrate on lower waist. The patients use abdomen as the support point, keep the front part of the trunk and upper limbs, the lower part of the trunk and lower limbs away from the bed like swallow walks on the water, upwarp upper limbs and lower limbs for 6 s, relax and lie down on the bed with abdomen. The patients inhale deeply and exhale slowly, and do the second training. The patients repeat the training for 6–8 times (Fig. 8.16). The training time is 15–20 min. There are 15 time in a therapy course (once a day).

8.2.6.3 Cautions in Self-Training

After the therapy of osteoarthritis, self-training or exercise can be instructed by rehabilitation doctor in hospital to master correct basic methods and key points of training. The training or exercise can be done according to movement prescription. There are some announcements in the training:

1. The training is mainly with active movement: During the therapy in hospital or at home after therapy, the patients should insist on active movement self-training or exercise for a long time.
2. Correct application of active movement training on the basis of regulation of mind and breath: The training is guided by Daoyin technique to exclude distracting thoughts and the patients can concentrate on training. The movements in the training should be easy and stable. After completion of every movement, the patients should go back to starting posture to obtain good therapeutic effect and prevent accident injury.
3. The difficulty of training or exercise should be increased step by step. The progress and effect cannot be chased one-sided in the training. The tempo should be from slow to quick. The

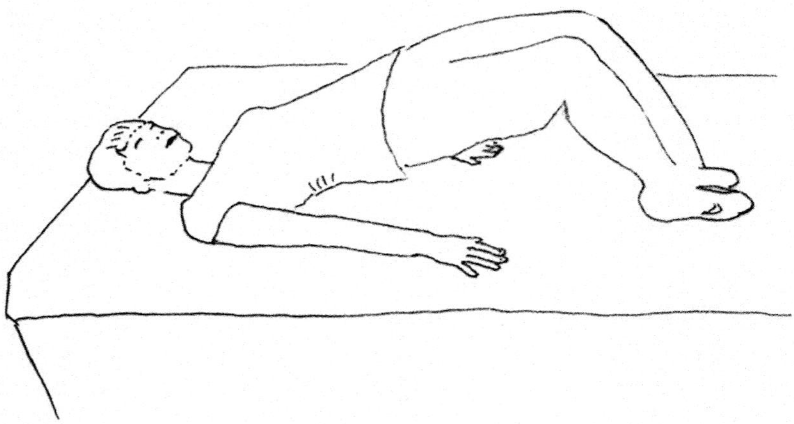

Fig. 8.16 Bridging training

amount of training and the range of joint motion should be from small to large in case of new injury.

4. Keep training record: under the premise of guaranteeing the amount and quality of training, the patients should do the training continuously and record the time, the amount, effect and problems of every training. Timely summarization and improvement are good for accumulation of experience.
5. Find the problems and rectify them timely: in the training or exercise, if there is any pain, dizziness or other discomfort, the patients should stop the training, seek the reason and adjust themselves. If the discomfort cannot be eliminated, the patients should go to hospital for therapy.
6. The patients should keep touch with the doctor and obtain training instructions. The patients should keep touch with the doctor during rehabilitation training in hospital and report their training conditions in order to obtain technique instructions. If necessary, the patients can go to rehabilitation department for help in order to adjust training or exercise schedule timely and obtain better effect.
7. The patients can control the training time by themselves. There are 15 times in one therapy course (once a day). After 2 days' rest, the patients do the next training. It can be treated as life cultivation and health preservation and the patients can keep on it.

8.2.6.4 Precautions of Joint and Muscle Injuries

Precaution is more important than treatment. Once there are bony joint, muscle injury and inflammation, there will be sequelae to a certain extent such as tissue adhesion, hyperostosis, low muscle strength or low local resistance. Even if the patients can be cured, it takes a long time. Therefore, in daily life, work and labor, the patients should protect bony joint and muscle in order to avoid injury and osteoarthritis.

1. Emphasize early treatment and try to cure the disease without future trouble: In the early phase of scapulohumeral periarthritis, lumbar sprain and osteoarthritis, the patients should go to standard hospital for therapy and try to cure it. The patients should take a rest until it is cured in case of chronic disease that creates great trouble for successive therapy.
2. Avoid cold-dampness and pay attention to changes in temperature: In daily life, the patients should increase and decrease clothing according to climate. The patients should clean the body after sweating and change clothes. The patients should avoid cold bath or air-conditioning cooling.
3. Emphasize labor hygiene: in the labor, especially heavy physical labour, the patients should pay attention to waist and joint. The patients should do exercise according to their abilities in case of overwork that can lead to damage of

organ and tissue. The patients should alternate work with rest in work or labor.

4. The patients should wear labor protection tools: if the condition is permissive, the patients should wear labor protection tool such as waist support, wide belt and glove.
5. Warm-up before exercise: in any labor or physical exercise, especially aggravating activities, the patients must do warm-up, preheat muscle, tissue and joint in case of injury.
6. Control body weight: Obesity gives too much pressure on waist and lower limbs joint and induce injury. Therefore, the patients should do exercise and control diet in case of obesity.
7. Rectify bad posture: Abnormal posture is the common reason to induce tissue injury. Therefore, in daily life, the patients should avoid keeping a posture for a long time such as long-term stoop or long-term bending over a table. If the time of maintaining a posture exceeds 20 min, there will be muscle tension. If the time is prolonged, there will be injury such as stiff neck. Stiff neck is because after excessive fatigue brain cannot perceive long-term traction of sternocleidomastoid and it can lead to injury of sternocleidomastoid at the end.
8. Strengthen physical exercises: Physical training can make muscle, ligament and joint capsule in healthy and well developed state. The patients with good myodynamia and elastic ligament are difficult to be injured.
9. Reinforce protection and avoid injuries: In daily life and labor, there are dangerous factors everywhere so that it is necessary to enhance protection consciousness. For example, when taking a bus, do not stand still or sit still in case of the injuries of centrum and joint due to accident turbulent jolt. The person should use hands to grasp the reel and the legs should be curled slightly to buffer impact force to bony joint. When walking, the person should look around in case of object falling from high altitudes and vehicle, etc.

In a word, pain, limitation of motion and adhesion in osteoarthritis should be considered at the same time in therapy. Interventional therapy of physical agent can alleviate pain, joint lessening can increase motion range and self-training or exercise can prevent relapse. Close combinative application of the three is the common effective method to treat scapulohumeral periarthritis, lumbago-leg pain and pain due to osteoarthritis and muscle injuries.

References

1. Yupu L, Xiaoting X, Baofeng G, et al. Practical bone science [M]. 1st ed. Beijing: People's Military Medical Press; 1995.
2. Hua Z. Orthopedic rehabilitation medicine. Shanghai: Shanghai Medical University Press; 1999.
3. Shifang Z, Fan Z. Practical rehabilitation medicine. 2nd ed. Nanjing: Southeast University Press; 1998.
4. The Medical Department of Ministry of Health of the People's Republic of China. The Medical Department of Ministry of Health of the People's Republic of China. First volume. Beijing: Huaxia Press; 1998. p. 1–2.
5. Aiguo Z, Yanchun W, Qun C, et al. In vivo near-infrared photodynamic therapy based on targeted upconversion nanoparticles. J Biomed Nanotechnol. 2015;11(11):2003–10.
6. Pantiushenko IV, Rudakovskaya PG, Starovoytova AV, et al. Development of bacteriochlorophy lla-based near-infrared photosensitizers conjugated to gold nanoparticles for photodynamic therapy of cancer. Biochemistry (Mosc). 2015;80(6):752–62.
7. Dongmei L, Shuang L, Xiuhua F, et al. Study and fabrication of broad band-pass filters in infrared therapy apparatus. Acta Photon Sin. 2015;44(3):331001–6.

9 The Application of Rehabilitation Medical Engineering in Neurological Training

On the basis of modern engineering technique, according to the principle of compensation and adaption, rehabilitation medical engineering is a subject that can design and produce assistive devices to help the disabled to improve their independent life ability.

Orthotics is an important content in rehabilitation medicine, which belongs to rehabilitation medical engineering. The purpose of orthotics is to prevent and rectify the deformity of the trunk and joint, protect lesion tissue, prevent limbs disuse, improve or compensate the lost functions [1], which is essential for clinical rehabilitation medicine and is widely used in clinic.

There are many types of orthotics. According to material type, it is divided into plastic orthotics, metal orthotics, metal framework orthotics and so on. According to therapeutic goal, it includes orthotics for medicine, temporary orthotics for medicine and orthotics for rehabilitation. The manufacture of artificial limbs and walking assistive devices are complicated, which require special equipment and technique and are hard to be developed in normal hospital. Therefore, we don't discuss it in this book.

In rehabilitation therapy of neurological training, in order to obtain better effect, except traditional orthotics, independent research and development orthotics material and orthotics are classified according to the prevention, rectification and function of orthotics. We discuss them separately.

9.1 The Research and Development of Preventive Orthotics

9.1.1 Semi-Finished Product Macromolecule Orthotics Material

Orthotics for medicine is external fixation support equipment that can relieve dysfunctions of bone and muscle of injured limbs through restricting and assisting body movement or changing body force line [2].

From the wearing comfort and functional reliability, the characteristics of ideal orthotics material are as follows:

- It is easy to process, mold and manufacture. Air permeability is good. It is sturdy and durable.
- It is in light weight and it is non-poisonous, tasteless and hurtles.
- It is radiolucent and it cannot affect the X ray examination quality when wearing orthotics.
- It is easy to use and comfortable to wear.

At present, orthotics materials widely used at home and abroad include high temperature thermoplastic plastic plate, resin matrix composite and low temperature thermoplastic material.

1. High temperature thermoplastic plastic plate:
   The characteristics of it is that it can go soft

W. Zhao, *Rehabilitation Therapeutics of the Neurological Training*,
https://doi.org/10.1007/978-981-13-0812-3_9

under high temperature (180 °C). Not only the processing requires special equipment, but also the working procedure is complicated. Generally, the working procedures include negative plaster model, positive plaster model, model patching, plate clipping, heating, moulding, cooling, patching, fitting, re-patching, pasting body limbs sponge, drilling sweat pore, fastening fixing band, polishing and truing. Technical requirements to orthotics master are high. In the non-rehabilitation hospitals such as normal hospital, county hospitals, community and country health-center, it is hard to carry out the work and influence the application range.

2. Resin matrix composite: it is fiber reinforced material on the basis of organic polymer, which includes glass fibre, carbon fibre or aramid fiber. They are widely used in aviation, automobile, marine industry and medical science. Reinforced polymer composites include epoxy resin and unsaturated polyester resin. The common used resins include thermosetting resin, thermoplastic resin and various kinds of modified or alloying matrix. Thermoplastic resin can dissolve in the solvent. It can soften and fuse into viscous liquid when heated and also harden after cooling. Thermosetting resin can be heated and be molded once. It can solidify in the processing and become networking macromolecule chemical compound that is non-melt and insoluble. Therefore, it cannot be regenerated.
3. Low temperature thermoplastic material: The characteristics of it is that it can soften in the hot water (60–80 °C). It can be molded in the body limbs. After solidification, the strength of this material is limited so that the application is confined. Moreover, in the limbs with severe deformity (hand palmatum in the hemiplegic patients), it is difficult to be molded directly. It is easy to attend to one thing and lose another and it is difficult to produce the ideal orthotics that meets the requirements. It is easy to influence the quality and dressing effect and may waste the materials.

In addition, the basic material of high and low temperature thermoplastic material are plastic. The material can increase the weight of the orthotics, but is not with air permeability. It requires drilling a pore to increase air permeability. The number of the pores is small, which cannot reach the requirements of air ventilation. The number of the pores is big, which can affect the strength of the orthotics.

Because the processing of orthotics is complicated at present, many hospitals cannot develop it due to the limitation. It only can be processed in the orthotics manufacture factory in big city and rehabilitation medical engineering department or orthotics production room of several hospital so that many patients cannot wear orthotics timely because this is no opportunity. It can induce deformity of joint and abnormal motor pattern, and then affect the recovery of body limbs function.

Therefore, it is easy to be studied and developed. The tenacity is good and the intensity is strong. Air permeability is good and is not radio parent. Through slight modification, semi-finished product macromolecule glass fiber orthopedic material can be used for different levels hospitals in basic level and city, which has important clinical significance. We introduce several types of new orthotics materials and orthotics invented by the author and applied in clinic.

1. Making and processing: macromolecule glass fiber is adopted. According to the shape of different part and functional requirements, the materials are prefabricated to material plates with different size and thickness. After dip in solidification liquid, the materials are sealed and enveloped. We select PEISS 020 antiseize non-woven fabrics (the thickness is 0.12 mm) and cut it into pieces that is bigger than macromolecule glass fiber plates. We use normal saline to soak it and seal the envelope. Dry non-woven fabrics with same size are enveloped. Six fixing bands, several rivets and lining cloth inside and outside are separately enveloped. All the goods mentioned above are sealed package with external packing (Fig. 9.1).

   Semi-finished product medical macromolecule glass fiber material is as soft as mud in the airtight state, which cannot turn bad in 2 years. After sealing off, water in room tem-

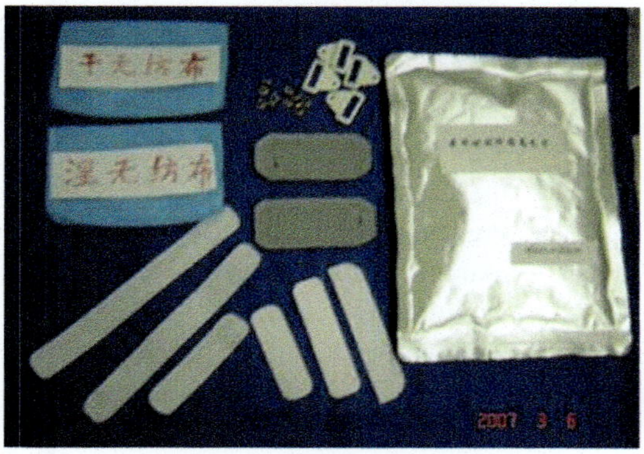

Fig. 9.1 Constitutional diagram of semi-finished product macromolecule fabric orthotics material

perature is used to soak it for 6 s and it can be molded at will. Six minutes after that, it can be solidified. After molding, the strength is high and the tenacity is good. Three layers can be used for upper limbs and six layers can be used as back dry frame material. After molding, it is showed as micro grid with good air permeability and without artificial punching. It is absorbent and moisture resistance. It can be washed for many times without metamorphosis or molding. It is light, non-poisonous, tasteless and easy to dress, which cannot affect X-ray examination.

2. Method of application: According to the body part of orthotics and somatotype of the patients, suitable sized semi-finished product macromolecule glass fiber orthotics material bag is selected. The therapists prepare for it such as half basin water in room temperature and temporary binder. In a warm room, the patients expose their body part for orthotics and open the external packing of semi-finished product macromolecule glass fiber orthotics material bag. Dry non-woven fabrics soak into warm water, are squeezed out excessive liquid and put on the limbs skin surface. At this time, the assistant should keep the limbs in functional position, open external packing of macromolecule glass fiber material plates, fold macromolecule glass fiber and dip them into water for 6 s. The assistant should press them on the plate as soon as possible until there is no bubble between layers, stretch it to the flat, put it on the wet non-woven fabrics of the body limbs, press them slightly until they fit with each other perfectly, put dry non-woven fabrics on it, use temporary binder to bind them up around for 6 min. After that, the assistant check the border of macromolecule glass fiber material and get them down if they are solidified and molded. At this time, because macromolecule glass fiber material is still not solidified, the assistant can use hands to mold specific unideal part and wash it with water to promote solidification process. After complete solidification, scissors or electric saw are used to cut off marginal excessive materials. Three hours later, grinding wheel or abrasive paper is used to polish the margin until it is smooth. The assistants use fine grit sandpaper for sanding or use polisher for polishing. Spare rivets are used to fix the fixing band and then the orthosis can be tried on. If there is no modification, the patients can try it on directly or put neck bush and dress it when the two sides are connected. Neck push can be removed periodically for washing or change. If the deformity of the patients is severe, negative plaster model can be done first and then can be made to positive plaster model. After molding modification, it can be made through the method of macromolecule glass fiber material molding.
3. Types and models of semi-finished product macromolecule glass fiber orthotics materials: According to body limbs part and function, semi-finished product macromolecule glass fiber orthotics materials are divided into orthotics material of the trunk, functional position orthotics material of wrist-hand, functional position orthotics material of elbow-wrist-hand, functional position orthotics material of knee joint, functional position orthotics material of foot-ankle, overhang support material of upper limbs and cervical gear material. Every kind can be divided into three types such as adult type, children type and special type. Every type includes three sizes such as big, middle and small size.
4. Clinical application: From April 2006 to April 2007, semi-finished product macromolecule

glass fiber orthotics are used to make orthotics in 115 patients who are all at hospital or out patients in Beijing Tongren Hospital affiliated to Capital Medical University. There are 69 cases of functional position orthotics of wrist-hand, 33 cases of functional position orthotics of foot-ankle, ten cases of orthotics of trunk and three cases of cervical orthotics. They are all one-stage molding and the rate of finished products is 100%. It is in light weight, non-poisonous, tasteless and is with good air permeability. It is strong but pliable in texture and it cannot affect the X ray examination quality when wearing orthotics. Semi-finished product material is used to make orthotics. The manufacturing operation is simplified obviously and the rate of finished products is increased. Manufacturing time is shortened to 4 h from 3 days, which alleviate labor intensity and simplify manufacturing process.

5. Functions and indications: Except individual joint, the effects and indications are the same as these of orthotics made from high temperature thermoplastic plate materials.
   (a) Functions: Except for foot-ankle orthotics, effects of macromolecule glass fiber orthotics are the same as that of orthotics made from high and low temperature thermoplastic plates.
      - Prevention and rectification of joint deformity and prevention of tendon, muscle spasm and the formation of abnormal motor pattern
      - Fixing function
      - Movement or walking assistance function to help the patients move body limbs
      - Protection function
      - Load-bearing and supporting functions
   (b) Indications: This material is suitable for preventing abnormal position of joint and trunk with orthopedic functions.
      - It is necessary to restrict abnormal movements of joint and limbs in order to stabilize joint, alleviate pain or recover the function of load-bearing such as manufacture of knee-ankle-foot orthotics used for poliomyelitis.
      - It is necessary to fix and protect injured limbs or joints in order to promote manufacture of orthotics for healing such as various kinds of orthotics for the therapy of bone fracture.
      - Prevention of limbs deformity such as manufacture of orthotics used for congenital talipes equinovarus, gonyectyposis and genu valgum.
      - It is necessary to alleviate load-bearing of long axis of limbs or the trunk such as load-bearing of ischium of orthotics for aseptic necrosis of head of femur.
      - It is necessary to control abnormal movements of joint to decrease muscle spasm during standing and walking such as ankle-foot orthotics used for the patients with cerebral palsy to alleviate spasmodic talipes equinovarus during walking and improve walking function of ankle-foot.
      - It is necessary to improve the patients' daily life movements and working ability such as wrist-hand orthotics to improve defects of holding functions of hand.
6. Cautions
   (a) When use water to steep it, the therapists should immerse macromolecule material into water and stir it slightly until soaking degree is even because materials with different hardenability can affect the quality of orthotics.
   (b) After the material is totally solidified, the therapists cut it and polish it in case of low strength due to interlaminar separation.
   (c) After orthotics molding, sandpaper is used to polish inside and outside of orthotics in case that it abrades clothes.

Semi-finished product macromolecule glass fiber orthotics material is easy to use and can simplify the manufacturing process of orthotics. It can meet requirements of high quality without special and can be used in orthotics factory of big city and orthotics department of big hospital or small and medium hospitals and basic health organizations.

Cooperated with former of orthopedic brace made from macromolecule materials, it is easy and comfortable to make orthotics from macromolecule glass fiber orthotics materials, especially for severe deformity such as chicken feet. However, macromolecule glass fiber material molding is used for foot-ankle orthotics for walking. The heel part of orthotics should be flapped repeatedly in order to make the solidification liquid to fill in mesh of the materials to increase the strength of this part after solidification in case that there is no effect due to inadequate strength. Semi-finished product macromolecule glass fiber orthotics materials are used to make ankle-foot functional position orthotics and wrist-hand functional position orthotics (Fig. 9.2).

9.1.2 Former of Orthopedic Brace

At present, at home and abroad, the manufacturing processing of orthotics is complicated, which is associated with poor suitability and material loss because it is impossible to be molded in the body or molded directly. It affects the quality of orthotics and their wide clinical application. Therefore, development of processing technic and methods that can mold the materials directly or in human body can simplify the manufacturing processing of orthotics, decrease orthotics material loss and increase suitability of orthotics, which can make orthotics be widely applied in city and primary hospital.

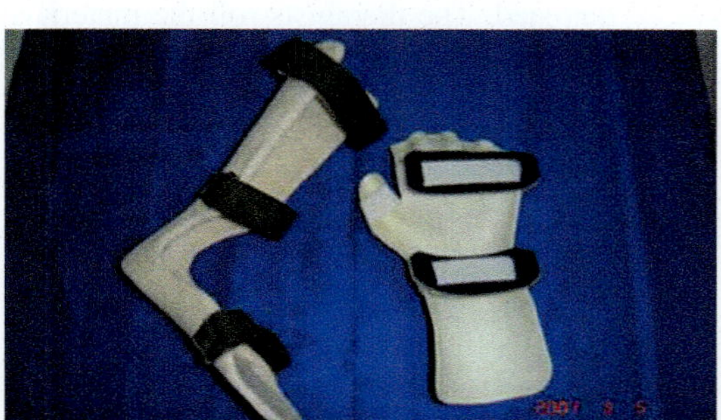

Fig. 9.2 Ankle-foot functional position orthotics and wrist-hand functional position orthotics made from macromolecule materials

On the basis of developing semi-finished product macromolecule glass fiber orthotics materials, in order to cooperate with clinical application of this material, according to the mooncake mould and different shape of different body parts, the author developed a series of former of orthopedic brace. After actual clinical application, the effect is satisfying.

1. Material: Macromolecule glass fiber material or other material is used and the thickness is six layers. The material in sealed package is as soft as mud. After unsealing, the therapists steep it into cold water for 6 s and solidify it for 6 min. After solidification, it is with good air permeability and radio transparent. The tenacity and strength are good. It can resist to moisture. It can be used for a long time without metamorphism and deformation.
2. The structure and function of former: Except for shape, side and size, the other structures of it are the same. We use wrist-hand functional position brace former as an example to introduce basic structure and functions.

   Wrist-hand functional position brace former is composed of main body, fixing band and sponge slice (Figs. 9.3 and 9.4).

   (a) Main body: Forearm end is an arc groove that is adaptable to human forearm. It is the forearm part of molded orthotics brace. Wrist part is a groove that is adaptable to the shape of wrist and palm. It is the wrist part of molded orthotics. The finger end is a groove that separates index finger, middle finger, ring finger and little finger and bends laterally to palm. It is the

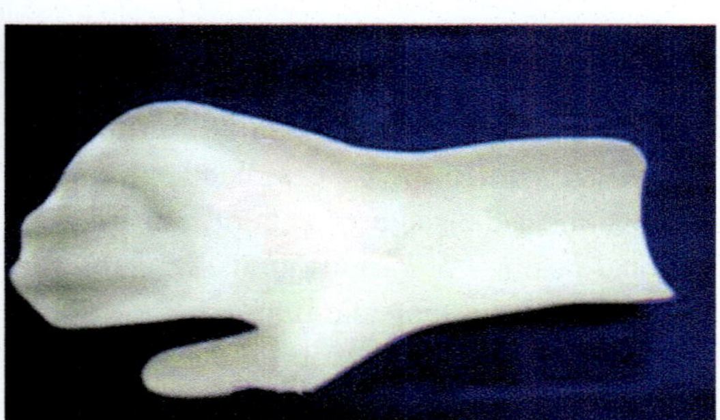

Fig. 9.3 Former of orthopedic brace

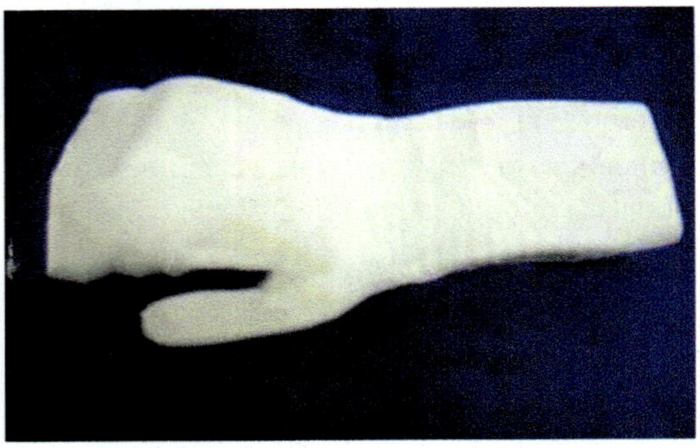

Fig. 9.4 Fixing band of former of orthopedic brace

part from index finger to little finger of molded orthotics. The thumb end is thumb part of molded orthotics. The comprehensive effect can make the wrist joint be in 30° dorsiflexion position. The functional position is that five fingers bend to palm and it is in a teacup state.

(b) Fixing band: It is made from elastic band with different width, which includes fixing band of forearm, fixing band of wrist-hand and fixing band of thumb. The son button nylon thread gluing at two ends can be compressed and fixed on the mother thread of nylon thread gluing on the lateral wall of former. Its role is to compress materials in the condition of unmanned compression and fixation in order to mold it inside the former according to limb shape.

(c) Sponge slice is soft sponge slice with thin layer. Its role is to increase adaptation of former. If the therapists don't find former with proper type, they can use sponge slice of one layer or two layers to fill in order to make the orthotics adapt to the outline of limbs.

3. Manufacture method of former of orthopedic brace: In order to make molded orthopedic brace meet the requirements of human functional position of various joints. Manufacture of former of orthopedic brace should choose normal people in different age and different posture as the model. Functional position of every bilateral joint is chosen for negative plaster model. According to negative plaster model, positive plaster model is duplicated. After that, on the basis of positive plaster model, former of orthopedic brace is made according to following technological process (Fig. 9.5). Orthotics should be made uniquely for the patients with special body type.
4. The kinds and types of former of orthopedic brace: According to the body parts, former of orthopedic brace is classified, which includes wrist-hand former of orthopedic brace in functional position, elbow joint former of orthopedic brace in functional position, neck former of orthopedic brace, the trunk former of orthopedic brace, knee joint former of orthopedic brace and foot-ankle former of orthopedic brace. Except for the trunk and cervical vertebra, every kind is divided into two types and every type is divided into two models. There are six different sizes in each model and 12 models in two sides. Together with six thin layer sponge slices, they are stored in special tool box for orthotics manufacture center or studio.
5. Clinical application of former of orthopedic brace: According to processing norm, former of orthopedic brace is used to process and mold orthotics.
   (a) Model selection: According to body part that requires orthotics, side and size, former with proper model is selected.
   (b) Processing and molding: The procedures are as follows: Macromolecule glass fiber orthotics materials are soaked into cold water for 6 s, taken out, squeezed out excessive water, pressed on the plate and flattened. The therapists roll the materials out in the former and spread a layer of drenched non-woven fabrics on it. The therapists put limb part into the mould, press it slightly until the body part perfectly matches the former. The therapists stretch the fixing band of the former tightly and fix it on the outside of the other end of the former around the body. Tensile force of fixing band should be equal to avoid impression after the molding of former. The impression can affect the beauty or can induce pression phenomenon after

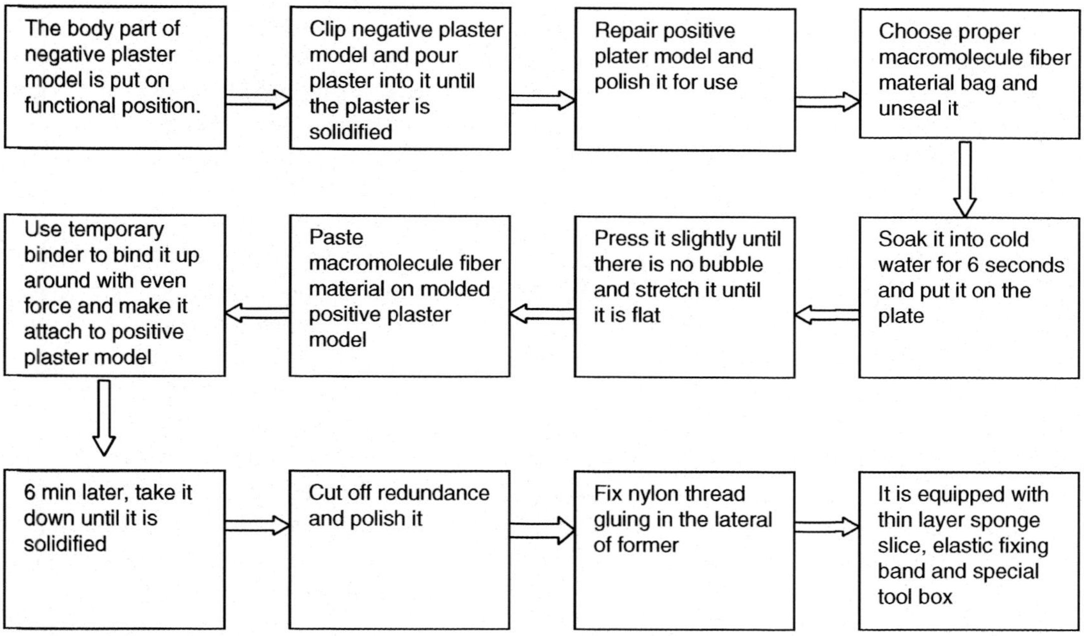

Fig. 9.5 Flow chart of former of orthopedic brace

dressing it. The materials are fixed for 6 min until macromolecule glass fiber material is solidified. After that, the therapists loose fixing band and take it from the former carefully. Water washing can accelerate the solidification process of macromolecule glass fiber material. The therapists clip excessive materials on the margin of orthotics brace, use fine sandpaper to polish it, add lining, fix the fixing band and then use it for the patients.

The therapists can wash the former, dry it in the air and put it into tool box for standby application.

(c) Clinical application: from April 2006 to February 2007, there are 54 patients who use orthotics made from former of orthopedic brac. They are all the inpatients of rehabilitation. There are 23 cases of wrist-hand orthotics in functional position, 20 cases of orthotics in functional position orthotics, eight cases of the trunk orthotics and three cases of cervical orthotics. They are all one-stage molding, but there are three patients who use wrist-hand orthotics in functional position and feel pressed in the inside of thumb. The feeling can be relieved after stiff paper sponge is pasted on the inside of thumb. In one case of foot-ankle orthotics in functional position, after dressing it for several days, materials problems lead to layering and low strength in the lateral of ankle. In two cases of the trunk orthotics, after dressing it, the patients feel pressed in iliac crest and can be relieved through clipping. If there is no material loss, the rate of finished products is 100%. Plaster model is unnecessary in the process that former is used to make orthotics, which can simplify manufacturing operation and decrease manufacturing cost. The manufacturing time is shortened to 4 h from 3 days, which decrease labor intensity of the staff obviously. Because the solidness, tenacity and air permeability of materials are good, these characteristics increase the quality of orthotics and dressing comfort obviously. The method doesn't need many equipment so that it can be used in village, community health center, big hospital in city, and special orthotics manufacture factory.

6. The advantages of former of orthopedic brace: although macromolecule glass fiber material is as soft as mud in airtight condition, the materials can be molded at will and solidified in 6 min after unsealing. However, soft materials don't mean that they are easy to be made to qualified orthotics brace. In the process of manufacturing wrist-hand orthotics in functional position for the hemiplegic patients with severe deformity (chicken feet), severe spasm of flexor carpi and all digital flexor tendon make it difficult for the molding of the materials on the limbs. If the wrist is fixed, the finger cannot meet the requirement and if the thumb is in functional position, the other four fingers cannot meet the requirements. Molded orthotics with too strong press are easy to sunk inside and are difficulty to be made to satisfying orthotics, which may lead to material loss. The idea of former of orthopedic brace is enlightened from mooncake mould and auto wrench tool box. Through repeated trial-manufacture and modifications, a series of molded former of orthopedic brace are developed according to different parts of limbs. Orthotics made from macromolecule materials reduce the difficulty of orthotics, shorten manufacture time, increase comfort of dressing brace. Which provides advantages for the increase of quality of orthotics and wide application.

9.1.3 Retainer of Joint in Functional Position

In clinic, unmovable limbs due to coma, hemiplegia after central nerve injury, paraplegia after spinal cord injury, injury of bone, joint and muscle and extremely weakness, not only lose autokinetic movement ability, but also lead to abnormal joint positions because the paralyzed muscle is lack of tension such as foot drop, strephenopodia, hypertension of knee joint, elbow and wrist joint flexion. Therefore, it can induce abnormal motor pattern of limbs. Limbs are at the poor joint function position for a little long time, which can lead to extension of muscle, tendon, ligament and joint capsule in paralyzed side. Limbs are shortened at the muscle spasm state, which can make the muscle be in an improper initial length state and can induce adhesion of muscle, ligament and joint capsule and tendon contracture. In severe cases, there is joint deformity, which can affect motor function of joint and limbs.

The research demonstrated that if shoulder joint of normal person is fixed for 1 day, it may take 7 days to loose adhesion induced by immobility of muscle and soft tissue. If the joint is fixed for 3 weeks, it may take 300 days to loose adhesion. If the fixing time is longer, it can lead to joint congelation, joint rigidity, even irreversible disability such as fibrous ankyloses or bony ankyloses due to loose difficulty. Once the deformity is formed, through therapy, neural function can be recovered, but motor function of limbs is hard to be recovered because of joint deformity. Therefore, the patients' daily life ability is affected. In order to prevent this situation, it is necessary to put limbs in good position and do joint movements in clinic.

Good limb position is different from functional position. Good limb position is temporary body position from therapeutic angle. For example, after reduction of humerus surgical neck fracture, shoulder joint is necessary to be fixed at 45° abduction position temporarily for the healing of bone fracture. However, if there are joint spasm, adhesion or rigidity, they can affect greatly motor function of shoulder joint.

Functional position is the angle and position at which the limbs and joints can play roles. In this angle and position, even if there is joint spasm or rigidity, the functions of limbs can be developed. For example, the functional position of ankle joint is at 90° position, which means that the planta pedis is parallel to the ground. If the ankle joint is fixed in this position, the patients can walk.

Regardless of functional position or good limb position, the purpose of them is to maintain the limbs and joints at the position that is good for complications prevention and functional recovery in the future. The bad position that leads to complications and affects joint functions is easy to increase muscle spasm. After joint adhesion in this position, the joints cannot exert functions. Therefore, the purpose of limbs in functional position is to prevent joint adhesion not in functional position, prevent loss of suitable initial length required for joint motion because of passive stretching of paralyzed muscle, ligament, tendon and joint capsule and avoid increasing muscle spasm (antispasmodic position).

From the goals mentioned above, in clinic, the place of functional position of limbs should inhibit spasm pattern and be in accordance with the principle of functional position. Meanwhile, the therapists should realize that place of functional position is not equal to prevention of tissue adhesion. Joint adhesion in functional position can affect joint functions in a certain extent. There should not be complications. Therefore, during the process of placing limbs in functional position, the patients should do rehabilitation therapy in early phase such as active and passive joint motion, which can promote blood circulation, prevent muscle spasm and adhesion of joint and soft tissue, provide basis for motor function recovery of limbs.

9.1.3.1 Common Place Method of Good Limb Position

At present, in clinic, the medical staff don't emphasize on good limb position and functional position of limbs. Some simple supplies such as soft cushion, pillow, quilt and position retaining appliance of individual joint can keep the joint in good limb position. These supplies not only cannot prevent joint deformity, but also should be rearranged to keep good limb position due to the body position change because the patients in bed should frequently turn over (at least once in every 2 h). It is tedious and the effect is not reliable.

At present, in clinic, the place method of good limb position is summarized as follows:

1. Place of good limb position with the help of underbed means pillow, cotton cushion, quilt and sandbag are used to keep the joint and limbs in a position where the limbs can exert function and the complications can be prevented.
   (a) Supine position: The head is put on the pillow to the uninjured side and the face is to injured side. The altitude of the pillow is proper without flexion of thoracic vertebra. Hip in the injured side is cushioned with a pillow to put forward the pelvis in order to prevent over flexion and extorsion of joint. Shoulder joint in injured side is cushioned with a small pillow to put forward the scapula. Elbow joint of upper limbs is extended and is put on the pillow. Wrist joint is dorsiflexed and finger is extended. Two sandbags are separately put on the lateral of thigh and the middle of shank to prevent abduction and extorsion of hip joint. Popliteal space is cushioned with a small pillow to prevent hyperextension of knee joint.
   (b) Lying position on uninjured side is the lateral position on the injured side. The specific method is that upper limb in injured side stretch out forward, shoulder joint flex 90°, pillow is used to support the joint and upper limb in uninjured side can be put at will. Hip and knee joints flex and are put on the pillow. Hip joint in uninjured side is extended and knee joint is slightly flexed. There is a pillow on the back to make the trunk in a relaxed state.
   (c) Lying position on injured side is the lying position method above the injured side. The specific method is that shoulder girdle in injured side stretch out forward, shoulder joint flexes, elbow joint extends, wrist joint dorsiflex and the finger is like grasping a teacup. Lower limb in injured side extends and knee joint slightly flexes. Hip and knee joints flex and a pillow is below them to prevent oppressing the lower limb in injured side. There is a pillow on the back to be lied with the trunk in order to relax the body.
2. The place of good limb position with the help of appliance is used for keeping the body in good limb position to prevent complications and make the body to exert functions.
   (a) Ankle-foot orthotics brace can strictly immobilize ankle joint to prevent foot drop and talipes varus and valgus. It is easy to dress and cannot be affected by turning over.

(b) T-Shaped board shoes: in the heel of the foot, 20 cm plank is nailed into the shoes, which is vertical to the long axis of the shoes and T-shaped. The patients in supine position wear shoes to prevent foot drop and internal and external rotation of lower limbs.
(c) Mattress and tail board are used to prevent foot drop. The patients lie on their back in the bed. There is a 15 cm space between mattress and tail board. The patients put heel into this space and make pelma close to baseboard to make foot in a 90° dorsiflexion position. It can prevent pressure sores due to oppression of heel and prevent foot drop.

9.1.3.2 Retainer of Limbs Joints in Functional Position

Macromolecule glass fiber orthotics materials with air permeability and radio transparent are developed to a series of retaining appliances of limbs joints in functional position according to different sides, shape, part and age, which are suitable for the coma patients and the maintenance of joint functional position of paralytic limbs. Once in hospital, the patients wear it from the early phase to prevent muscle spasm and joint deformity [3] of paralytic limbs effectively.

1. Machine shaping: Macromolecule glass fiber material is used to make the orthotics according to the requirements of normal functional position of all joints. Normal orthotics materials can also be selected.

   According to normal person in different age and posture and the shape of limbs joints, positive plaster model is prefabricated. Macromolecule glass fiber orthotics materials with 3–6 layers are used. Before solidification, it is as soft as mud. It is sealed. After unsealing, the materials are soaked in water at room temperature for 6 s and be solidified for 6 min. After solidification, the materials are not only with good air permeability and radio transparent, but also with good tenacity and solidness, strong waterproof and anti-dampness ability. It can be used for a long time without metamorphism and deformation.

   The structures of retaining appliances of all joints in functional position are the same, which include the main body, fixing band and sponge slice.
   (a) The main body is arc groove and is adaptable to human joint. Its role is to keep the joint in functional position.
   (b) Sponge slice: The role of soft sponge slice with thin layer is to increase adaptability of retaining appliance of joint in functional position. If there is no proper retaining appliance of joint in functional position and the existing retaining appliance is too big, sponge slice with one layer or multiple layers can be used for filling. It can better adapt to the outline of the body and play a fixed effect.
   (c) Fixing band is made from elastic band with different width. Its role is to fix retaining appliance of joint in functional position on limbs.

   Retaining appliance is easy to dress, light, fragrant, non-toxic, air permeable, radio transparent. It is convenient for the patients to do X-ray examination in bedside. Except for retaining appliance of shoulder abduction and hip abduction in functional position, the others are not affected by the body position change of the patients. All the joints can be maintained in functional position to prevent joint deformity effectively, which provides advantages for functional recovery in the future.
2. The types of retainers of limbs joint in functional position
   (a) According to body parts, it is divided into retaining appliance of shoulder joint, elbow joint, wrist-hand joint, hip joint, knee joint and ankle joint in functional position.
   (b) According to the size, it is divided into the adult type, the children type and special type.
   (c) According to the body side, it is divided into upper limb, the trunk and lower limb or right side and left side.

   The adult type retaining appliance of the joint in functional position refer to Fig. 9.6, 9.7, 9.8, 9.9, 9.10, and 9.11.

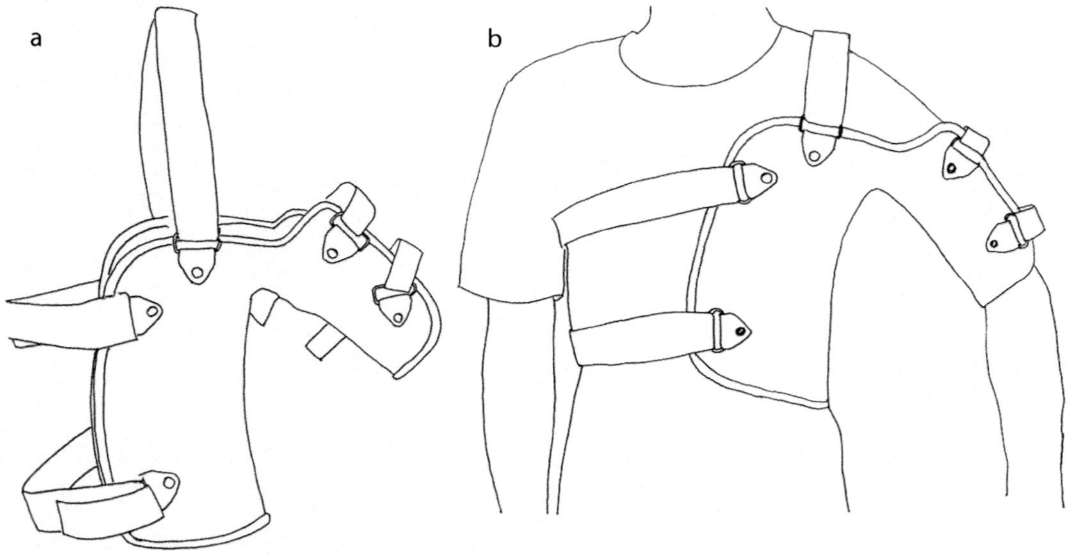

Fig. 9.6 (**a**) Brace of shoulder joint abduction in functional position. (**b**) Dressed brace of shoulder joint abduction in functional position

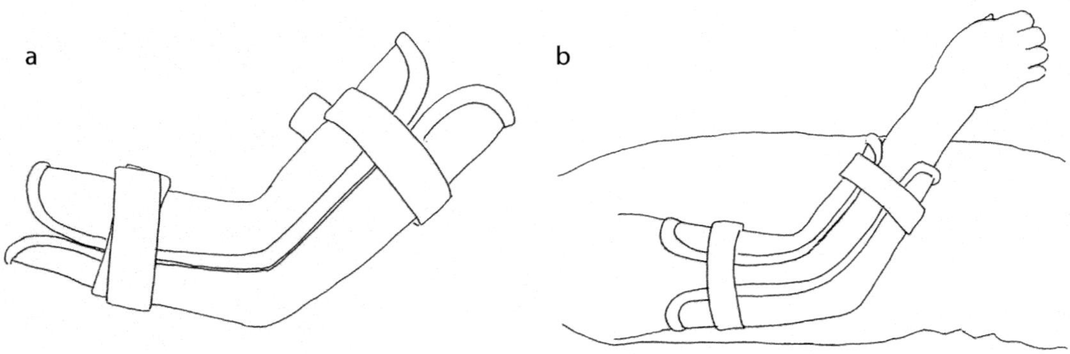

Fig. 9.7 (**a**) Retaining appliance of elbow joint in functional position. (**b**) Dressed retaining appliance of elbow joint in functional position

3. Indications and contraindications: Retaining appliance of limb joints in functional position is widely applied.
   (a) Indications: It is suitable for the patients with motor function loss of limbs due to coma or various causes such as quadriplegia, hemiplegia, cerebral palsy, child cerebral palsy and paraplegia due to low conscious state, CNS injuries, and injuries of bone, joint and muscle.
   (b) Contraindications: it is not suitable for the patients with unhealed local skin injuries such as burn, scald and openness injury. The patients with severe edema of joint and limbs should use it with caution.
4. Cautions of clinical application: The therapists should realize that maintenance of functional position is not equal to prevention of tissue adhesion. Joint adhesion in functional position may affect joint functions, which is the complication that should not occur. Therefore, during the process of keeping joint in functional position, the patients should emphasize on rehabilitation training. The patients undress retaining appliance of joint in functional position and do active and passive training of joint.

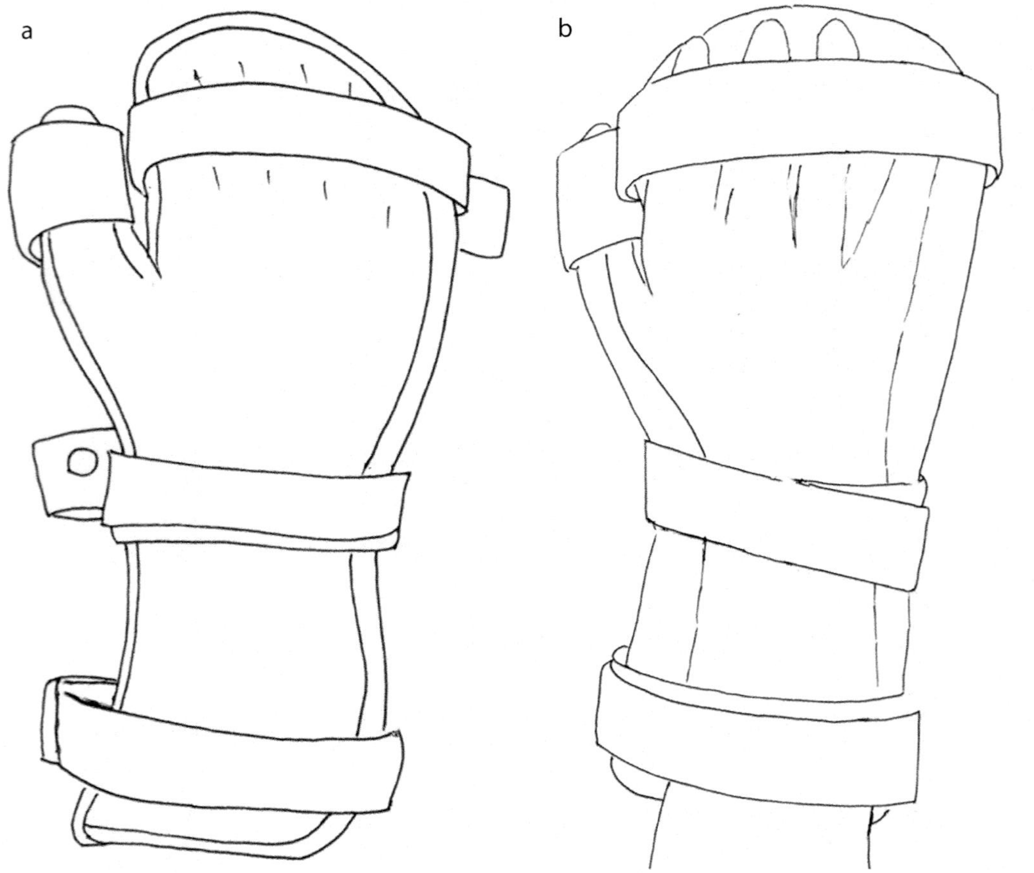

Fig. 9.8 (**a**) Retaining appliance of wrist-hand in functional position. (**b**) Dressed retaining appliance of wrist-hand in functional position

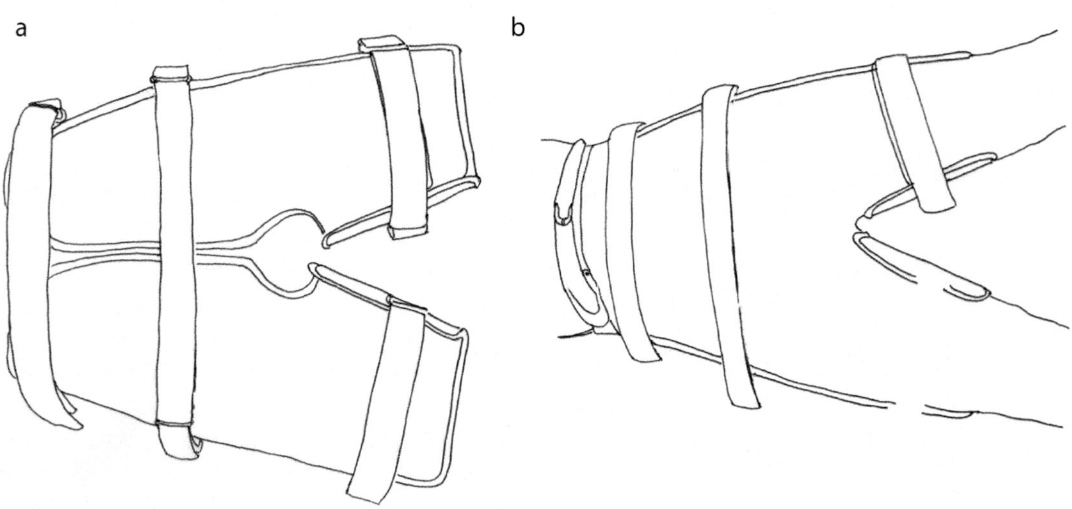

Fig. 9.9 (**a**) Retaining appliance of hip joint in functional position. (**b**) Dressed retaining appliance of hip joint in functional position

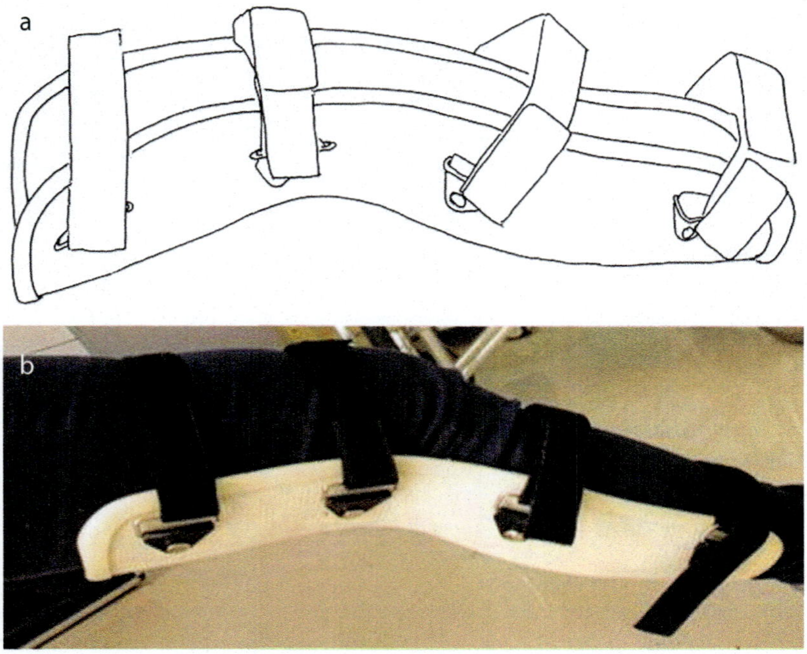

Fig. 9.10 (**a**) Retaining appliance of knee joint in straight position. (**b**) Clinical application of retaining appliance of knee joint in straight position

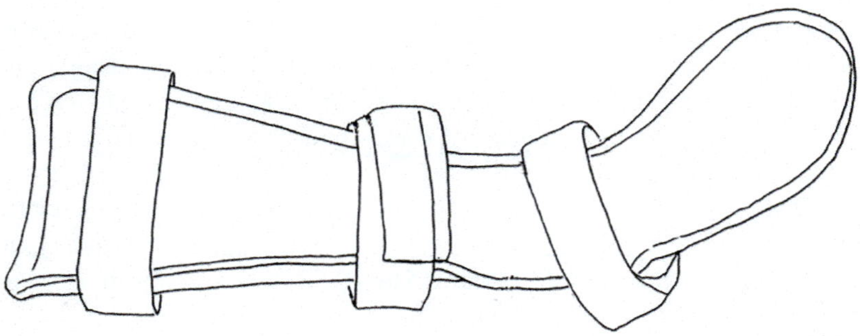

Fig. 9.11 Retaining appliance of foot-ankle joint in functional position

The training time is 10–15 min per time (1–2 times a day) to prevent adhesion of joint and soft tissue. Physiotherapy can be used to promote blood circulation in order to increase therapeutic effect.

5. Functional position of all joints (Table 9.1).

9.1.4 Convenient Turning-Over Device to Prevent Pressure Sores

Pressure sores have affected human society for centuries. Although there are progresses in the wound formation and therapy, the number of the patients with pressure sores is big and the cost is extremely high. It not only can increase the hospital day, the time back to family and work time, but also increase occurrence rate of other complications evidently. In 1992, clinical guideline established by American health care policy and research institute regards pressure sores as one of the seven medical problems needed to be solved and confirmed that pressure sores can be prevented.

9.1.4.1 The Definition of Pressure Sores

Pressure sores is that in a certain area, especially constant pressure of osseous process induces tissue ischemia, cells death and tissue necrosis and

Table 9.1 Functional position of all joints

Joint	Functional position	Angle (°)	Supporting detail
Shoulder joint	Abduction	45–75	
	Anteflexion	30–45	
	Extorsion	15–20	
Elbow joint	Flexion	70–90	Neutral position of forearm
Wrist joint	Dorsiflexion	30	
	Ulnar deviation	5–10	
Thumb joint	Palmar opposition		
Finger joint		140	
Metacarpophalangeal joints		140	
Near interphalangeal joint		130	
Far interphalangeal joint		150	
Hip joint	Abduction	10–15	
	Anteflexion	15–20	
	Rotation	0	
Knee joint	Flexion	5–20	
Ankle joint	Foot dorsiflexion	90	

it is commonly seen in bedrid patients so that it is called decubitus ulcers or bedsores. Decubitus is Latin, which means lying down and the ulcer is induced by long time in bed. Constant pressure of any part for a long time can induce it so that the name of pressure sores is more precise, which indicates that the pathogenesis of pressure sores is constant pressure that induce tissue ischemia and necrosis but not simple special body position.

9.1.4.2 Epidemiology of Pressure Sores

In the emergency medical establishment, the occurrence rate of pressure sores is 15–18.3%. Some people do study of nursing in acute stage on large sample about 148 hospitals and found that the occurrence rate of pressure sores is 9.2%. The occurrence rate of pressure sores in the patients in a long period of hospitalization is 3.5–29.5%. In skilled nursing facility and sanatorium, the occurrence rate of pressure sores is 2.4–23%.

Occurrence rate of pressure sores differs in different population and organizations. In acute nursing institute, the occurrence rate is 3–40%. Allman found that at least 7.7% of inpatients are diagnosed with pressure sores 3 weeks after admitted to hospital. In special crowd, such as the patients with senile diseases and orthopedic department of orthopaedics, the occurrence rate reaches 24–59%. Young and Burns found that the occurrence rate of the patients in acute phase and in rehabilitation hospital is 40%. In the follow-up visit of every 5 years, the occurrence rate is 30%.

9.1.4.3 The Causes of Pressure Sores

There are many causes of pressure sores. Pressure, shear force and friction force are the three primary factors. The most important is pressure. Secondary factors include state of motion, sense-motor function, state of nutrition, age, blood system change, diabetes mellitus, circulatory disturbance and gatism [4].

1. Pressure: There are three important factors related to pressure, which include intensity, time of duration and the tolerance of tissue to pressure.

Pressure has negative relation with time, which means high pressure in a short time and low pressure in a long time do the same harm to the tissue. The research found that 70 mmHg pressure for 2 h can lead to pathological change of tissue. The tolerance ability of tissue to intermittent pressure is stronger than the tolerance ability of tissue to constant pressure. For example, if the pressure is removed every 3–5 min, the tissue can tolerate higher pressure. Therefore, pressure must be removed regularly to reduce pressure on the skin surface.

In clinic, one turning over every 2 h and frequent posture change can relieve pressure, which is based on these researches. Compared with skin, muscle is more sensitive to pressure. Pressure can be transmitted from body surface to the bone under it. Because of counter-acting force, the tissue on the bone bears more pressure. Therefore, the pressure distributes like a cone shape. Basis pyramidis is the body surface under pressure, which lead to slight skin injury and severe subcutaneous injury.

In 1930, through microinjection, Landis proved that the average pressure of the part from artery to capillary is 32 mmHg. In the terminal of vein, the pressure is decreased to 12 mmHg. The average capillary pressure is about 20 mmHg. Therefore, in clinic, the therapists should seek bearing surface that can decrease pressure to below 32 mmHg in order to decrease the harm of the tissue due to constant pressure for a long time. Constant low pressure does more harm than high pressure for a short time.

2. Shear force: When the skin touches the bed and they are immobile, subcutaneous tissue is moved because of some kind of cause, which can induce shearing phenomenon [5] between subcutaneous tissue and skin. For example, the occurrence of pressure sores in pars sacralis is related to this. When the bedside is elevated, the pressure of tissue in the back of sacrum is stronger than that in normal time. Although skin of sacrococcyx is attached to bed sheet, the body slides to the bedside and subcutaneous tissue moves with it, which induce shearing phenomenon. The artery from subcutaneous fascia and muscle to skin is pressed and it leads to ischemia and then necrosis, which easily induce shearing ulcer with wide base area.

The common causes that induce shearing include spasm, bad sitting position, bad prone position and sliding in transfer.

3. Force of friction: The movement of skin on the bearing surface can generate friction force. Excessive friction force can lead to skin tear. Damaged extent is confined to epidermis and corium layer. If there are pressure and shearing force, the harm induced by friction force is bigger. If there is friction force, minor skin pressure can induce pressure sores [6].

The degree of spinal cord injury is not obviously correlated with the severity of pressure sores. If medical history of the patients is more than 3 years, the concentration of proline, lysine and hydroxylysine of the skin under the paraplegia level is decreased. Because these substances are related to skin tension and can resist pressure, possibility of pressure sores is high.

9.1.4.4 Common Body Parts of Pressure Sores

More than 95% of pressure sores occurs in osseous processes of bottom half of the body. Sixty-seven percentage occurs around hip and haunch. Twenty-nine percentage occur in lower limbs. The most common parts are ischium, sacrum, greater trochanter of femur and heel. It can also occur in any part of the body where soft tissue is pressed, which includes the oppression from splint, orthotics or orthopedic fixity. The most common part of pressure sores is sacrum in the patients with spinal cord injury. The more time the patients spend in the wheelchair, the higher the occurrence rate of pressure sores in ischial tuberosity and heel is. In the children patients whose age is from 10 to 13, the common part of pressure sores is occipitalia. With age, pars sacralis is the common part.

9.1.4.5 Prevention of Pressure Sores

The prevention of pressure sores is based on the understanding of etiology. The key point of prevention is to eliminate the dangerous factors that can lead to injury such as pressure, friction force and shearing force. They can be summarized as follows.

1. Body posture adjustment can relieve local tissue oppression. According to the oppressed body part, when the pressure reaches 70 mmHg for 2 h, pathological changes of tissue occur. The following measures can be

used to decrease the oppressed intensity and duration time.

(a) Timing turning over: for the patients with dyskinesia, body elevation and turning over is the simplest, most common and most effective method [5] to avoid constant oppression. The patients who lie in bed should be turned over once every 2 h, which is widely accepted in clinic, but the therapists should examine the skin carefully. If there is any problem, it should be solved in time.
(b) Frequent body position change: the main position is divided into supine position, prone position, right lateral position and left lateral position. Lateral position should avoid the direct pressure on greater trochanter. Seiler suggested that in lateral position it is suitable to incline the body at 30° to decrease the pressure on the skin of greater trochanter.
(c) Preventing the pressure on osseous process and heel: Wedge or pillow can be used to prevent the oppression of osseous process. The device that can lift the feet away from the ground is used, which is an effective way to prevent pressure on heel.
(d) Preventing shearing injury of skin friction and subcutaneous tissue: when the therapists take the patients away from bed or wheelchair, they should try to decrease the friction force and shearing force between body and bed or wheelchair.
(e) Decreasing pressure on hip in wheelchair: when the patients go out with wheelchair, the sitting posture must be right. Footboard should be put in the altitude that can make the thigh bear load to decrease the load bearing of ischium. Moreover, the posture should be changed every half an hour such as inclining backward, inclining laterally or elevating the body.
(f) The therapists should examine the oppressed body part frequently: the therapists should examine the body part at least two times a day including skins, especially the skin in osseous process.

2. Improving bearing surface to decrease intensity of pressure of the oppressed tissue: The bearing surface can decrease the pressure on osseous process through the closest touch and the weight redistribution in a larger area. In the bearing surface applied at present, bearing surface in bed, removable mattress and tailor-made bed have effects [7].

Low air consumption system can supply flow air around skin except air filling channel to make the skin keep dry, which is good for decreasing friction force and shear force in the movement.

Tailor-made bed can relieve pressure, decrease shear force and friction force, prevent dampness, which includes entrained-flow bed, low air consumption bed and tailor-made power bed. Entrained-flow bed contains airflow bubble. Bed is covered with osmotic nylon textile and human float on the bed to decrease skin pressure, which is good for wound drainage.

At present, at home and abroad, the types, advantages and disadvantages of the common bearing surface refer to Table 9.2.

9.1.4.6 The Composition and Function Mechanism of Convenient Turning Over Device to Prevent Pressure Sores

Although at present the measures have an effect on preventing pressure sores, there are some obvious shortcomings.

1. No obvious effect of soft bearing surface on decreasing the intensity of pressure: Bearing surface in soft bed can be used to enlarge the contact area between skin and bearing surface. It can induce the weight distribution to a certain extent and decrease the intensity of pressure in osseous process. Because the pressure from osseous process on upholder is bigger than that in other body parts, the bigger the pressure on upholder is, the bigger the bounce from upholder is. Therefore, it cannot decrease the pressure on osseous process effectively. This is why in clinic it is necessary to turn over the body regularly on the condition of using bearing surface in soft bed.

Table 9.2 The types, advantages and disadvantages of the common bearing surface

Support device	Type	Advantage	Disadvantage
Static upholder (bed or cushion)	Foam	Cheap, light, multiple-purpose uses	Absorb liquid with odorous, short service life
	Air	Light, good decompression, easy to clean	Easy to pierce, unstable air inflation, expensive
	Floating body (gel and water)	Good decompression, easy to move and adjust	Heavy, expensive, heat collector
	Recombination cushion (foam and gel)	Convenient for body placement and decompression	Heavy and expensive
Dynamic upholder in bed	Mattress	Portable, clean and easy to control humidity	Force requirement, expensive, noisy
Upper upholder	Low air consumption bed	Good decompression, easy to control humidity, move and decrease friction force and shear force	Expensive
	Replaceable mattress in hospital	Inner decompression, low supporting cost	High initial cost
Breeze bed		Good decompression, antibacterial glass ball, absorb liquid and dampness	Expensive, hard to carry, affecting sense and dehydration

2. It is effective to turn over the body but the labor intensity is high. Turning over once every 2 h is the effective measure to prevent pressure sores and is the clinical care routine of the patients with pressure sores. However, the labor intensity of turning over the patients, especially the patients with coma or heavy body weight is big, which can increase the nursing difficulty and workload.

The key point of preventing pressure sores is to eliminate pressure, friction force and shear force. If the bearing surface in bed is changed to hardness from softness, the osseous process cannot bear pressure, but can eliminate friction force and shear force effectively. It can maintain ventilation of skin and avoid dampness. It is convenient for the turning over of the patients and decrease nursing difficulty and intensity. During the process of preventing pressure sores, it helps the patients to turn over their body. Hard bearing surface with air permeability molded according to the body outline can enlarge the contact area between skin and bearing surface and decrease the intensity of pressure of skin without the counter-acting force generated from the pressure of the body on upholder. Through machine shaping technology, the osseous part is suspended so that it doesn't bear pressure, which is good for prevention of pressure sores.

Hereunder, the raw material is hard bearing surface. The author developed a turning over device that can prevent pressure sores effectively, is easy for turning over and is convenient for the patients to defect, which is called convenient turning over device to prevent pressure sores.

1. The composition of convenient turning over device to prevent pressure sores: The device is made from macromolecule glass fiber orthotics materials with six layers. According to molded arc-shaped body from back and waist-hip to anterior axillary line, osseous process protrudes outside and hangs inside, which includes sacroiliac part, spinous process of the seventh cervical vertebra and bilateral greater trochanter. The back of arc-shaped body is pasted with four arc hollow strips molded form macromolecule glass fiber material, which adapts to arc-shaped body. Four arc hollow strips of arc-shaped body touch the bed. The inner face of arc-shaped body is pasted with ventilated sponge with thin layer. The two sides of arc-shaped body are fixed fixing band. When dressing, it can be pasted and fixed with nylon thread gluing in the end, which is convenient to put

on or off. The patients lie inside and only one person slightly pushes this device to make the patients turn over and change the oppressed part of the body. Wedge-shape cushion or thin cushion is cushioned outside of turning over device to fix the patients' body position. There is herringbone nursing opening in the hip for the nursing of the patients' urine and stool.

2. The function mechanism of convenient turning over device to prevent pressure sores: The difficulty in turning over is that the patients cannot turn over timely so that pressure sores are formed. The difficulty in turning over is common in the patients with severe state of illness and heavy body weight. Sometimes, it requires 2–4 people to help the patients to turn over. In clinic, soft substances such as air cushion, sponge cushion and water bed are usually used to decrease the pressure on skin from body weight through buffer action in order to prevent pressure sores. These materials are airtight and can make the bed surface damp. The elasticity of the upholder materials is proportional to pressed degree of the skin. The bigger the pressure of local part is, the bigger the bounce is. Therefore, the stress of osseous process is big and the risk of pressure sores exists. Convenient turning over device to prevent pressure sores adopts suspension technique of hard bearing surface in osseous process. The functions are as follows:
   - Osseous process cannot bear load.
   - The drawback that the more the soft bearing surface is pressed, the bigger the bounce is avoided. The force is uniformly distributed in all the contact surface to decrease the intensity of pressure effectively.
   - Bearing surface is ventilated to prevent local skin temperature increase, exhaust dampness and keep the skin dry.
   - The arc and four arc hollow strip of convenient turning over device to prevent pressure sores can help the patients inside it turn over easily through rolling this device.
   - This device's lining is ventilated sponge with thin layer, which is good for skin ventilation and keeping the skin dry to increase the comfort of using it.

In addition, convenient turning over device to prevent pressure sores materials are fragrant, adaptable, firm and ductile. The patients lie inside it. The entire is hard but the osseous process is suspended to avoid pressure. Radio transparent characteristic is convenient for the patients to do X-ray exam in bedside. There is herringbone nursing opening in the hip for the nursing of the patients' urine and stool.

Hard inner face can enlarge the contact area between the body and the device and lining sponge has a buffer action, which can enlarge the stress area of the body and decrease the intensity of pressure obviously. It makes the device comfortable and reduces the pressure on the body tissue.

3. The manufacture and application method of convenient turning over device to prevent pressure sores According to the shape of human back and waist-hip and the level of anterior axillary line, positive plaster model is duplicated from negative plaster model. After modification, proper macromolecule glass fiber material with six layers is taken out, unsealed and soaked into cold water for 6 s. After that, it is flattened in the operating floor and is pasted on positive plaster model. It requires 6 min to mold and solidify. Arc-shaped body is molded according to the shape of human back and waist-hip and the level of anterior axillary line, osseous process protrudes outside and makes inside suspended, which includes sacroiliac part, spinous process of the seventh cervical vertebra and bilateral greater trochanter. Four arc hollow strip are formed of four arch apophysis that are made from macromolecule glass fiber material with the same thickness outside of convenient turning over device to prevent pressure sores on the basis of plastic tube (the diameter is 5 cm). The periphery of it is fixed on arc-shaped body with rivet. The back of arc-shaped body is pasted with four arc hollow strips molded form

macromolecule glass fiber material, which adapts to arc-shaped body. Four arc hollow strips of arc-shaped body touch the bed (Fig. 9.12). After solidification and modification, the inner face of arc-shaped body of turning over device is attached with artificial limb sponge with thin layer (Fig. 9.13). The two laterals are pasted with fixing band with nylon thread gluing. The device can be divided into big, middle and small size. The device should be made uniquely for special body type.

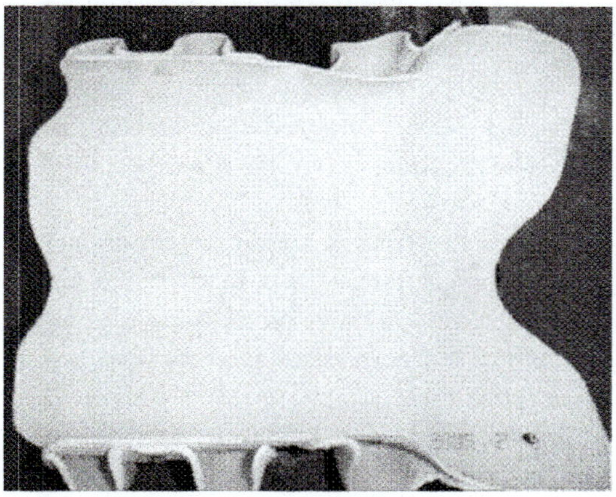

Fig. 9.12 Inside view of convenient turning over device to prevent pressure sores

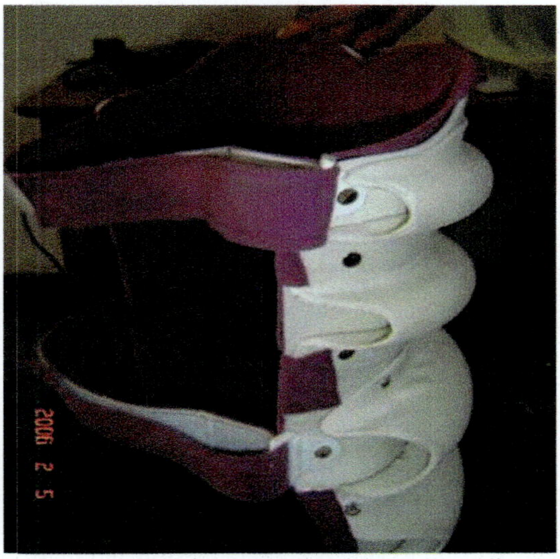

Fig. 9.13 Convenient turning over device to prevent pressure sores with lining

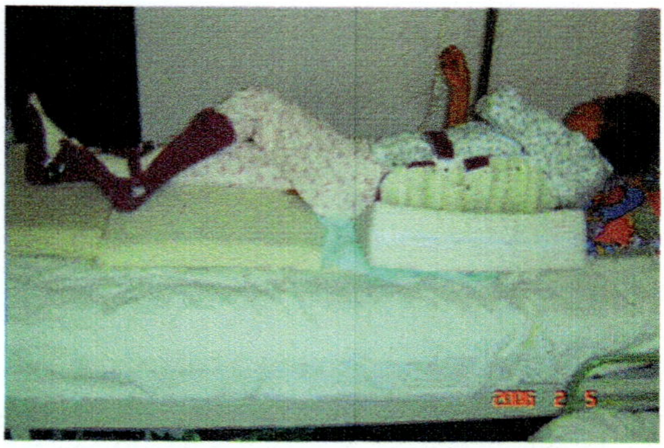

Fig. 9.14 Clinical application of convenient turning over device to prevent pressure sores

When dress up, the patients turn over to one side slightly, place convenient turning over device to prevent pressure sores, change to flat-on position and fasten fixing band. The therapists can make the patients turn over to the left or the right as needed and adjust the angle of turning over through the inserted depth of wedge-shape cushion from the bottom of the device (Fig. 9.14).

After dressing convenient turning over device to prevent pressure sores, the nurses and family of the patients with high paraplegia can change the turning over degree of the patients as needed and use wedge-shape cushion to keep the changed position.

4. Clinical indications and contraindications of convenient turning over device to prevent pressure sores
   (a) Indications: it is suitable for the long-term bed patients with coma, paraplegia, myasthenia gravis, severe bone fracture or dyscrasia.
   (b) Contraindication: it is forbidden in the patients with burn of neck-back and waist-hip or unhealed wound.

9.2 The Development of Orthopedic Orthotics

In clinic, because of short of consciousness and methods of early rehabilitation intervention or the development and prognosis of the disease, there always are abnormal joint position, rigidity even bony ankyloses. The therapy is difficult and it affects motor function recovery of the patients' limbs and promotion of life quality. In order to solve these problems, not only rehabilitation consciousness should be enhanced, the joints are kept in good limb position or functional position in early phase and rehabilitation training should be done, but also the abnormal should be rectified through requisite measures for the rigidity joint in abnormal position. It provides conditions for rehabilitation training and functional recovery of limbs.

9.2.1 Ankle Orthotics of Controlled-Release Force

In clinic, foot drop is the most common joint deformity due to improper handling. Tibialis anterior muscle paralysis due to coma, central nerve injury and peripheral nerve injury induces foot drop because of plantar flexion of ankle joint. If there is no rehabilitation consciousness and the patients don't do good limb position placement and passive joint motion in the early phase, contracture of Achilles's tendon and musculus gastrocnemius, fibrous adhesion of ankle joint can be induced for a longer time. For a long time, fibrous rigidity and bony ankyloses of ankle joint are formed, which bring about great difficulty to the training of functional recovery. Therefore, difficult orthotic foot drop is related to long-term immobilization and disuse [8].

In the early phase of foot drop formation, passive joint motion can stretch contracture of musculus gastrocnemius and Achilles's tendon and loose adhesive ankle joint. Orthotics is kept in functional position to make the adhesion occur in functional position even if there is adhesion [9], which can assure the basic functions of the joint. However, if the opportunity of early rectification is lost, the relievable foot drop may become irreversible [10], which brings about further difficulty to rehabilitation therapy and has a strong impact on functional recovery of the standing and walking [11, 12] of the patients. General conditions of rehabilitation training are even lost such as severe foot drop of fibrous rigidity.

For foot drop with severe contracture of musculus gastrocnemius and Achilles's tendon, fibrous rigidity and bony ankyloses of ankle joint, it is understandable to be rectified by operation [13]. For the foot drop with passive joint range of motion, the operation therapy should be careful. The foot drop of the patients with coma and low conscious state cannot rectified by operation because there are no indications. Extremely plantar flexion of ankle joint lead to unable standing training and long-term bed, which induces a series of complications of respiratory, urinary, cardiovascular and digestive system, even life danger and losing the hope of functional recovery. It is the problem that to be solved in clinic.

At present, there is seldom report about the rectification therapy of this kind of foot drop. Although there are many types [14, 15] of ankle orthotics at home and abroad, there is no report about orthotics of controlled-release force.

The stretched length of slow traction of rubber band is longer than that of quick traction of rubber band. Strong traction of foot drop easily induce pressure ulcer and make it difficult to loose contracture of musculus gastrocnemius and Achilles's tendon. Through the bounce of orthotics elastic band of controlled-release force and hinge design of ankle joint of foot tray, elastic band tracts the pelma part of orthotics to increase dorsiflexion angle of ankle joint. Through slight and slow traction, contracture of musculus gastrocnemius and Achilles's tendon, fibrous adhesion of ankle joint receives progressive loosing and stretching to increase the motion range of ankle joint and rectify foot drop without inducing micro injury condition of muscle spasm. It creates conditions for decreasing complications and promoting functional recovery.

Ankle orthotics of controlled-release force in accordance with the principle of slight and constant traction is developed using elastic recoil of elastic band to slowly loose adhesion and rectify joint deformity, which can provide conditions for rehabilitation training and joint function recovery.

9.2.1.1 Basic Structure and Functions

Ankle orthotics of controlled-release force is composed of the main part and traction part of controlled-release force. The main part is that moveable ankle orthotics of ankle joint is made according to the shape of facies cruralis posterior and foot of the patients. Its role is to fix shank and pelma. Meanwhile, exogenous process is used to generate dorsiflexion of ankle joint to loose contracture of musculus gastrocnemius and Achilles's tendon. Traction part of controlled-release force is that elastic band is used to connect toe and the front of tibia. Through the bounce of elastic band, slight and slow traction can stretch contracture of tendon and muscle to loose the adhesive joints.

9.2.1.2 Materials and Manufacture Method

1. Materials: Macromolecule glass fiber material or high temperature thermoplastic plate is used. The characteristics of the materials are as soft as mud before solidification, adaptable and easy to be molded. After solidification, they are with good air permeability, light, strong but pliable in texture, radio transparent and easy to dress.
2. The manufacture of ankle orthotics of controlled-release force: We use semi-finished product macromolecule glass fiber material as an example. The therapists select ankle orthotics materials in functional position, open packing bag, take out macromolecule glass fiber material slice, soak it into water of room temperature for 6 s, flatten it, use it to cover the ankle and facies cruralis posterior of the patients. The materials are pressed evenly and fixed for 6 min. Until macromolecule glass fiber materials are solidified, the therapists take it down, cut the edge and make the vertical plane projection of shank margin and tibia ridge are at the same altitude. The therapists cut two wedge-shape slices from the two sides of rotation center of ankle joint and use it as an axis with the function of hinge. There is a bordure (2 cm height) in outside of foot. The therapists use the inside to encase longitudinal arch and polish it. The therapists punch a hole in shank and ankle, use hollow rivet to fix fixing band and paste artificial limb sponge slice with thin adhesive sticker layer to the inner face for fitting. During the process of fitting, the technicians select elastic traction band with proper elasticity with one end fixed on the toe of orthotics and the other end fixed on the upper end of shank of orthotics from anterior tibia. The technicians adjust the length of elastic traction band and fix it. Through traction of elastic band, the angle of foot dorsiflexion is increased gradually.

9.2.1.3 Clinical Application

1. Clinical test results: Macromolecule glass fiber material is used to make ankle orthotics of controlled-release force. Because of good air permeability and better body limb adaptation, it is comfortable to dress and there is no pressure ulcer in all the ceases. Elastic recoil of elastic band of orthotics has a slight and slow traction effect persistently.

In 22 patients with foot drop who are rectified by orthotics of controlled-release force, there are 18 males and four females. There are 13 patients with low conscious state and nine patients with spinal cord injury. Passive motion range of ankle joint is $3.54° \pm 1.63°$. The average of fixing angle of plantar flexion (the minimum angle of plantar flexion of passive motion of ankle joint) is $44.91° \pm 5.35°$. the patients cannot do standing training. The patients receive orthotics therapy of controlled-release for four weeks and the passive motion range of ankle joint is $28.09° \pm 9.26°$. There are 16 patients whose passive motion range of ankle joint is equal or more than 32.5°. The average of plantar flexion recovers to $17.59° \pm 10.04°$. there are four patients who are at 25° plantar flexion, but they can basically meet the requirements of standing bed training. There are two patients whose functions are not improved because of ossifying ankle joint, contracture of severe Achilles's tendon and ankle joint adhesion.

Before and after rectification, the data of fixing angle of plantar flexion of ankle joint and passive motion range are analyzed by SPSS12.0 software with T-test. There is significant differ-

Table 9.3 Before and after rectification, the data comparison of fixing angle of plantar flexion of ankle joint and passive motion range (X ± S)

Angle of ankle joint	Case number	Before therapy (°)	After therapy (°)
Fixing angle of plantar flexion	22	44.91 ± 5.35	17.59 ± 10.04*
Passive motion range of ankle joint	22	3.54 ± 1.63	28.09 ± 9.26*

*$p < 0.05$

ence before and after rectification ($p < 0.05$, Table 9.3). Ankle orthotics of controlled-release has a good effect on foot drop with contracture of musculus gastrocnemius and Achilles's tendon and fibrous adhesion of ankle joint, but has no effect on severe fibrous adhesion or ossification stiffness.

2. Clinical indications, contraindications and cautions
   (a) Indications: it is suitable for the patients with foot drop due to various causes, especially accompanied with contracture of Achilles's tendon and musculus gastrocnemius, fibrous adhesion of ankle joint.
   (b) Contraindications: all the following cases are not suitable for application of Ankle orthotics of controlled-release force.
      - Foot drop induced by scar contracture after burn of shank and ankle part
      - Joints with severe contracture of Achilles's tendon and musculus gastrocnemius; immobile joints in passive movements
      - Ankle joint with fibrous rigidity or ossification stiffness
      - The patients with ankle ulcer, thrombus of lower extremity veins or severe varicosity
   (c) Cautions: in clinical application, local pressure ulcer should be prevented strictly. Because this kind of patients have not good enough feelings or any feeling of the limbs. Therefore, it should be watched carefully in application. In the first 3 days, the patients should undress orthotics every 2 h to examine if there is red and swollen and pressure ulcer in ankle part or not. If there is no pressure ulcer, the patients can wear it day and night.
   (d) Other cautions: orthotics of controlled-release force can be made from high temperature thermoplastic plate. The characteristics are that it becomes soft when heated at 180 °C. After molded, it is smooth, with good tenacity and strength. It can be repeatedly heated and modified. High temperature thermoplastic plate is used for machine shaping and its process is complicated. Positive plaster model should be made first and flat heater is required. Moreover, this material is not with air permeability so that the technicians should punch a hole. It is heavy and uncomfortable to dress. In the manufacture, the technicians clip high temperature thermoplastic plate with proper size, put it into flat heater for 10 min at 180 °C, paste positive plaster model and drain it after the board becomes soft. The plate is completely pasted to positive plaster model. After solidification, the technicians take it down. The other procedures are the same as the method that macromolecule glass fiber materials are used to make orthotics.

In addition, this kind of orthotics can also be used for orthotics of other joints. According to the shape of orthotic joints, the orthotics is processed and molded to increase compatibility and decrease complications.

9.2.2 Antispasmodic Dynamic Joint Position Retainer

There is spastic hemiplegia in the hemiplegic patients with stroke. Spastic hemiplegia. Generally, spastic hemiplegia is transformed from flaccid hemiplegia, but in some subacute or chronic patients, spastic hemiplegia can be formed without flaccid paralysis.

The characteristics of spastic hemiplegia are the paralysis of upper limb extensor and lower limb flexor, especially hands and feet. Moreover, the upper limb is more severe than the lower limb. There are paralysis of flexor of upper limbs and extensor of lower limbs to varying degrees in hemiplegic side, which can lead to obvious weakness or total loss of motor function.

Spasm of flexor of upper limbs makes elbow joint in passive flexed position. The wrist and finger are in flexed state, which make upper limb like carrying basket in paralyzed side. Spasm of extensor of lower limbs induces hyperextension and extorsion of knee joint. Meanwhile, there are foot drop and strephenopodia, which make the foot like talipes equinus. When the patients step forward and lift injured limbs away from ground, the patients with foot drop must incline the body to the offside and put forth their strength to lift hip so that the lower limbs can be lifted upward. The patients step forward in an arc and step down in front of the body to complete stepping movements, which is called circle. Result from the joint effects is that abnormal motor pattern, circle gait, is formed, which is the most common abnormal motor pattern of hemiplegia.

In order to prevent spasm position in hemiplegic side. In clinic, the prevention method is to keep antispasmodic position. The posture in antispasmodic position of upper limb is as follows:

- In supine position, the head is on the pillow and there is no hyperextension and hyperflexion. Injured shoulder is cushioned in case of shoulder retraction and injured upper limb extends and slightly abducts. The forearm supinates backward and the thumb points to outside.
- In lateral position in uninjured side, the head is supported by pillow in case of turning backward. The trunk is vertical and injured shoulder girdle extends forward fully. Shoulder flexes 90–130° and elbow and wrist extend. Upper limbs are on the front pillow.
- In lateral position in uninjured side, the head is supported by pillow. The trunk fade away slightly and is cushioned with pillow in case of downward of injured shoulder. Injured shoulder girdle extends forward fully. Shoulder flexes 90–130° and injured elbow extends. The forearm supinates backward and the hand is in dorsiflexion position without grasping something.

However, these placements of antispasmodic position can be used without hard constraints for the patients with coma or no voluntary movements through pillow, soft cushion or nature placement. If they are used for the sober patients who can move their limbs, it is hard to keep antispasmodic position. Because spasm of flexor of upper limbs is severe, without hardness restricted device, only pillow and soft cushion are difficult to keep injured elbow in extension and forearm supination position. For the patients with spasm of flexor of upper limbs and extensor of lower limbs, non-hardness restricted position placement is difficult to relieve the spasm.

However, in paralyzed side, the spasm of flexor of upper limbs lead to abnormal motor pattern of carrying basket, which not only easily induces adhesion of muscle fiber and other tissues, contracture of tendon because of long-term spasm of flexor of upper limbs in injured side, but also induce uncoordinated swing of upper limbs in walking and more energy consumption. Therefore, prevention and rectification of spasm effectively are the key points to prevent complications, joint deformity and recover autonomic nerve innervation of spasm muscle. It is a problem to be solved in clinic.

The development of retaining appliance of antispasmodic dynamic joint position is to rectify spasm of flexor of upper limbs and extensor of lower limbs effectively in paralyzed side to keep the joint in functional position, which don't affect autonomic flexion and extension of joints obviously. After clinical application, there are good therapeutic effects.

Retaining appliance of antispasmodic dynamic joint position includes retaining appliance of dynamic elbow joint in straight position and retaining appliance of dynamic knee joint in flexed position.

9.2.2.1 Basic Structure of Antispasmodic Retainer of Dynamic Elbow Joint in Straight Position

Retaining appliance of dynamic elbow joint in straight position is mainly composed of angle adjustable artificial assistive elbow joint and branch, elastic traction belt and elbow support (Fig. 9.15). Bilateral angle adjustable artificial assistive elbow joint and branch can restrict flexion of elbow joint in necessity. Fixing plate of upper arm and fixing plate of forearm are connected to branches, which make the bilateral branches connect to upper arm crossing elbow joint. Fixing plate is made from macromolecule glass fiber material according to the shape of upper arm and forearm. Elbow support is fixed on the back of elbow through fixing band of elbow support. The function of it is to prevent friction of the back of elbow joint by elastic traction belt. The upper and lower end of elastic traction belt are separately fixed on fixing ring of the upside of fixing plate and elastic band in the back of fixing plate in forearm.

According to the specific condition of spasm of flexor of upper limbs, elastic bands with different width and strength are selected. Elastic band is strained to make elbow joint in 120–150° straight position and make the patients can flex elbow actively if the elbow flexion ability is not lost. After strength adjustment, elastic band is fixed through fixing ring of elastic band in upper and lower end.

9.2.2.2 Basic Structure of Antispasmodic Retainer of Dynamic Knee Joint in Flexed Position

Retaining appliance of dynamic knee joint in flexed position is mainly composed of angle adjustable artificial assistive elbow joint and branch, elastic traction belt and knee support. Bilateral angle adjustable artificial assistive elbow joint and branch can restrict hyperflexion of knee joint in necessity. Fixing plate of thigh and fixing plate of shank are connected to branches, which make the bilateral branches be fixed crossing knee joint. Fixing plate is made from high temperature thermoplastic plate according to the shape of thigh and shank. The upper and lower ends of elastic traction belt are separately fixed on fixing plate of thigh and fix-

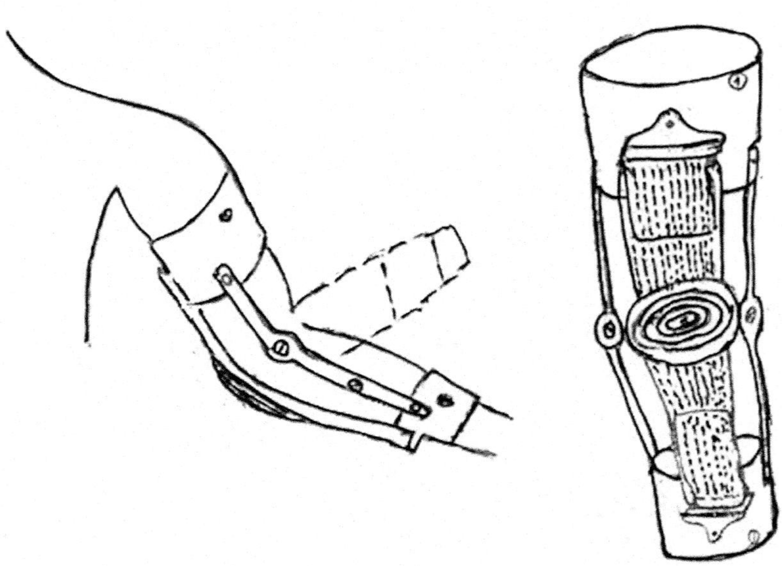

Fig. 9.15 Antispasmodic retainer of dynamic elbow joint in straight position. (1) Angle adjustable artificial assistive elbow joint and branch. (2) Elbow support. (3) Elastic traction belt. (4) Fixing board of forearm. (5) Fixing board of upper arm. (6) Fixing band of elbow support. (7) Posterior view. (8) Fixing ring of upper arm of elastic band. (9) Fixing ring of forearm of elastic band

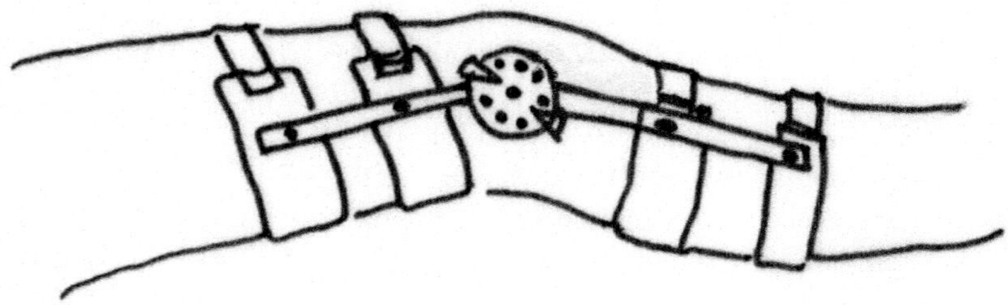

Fig. 9.16 Dynamic knee joint position holding appliance in straight position

ing ring of elastic band in the back of fixing plate in shank. Because the strength of extensor of lower limbs is big so that fixing plate of thigh and shank is double plate structure to increase strength.

According to specific condition of spasm of the patients' extensor of lower limbs, elastic bands with different width and force are selected. Meanwhile, elastic bands are stretched to keep knee joint in 20–30° flexion position until the patients can extend knee actively. The technicians adjust the intensity and use fixing ring of elastic band in upper and lower end to fix elastic band (Fig. 9.16).

9.2.2.3 Clinical Application of Antispasmodic Dynamic Joint Position Retainer

Because abnormal joint position due to muscle spasm is very common, clinical application of antispasmodic dynamic joint position holding appliance is wide. During the process of clinical application, the therapists should pay attention to complications.

1. Indications: It is suitable for the patients with flexion spasm of upper limbs in hemiplegic side and hyperextension of knee joint. The patients can dress it when they don't do rehabilitation training, even at night. The force of elastic traction belt shouldn't be too strong so that the joint can be kept in 120–150° straight position and the patients can flex or extend it actively.
2. Pay attention to avoid soft tissue injury: The therapists should inspect if there is bruise or uncomfortableness regularly. Once found, the therapists should adjust or modify it immediately.
3. Manufacture according to standard process: in order to dress is comfortably and prevent complications, the manufacture of retaining appliance should be specific. Negative plaster model should be made first and then positive plaster model is duplicated and modified. After that, on the basis of positive plaster model, it is processed and molded according to standard process.
4. To obtain better effects with the help of orthotics: If simple application of antispasmodic dynamic joint position holding appliance cannot rectify deformity of joint position completely such as waist, hand, finger and foot, the patients should wear wrist-hand or foot-ankle orthosis in functional position to obtain anticipated effect with retaining appliance in joint position.
5. To cooperate with other methods: For the patients with severe limbs spasm in paralytic side, antispasmodic dynamic joint position holding appliance use elastic band as traction force and is hard to keep the joint in the necessary position. Therefore, metal or high temperature thermoplastic plate are used to make restrictive orthotics to keep the joint in functional position. Through rehabilitation training or drug therapy, after alleviation of muscle spasm, antispasmodic dynamic joint position holding appliance is used to keep the joint in functional position and to move joint, which is good for functional recovery of the joint.

9.3 The Development of Functional Assistive Device

Functional assistive device is the device that can make the patients complete unaccomplished joint motion before or difficult joint motion and limbs movements in order to increase original functions obviously.

9.3.1 Elastic Band Orthosis of Lower Limbs

Elastic band orthosis of lower limbs is designed for the patients who are difficult to lift lower limbs because of inadequate strength of hip flexion and cannot complete walking movement. Through retraction force of elastic band that is fixed on the waist, the patients can easily lift lower limbs and lower it down to the ground stably. It is a simple assistive device for completion of walking.

9.3.1.1 Basic Structure of Elastic Band Orthosis of Lower Limbs

Elastic band orthosis of lower limbs is composed of three main parts such as waistline, elastic band and knee joint fixing band. Waistline can be hard wide belt or high temperature thermoplastic plate molding waistline to increase area of thrust surface and decrease local skin pressure. Knee joint fixing band made of soft cotton tape (5 cm wide) is groined. Patella is fixed on the back of knee joint. According to actual ability of hip flexion of the patients, the force can be calculated and elastic band with proper elastic force can be selected. The upper end is connected to midline of lower limbs of waist. The lower end is fixed on the upper end of the front of knee joint fixing band. In the trial walking, the retraction force of elastic band should be adjusted to make the patients lift lower limbs easily and touch the ground easily in straight position when the lower limbs are falling down. Elastic band is fixed (Fig. 9.17). After walking training for a period, the patients can gradually adapt to walking with the help of elastic band orthosis of lower limbs.

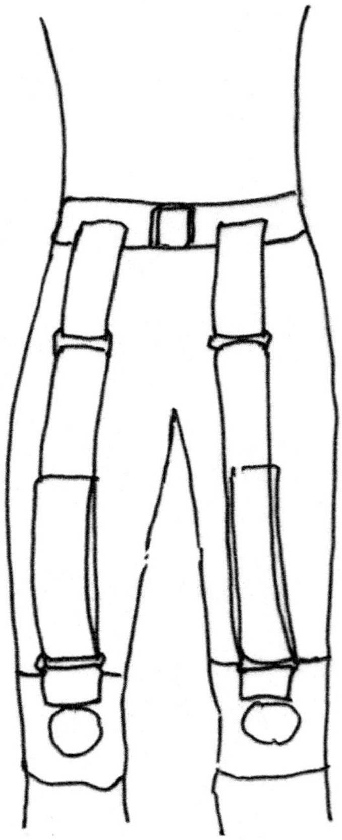

Fig. 9.17 Schematic diagram of elastic band assistive walking device of lower limbs

In the process that the patients use elastic band to walk with the help of orthosis of lower limbs, hip flexor can be strengthened and the myodynamia is enhanced until the patients can flex hip joint autonomously and easily.

9.3.1.2 Indications and Contraindications

1. Indications: it is suitable for the patients with incomplete paraplegia, hemiplegia and myasthenia, myodynamia of hip flexor (grade II–III), autokinetic movement of lower limbs with hip flexion difficulty.
2. Contraindications: the patients with soft tissue injury of waist and pelvis or unhealed bone fracture in pelvis, soft tissue injury of knee joint or unhealed bone fracture, deep venous thrombosis of lower limbs and limb swelling, severe varicosis of great saphenous vein

9.3.2 Assistive Walking Device of Complete High Paraplegia

In tradition, high paraplegia is the transverse injury in the high level of spinal cord. Generally, paraplegia due to transverse injury of spinal cord above the second thoracic vertebra is called high paraplegia. Paraplegia due to transverse injury of spinal cord below the third thoracic vertebra is called paraplegia of the lower part of the body (low paraplegia).

There is usually quadriplegia in high paraplegia. The sensory, motor, sphincter vesicae and sphincter and functions are totally lost in the spinal cord injury under transverse plane without reflex, which is called complete paraplegia. After cervical spinal cord is damaged, there is neurological dysfunction in double upper limbs, which is called quadriplegia.

Paraplegia is one of the most severe dysfunction in motor function. There are complete or partial autonomous motor function loss and standing and walking ability loss to varying degrees in the patients whose standing and walking ability can be recovered through assistive walking device.

From the power producer, the orthosis that help the patients with paraplegia to walk can be divided into unpowered orthosis and powered orthosis. Unpowered orthosis is without external human power producer and with the own stamina such as hip-knee-ankle-foot orthosis (HKAFO), knee-ankle-foot orthosis (KAFO), walkabout orthosis (WO), reciprocating gait orthosis (RGO), advanced reciprocating gait orthosis (ARGO), isocentric reciprocating gait orthosis (IRGO) and so on. HKAFO and KAFO are used to restrict range of joint motion. Meanwhile, crutch is used to support the body weight and keep the balance of the body when the center of gravity is shifted, which is widely used for rehabilitation training of the patients with paraplegia. The patients can obtain standing ability but cannot step [16] forward alternatively with two lower limbs.

WO, RGO, ARGO and IRGO are the best no-power orthosis. In design, WO is divided into two parts. Interactive hinge device is the key part of the equipment. Through using gravitational potential energy, it can provide power for alternative walking. KAFO is used for supporting double legs and provide essential guarantee for supporting standing balance. Operating principle of clock pendulum is used to realize passive forward and backward movement of paralytic limbs with the help of interactive hinge device that is installed in bilateral thigh when the weight of the patients is shifted. When the trunk of the patients inclines the center of gravity to the left, WO drives the right lower limb to get off the ground and the center of weight move forward. Under the action of gravity, with the help of interactive hinge device, suspended right lower limb can move forward with the center of weight. After that, under the action of inertia, the patients swing leg forward and complete stepping with right leg. When in standing and walking, the patients need the help of double crutches.

The hardcore of RGO includes two highwires that connect to hip joint and a pair of hip joints. In addition, it still has associated the upper part of the trunk and the lower part of thigh. The upper and lower lattice framing of hip joint can be separately combine the trunk with thigh. The trunk part is composed of lateral lattice framing, the belt that fix the trunk and pelvis hipline. There is no inside lattice framing in the lower part of thigh. Ankle-foot orthosis (AFO) made from polypropylene plastics wraps knee joint and malleolus medialis to increase stability.

Action principle: Through guide lock, hip joints of orthosis are connected. When hip joint in one side is over extended, through the movement of guide lock, hip joint in the other side can be flexed opposite to hip extension in order to move two legs forward alternatively so that the patients with paraplegia can do functional walking.

ARGO is mainly suitable for the patients with paraplegia due to injury of T_5–L_2. It is possible to realize practical walking. Structural features of walking assistive device not only include mobility-assisted function in walking, but also can directly stand up or sit down without using hands to manipulate hinge lock if knee joint in the switch between sitting position and standing position. Because of spring in knee joint, the patients can get support in position interchange. It can save labor and easy to be manipulated and dress. Compared with traditional orthosis, it can better improve the standing and walking function of the patients and decrease the energy consumption of the users, but it is expensive.

IRGO is a modified type of RGO. Its structural characteristic is to use connecting rod equipment that connects to bilateral hip joint to replace wire of RGO for better assistive movement function. This kind of connecting rod equipment is more durable than wire of RGO. Its action principle is to flex hip joint in one side and extend hip joint on the other side through moving bilateral hip joint alternatively.

KAFO, HKAFO, WO, RGO, ARGO or IRGO are applied for the patients with paraplegia (T_4–L_2). Its clinical indications and functions are different. KAFO is suitable for the patients with complete spinal cord injury (below L_1). WO is applied for the patients with complete spinal cord injury (below T_{10}). Swing equipment inner thigh is closely connected with KAFO of two legs and the coronal plane of lower limbs is increased relatively. RGO, ARGO and IRGO can connect upper and lower lattice framing of the trunk with thigh orthotics through hip joint. Compared with WO, no matter in coronal plane or vertical plane, they provide more ideal stability for the walking of the patients with paraplegia. For the patients with high paraplegia and paraplegia (below T_4), there are some reports that RGO is used for therapeutic walking successfully. However, in most cases, it is difficult to use existing walking assistive device to realize functional walking. When walking, because it is impossible to do hip and knee flexion, the patients cannot lift lower limbs and can only move forward in the slippery ground difficultly. Therefore, at present, walking assistive device that is applied in the patients with high paraplegia cannot realize actual walking of the patients.

Power orthotics is the orthotics driven by human external power. At home and abroad successfully developed motor direct-drive unidirection double joint walking device, electric drive bidirection paraplegia walking equipment, and direct current power producer actuator are embedded in hip and knee joint of ARGO, which can produce external power producer gait orthotics of hip and knee joint.

These kinds of orthotics are only suitable for the patients with walking rehabilitation training. They can make the patients move passively, but this is not the walking in real sense, even not active walking. They are expensive and the family cannot afford it. In addition, there is still functional electrical stimulation (FES) orthotics. Through electric stimulation, the patients with paraplegia who lose motor function of lower limbs can walk with orthotics. In the paraplegia due to spinal cord injury of cervical cord or upper thoracic cord, because it is difficult to obtain stable gait with unstable trunk, it is not suitable for FES orthotics. Only in the spinal cord injury below lower waist, when the muscles that control standing and walking can response to electric stimulation, it is suitable for FES orthotics.

Although various walking assistive devices cannot be used for the patients with paraplegia to walk in reality, the walking without true sense of the patients with paraplegia is significant, especially in the prevention of complications [17].

9.3.2.1 Preventing or Decreasing Complications Effectively

1. Decreasing pressure sores: Because sensory and motor function under paraplegia plane are totally lost, the position of the patients with complete high paraplegia cannot be moved at will. The skin and subcutaneous tissue of apophysis are oppressed and are turned into necrosis, which can form pressure sores. Because the nerve that dominates skin is injured, it leads to decrease of local neurotrophy function. Once there is pressure scores, it is difficult to be cured. The standing and walking with assistive device can obviously decrease bedtime and prevent pressure scores.
2. Promoting digestive system function: After spinal cord injury, there are dysneuria of the body, imbalance of autonomic nervous function and digestive tract disorder. There are abdominal distension and hypoactive or eliminated bowel sounds in the patients with complete paraplegia, which make diaphragm rise and affect breath. In the standing and walking with assistive device, enterocoelia content is decreased and diaphragm declines, which

increase thorax volume and are good for recovery of respiration function. Exercise can promote gastrointestinal peristalsis and evacuation of intestinal content, which can eliminate abdominal distension and promote recovery of digestion-absorption function.

3. Preventing respiratory tract infections: there are intercostal muscle paralysis, small vital capacity and respiratory secretions in the patients with high paraplegia, which lead to pulmonary infection. Standing and walking are good for increasing vital capacity, which can promote elimination of secreta and then prevent pulmonary infection.
4. Preventing joint adhesion, amyotrophy and osteoporosis: The standing and walking can give pressure on paralyzed or spasmodic limbs and move the joints, which can prevent effectively disuse amyotrophy, osteoporosis, joint and soft tissue adhesion, even joint deformity.

9.3.2.2 Promoting Motor Function Recovery and Improving General Conditions

1. Promotion of possible motor function recovery: There is little possibility that motor function of spinal cord injury is recovered completely. However, incomplete spinal cord can be further recovered through rehabilitation training. The standing and walking training with walking assistive device is one of the best methods to promote motor function further or make maximum use of residual function.
2. Increase of metabolism after spinal cord injury, neurotrophy function is decrease and cardiovascular stress response ability is decreased, which can affect the metabolism of entire blood circulation, tissue and organ greatly such as postural hypotension, even shock due to improper standing. The standing and walking training with walking assistive device can enhance cardiovascular stress response ability, promote blood circulation and metabolism, which are good for complications prevention and functional recovery.

9.3.2.3 The Significance of Preventing Complications

Through standing and walking training of walking assistive device, the complications of the patients with high paraplegia can be prevented. The body and organ can be maintained in a good state and it is significant.

1. Creating conditions for realizing independent life and improving life quality: Standing and walking training with walking assistive device can effectively prevent complications. The patients' body is in good state, which can create basic condition for shifting training. Through the training, development and utilization of residual functions of the patients, in the condition of with or without assistive device, the patients recover transfer capability from bed to wheelchair and from wheelchair to potty chair and daily life ability by themselves to increase the patients' life quality.
2. Waiting for better therapeutic method and creating conditions for recovering lost functions: At present, the development of science technology is fast and changed quickly, especially in the repair of neural functions, which includes medicine, neural transplantation and neural stem cells transplantation. Although some technologies such as neural stem cell transplantation are not immature, there are new theories and therapeutic methods for clinical application. Only with good bone and muscle system, the patients can receive the therapy of new method and is possible to be recovered.
3. Changing thinking and creating condition for returning to the society: With the development and progress of technology, the disabled can earn their own living and contribute to the society through different ways. A famous British physicist Stephen Hawking who is severely disabled and no one can compare with him, contribute a lot to the development of physics. The people should take this as a warning and change thinking. They should re-recognize that the disabled is not disabled. They should use Stephen Hawking as an example and apply modern technique apparatus and

procedure to go back to the work and society in different extent and depth. No matter how severe the paraplegia is, with normal brain function and intelligence, the disabled can contribute to themselves, the family, the society and human.

Therefore, research and development help the patients to walk independently with the help of walking assistive device.

9.3.2.4 Walking Assistive Device of Rollerskate

As mentioned above, at present, walking assistive device used by the patients with paraplegia, no matter walking assistive device of hip knee ankle (HKAFO), reciprocating walking assistive device (RGO), or central reciprocating walking assistive device (IRGO), with the help of other assistive device such as balance bar and double crutches, through shifting of weight and swing training, the trunk shakes to make lower limbs move forward. Because of hip and knee flexion, lower limbs cannot be lifted so that it only can move in slippery ground difficultly, especially in the patients with complete high paraplegia. It is difficult to move forward through shifting of weight and swing forward. It cannot be completed alone and the patients can swing forward slowly with the help of others.

Walking assistive device of rollerskate can help the patients with high paraplegia to slide forward independently with the help of walking assistive device and assistive standing device such as double crutches and rectification weight support walking training device of abnormal gait.

1. Basic composition: The device is composed of foot orthosis, spring column, pulley and fixing band. Foot orthosis is cut out from steel plate (2 mm) according to pelma shape, which is divided into half sole part, heel part and middle part. The above of foot orthosis is pasted with a layer of stereoplasm sponge and the below of foot orthosis is pasted with rubber non-slip mat. Four spring columns are composed of axle sleeve and axostyle. Four columns are made of steel and are separately fixed on four corners of foot orthosis. The upper end of axostyle is equipped with spring. It is enveloped into sleeve with axostyle. The lower end of axostyle is equipped with pulley. Fixing band is made of backpack strip and is connected through snap joint. Its tightness can be adjustable (Fig. 9.18).
2. Design principle and method of application: After wearing the walking assistive device and bilateral pulley, the patients can stand up with the help of assistive device such as double

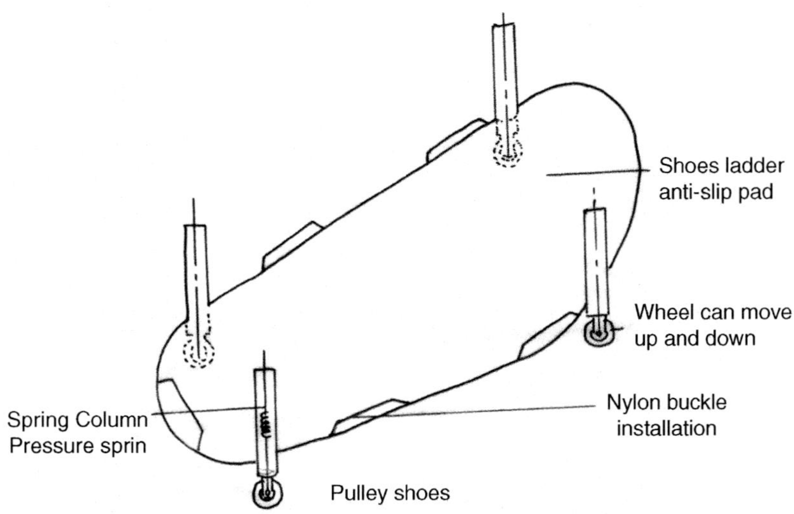

Fig. 9.18 Sketch map of walking assistive rollerskate

crutches, rectification weight support walking device of abnormal gait. At this time, foot orthosis of two feet is stressed. Because the spring is compressed when the force is no less than 20 kg, the foot orthosis touches the ground and the pulley in the rollerskate cannot move forward. When the patients try to step forward, the body weight center moves to offside. When the patients prepare to move the limbs forward (the weight is less than 20 kg), the spring can bounce the foot away from the ground. Through swing force of the trunk, the pulley move forward and the body move forward with it. When lower limb in one side slides forward, the body weight center moves to this side. When the weight is no less than 20 kg, the spring is oppressed and retracts. The foot orthosis touches the ground and the lower limb in this side bears load. Foot orthosis in the other side is bounced by the spring and slides forward. The body moves forward with it. The training is repeated and the patients can slide ahead (Fig. 9.19 and 9.20).

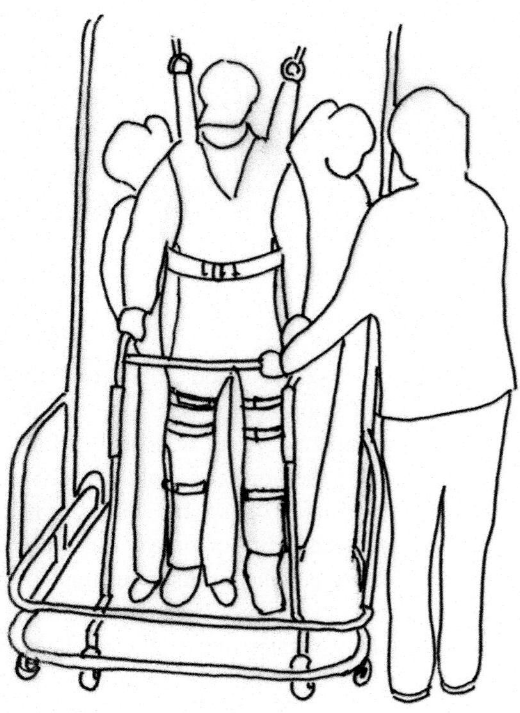

Fig. 9.19 The patients with high paraplegia can move forward with the help of two people

3. Indications and Contraindications
   (a) Indications: It is suitable for the patients with complete or incomplete high paraplegia to stand and step forward and the patients with low paraplegia to walk in the early phase with assistive device.
   (b) Contraindications: the patients should prepare the safeguard procedures of falling damages, especially for the patients with high paraplegia and upper limbs paralysis. Mobile weight support walking device can lose weight and protect the body, especially for the patients with high paraplegia in standing and walking training.

9.3.2.5 Walking Assistive Device of Shoulder Power

No matter walking assistive device is advanced or so expensive, they swing forward through waggling the trunk but not step forward in a real sense. Walking assistive device of shoulder power developed by the author is active walking device of high paraplegia that is formed by that using self-shrug power as power producer and locking joint to make the lower limbs bear load in standing position, the trapezoid self-locking hip and knee joint can allow joint motion and lift legs in stepping. With the help of this device, the patients with high paraplegia are able to lift lower limbs and step forward by themselves. So far, there is no report using shrug force as the power producer to make the patients with paraplegia walk independently.

1. Feasibility study that human shrug force can lift lower limbs: The main muscles of shrug are trapezius and musculus levator scapulae. Trapezius is dominated by accessory nerve that belongs to the 11th brain nerve. Even in high level spinal injury, generally, it cannot hurt this nerve. Therefore, the patients with high paraplegia are able to shrug and can obviously increase myodynamia of this muscle through training.

   The actual test demonstrated that the normal people's shrug force is twice of lower

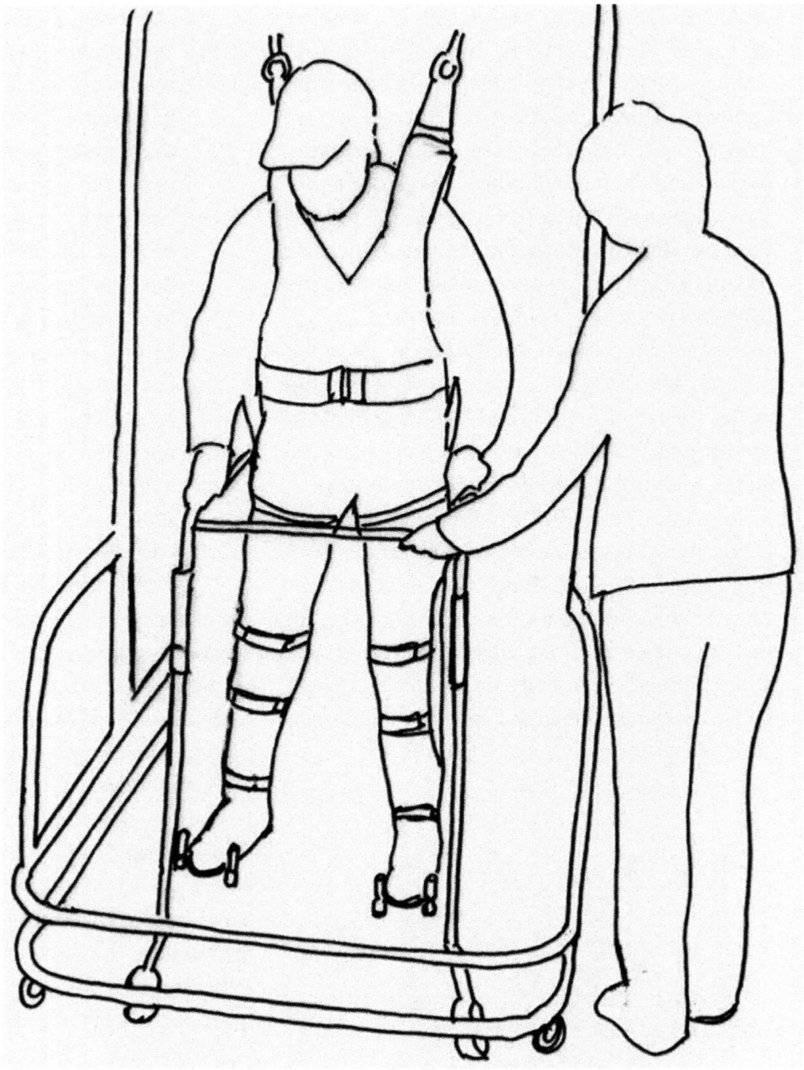

Fig. 9.20 The patients can slide forward with walking assistance pulley independently

Table 9.4 Experimental results of comparison of shrug force and lower limbs weight

Gender	Shrug force (kg)	Lower limbs weight (kg)	Force weight ratio
Male	33.45	14.41	2.32
Female	23.97	14.82	1.62
Mean value	28.71	14.62	1.97

limbs weight when shrugging (Table 9.4) and is able to lift lower limbs. With the help of mechanical saving labor equipment, through shrug, the patients can life lower limbs easily and complete stepping movement. Through training, shrug force can be increased obviously, which is good for completing movement of stepping forward.

The experimental result demonstrated that shrug force of the normal people is twice of lower limbs force. It can life lower limbs. Shrug force can be obviously increased through training. The realistic example is bearer in the mountain. The normal people can bear 25 kg water and walk, but bearer through training can bear 50 kg goods or even more heavier and climb the mountain. Therefore, the person uses shrug force to lift lower limb. It is possible in theory.

2. Basic composition of walking assistive device of shoulder power: The equipment is composed of waistcoat of shoulder power, power conduction system and self-locking system of assistive device joint.
   (a) Waistcoat of shoulder power is composed of shoulder pocket, support rod, dead plate and corsage. Shoulder pocket is made from cattlehide or canvas. The outer is enveloped in L shape extremitas acromialis of support rod, which can reach the middle of clavicle. The anterior part of shoulder pocket is long and is with slidable power line connection equipment, which can be connected to back part through bayonet. The length in oxter can be adjustable to the patients with different shoulder breadth. The extremitas acromialis of support is L shape, which is connected with the external of shoulder pocket. Spinal terminal of support is sphere, which can be adjustable to hemispheric glenoid fossa of dead plate. It can make support rod like shoulder joint that can move to all directions. The role of support is to prevent that sternoclavicular joint cannot move upward because acromion move upward when shrugging. It will make an incline that is higher in outside and lower in inside. Because shoulder pocket slides inside, it can affect the strength of shrug. Hemispheric glenoid fossa of dead plate can accommodate spherical head of support rod. When shrugging, it drives support rod and moves with it with sliding inside. Dead plate is fixed on thoracodorsal part through double team way using corsage. Corsage is made from double canvas. The inside is coated with thin layer sponge and is fixed with nylon thread gluing.
   (b) Power conduction system is composed of pull wire, movable block and standing valve. Pull wire is brake cable of bicycle. Pull wire is coated with plastic drivepipe in case the slide of pull wire abrase clothes and skin. In the two side of high temperature plastic plate of waist and corsage in the chest, there are standing valves of brake cable. Its role is to prevent stretching tight of pull wire when shrugging so that it is not appropriate to wear inside the clothes. Movable block is fixed in plastic drivepipe in the chest part of pull wire. Its role is to save the force of lifting body limbs. The upper end of pull wire is connected to bayonet of pull wire in oxter of shoulder. The wire penetrates into plastic drivepipe and invert upward bypassing movable block. Out of plastic drivepipe, it is connected with the bayonet on the side wall of corsage. There is ring loop in movable block and there is bayonet in ring loop. Bayonet is connected to pull wire in the below. The below pull wire is fixed on lock cylinder of self-locking system of hip and knee joint of assistive device and lifting leg point of strength above knee joint of walking assistive device when out of plastic drivepipe.
   (c) Self-locking system of assistive device joint: An important part of a walking assistive device of shoulder power includes a upside-down trapezoid metal lock sleeve and a metal lock cylinder compatible with trapezoid metal lock sleeve. The above mouth of trapezoid metal lock sleeve is open, which can contain metal lock cylinder. The below mouth is sealed with a small pore. The upper end of lock cylinder is connected with pull wire of shoulder power. Spring is fixed on the bottom of lock cylinder, which can penetrate the small pore of trapezoid metal lock sleeve and is fixed on the lattice framing of walking assistive device. Its effect is to use the retraction of spring to pull down lock cylinder to complete self-locking. This self-locking system are separately fixed on the hip joint and knee joint of walking assistive device. The above mouth of trapezoid metal lock sleeve is parallel to the axis of knee joint and artificial hip of walking assistive device. Two centimeter above lattice framing knee joint of walking assistive device of leg, the bracket that protrude 5 cm upright forward is installed.

The end of bracket is connected with the terminal of pull wire of shoulder power. Its effect is to increase the arm of force of point of strength to make the patients be easy to lift lower limbs and step forward through shrug. Drop ring lock of hip and knee joint in walking assistive device is eliminated to make hip and knee joint in a free movement state.

After dressing walking assistive device of shoulder power, in standing position, because of trapezoid lock cylinder of self-locking joint, the weight of limbs falling to the ground and traction of spring below lock cylinder can make lock cylinder slide downward in lock sleeve until it fills in the whole lock sleeve in an entirely dead lock condition to support hip and knee joint in an upright position so that the patients can stand still. When walking, the patients shrug actively. The upward force of shrug can lift lock cylinder upward of self-locking system in hip and knee joint through power conduction system. The higher the lock cylinder is lifted, the bigger the space between lock cylinder and lock sleeve is. The motion range of hip and knee joint is increased accordingly. The patients flex hip and knee joint and lift lower limbs. Meanwhile, the patients antevert the body to form stepping forward position. When the patients stop shrug and the lower limbs touch the ground, lock cylinder is on the double inclined plane in trapezoid lock sleeve. The body weight and traction of spring below lock cylinder can pull it down. The longer the lock cylinder descends, the smaller the space between lock cylinder and lock sleeve is. The motion range of hip and knee joint is decreased accordingly. Finally, it is in a dead lock condition. Hip and knee joint is locked extending state. With the help of steel walking assistive device lattice framing, the body weight can be supported to stand still.

The results of comprehensive effect make the patients walk independently. The patients repeat the above process in offside limbs and alternate the two sides until the process of stepping and walking is completed (Figs. 9.21, 9.22 and 9.23).

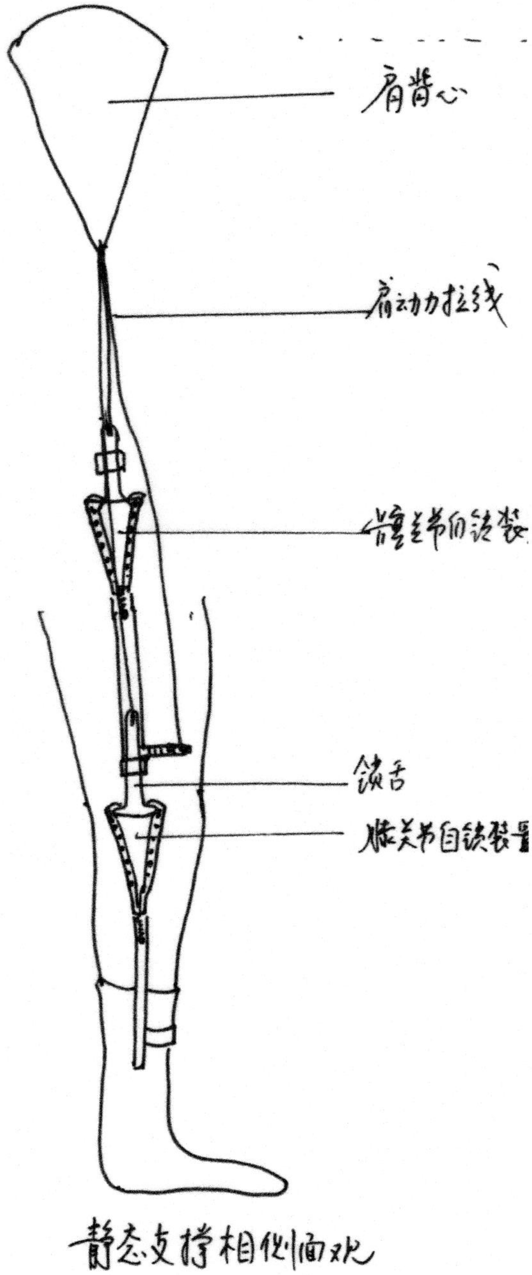

Fig. 9.21 Sketch map of standing position of walking assistive device of shoulder power

3. Clinical indications, contraindications and cautions of walking assistive device of shoulder power
   (a) The patients with high paraplegia should meet the following requirements to use walking assistive device of shoulder power:

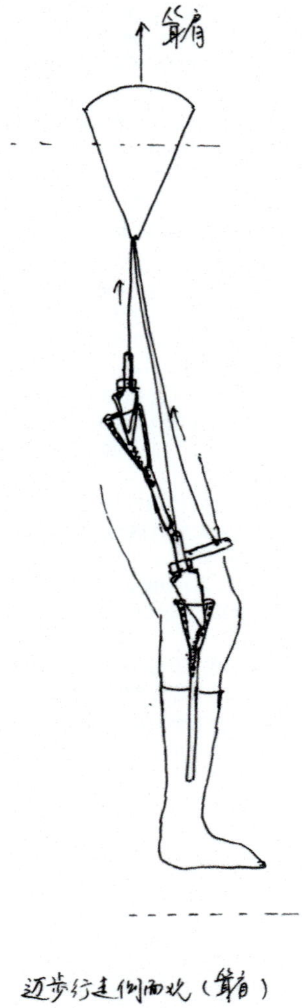

Fig. 9.22 Using shoulder power to lift lower limbs and walking with the help of assistive device

- Shrug force is basic normal.
- The patients are able to shift their weight.
- The patients with paraplegia can use it without hip flexion.

(b) Contraindications:

- The patients with poor cardiovascular stress response or postural hypotension in standing position;
- The patients with unhealed bone fracture or unstable internal fixation;
- The patients with unhealed rib fracture or unhealed soft tissue injury of chest or pelvis

Cautions: Before using this device, the patients should do the training step by step such as standing bed training and development of lower limbs potential and notice the protection in case of falling damage. If necessary, the patients can use axillary crutches, walking stick or personal mobile weight support walking device to help walking for assurance.

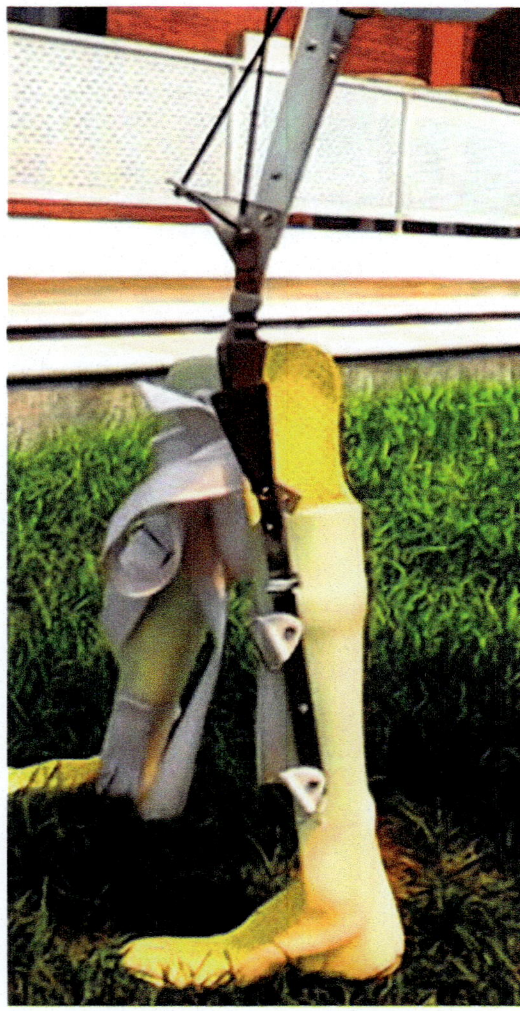

Fig. 9.23 Real products of walking assistive device of shoulder power

References

1. Hongtu W, Dongfeng H, Peng L, et al. AFO early intervention for cerebral apoplexy patients daily living activity and the influence of the quality of life. Chin J Phys Med Rehabil. 2007;29(1):41–4.
2. Maobin W. Rehabilitation of cerebral apoplexy. Beijing: China Science and Technology Press; 2006. p. 212–486.
3. Changshui W, Huaimin G, Jun X. Effects of lower extremity orthopedic therapy on function recovery of stroke patients with severe hemiplegia. Chin J Rehabil Med. 2002;17(3):159–61.
4. Chunjing Y, Jie H, Guorong H. Application of reciprocating gait orthosis in the rehabilitation of patients with paraplegia. Chin J Phys Med Rehabil. 2002;24(1):435–6.
5. Caifeng W, Xiangqian W. Research progress in mechanism of pressure ulcer. J Nurs Sci. 2007;22(1):74–5.
6. Cannon BC, Cannon JP. Management of pressure ulcers. Am J Health Syst Pharm. 2004;61(18):1895–905.
7. Yixia G, Donghong X, Yiming L. The study on the relationship between the time interval and pressure ulcers in subhypothermia treatment of craniocerebral injury. Nurs Res. 2008;22(8A):2024–5.
8. Liping J, En Z, Luo X. Evidence evaluation of supporting tools in the prevention and control of pressure sores. J Nurs Chin. 2009;44(12):1148–50.
9. Tong W, Yong Z, Tao L, et al. Analysis of the effect of ankle foot orthosis on the function of lower extremity of foot droop. Chin Rehabil Theor Pract. 2004;19(1):30–1.
10. Kemin L, Shouchang C, Watanabe K. Orthopedic treatment of ankle dysfunction. Chin Rehabil Theor Pract. 2003;9(6):358–60.
11. Yuanming S, Patriotic C, Xiaoping Y, et al. Prevention of pronation and ptosis in hemiplegia patients. Mod Rehabil. 2000;4(4):590.
12. Hongtu W, Dongfeng H, Peng L, et al. The effect of early AFO intervention on the daily life activity and quality of life of stroke patients. J Chin Phys Med Rehabil. 2007;29(1):41–4.
13. Nan Y, Bingshui W, Ling L, et al. The production and application of dynamic ankle orthotics for adult hemiplegia patients. J Chin Phys Med Rehabil. 2002;24(4):232–4.
14. Xinlu J, Zhenfeng Y, Dawei W. Posterior tibial tendon metastasis is treated with ptosis. Chin Orthopaed Surg J. 2000;7(2):205–6.
15. Lin S, Shumei Z, Jiading Z, et al. Improvement and application of ankle foot orthotics. Chin Rehabil Mag. 2005;20(1):64–5.
16. Dawei Z, Jiankun Y. Effect of fixed ankle foot orthotics on lower limbs. Chin J Rehabil Med. 2006;21(9):829–31.
17. Huaimin G. Progress of walking aid appliances and orthosis on walking training. Mod Rehabil. 2000;4(7):964–5.

10 Rehabilitation Therapy of Neurological Training of Hemiplegia

Hemiplegia is also known as paralysis of half of one's body, which means motor function loss to varying degrees in one side of the body includes the trunk, upper limbs and lower limbs. It is induced by lesion to varying degrees of brain tissue in offside of the hemiplegic side. Ninety percent is cerebrovascular accident hemiplegia. It is the common sequelae of stroke, which includes cerebral thrombosis, cerebral infarction, cerebral hemorrhage and subarachnoid hemorrhage accompanied with central nervous system injury diseases such as cerebral trauma and brain tumor. The morbidity in China is about 0.55%. There are more patients in the North than in the South. There are more male patients than female patients and there are elder patients than adolescent patients [1]. Hypertension, heart disease, diabetes mellitus, hyperlipemia and smoke are risk factors of stroke.

The prognosis of the patients with stroke is related to illness degree, concomitant disease, therapy time, age, physical condition before the disease, the patients' rehabilitation desire and the effect of rehabilitation method. It is reported that in the 6 months after disease, about one to third of the patients recovered hand functions and 70–90% of the patients recovered walking ability, but accompanied with abnormal motor pattern. About 50% of the patients recovered daily life self-help ability and 30% recovered partial working ability. Only 24% of limbs movement functions are recovered to basic normal level.

Clinical observation found that if in 1 month after the disease the patients' finger can complete coordinated flexion and extension movements in full range of joint motion, most of the functions can be recovered to practical hands. If in the early phase after cure the patients in supine position can keep lower limbs at hip flexion position (more than 45°) and knee flexion (90°). There is no plantar flexion of foot and the injured leg doesn't incline to one side. About 90% of the patients can recover walking ability. In the early phase after cure, there is no autonomic movement of the injured leg. If the physiological reflex exists such as patellar tendon reflex and Achilles tendon reflex without obvious pathological reflex, through proper training, most patients can recover autonomic movements, even walking ability.

Epidemiological investigation data demonstrated that in the patients who survive after stroke, about 70–80% are disabled to varying degrees. The patients who cannot take care of themselves account for 42.5%, which bring about heavy burden on the family and the society. Therefore, correct rehabilitation therapy in early phase [2], especially rehabilitation method with good therapeutic effects to promote CNS plasticity and functional reorganization, is of great

W. Zhao, *Rehabilitation Therapeutics of the Neurological Training*,
https://doi.org/10.1007/978-981-13-0812-3_10

significance to motor function recovery of the patients, increase of daily life self-care ability and return to the society maximally.

At present, at home and abroad general applied facilitated rehabilitation technique is used to recover motor function of the patients with stroke, which begins in several days after the disease. In 1–3 months, it can be recovered at the greatest extent. Individual patient's recovery can last more than 1 year, but seldom more than 2 years. In the patients characterized by apraxia, even if the disease time is long, the functions can be further improved through training.

It is generally acknowledged that at present facilitated rehabilitation technique is applied in 6 months after the disease, which is the best opportunity of rehabilitation. Six months later, because there are complications such as amyotrophy, joint adhesion and tendon contracture, it is difficult to obtain obvious functional recovery although rehabilitation training has some help. Therefore, most scholars regarded the 6 months after the disease as the time point of final prognosis.

However, functional recovery in the early phase (during the 6 months after the disease) is not completely the effect of rehabilitation training. Partial functional recovery is achieved through medicine or surgery to eliminate hematoma, decrease intracranial pressure, dredge blood vessels, decrease serum fat, control hypertension and diabetes mellitus. The functions of undead brain cells in injured area are recovered. Therefore, rehabilitation training to recover motor function after CNS damages is the training to recover residual functions and make full use of it.

Clinical practices proved that rehabilitation technique of neurological training whose basic theory and training method are neural potential development, motor program reestablishment and motor pattern remodeling is not restricted by disease time of the patients with stroke. In the patients have been sick for more than 2 year, this method can help to obtain better functional recovery. Therefore, in clinic, we cannot lose confidence of rehabilitation training and functional recovery because of long disease time.

10.1 Dysfunction Type and Rehabilitation Stage of Hemiplegia

10.1.1 Dysfunction Type of Hemiplegia

According to the injured part, range and degree of the patients, the types of dysfunction are different include the symptoms of pyramidal system injury, extrapyramidal system injury and cranial nerve injury.

10.1.1.1 Motor Dysfunction

The manifestations of motor dysfunction are muscle paralysis and increase of reflex tension.

1. Pyramidal system signs: paralysis and atony of limbs to varying degrees.
2. Extrapyramidal system signs: various kinds of involuntary movements, increase of reflex muscle tension, coordinated movement ability and balance function disorder.

10.1.1.2 Cranial Nerve Dysfunction

The manifestations are hemianopsia, facioplegia and bulbar paralysis.

1. Hemianopsia and quadrantanopia: it is induced by injuries of optic radiation and occipital cortex. When there is bilateral occipital lobe lesion, there is cortical blindness, which means vision loss of two eyes induced by bilateral lateral geniculate body, posterior limb of internal capsule, optic radiation or visual cortex of occipital lobe with light reaction.
2. Facial nerve dysfunction: The manifestations are disappearance of frontal line, distortion of commissure and shallow of nasolabial groove due to motor dysfunction of mimetic muscle. The manifestation of supranuclear facial paralysis is dyskinesia of mimetic below palpebral fissure, which can influence pronunciation and diet.
3. Bulbar paralysis includes true bulbar paralysis and pseudobulbar paralysis. Pseudobulbar paralysis is common. The manifestations of it

are disorders of swallowing function, articulation and emotion.

10.1.1.3 Sensory Disturbance

It includes deep sensation disorder (proprioception) and superficial sensation disorder. The manifestations of it are decrudescence or loss of deep and superficial sensation accompanied with hyperesthesia or paresthesia, even severe pain.

10.1.1.4 Speech Disorder

It includes dysarthria and aphasia. Dysarthria is induced by motor muscle paralysis or coordinated movement disorder of articulators. The main manifestations are unclear pronunciation and low volume. Aphasia is due to speech area injury of cerebral hemisphere (dominant hemisphere). The manifestations are loss or disorder of listening, speaking reading and writing ability.

10.1.1.5 Agnosia and Parectropia

Both are the common dysfunctions in stroke, especially in acute phase. Diseased region is in cerebral cortex. Agnosia is the cognition and identification disorder of sensory stimulus with the integrated sensory input system. For example, without visual field deficiency, the patients cannot see objects in left half visual field. With normal vision, the patients cannot distinguish the name and use of what they see and only can tell the shape, but they can tell the name and use once they touch it.

Agnosia includes visual agnosia, tactile agnosia, auditory agnosia, body neglecting, body dysmorphic disorder and anosognosia. Apraxia is that the patients without motor and sensory disorder cannot complete conscious movement, but can do some unconscious movements. For example, the patients cannot execute oral instructions of movements and cannot imitate other's movements such as dressing. The common types include motor apraxia, ideational apraxia, ideational motor apraxia, structural apraxia, dressing apraxia, walking apraxia and verbal apraxia.

10.1.1.6 Other Disorders

Other disorders include mental retardation, mental disorder and sphincter disturbance. When the patients are with dysfunction mentioned above, there are self-care ability losses to varying degrees. Long-term lying in bed can induce apraxia syndrome such as pressure sore, pulmonary infection, tendon contracture, amyotrophy, osteoporosis, postural hypotension, heterotopic ossification, decrease of cardio-pulmonary function and melancholy.

In this chapter, we mainly introduce rehabilitation method to recover motor function of the patients with hemiplegia through neurological training and rehabilitation therapy of other sequelae after CNS injury.

10.1.2 Rehabilitation Stage of Hemiplegia

What is acute phase and recovery phase of stroke and what is early rehabilitation and convalescence rehabilitation? The definition is unclear, plentiful and without single standard. For example, someone deemed that the acute phase is 3 days after stroke. Some reports demonstrated that two weeks after stroke is acute phase. It is generally acknowledged the rehabilitation in 3 months after brain injury is early rehabilitation and convalescence rehabilitation is the rehabilitation after 3 months after stroke.

Hemiplegia has its unique recovery mode. According to the specific pathological process and motor function evaluation after hemiplegia, some reports think that Brunnstrom, the physical therapist in Sweden, suggested in six-phase recovery process of hemiplegia (Table 10.1), phase **I** is acute phase (during 14 days after stroke) and phases **II–IV** are the middle and later phases (after 14 days after stroke).

The patients who are diagnosed and receive therapy in rehabilitation department of specialized rehabilitation hospital are transferred from related clinics such as neurology department, surgery department and department of orthopaedics department in the same hospital or other hospital. Their vital signs are stable after therapy in acute phase. The patients who are transferred from related clinics in the author's hospital have access to clinical departments for early rehabili-

Table 10.1 Six-phase evaluation method of Brunnstrom

Phase	Characteristic	Upper limbs	Hand	Lower limbs
I	No voluntary movement	No movement	No movement	No movement
II	Can induce united movements	Only synergic movement	Impalpable flexion movement	Only seldom voluntary movement
III	Random associated movement	Synergic movement at will	Can be hooked grip, but can not catch food	In sitting and standing position, there is synergic flexion of hip, knee and ankle
IV	Common motor pattern is disrupted and there is separation movement	There are movements separated form synergic movements. In the condition that shoulder is at 0° and elbow flexes 90°, there is pronation and supination of forearm. Shoulder can flex forward at 90° with straight elbow. The arm can touch lumbosacral portion	The patients can hold thumb between the fingers and loose it with half optional extension in a small range	In sitting position, knee can flex more than 90° and foot can slide backward. Ankle can dorciflex when the foot root touches the ground
V	Muscle tension is recovered gradually and there is separation fine movement	There are movements separated form synergic movements. The shoulder can abduct 90° with straight elbow. In the condition that elbow is at straight position and shoulder flexes 30–90°, there is pronation and supination of forearm. In the condition that elbow is at straight position and forearm is at neutral position, the upper limbs can be lifted overhead	Globular and cylinder grabing and grasping. The five fingers can extend at the same time, but cannot extent separately	The injured leg can flex knee at first and then extend hip when the uninjured leg is in standing position. The ankle can dorsiflex when the knee is in extension position
VI	Approximate normal level	Motor coordination approximate normal level. There is no obvious dysmetria when using finger to point nose, but the speed is slower than the uninjured side (less than 5 s)	The patients can complete all the grabing and holding but the speed and accuracy are worse than the uninjured side	In standing position, hip can abduct to the range that the pelvis is elevated. In sitting position, the patients can extort and intort lower limbs with talipes varus and valgus when knee is in straight position

tation training in bedside. Others all enter into convalescence rehabilitation.

Therefore, in department of rehabilitation medicine, according to the classification of acute phase and convalescence phase, targeted rehabilitation training has significance, but there is no actual meaning because there are no patients in acute phase received by rehabilitation department. If the early phase and convalescence phase are classified according to the time point (3 months) in traditional significance, there is still no obvious actual meaning because 3 months after stroke is not the early phase of rehabilitation.

Ultimate goal of rehabilitation of neurological training is recovering normal motor pattern. According to the patients have already got out of bed or not, the classification may be of practical clinical value and guiding significance. Because, under general circumstance, the patients who don't get out of bed are patients in acute phase except some in severe conditions or coma. There is no abnormal motor pattern in these patients because of not getting out of bed. For the patients who already get out of bed and do exercise, most of them are the patients with stable condition after acute phase. However, there is abnormal motor pattern to varying degrees in these patients because the functions of paralytic muscles are compensated by other muscles due to too early or incorrect off-bed activity except case-by-case.

Therefore, the time of off-bed activity is the limit used for rehabilitation phase. It not only can reflex the length of disease time and the severity of the disease after stroke, but also can reflex there is abnormal motor pattern in the patients or not, which has practical guiding significance to the design of rehabilitation therapy schedule and adopted basic rehabilitation method. According to the time of off-bed activity, rehabilitation of neurological training can be divided into "rehabilitation lying in bed" and "rehabilitation off bed".

10.2 Rehabilitation Therapy of Hemiplegia

10.2.1 Rehabilitation Therapy in Bed

10.2.1.1 Definition

Rehabilitation lying in bed in rehabilitation of neurological training means rehabilitation training methods used for the patients who cannot yet get out of bed after stroke or cannot get out of bed due to disturbance of consciousness or severe condition. For discussion, the author called the former convalescence patients lying in bed and the latter severe patients lying in bed.

10.2.1.2 Rehabilitation Therapy

Rehabilitation therapy lying in bed includes rehabilitation therapy in the initial department before entering into rehabilitation department or rehabilitation therapy in rehabilitation department with maintenance treatment such as medicine therapy for hypertension and diabetes mellitus and without follow-up therapy after acute phase. In this kind of patients, most are convalescence patients lying in bed who are stable and want to do rehabilitation training for further functional recovery. Small parts are severe patients lying in bed who are severe and cannot do exercise out of bed, but the vital signs are stable and the internal and surgical therapies are completed.

Therefore, rehabilitation therapy lying in bed is divided into rehabilitation therapy in the early phase of lying in bed and earlier phase before off-bed.

1. Rehabilitation therapy in the early phase of lying in bed takes bedside rehabilitation training as the principal thing, which is suitable for all the patients lying in bed.

   Bedside rehabilitation training can be done without affecting the rescue treatment of the patients. In fact, rehabilitation training can be done as soon as possible, which not only don't affect rescue treatment in acute phase, but also can prevent complications and increase internal and surgical therapeutic effect [3]. It is a pity that at present most of clinical doctors doesn't recognize it so well, which lead to complications and antibiotics abuse. For example, after urinary system infection due to long-term indwelling catheter, large dose antibiotic is usually used to control infection. Long-term bed without joint motion and muscle massage, especially in the coma patients, usually lead to foot drop and joint deformity and tissue adhesion in knee flexion position, which brings about big problem to sequential treatment.

   Rehabilitation therapy in the early phase of lying in bed includes retaining joints in functional position, passive movements and active motor function training.

   (a) Placement of limbs in good limb position and retaining joints in functional position: Good limb position is temporary position from clinical therapy. However, if there is joint contracture in this position, it still affects motor function of limbs. Functional position is the angle and place required for the limbs and joints to play functions. In this angle and place, even if there is joint contracture or joint rigidity, it can still keep the basic functions of the limbs. The purpose of the two positions is to keep the limbs and joints in the position that is good for complication prevention and functional recovery in the future. In the hospitals or departments with good condition, it is best to use retaining appliance of joint in functional position and keep the joint in functional position. At least twice a day, the patients undress retaining appliance of joint in functional position and do active or passive joint motion and muscle massage (10–15 min per time). In the hospitals or departments without retaining appliances, the therapists can use pillow or cushion to keep the joints in good limb position and do active, passive movements of joint and muscle massage.

The placement of limbs in good limb position and retaining joints in functional position are one of the important content in the early rehabilitation of the patients lying in bed.

(b) Position change: The purpose of position change is to prevent pressure sores. In addition, because supine position strengthens extensor, lateral position in uninjured side strengthen flexor in injured side and lateral position in injured side strengthen extensor in injured side. Constant position change can make muscle tension of extensor-flexor in a balanced state. It can prevent spasm pattern to a certain extent (position change per 60–120 min).

(c) Passive movements of limbs and joints: The purpose of passive limb movement and joint motion is to prevent adhesion of joint and soft tissues such as muscle, tendon contracture and joint deformity, which can increase limbs bold circulation, prevent deep venous thrombosis and increase sensory input. It is suitable for the patients with low conscious state or complete or partial loss of limbs active movements.

When doing passive joint motion, whether the patients is conscious or not, six-step Daoyin technique can be used to do active and passive joint motion. For conscious patients, the patients are guided to do regulation of mind and breath and do single joint motion. Anti-resistance training can increase potential development. The patients with low myodynamia who cannot complete joint motion autonomously can adopt auxiliary active joint motion for training. The therapists use Daoyin technique to guide the patients to do regulation of mind and breath with speeches. In the process that the therapists help the patients to do autonomous joint motion, the therapist not only encourage the patients to increase the range of joint motion, but also exert resistance intermittently to induce natural anti-resistance response of the patients' body and make the patients find the signal orientation, which is good for the recovery of autokinetic movement.

For the patients with low conscious state, the patients are guided to do regulation of mind and breath with speeches. After that, in the process of passive joint motion, the therapists exert resistance in the right-about suddenly to induce natural anti-resistance response of the patients and use speeches to encourage the patients to do anti-resistance training in order to promote awakening. The patients are diagnosed with low conscious state in clinic, which doesn't mean they have no deep subconsciousness. For this kind of patients, the therapists should emphasize on massage of muscle and soft tissue.

According to the sequence from proximal end to the distal end of the limb, passive joint motion training should be started from uninjured side and then to the injured side in accordance with range of joint motion in uninjured side. The movement should be soft and slow. The key points are abduction, extortion, protraction, rear protraction and cyclovergence of shoulder joint, elbow extension, wrist and finger extension, abduction and extension of hip joint, flexion and extension of knee, foot dorsiflexion and strephexopodia. There are six time in a trial and two trials a day for each joint. With the improvement of the disease and consciousness recovery, the patients are recovered to do active and passive joint motion by themselves (once a day).

(d) Mechanical device is used to do passive joint motion. In a certain motion range, continuous passive motion can drive joint to do passive joint motion is a certain time through mechanical transmission continuously, which can prevent joint adhesion, promote blood backflow, relieve limb edema, prevent ankyloses and relieve pain, improve range of joint motion and decrease bedside complications [4].

Application method: according to the tolerance condition of the patients, one cycle is 1–2 min and the movement time is 1 h (1–3 times a day). According to the specific condition of limbs dysfunction, different kinds of CPM can be used for passive motion of upper limbs, lower limbs, wrist, hand and ankle joint.

(e) The application of vapour-pressure type blood circulation driver: for the long-term bed patients, because they lose the ability of the muscle contraction to push the blood back to the heart, blood flow is slow and visible component of the blood can precipitate and attach to the vascular wall. It develops gradually and the thrombus is formed finally. Blood backflow is obstructed and there is edema of distal limbs. Once the thrombus fall off, there may be pulmonary vascular embolism and cerebrovascular embolism, even mortal danger. For long-term bed patients, if rehabilitation training is not done timely, the occurrence of deep venous thrombosis of lower limbs is 40–70%.

There are many types of vapour-pressure type blood circulation driver. The best function is to squeeze muscle belly. Gasbag pressure is 8–12 kPa (60–90 mmHg) in upper limbs and the time is 12–15 min. Gasbag pressure is 10.7–14.7 kPa (80–110 mmHg) in lower limbs and the time is 15–20 min. There are two times a day and 7–10 days in a therapy course. If there is no adverse reaction, it can be used for a long time.

(f) Physiotherapy: The purpose of interventional therapy of physical agent is to relieve pain, increase blood circulation of limbs, alleviate edema, relieve spasm and increase tension of paralytic muscle. The main methods are far infrared ray, medium frequency electrotherapy, interference electricity, laser, kerotherapy, ultrashort wave, decimeter wave, centimetric wave and millimeter wave, medical massage, traction.

(g) Active movement training: Retaining limbs in functional position, turning over and passive joint motion can prevent pressure scores and contracture of soft tissue and joint, but they cannot prevent apraxia syndrome such as apraxia amyotrophy and cannot promote CNS function recovery directly. Therefore, active movement training should be done as soon as possible.

In principle, if the patients are conscious, with stable vital signs and the disease condition is not aggravated progressively, this training can be done. For the stroke patients with mild symptoms and without disturbance of consciousness, active movement training can be started with vital signs (breathing, blood pressure, pulse and ECG) monitoring in the second day after stroke. The training should be progressive and be started with low amount of training. According to the disease condition and tolerance degree of the patients, the amount of training can be increased or decreased gradually.

The purpose of active joint motion training is to develop CNS potential, promote undead brain cells to recover function in CNS injury zone, induce autonomous muscle contraction and joint motion. It is suitable for the conscious patients with incompletely lost autokinetic movement of limbs.

According to neural development, sequential training should be done for better recovery of motor function. The recovery sequence of motor function of the trunk is the trunk, shoulder girdle and pelvic girdle in sitting position, knee standing position and walking. The recovery sequence of motor function of the limbs is from proximal end to distal end. Because functional recovery of ankle joint, toe and thumb takes a long time and are difficult.

The main content of active movement training is as follows:

Turning over training in bed: it is the basic functional training of the trunk. The patients cross fingers, extend upper limbs, lift it forward and extend to the lateral. During turning over, crossed hands extend to the turning over side and the flexed legs swing to this side until the patients are in lateral position. The patients go back to supine position and then turn over to the other side. There are several time in a day and the trainer should help the patients as needed. During turning over, the head should turn to the turning over side firstly.

Bridge-style movement: its purpose is to training hip extension. The patients are in supine position, flex two legs, use foot to step on the bed, lift hip for a while and put it down slowly (double bridge-style movement). If the patients can easily complete double bridge-style movement, the patients suspend leg in uninjured side, only flex injured leg, use foot to step on the bed and lift hip (single bridge-style movement). In the early phase of training, is necessary for the trainer to help the patients to fix injured leg and stimulate thigh contraction to complete the movement.

Leg lock movement: the purpose is to train intorsion and adduction of injured hip to prevent extorsion gait of injured leg in walking. The patients are in supine position, flex two legs, use foot to step on bed and separate two knees in extorsion position. The patients actively fold two knees. Meanwhile, the trainer exert resistance on uninjured leg of the patients to prevent intorsion and adduction in order to induce intorsion and adduction of injured leg through associated movement. If the patients can easily complete the movement, the patients can extend leg in uninjured side and only do intorsion and adduction training of injured leg.

Sitting position training: sitting position is the easiest position to be completed by the patients and is the necessary movement to prevent postural hypotension, standing, walking and daily life movement. Because postural hypotension usually occur in the elder and long-term bed patients, when the patients are in sitting position for the first time, they are inappropriate to sit up-right (90°). The trainers can use standing up platform or back rest and are sequentially in 30°, 45°, 60° and 80° sitting position. If the previous position can be maintained for 30 min and there is no obvious postural hypotension, the patients can transmit to the next position. If the patients can be maintained in 80° sitting position for 30 min and the vital signs are stable, there is no postural hypotension when the patients are in sitting position.

Sitting position training includes sitting position balance and tolerance training. During the process of balanced training, endurance can be increased. This training should be better if there is no support and assistance.

In static balanced training, the patients are required to sit on the bed or chair without support and flex hip joint, knee joint and ankle joint in 90° flexion position. If the foot cannot step on the ground, the trainers can use pedal or low stool to keep it in 90° dorsiflexion position. The space between the two feet is as width as the shoulder and the hands are on the knees. The trainers adjust the trunk and head of the patients to the center and loose their hands when they don't exert force. The patients are required to keep in this position as long as possible. The trainers can use count method to encourage the patients. When the patients' bodies incline to one side, the trainers require the patients to adjust their body back to home position. If the patients cannot do this, the trainers should help them.

If the patients meet the requirements of static balanced positions, balanced training in dynamic sitting position can be started. the patients cross fingers and move forward, backward, left, right, upright and downward with center of gravity. If the patients can keep balance on the condition of sudden push or pull, it demonstrates that the patients are able to keep balance in sitting position and they can do endurance training in sitting position.

During the process of sitting position training, transition training between sitting position and lying position helps the patients to sit up by themselves. This training includes sitting up from uninjured side and sitting up from injured side.

Sitting up from uninjured side: The patients are asked to turn over to the uninjured side, flex upper limb in uninjured side below the trunk of uninjured side, hand two legs down the bed, rise head and the trunk to injured side, use upper limbs in uninjured side to support the trunk and sit up with the trunk in 90° neutral position.

Sitting up from uninjured side: The trunk rotates to semipronation. The upper part of the body straighten to uninjured side and upper limbs in uninjured side support the trunk to sit up. This movement is opposite with the movement from sitting position to lying position. It is more difficulty to sit up from injured side than to sit up from uninjured side.

(h) Bedside rehabilitation training of neurological training: In the rehabilitation training in bed, neurological training technique is used to do bedside rehabilitation training. Because the sensitivity of neurological training instrument is high, it can detect very weak motor program signal. It not only can set surpassing goals for the patients' training, but also can increase therapeutic interests to motivate rehabilitation confidence and desire of the patients.

Single channel is usually used in the training. The therapists use Daoyin technique to guide the patients to give out signal to agonistic muscle of movable joint. Neurological training instrument can display this signal on fluorescent screen in curve form. After explaining the significance and functions of this signal to the patients, the therapists use this signal intensity as a standard and mark it in a transverse line that is the surpassing goal of the next training of the patients. The therapists use new signal intensity as a baseline and guide the patients to surpass it. The rest can be done in the same manner. The patients can recover functions in carefree training.

According to specific condition of motor dysfunction of the patients, the therapists can design training schedule. The main training is the training of agonistic muscle but not the proportion of motor program signal.

There are 30 min in one training (once a day) and there are 30 times in a therapy course.

(i) The training of virtual reality: Cooperated with virtual reality training instrument of neurological training of guiding collaterals through meridians, the method is the same as rehabilitation training of neurological training. It is best to do the training accompanied with neurological training instrument. Virtual reality can make the patients know the actual conditions of motor program and instruct the training. The defect that the actual motor program signal cannot be increased for a long time and can affect therapeutic enthusiasm of the patients can be compensated by virtual reality training.

In the virtual reality training in bed, there are 30 min in one training (once a day) and there are 30 times in a therapy course. One of the key points of training lying in bed is to prohibit the patients to walk out of bed in case of abnormal motor pattern.

2. Rehabilitation therapy in the early phase of off-bed: it means preliminary training before overall training that the patients with stable disease condition are ready to do in rehabilitation hall, which includes the patients with consciousness and disturbance of consciousness.

Through further medicine therapy and rehabilitation training lying in bed, the disease condition of most patients is stable and functions are recovered to a certain extent. According to the disease condition, this part of patients can be divided into three types.

(a) The patients with consciousness and partial recovery of motor function: This kind of the patients usually is diagnosed with slight brain injury. For this kind of patients with hypertension and diabetes mellitus, if the therapy is in time and proper with symptomatic medicine, they can be maintained in basic normal level. Although there is motor dysfunction of limbs in one side, the active movements can still be maintained to a certain extent, physiological reflex exists in physical examination and pathological signs are not obvious or slight.

(b) The patients with consciousness but obviously or completely motor dysfunction of limb in one side: This kind of the patients usually is diagnosed with severe brain injury. For this kind of patients with hypertension and diabetes mellitus, even if they are treated with symptomatic medicine, they cannot be maintained in basic normal level. The patients are conscious but with cognitive, speech, emotional and mental disorders. The myodynamia of limb in hemiplegic side is very weak or zero. It is usually with severe muscle spasm, obvious hyperfunction of physiological reflex and obvious pathological signs.

(c) The patients with unconsciousness: It is usually seen in the patients in coma after severe brain damage. It can be developed to low conscious state (vegetative state).

According to training procedures and requirements of neurological training, regardless of the type of the patients, they all should do neural potential development training that includes CNS potential of upper limbs, lower limbs and the trunk. Because the training intensity is strong, cardiovascular stress response ability must be increased before this training to keep enough blood supply of tissues and organs in order to prevent postural hypotension effectively. Therefore, the increase of cardiovascular stress response ability is the main content of rehabilitation training in the early phase of off-bed.

(a) Standing bed training: long-term in bed can lead to a series of problems such as pressure scores, urinary and digestive system functions disorders, hypostatic pneumonia, osteoporosis, amyotrophy and muscle apraxia. The leading problem is the decrease of cardiovascular function. When the body position of the patients is changed, blood gravity can easily lead to insufficient blood supply of brain tissue and there will be orthostatic hypotension, even shock.

The research demonstrated that in standing position, most of capacity vessels are below the heart plane. If a person stands still, the veins in lower part of the body are expanded and they content 400–600 ml blood than that in lying position, which can lead to blood volume redistribution among different organs. It can decrease temporary returned blood volume and central venous pressure. Cardiac output is decreased 25% in standing position than in lying position. Finally, blood pressure is decreased and there are a lot of symptoms.

Normally, the reason why people cannot have postural hypotension is related to cardiac muscle contraction and squeezing action of skeletal muscle to blood vessel in movement. The contraction effect of cardiac muscle: The stronger the cardiac contraction is, the more completely the ventricle evacuate after cardiac ejection. The more obviously the intraventricular pressure decreases in diastolic phase, the bigger the effect of promoting blood flow of atrium and vena cava are. Squeezing action of skeletal muscle: in walking, alternative contraction of muscles in lower limbs squeeze intramuscular veins and veins between muscles to accelerate blood flow in vein. Valves of veins in lower limbs make the blood only flow to the heart. Therefore, skeletal muscle and vein valve make the blood flow back to heart. The effect of muscle pump is important for decreasing lower limb peripheral venous pressure in standing position and blood retention in veins in lower limbs. For example, when the person stand still, venous pressure in foot is 12 kPa (90 mmHg) and decreased below 3.3 kPa (25 mmHg). In running, muscle pump of lower limbs can squeeze several litres of blood per minute. In this case, muscle pump of lower limbs accelerates blood circulation of the whole body to some extent and pumps the blood back to heart. However, if rhythmic relaxation and contraction of the muscle is not normal, constant tonic contraction can press veins continuously and decrease returned blood volume.

The tonicity of venous blood wall in long-term bed patients is low, the expansibility is high, the myocardial contractility decreases and contraction power of abdomen and lower limbs' muscle weakens. After that, the squeezing effect on veins is weakened. When the patients are from horizontal lying position to standing position suddenly, blood retention in lower limbs can decrease return blood volume and induce blood pressure drop, even faint. The normal people squat for a long time and stand up suddenly, which can lead to insufficient blood supply of brain such as dizziness and seeing the stars.

The leading function of standing bed is keeping the patients in 0–90° passive standing position through mechanical device. It is the preliminary training of doing other rehabilitation training.

The mechanism of standing training: when the people stand up, blood gravity make the blood accumulate in lower limbs and return blood volume is decreased, which stimulate baroceptor of internal carotid sinus and arcus aortae, decrease inhibitory impulse from these areas to vasomotor center and induce excitability increase of adrenergic sympathetic nerve reflexively. The content of noradrenaline in blood are increased, which lead to arteriole contraction and heart rate increase. In addition, baroreceptor of blood vascular system is stimulated after venous passive congestion and then induces vasoconstriction, tension increase and isometric contraction of muscle in lower limbs, which make the blood flow back to heart and stop the sudden decrease of cardiac output. These mechanisms can increase cardiovascular stress ability and there is no obvious blood pressure decrease in standing position.

In standing position, the broken ends of fractured bone, normal bones and joint surface are pressed, which are good for calcareous deposit, regeneration of osteocytes and bone reconstruction. The researches demonstrated that with the increase of pressure stress, piezoelectric effect is increased. When stress level of fracture end is coordinated with stimulation of histological differentiation, it can promote fracture healing.

The method of standing bed training: Standing bed includes automatic and manual types, but their functions are the same. There are several points that should be paid attention to:

Step-by-step principle: The patients are transferred from supine position to standing bed. The safety belt is fixed, lifting button of standing bed is pressed or the standing bed is elevated manually. The therapists should observe the patients' reaction. When the patients feel discomfort, the patients should stop the training and decline gradually until there is no any discomfort.

The standing training should be done under electrocardiograph monitoring. For example, if the patients are in a critical condition, especially for the severe patients who just start to do this training, the training should be done under electrocardiograph monitoring to keep safe.

The effect of active training can be increased. For the patients with consciousness and stable condition, the therapists instruct the patients to slightly flex knee joints intermittently in standing in order to make themselves stand up, which can promote CNS plasticity.

According to the specific condition of the patients, standing angle and time are increased gradually.

There are 1–2 trainings in a day (30 min per time). If the patients cannot hold on, they can rest for 1–2 times (5 min per time).

When the patients can stand up erectly (900) for 30 min without discomfortableness and vital signs are normal, the goal of standing bed training is achieved. Stronger training items such as potential development can be done.

(b) Vapour-pressure type blood circulation driver: Because vapour-pressure type blood circulation driver can replace muscle contraction to promote blood back to heart and increase return blood volume and contractility ventricular muscle.

In rehabilitation training of lying in bed, the patients are forbidden to do exercise out of bed, which is the important measure to prevent abnormal motor pattern. The patients who can receive standard rehabilitation training in the early phase, the rate of functional recovery is high and disability rate is low. Moreover, except for the patients with severe brain damage, motor pattern of most patients can be recovered to normal level, which is good for increasing the patients' life quality, returning to family, work and society.

10.2.2 Rehabilitation Therapy Out of Bed

Rehabilitation therapy out of bed is for the patients who can do exercise out of bed. This part of patients includes the patients who don't do exercise out of bed through rehabilitation training of lying in bed. These patients mostly come from associated departments of the hospital and complete rehabilitation training of lying in bed according to training schedule, but don't do exercise out of bed. This part of patients also includes the patients who already do exercise out of bed without doing rehabilitation training of lying in bed. These patients mostly come from associated departments of other hospitals or society and don't receive standard rehabilitation training, but they start to do exercise out of bed.

Because these patients' conditions are stable and cardio-pulmonary function are normal, the can tolerant strong rehabilitation training. Because the former don't do exercise out of bed, there is no abnormal motor pattern. The main goal of rehabilitation training is to recover normal motor pattern directly. The training time is short, the therapeutic effect is good and there is no abnormal motor pattern. Because the latter already do exercise out of bed with abnormal motor pattern to varying degrees, the main goal of rehabilitation training for these patients is to rectify abnormal motor pattern and then remodel normal motor pattern. The training difficulty is big and takes a long time. It is hard to recover normal motor pattern without orthotic assistance device. In the early phase, correct rehabilitation method is adopted for training in case of abnormal motor pattern and has an important effect on recovering and reestablishing normal motor pattern.

10.2.2.1 Functional Assessment of Rehabilitation Training Out of Bed

Detailed and correct functional assessment is the basis of formulating anticipated rehabilitation goal, ascertaining entire rehabilitation principle and specific rehabilitation schedule, which can directly influence the effect of rehabilitation training.

1. Detailed functional assessment is used to find the main dysfunction point.

   There are two kinds of functional assessments: The first is the assessment of survival capability after dysfunction. This kind of assessment method accounts for the most of functional assessments such as ability of daily living (ADL), Brunnstrom functional assessment and so on. This kind of method usually uses comprehensive abilities as assessment indicators such as clothes, going to toilet and walking up and down stairs. These methods can reflex comprehensive abilities of the patients that are good for identification of degree of disability and assessment of therapeutic effect. Therefore, the therapists can know the effectiveness of these methods. However, because this kind of assessment cannot explain the cause of motor dysfunction of specific muscle, it is difficult to design targeted rehabilitation therapy schedule according to this. The second is the assessment of dysfunction cause and degree. Whether the patients are severe or not and whether motor dysfunction is severe or not, abnormal motor pattern was formed. It is necessary to do detailed assessment. Under general circumstance, not all the muscles are paralyzed in paralytic limbs. The cause of abnormal motor pattern is usually one or several paralytic muscles. If there is no detailed functional assessment, it is hard to find out the main obstacles of abnormal motor pattern and therapeutic schedule is blind. Therefore, the purpose of rehabilitation training is not specific. The normal training not only wastes time, but also affects training effect.

   For the formulation of therapeutic schedule, the functional assessment methods that can ascertain the cause of motor dysfunction and abnormal motor pattern are more valuable in clinic.

   One of external manifestations of CNS injury is motor dysfunction. The method to recover CNS functions through promoting CNS plasticity is achieved through recovering autonomous muscle contraction, single joint motion and limbs movement. Therefore, if the therapists can definitely evaluate muscle functions, single joint motion and the entire motor function of the trunk and limbs, it can help to formulate rehabilitation therapy schedule and is the most valuable assessment item. It is not the functional assessment method that us only suitable for therapeutic effect evaluation.

For the condition of motor function, Lovett MMT muscle test, range of motion (ROM), motor program signal intensity and proportion exam, balance function assessment, spastic degree assessment of muscle and gait assessment, cognitive and speech function assessment are usually used. In addition, the entire body function conditions should be evaluated such as vital signs, visceral functions, nutrition condition and emotion, therapeutic alliance.

For example, a patient with right cerebral hemorrhage and left hemiplegia walk with circle gait and the main obstacles of the patients are paralysis of tibialis anterior muscle and peroneus longus and brevis muscle induced by injury of right brain tissue that dominates these muscles. A patient with left cerebral hemorrhage and right hemiplegia walk with circle gait and the main obstacles of the patients may be paralysis of hip flexor induced by injury of left brain tissue that dominates these muscles.

The main obstacle provides basic situation for formulating specific therapeutic schedule, which is good for all the rehabilitation therapy items that can be used in one point such as tibialis anterior muscle or hip flexor in order to increase therapeutic effect and save therapy time.

2. Establishing the types of motor function for formulating anticipated rehabilitation goal and overall rehabilitation principle.

   In order to formulate specific rehabilitation goal and principle, the motor function of the patients can be divided into three types.

   (a) The type of the patients who don't do exercise: This type includes the patients who don't do exercise out of bed and are transmitted from rehabilitation training in early phase. Therefore, although this kind of patients is with motor dysfunction to varying degrees, there is still no abnormal motor pattern. This kind of patients includes ordinary type of motor dysfunction and severe type of motor dysfunction. Ordinary type: after rehabilitation training of lying in bed, motor function of limbs is recovered to a certain extent, muscle spasm degree is no more than grade II and there is no obvious mental retardation and affective disorder. This kind of patients account for a great portion and the prognosis is good. Severe type: the patients are diagnosed with severe motor dysfunction. There is no autokinetic movement of limbs accompanied with severe muscle spasm and cognitive disorder. Muscle spasm degree is more than grade II. This kind of patients account for a small portion and the prognosis is not good.
   (b) Localized type: Motor dysfunction of this kind of hemiplegic patients is slight, usually localized in one joint motion or the patients feel fatigue, sore or discomfort in limbs. The patients cannot complete individual movement such as squat completely or stand up after squatting. There is no obvious abnormal motor pattern in this kind of patients and the prognosis is good after training.
   (c) The type of abnormal motor pattern: The disease history of this kind of patients is long. The patients are those who walk out of bed without standard rehabilitation training or walk too early or incorrectly after rehabilitation training with abnormal motor pattern in different degree and types. The common abnormal motor pattern includes hemiplegic gait (circle gait and drag gait) and myasthenic gait (tibialis anterior muscle gait, quadriceps femoris gait and gluteus maximus gait).

The muscle spasm degree is uncertain and there may be chicken hand and genu recurvatum in severe patients. This kind of patients is divided into ordinary type of motor dysfunction and severe type of motor dysfunction. The prognosis of ordinary type is better. Severe type requires a longer time and functional recovery is not good enough.

10.2.2.2 Establishing Anticipated Rehabilitation Goals and Overall Rehabilitation Principle

1. Ascertaining rehabilitation goal to fight for better therapeutic effect: through detailed functional assessment, the therapists find out the main functional obstacle of the patients and formulate individual anticipated rehabilitation goal according to the actual condition of the patients. This goal is a comprehensive possible result according to dysfunction part, degree, cognitive condition and the effect of rehabilitation method of the patients and is the internal material for rehabilitation staff, but not the goal that definitely will be achieved. Therefore, the therapists don't need to tell the patients and their family the goal as the definite therapeutic effect.

   Therefore, according to the degree and type of motor dysfunction of individual patient, cognitive dysfunction degree and general physical condition, anticipated rehabilitation goal is formulated through comprehensive analysis.

   (a) The type of the patients who don't do exercise: This type includes the patients who don't have abnormal motor pattern and may recover motor function through standard three-stage rehabilitation training of neurological training. Ordinary type: the patients have good functional recovery after the third stage of rehabilitation method training of neurological training. In the premise that there is no obvious cognitive dysfunction, rehabilitation goal may be to recover independent ambulation and self-care. If there is cognitive dysfunction, the effect can be influenced. Severe type: Degree of brain injury of the patients is severe accompanied with cognitive and emotional disorder. Motor function of limb in hemiplegic side is almost lost, there is no autonomous muscle contraction, physiological reflex disappears and pathological signs are positive. This kind of the patients is not suitable to receive three-stage rehabilitation method training of neurological training, because they are difficult to recover the degree required for the third stage of rehabilitation training. This kind of patients recovers partial functions through comprehensive training. During the process of potential development, they start to do abnormal gait rectification weight support walking training. The training is difficult and requires 2–3 therapists to help the patients to complete walking training. Moreover, at the end they need assistance device such as walking assistance device, foot tray or crutch to stand and walk. Therefore, anticipated rehabilitation goal of this kind of patients should be formulated according to the specific condition of the patients. Generally, after rehabilitation, with the help of assistance device, the patients are able to stand independently and walk.

   (b) Localized type: Because the dysfunction of this kind of patients is slight and it only affect single joint (slight strephenopodia) or the fatigue of limbs is the major manifestation, they have good functional recovery through rehabilitation training of neurological training. Therefore, for this kind of patients, rehabilitation goal is to recover motor function to normal level without cognitive dysfunction.

   (c) The type of abnormal motor pattern: The disease history of this kind of patients is long. They have abnormal motor pattern to varying degree although they are able to stand and walk with assistance or independently. Ordinary type: The patients' abnormal motor pattern is slight, which is induced by foot drop or circle gait due to strephenopodia, genu recurvatum due to increase of extensor tension. This kind of abnormal motor pattern is restricted to one or two groups of muscle. Rehabilitation training is easy and anticipated rehabilitation goal is to rectify abnormal motor pattern and gait to normal level with the help of foot tray to prevent foot drop or talipes varus and valgus. Severe type: the abnormal motor pattern of this kind of patients is severe accompanied with various kinds of abnormal motor pattern. For example, abnormal motor pattern such as circle or carrying basket is usually accompanied with gluteus maximus gait, which is the stretching the chest and expanding the belly posture due to myasthenia of hip extensor or wiggly duck gait due to paralysis and fatigue of gluteus medius. The disease condition of this kind of patients is complicated and the therapy time is long. Anticipated rehabilitation goal is to rectify abnormal motor pattern effectively and improve walking ability obviously through assistance device after training.

2. Establishment of overall rehabilitation principle to realize anticipated rehabilitation goal: Overall rehabilitation principle is the major principle of rehabilitation for anticipated rehabilitation goal but not specific rehabilitation training schedule and method according to individual dysfunctions and general physical condition. According to the common abnormal motor pattern of hemiplegic patients, from the view of reestablishing normal motor pattern, the adopted overall rehabilitation principles are different.

   With recovering functions as much as possible, recovering normal motor pattern is the final rehabilitation goal. In the premise of this, according to practical functional condition and requirements, overall rehabilitation principle to realize rehabilitation goal includes four aspects: three-stage rehabilitation training method principle; movement coordinated training principle; training principle for different disease; training principle to recover main functions.

   Individual overall rehabilitation principle is formulated according to the final rehabilitation goal that is to recover normal motor pattern. Prevention and rectification of abnormal motor pattern is the premise of reestablishing. Three-stage training method of neurological training is standard training procedure of reestablishing motor pattern.

   The formulation of overall rehabilitation principle is based on this combined with appropriate adjustment and flexible application of individual dysfunction of the patients.

   (a) The type of the patients who don't do exercise: Ordinary type: Typical three-stage rehabilitation method is adopted for training. Severe type: rehabilitation principle of standing in early phase and recovering walking is adopted. During the process of implementing the first and the second stage training, the patients can do the third stage rehabilitation training. The principle of children is rehabilitation principle of standing in early phase and walking development.
   (b) Localized type: Atypical three-stage rehabilitation principle is adopted. On the basis of potential development and proper adjustment of motor program, the motor pattern remodeling training in the third stage is done.
   (c) The type of abnormal motor pattern: Ordinary type: typical three-stage rehabilitation method principle is used to do the training sequentially. Severe type: rehabilitation principle of standing in early phase and recovering walking is adopted. During the process of implementing the first and the second stage training, the patients can do the third stage rehabilitation training. The principle of children is rehabilitation principle of standing in early phase and walking development.

10.2.2.3 Formulating and Implementing Rehabilitation Therapy Schedule According to Overall Rehabilitation Principle

According to overall rehabilitation principle based on the individual condition of the patients, corresponding rehabilitation training schedule is formulated and put into practice. After therapeutic schedule, it is forbidden for the doctors to show no interest in the patients and for the therapists to implement it by them. The results don't meet the therapeutic requirements of the schedule. Moreover, the doctors should participate in actual rehabilitation training and explain the mechanism of rehabilitation therapy of neurological training to the patients. The doctors organize the exercise therapists in every therapy group to do the training in allusion to the main obstacles and pay attention to timely adjustment of therapeutic schedule, which can obtain anticipated therapeutic effect.

1. The type of the patients who don't do exercise includes the patients who cannot do exercise out of bed through rehabilitation training of lying in bed. It includes ordinary type and severe type. The therapeutic schedule is as follows:
   (a) Ordinary type: the training should be done restrict according to three-stage rehabilitation method, which is the training of neural potential development, motor program reestablishment and motor pattern remodeling. What calls for special attention is that the implement should be strict. It is forbidden to walk in the first stage and the walking is restricted in the second. In the third stage, the training should be done in the motor pattern molding instrument and transmitted to natural movement without help. If three-stage rehabilitation training is implemented actually, the patients' function can be recovered to the normal level.
   (b) Severe type: the symptom of this kind of the patients is severe and there is usually no autokinetic movement of limbs. If the training is done according to three-stage method, the therapy time is long and the anticipated goal is difficult to be achieved. The principle of standing in early phase and recovering walking or the principle of standing in early phase and walking development for child cerebral palsyis adopted in the training. During the process of implementing the first and the second stage training, the patients can do the third stage rehabilitation training. The practice has proved this method is good for recovery of motor function and consciousness of the patients. The principle of standing in early phase and recovering walking is the rehabilitation policy according to choosing the less of two evils. Through compulsory assistance walking, the patients can recover walking ability to a certain extent, but the motor pattern is not always normal. Compulsory assistance walking is better than standing and walking inability in decreasing complications and increasing life quality effectively.

According to rehabilitation training of standing in early phase and recovering walking or standing in early phase and walking development, the specific training method is the same.

(a) Potential development training: this training is particularly suitable for the severe patients with disturbance of consciousness. Potential development training device of upper limbs, lower limbs, and the trunk and tibialis anterior muscle is used for the training. Weight support system of the device is adjusted to support the patients' body weight. The weight loss should not be too big in case pectoral girdle oppresses the thorax and then affect breath. Because this kind of patients cannot cooperate with therapy actively, it requires two therapists or the family and nursing workers to do this training. There are 1–2 times a day (30 min per time) and there are 30 times in a therapy course.

Cautions: before training, the patients must do standing bed training. When they can stand erectly for 30 min with normal vital signs such as breath and blood pressure, the patients can do this training. Sudden position change is used to induce autokinetic movement, which plays an important role in this training. Because this kind of patients cannot cooperate with the training actively, self-potential cannot be developed if the training is done with the help of others. During the process of assistance, the therapists suddenly reduce assistance force for a while and use Daoyin speech to encourage the patients to overcome the drop of their position when the patients' position is decreasing such as "stand up, or you will fall down!". Self-response of the patients is activated to develop neural potential.

For the severe patients who cannot complete the training full time, the training time can be shortened or they can have 1–2 breaks during the training.

(b) Motor pattern remodeling training: In actual, passive or assistance walking training is done. Abnormal gait rectification weight support walking training device is used in the training. After the weight is adjusted, the therapists sit on plate in the front of training device, put training shoe cover on the ankle of paralytic lower limbs, tell the patients to step forward using uninjured lower limbs and move the training device forward. Daoyin technique is used to guide the patients to try to step forward using injured limbs. If the patients cannot complete it autonomously, the therapists help the patients to step forward using lower limbs. The rest can be done in the same manner and the patients can increase walking ability gradually (Fig. 10.1).

The walking training can be done when lower limbs can step forward. There is one time a day (30 min per time) and there are 30 times in a therapy course. The training can include many therapy courses.

(c) Motor program reestablishment training: the purpose of this training is to use neurological training instrument to receive motor program signal induced by joint motion and anti-resistance training of the patients. This signal is marked in transverse line and the patients can use this line as the surpassing goal to do repeated training. They can see their own progress that is good for enhancing rehabilitation confidence and interest. Position change can be used to induce motor program signal. For example, standing up and squatting can induce the drive signal from brain to quadriceps femoris.

There are 1–2 times a day (30–50 min per time) and there are 30 times in a therapy course.

(d) Physical exercise therapy of neurological training includes active joint motion induction, passive joint motion and loosening soft tissue adhesion. There are 1–2 times a day (45 min per time) and there are 30 times in a therapy course. The training can include many therapy courses.

In addition, CPM is used to do constant passive joint motion to prevent adhesion of joint and soft tissue. Physiotherapy such as medium frequency, interference current, far infrared and ultrashort wave are used to increase blood circulation of local tissue and promote metabolism.

For the patients with muscle spasm in paralytic limb, tendon contracture, joint and soft tissue adhesion, skin traction and manipulation loosen are used for therapy.

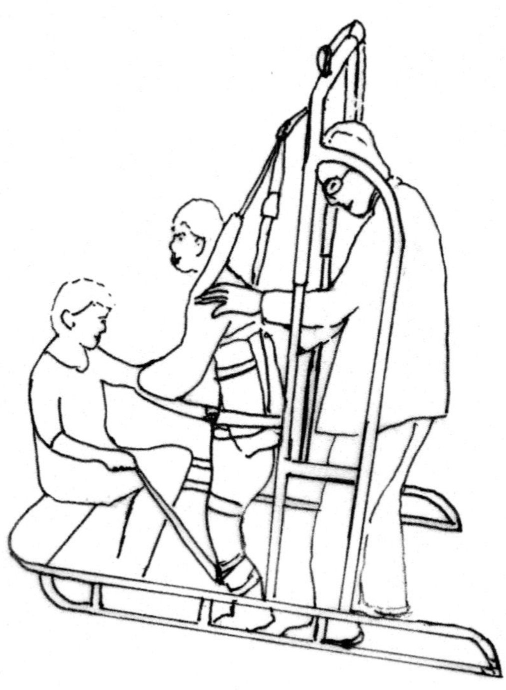

Fig. 10.1 Walking training of severe hemiplegic patients

2. Localized type includes the patients with local dysfunctions. For this kind of patients, atypical three-stage rehabilitation method is training principle. After a short time training of potential development and motor program reestablishment in dysfunction parts such as lower limbs with foot drop and tibialis anterior muscle, motor pattern remodeling training can be started. If there is no abnormal motor pattern, the walking should not be restricted.
   (a) Physical exercise therapy of neurological training: Bare-handed operation method of six-step Daoyin technique in traditional Chinese medicine is used. The therapists adopt proper position according to the muscle, usually supine position and sitting position. Excitatory anti-resistance of agonistic muscle and relaxation of antagonistic muscle are the main training. During training, manipulation massage is used to loosen the adhesion of muscle and soft tissue.

   There are 1–2 times a day (45 min per time) and there are 30 times in a therapy course.
   (b) Potential development training: According to the dysfunction part of the patients, corresponding potential development training is selected. Because there is certain muscle contraction ability of the patients, during potential development training, the therapist can exert resistance to increase the effect of potential development training that should be guided by Daoyin technique.

   There are 1–2 times a day (30–45 min per time) and there are 30 times in a therapy course.
   (c) Motor program reestablishment training: Under the guidance of animation light-spot blink indicator system of main and collateral channels guiding collaterals through meridians, neurological training instrument is used to receive and display the motor program signal form brain to agonistic muscle and antagonistic muscle real-timely. Through establishing target line with different altitude, the patients are guided constantly to increase signal intensity of agonistic muscle and decrease signal intensity of antagonistic muscle. During the process of developing central neural potential and increasing myodynamia, motor program of normal single joint motion can be reestablished. When the myodynamia is no less than grade **III**, motor program reestablishment training of associated movement can be done such as walking and grasping.

   The training mentioned above can be cooperated with virtual reality training instrument and it is better to be applied with neurological training instrument. Not only the therapists can know exactly the specific condition of motor program and guide the patients to instruct the training, but also it can overcome the defect that actual motor program signal cannot be increased for a long time and easily affect the therapeutic enthusiasm of the patients.

   There are 1–2 times a day (50 min per time) and there are 30 times in a therapy course.
   (d) Motor pattern remodeling training: Because the symptoms of this kind of patients are slight, when the myodynamia of the patients' dysfunction muscle is no less than **III** and agonistic muscle motor program signal intensity is no less than 160 μV, the training can be done. Meanwhile, the training of potential development and motor program reestablishment can also be done.

   There are 1–2 times a day (50 min per time) and there are 30 times in a therapy course. The patients can receive therapy courses repeatedly.

   In addition, other methods or physiotherapy such as massage, myodynamia enhancement training, ascending and descending the stairs training and middle frequency electrotherapy can be added to the training.

   The therapy course is 1 month. After one therapy course, the therapists evaluate the effect and do the second therapies course if necessary, but new therapeutic schedule should be formulated.

3. The type of abnormal motor pattern includes the patients who do exercise out of bed with abnormal motor pattern. According to the severity of abnormal motor pattern, it is divided into ordinary type and severe type. However, because this kind of patients can do joint motion actively, the adopted therapeutic schedule all are three-stage rehabilitation method. The differences between ordinary type and severe type are training time and assistance instrument.
   (a) Ordinary type: typical three-stage rehabilitation method is the principle for training. The training method is the same as the ordinary type of the patients who don't do exercise out of bed. Because there is abnormal motor pattern in the patients, especially the patients who have been sick for a year or more with solidified abnormal motor program, it is difficult to rectify it. Due to the limitation of hospital stay and family economic capability of the patients, the patients cannot stay in the hospital for a long time. Therefore, orthosis assistive device is used to rectify abnormal position of joint, which is good for abnormal motor pattern rectification and therapy time shortening.

   The common abnormal motor pattern of ordinary type of the patients is hemiplegic gait. Hemiplegic gait is usually due to parapysis of tibialis anterior muscle, especially paralysis of peroneus longus and brevis muscles. The paralysis of these muscles leads to foot drop and strephenopodia and then induce circle gait in walking. There are some difficulties in rectification therapy of hemiplegic gait. The first reason is that it is difficult to recover autonomous innervation of this muscle and it takes a long time. The second reason is that even if the functions of muscle innervation, strephexopodia and foot dorsiflexion in sitting position are recovered, but there is still strephexopodia or foot drop for a long time in walking. This is because the motor program of associated movement cannot be rectified and solidified. Under this condition, foot tray is temporarily used to rectify strephexopodia, which is good for the rectification of abnormal motor pattern. Motor program of associated movement can be reestablished in the second therapy course. The comprehensive results can shorten therapy course and get twofold results with half the effort.
   (b) Severe type: except abnormal motor pattern of limbs, the patients are accompanied with abnormal motor pattern of pelvis, the trunk and upper limbs. Because numerous abnormal motor patterns are hard to be rectified at the same time, on the basis of adopting three-stage rehabilitation training method, according to specific condition, the training time of every stage can be prolonged and the method of treating partial abnormality and rectifying partial abnormality through orthosis assistive device is used, which can decrease the therapy difficulty. For example, back bracket is made to rectify abnormal motor pattern of the trunk and motor pattern remodeling training device of upper limbs is used to make upper limbs swing coordinately. The key point is the rectification of abnormal motor pattern of lower limbs and it is easy to obtain training effect. After that, the patients can figure the uncoordinated motor problem of upper limbs.

   Skin traction and joint mobilization are the common methods to loosen adhesion of bone joint and muscle. For the therapy of tendon contracture, standing bed training, manipulation release and shake release of tremor equipment are used to loosen tendon contracture on the basis of heating (far-infrared irradiation and kerotherapy).

For severe joint deformity with a certain tenacity such as flexion deformity of knee joint, after it is loosened to a certain extent, plaster support fixation is used to keep the position and new loosen therapy is used on the basis of this in case joint retraction after therapy and during evening sleep affects therapeutic effect. If the range of joint motion is further improved, plaster support is re-made to fix limbs and joints until joint motion is loosened to functional position or maximally.

10.3 Solutions to Some Common Problems

10.3.1 Rehabilitation Method of Neurological Training of Zero Myodynamia

In clinic, zero myodynamia assessed from hand feeling is not equal to zero motor program signal, which is far on behalf of the total necrosis of central nervous cells that dominate the muscle. For limbs in the hemiplegic side with physiological reflex and unconspicuous pathological reflex, through training, most patients can recover autonomous motor function to a certain extent.

There is myospasm and pathological signs in paralytic limbs. Through a series of training such as potential development, it is possible to recover some functions and it takes a long time.

10.3.2 The Therapy of Myospasm

10.3.2.1 Functional Recovery of Motor Neurons in High Level Is the Fundamental Measure for the Therapy of CNS Myospasm Induced by CNS Damage

Myospasm is the syndrome of abnormal increase of muscle tension induced by CNS damage and is one kind of motor dysfunction due to excitatory increase of myotatic reflex. Spasm degree is positively correlated to stretch speed of the muscle.

Myotatic reflex is reflex contraction due to muscle traction induced by external force. Its reflex arc is located in spinal cord and the pathway is simple but controlled by higher center. When spinal cord is out of control, myotatic reflex is reinforced. Any motor neuron from brain cortex to spinal cord is damaged, which can lead to muscle spasm. The nature of spasm is different because of different injury part, but all spasms are induced by higher motor neuron injury. Therefore, the effective method to alleviate muscle spasm due to CNS injury is to recover functions of higher motor neuron.

In clinic, spasm is usually induced by stroke, cerebral palsy, brain trauma, disseminated sclerosis and spinal cord injury. The common myospasm pattern of hemiplegic patients are as follows (Table 10.2).

Spasm is a pathophysiological status, which can affect motor function of limbs and daily life ability to varying degrees. Movement resistance is increase to make the voluntary movement difficult to complete. Fine movement is difficult. Increased resistance leads to bradykinesia, movement control difficulties. Therefore, it is difficult to complete fine movement. The movement is uncoordinated. Energy consumption is huge and there may be accidents such as tumble and bruise. Abnormal motor pattern can affect gait and daily life activities.

Clinical therapy of muscle spasm due to CNS injury is difficult, but there are many therapy methods such as posture and position control, physiotherapies such as cold therapy, hydrotherapy, thermotherapy and electric stimulating therapy, orthosis and medicine such as dantrolene and baclofen, neural dissolution technique of peripheral nerve, chemical denervation technology (injection of botulinum toxin type A on motor point), selective posterior rhizotomy (SPR), tendon elongation and neurotomy and kinesitherapy. Kinesitherapy is to training antagonistic muscle of spasm muscle in order to decrease spasm degree through interactive inhibition. For example, active and anti-resistance contraction of triceps muscle of arm can be done after spasm of bicipital muscle of arm. EMG biofeedback training is to train antagonistic muscle of spasmodic muscle. In addition, Bobath, Rood and PNF technique are used to inhibit spasmodic pattern passively.

However, because the methods mentioned above are lack of the function of recovering higher motor neuron. The therapeutic effect is not ideal and it is necessary to explore new therapy method further.

Table 10.2 Typical myospasm pattern in hemiplegic patients

Part	Pattern	Manifestations
Head	Spasm in injured side	Head flex to injured side and face to uninjured side
Trunk	Spasm in injured side	The trunk lateral flex and rotate back
Upper limbs	Flexor pattern	Shoulder joint adduct and intort, flexion of elbow and wrist, flexion of elbow joint and forearm supination
Wrist-hand	Flexor pattern	Wrist joints flex and incline to ulnar side, fingers flex and adduct and thumbs flex and adduct
Lower limbs	Extensor pattern	Pelvis in injured side rotate back, lift hip joint, flex, adduct and intort it, flex and inverse knee joint
Ankle	Extensor pattern	Plantar flexion, strephenopodia, flex and adduct toe

Table 10.3 Improved Ashworth method for assessment of myospasm

Grade	Signs
1	Muscle tension is increased slightly and there is resistance suddenly in 50% of the range of joint motion. After that, there is minimum resistance after 50% of the range of joint motion
II	Muscle tension is increased obviously. Most muscle tensions are increased obviously in the range of joint motion, but the involved part can do passive motion easily
III	Muscle tension is increased severely and it is hard to do passive motion
IV	the involved part is in contracture state when in passive flexion and extension and cannot move

Table 10.4 Modified improved Ashworth method for myospasm assessment

Grade	Signs
I	There is suddenly slight reflexive myodynamia in the 50% range of joint motion. The reflexive myodynamia disappears with the increase of range of joint motion
II	There is strong reflexive myodynamia in most range of joint motion, but the involved joint can still do passive motion
III	There is strong reflexive myodynamia in most range of joint motion and the involved joint is difficult to do passive motion
IV	There is reflexive contracture in full range of joint motion. The involved joint is in contracture state and cannot move when in passive flexion and extension

10.3.2.2 Assessment Method of Myospasm

In clinic, the common assessment method of myospasm is improved Ashworth method. Muscle reflex contraction angle induced by passive flexion and extension of joint is the basis to evaluate the severity of myospasm. The smaller the joint motion angle of muscle reflex contraction is, the more severe the spasm is. The detailed assessment standard refers to Table 10.3.

Myotatic reflex is reflex contraction due to external traction of muscle, which is different from muscle tension. Muscle tension is the tensity of muscle in static relaxed state, which is the basis to keep various posture of the body and normal movement. Examination method is to touch the hardness of the muscle. Under normal circumstance, there is no obvious resistance of joint in passive motion.

In the improved Ashworth method for myospasm assessment, muscle tension is used to show the muscle contractility of myospasm induced by myotatic reflex, which is easily to be confused with the concept of normal muscle tension. Therefore, muscle tension of myospasm should be expressed as reflexive myodynamia to differentiate them distinctly. According to this principle, improved Ashworth method for myospasm assessment refers to Table 10.4.

10.3.2.3 Rehabilitation Therapy of Neurological Training of Myospasm

Myospasm induced by CNS injury is the result of higher central nervous injury. According to the mechanism that skillful use and dependence can promote brain plasticity and functional reorganization, rehabilitation method of neurological training is used to train normal central nervous cells. Through active movement, normal central nervous cells around injured area are trained and reserved conduction pathway is activated to reestablish motor program and then treat myospasm. There is some certain therapeutic effect after clinical application.

1. Neural potential development training is the training in allusion to spasmodic muscle to recover higher motor neuron function and conduction pathway.
   (a) Potential development training device is applied for the training: according to spasmodic part, regulating collaterals through meridians or normal six-step Daoyin technique is used to guide the patients to do neural potential development training of spasmodic muscles in upper limbs, lower limbs or the trunk. The specific method is the same as that in potential development training of spasmodic muscle.

   There is 1–2 times a day (30 min per time) and there are 30 times in a therapy course. The therapists reevaluate the results after one therapy course. The patients can do the training repeatedly.
   (b) Physical exercise therapy of neurological training: Daoyin technique is used for active movement, anti-resistance and relaxation training of spasmodic muscle. During the process, manual massage is used to loosen adhesion of muscle and soft tissue.

   There are 1–2 times a day (30 min per time) and there are 30 times in a therapy course. The therapists reevaluate the results after one therapy course. The patients can do the training repeatedly.
2. Motor program reestablishment: Contraction degree of agonistic muscle and antagonistic muscle is adjusted. Spasmodic muscles are mainly trained. In upper limbs, the training muscle usually is flexor, which means the training of elbow flexion, wrist flexion and finger flexion. In lower limbs, the training muscle usually is extensor, which means the training of hip flexion, knee extension, foot dorsiflexion and strephexopodia.

   According to the method of reestablishing motor program of single joint, receiving electrode of motor program is placed. Six-step Daoyin technique in traditional Chinese medicine of regulating collaterals is used to guide the patients to do active joint motion and to try to do anti-resistance. Motor program signal from brain to agonistic muscle and antagonistic muscle is received and displayed in a curve form. The signal is marked as transverse line. Daoyin technique is repeatedly used to encourage the patients to surpass the original goal and reestablish normal motor program. The effect of the training includes two aspects.
   (a) Development of central nervous potential: Daoyin technique and the training of surpassing goal constantly under anti-resistance condition are used to gradually develop the number of central nervous cells that dominate spasmodic muscle, increase the quality of developed central nervous cells to replace injured central nervous cells in order to alleviate muscle spasm.
   (b) Actual motor program training with direct vision: it can effectively regulate disordered motor program and reestablish it. Disordered motor program is one of the reasons of joint motion stagnation, and myospasm. Therefore, motor program reestablishment training can alleviate muscle spasm to a certain extent. There are 1–2 times a day (50 min per time) and there are 30 times in a therapy course. The therapists reevaluate the results after one therapy course. The patients can do the training repeatedly.

3. Motor pattern remodeling training is the training to increase movement flexibility and practical application ability.
   (a) Disintegrated movement training is the training that disintegrate an entire limb movement into several movements according to the sequence of joint motion to decrease the difficulty of limb movement and recover the entire movement ability of limbs gradually. Disintegrated movement of drinking through holding a teacup: the patients sit on a chair and put upper limbs on the desk. In front of them, there is a teacup. The therapists ask the patients to relax and do disintegrated movement training according to the sequence of shoulder joint protraction, elbow extension, grasping teacup and elbow flexion. The patients are asked not to overexert and to make joint motion orderly (Fig. 10.2a–c). Disintegrated movement training of walking: The patients relax mind and body, and stand up. The space between two feet is as wide as shoulder. The patients use upper limbs in the offside of the trained leg to grasp handrail in case of falling down and nervousness. After that, the patients do the following disintegrated movement:

Stepping forward: The training is done according to the sequence of hip flexion, knee flexion, foot dorsiflexion and heel landing (Fig. 10.3a–c). The patients firstly flex hip and make lower limb step forward, flex knee slightly, dorsiflex foot and then step downward to make the heel touch the ground.

Bearing load: at the position of heel landing, the training is done according to the sequence of hip flexion, knee flexion, foot dorsiflexion and foot flat landing (Fig. 10.4a, b). The patients firstly flex hip and make lower limb step forward, flex knee slightly, dorsiflex foot and then step downward in the lateral midline of the trunk to make the foot flat touch the ground.

Driving leg: at the position of bearing load, the training is done according to the sequence of hip flexion, knee flexion, foot dorsiflexion,

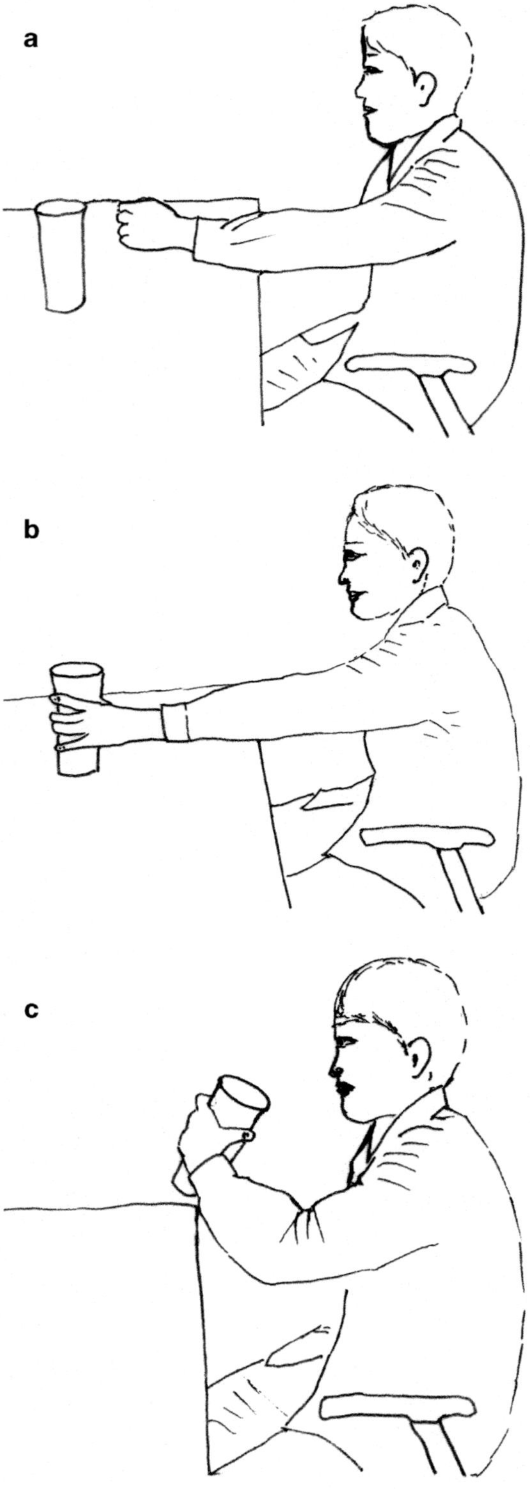

Fig. 10.2 (**a**) Drinking water through holding a teacup 1 (upper limbs protraction). (**b**) Drinking water through holding a teacup 2 (grasping a teacup). (**c**) Drinking water through holding a teacup 3 (grasping the handle of teacup)

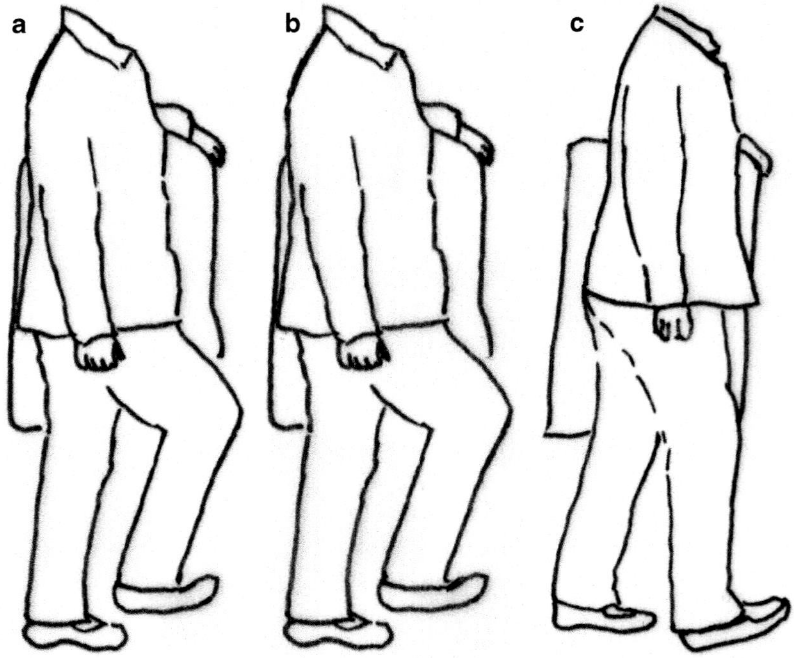

Fig. 10.3 (**a**) Stepping forward 1 (lifting lower limbs). (**b**) Stepping forward 2 (foot dorsiflexion). (**c**) Stepping forward 3 (heel landing)

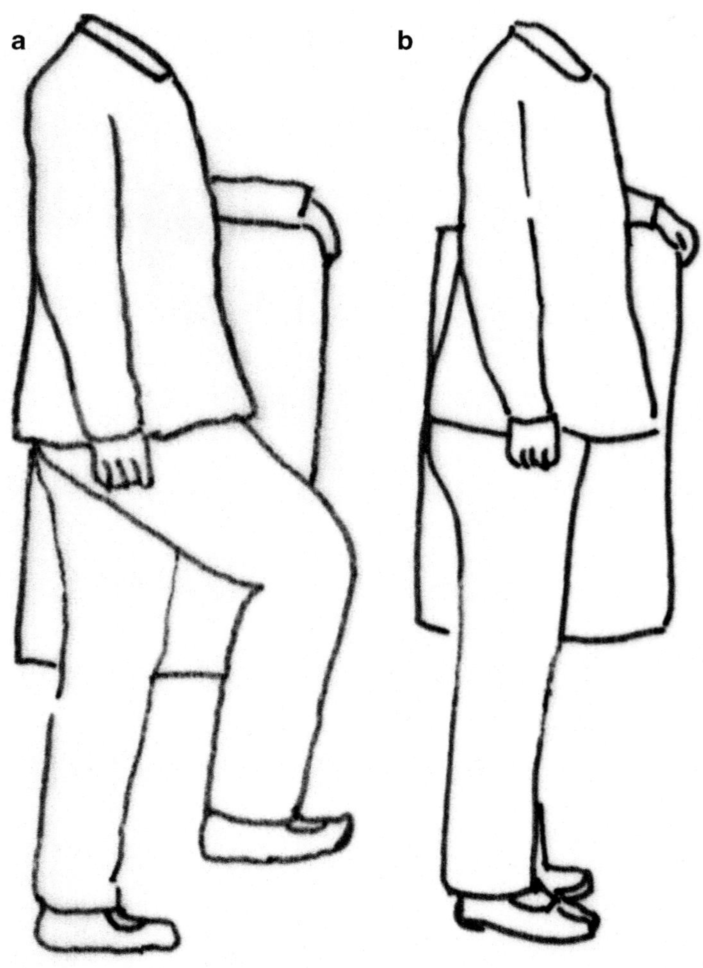

Fig. 10.4 (**a**) Bearing load 1 (lift lower limbs upward). (**b**) Bearing load 2 (foot flat landing)

toe landing and driving leg (Fig. 10.5a, b). The patients firstly flex hip and make lower limb step forward, flex knee slightly, dorsiflex foot and extend hip to make lower limb step backward, go across the lateral midline of the body, step backward in half step and make toe touch the ground like driving leg.

According to the principle mentioned above, the therapists can design different types of disintegrated movement training schedule according to the actual dysfunction of the patients. There is 1–2 times a day (30 min per time) and there are 30 times in a therapy course. The therapists reevaluate the results after one therapy course. The patients can do the training repeatedly.

(b) The integrated motor pattern remodeling training: lower limbs can be trained with the help of abnormal gait rectification weight support walking training device and upper limbs are trained with the help of upper limbs motor pattern remodeling training device. They can be separately used or used at the same time to recover the coordination of upper and lower limbs movement. Through using training, the control of central nerve to lower central nerve is recovered and finally muscle spasm is relieved. There is 1–2 times a day (45 min per time) and there are 30 times in a therapy course. The therapists reevaluate the results after one therapy course. The patients can do the training repeatedly.

4. Other therapies include the therapy methods such as traction to relieve myospasm, massage and physiotherapy.

(a) Skin traction: Small dose constant skin traction has a certain effect on relieving adhesion and contracture of muscle, tendon and other soft tissues. It can be done at night, which can figure out the problem that the therapists' manipulation loosen time is limited and traction in daytime affects other rehabilitation trainings.

The dose of skin traction is 3–5 kg. The time of one therapy course is 2–3 week. In the traction, the therapists should observe the patients at any time in case of skin pressure ulcer and affecting blood circulation.

(b) The application of temporary orthosis: through manipulation and traction, spasmodic muscle and adhesive tissue are partially loosened. In order to prevent retraction of spasmodic muscle at evening sleep, plaster support, macromolecule fiber orthosis and plastic orthosis are used to fix it temporarily. With the persistence of the therapy, the improvement of spasm and the increase of range of joint motion, new temporary fixator should be changed timely to keep therapeutic effect.

The application time of temporary orthosis should depend on the recovery degree of range of joint motion. When the range of joint motion is recovered to the possible maximum, the next therapeutic measures such as auxiliary autonomous joint motion, medicine, functional orthosis and surgery are decided according to actual situation. When tendon contracture or joint adhesion cannot be loosened effectively and myospasm cannot be relieved, which can affect motor function greatly, selective posterior rhizotomy can be applied.

(c) Physiotherapy: Thermotherapies such as infrared, kerotherapy and microwave can inhibit myospasm. Cold therapy such as long time cold compress and soaking in ice water can inhibit spasm. Because the elder is intolerant to the cold and cold has bad effect on the angiocarpy and kidney, it is not suitable for the elder. Electrical stimulation includes spasmodic muscle stimulation, antagonistic muscle stimulation and functional electrical stimulation. Low frequency electric stimulation is mainly used to induce intense muscle contraction and the muscle enters into refractory period, which can relieve spasmodic muscle. The refractory period sometimes lasts several hours. The effect of functional electrical stimulation is the best.

The therapies mentioned above can be done once a day (2–3 kinds of therapies a

Fig. 10.5 (**a**) Driving leg 1 (lift lower limbs backward). (**b**) Driving leg 2 (toe landing and driving leg)

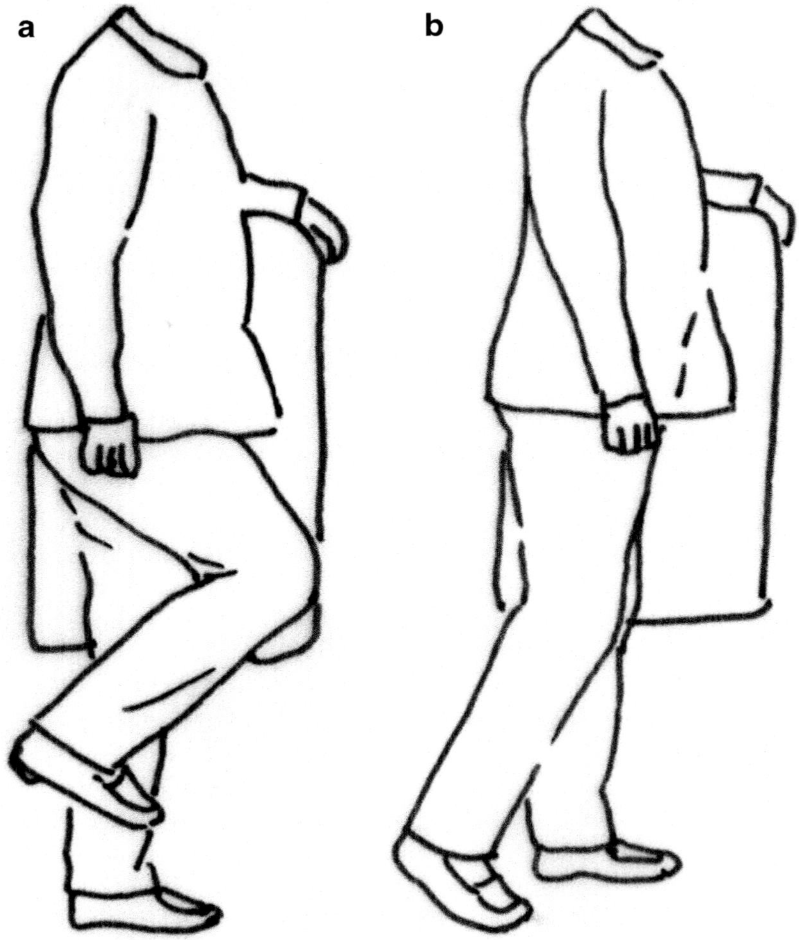

day) for three weeks according to the specific condition of the patients.

(d) Massage and acupuncture: massage and manipulation can loosen adhesion of muscle and soft tissue. Acupuncture can relieve muscle spasm to a certain extent.

The therapies mentioned above can be used as support measures of active movement training to improve the effect of active movement training. If they are used alone, the effect of relieving muscle doesn't last long. Only if higher CNS functions are recovered, muscle spasm due to CNS injuries can be relieved at last.

References

1. Zhaosu W, Chonghua Y, Dong Z. Epidemiological study of stroke morbidity and mortality in Chinese population. PLoS. 2003;24(3):236–9.
2. Dinghua F, Maobin W, Dameng H, Hu DM, et al. A study of early rehabilition of stroke. Chin J Rehabil Med. 2001;16(5):266–72.
3. Yongshan H, Yulian Z, Peijun Y, et al. The effects of early rehabilitation on motor function in hemiplegics after stroke. Chin J Rehabil Med. 2002;17(3):145–7.
4. Xiaohong W. The application of the continuous passive active activity trainer (CPM) in the lower extremity of the lower extremity in clinical rehabilitation. Chin Foreign Med Res. 2011;9(36):161–3.

Rehabilitation Therapy of Neurological Training of Facial Paralysis

11

11.1 Main Dysfunctions of Facial Paralysis

11.1.1 Pathogenesis and Dysfunction Characteristics of Facial Paralysis

Facial paralysis is vulgo of facial neuritis and facioplegia, which is also called Bell disease [1]. It is non-purulent inflammation of facial nerve, which usually occur in winter and spring. The pathological change is neural edema, degeneration of myelin sheath and axon to varying degrees. The patients are recovered to varying degrees in 2 months after disease attack and some patients are recovered 1 year later. Some got persistent sequelae.

1. Causes: Facial neuritis can be induced by various factors.

   Facial neuritis usually is induced by cranial nerve diseases. This may be because facial nerve canal is a long bony pipeline. If petrosal bone develops abnormally, there usually is facial nerve canal stenosis, which is the internal pathogenic factor of facial neuritis. The external pathological factor of facial neuritis remains unclear. The early pathological change is edema of facial nerve, degeneration of myelin sheath and axon to varying degrees. The reason may be that cold air blast induces nutritional microvascular spasm of facial nerve and then lead to ischemia and anoxia of local tissue. Someone think that it is related to virus infection [2]. However, until now, no one can isolate virus. In recent years, some reports think that it may be a immunoreaction. Ramsay-Hunt Syndrome is induced by infection of herpes zoster virus and inflammation of geniculate ganglion and facial nerve.

   In short, the factors that can affect functional nucleus of facial nerve and neural axon functions can lead to dysfunction of facial muscles dominated by them such as infectious, compressive, traumatic, physical and neurogenic factors.

   Infectious factor accounts for 42.5% of the total number. It is the herpes zoster virus in dormant state, which usually hides in sensory ganglion of facial nerve. The virus is activated when local immunity is low. It can also be induced by inflammatory diseases such as meningitis, mumps, influenza, scarlet fever, malaria, multiple cranial neuropathy, local infection and otogenic infection (otitis media, labyrinthitis, mastoiditis).

   Compressive factor can induce facial neuritis, which is usually observed in tumors such as acoustic neuroma, parotid gland and primary acquired cholesteatoma and accounts for 5.5% of the total number.

   The common traumatic factors of facial paralysis include temporal bone fracture, facial trauma, surgery and injection of

W. Zhao, *Rehabilitation Therapeutics of the Neurological Training*,
https://doi.org/10.1007/978-981-13-0812-3_11

neurotoxic drug in facial nerve distribution area and account for 8.2% of the total patients.

Neurogenic facial paralysis accounts for 13.5% of the total patients, which is usually induced by cerebrovascular disease, encephalic and non-traumatic neurogenic disease. If cold wind blows the face for a long time, undercooling in face can directly stimulate local nerve trophic vessels and induce spasm, which can induce ischemia and edema of neural tissue and dysfunctions. It is the common factor to induce facial paralysis.

In addition, poisoning, metabolic disturbance such as diabetes mellitus and vitamin deficiency, vascular function insufficiency and congenital facial nucleus hypoplasia is one of the pathological factors.

2. Types: Facioplegia is divided into peripheral type and central type. The majority is peripheral type.
   (a) Central type is paralysis of muscle in lower part of the face on the offside of lesion induced by injury of supranuclear tissue includes cortex, cortex and brainstem fiber, medullary triangle and pons, which are usually observed in cerebrovascular disease, brain tumor and encephalitis.
   (b) Peripheral type is paralysis of all facial muscles in the ipsilateral of the lesion induced by injury of facial nerve nucleus or facial nerve, which is usually observed in catching cold, ear or meninx infection, peripheral facioplegia induced by neurofibroma. In addition, there is dysgeusia in the front two third of tongue and unclear speaking.
3. Dysfunctions mainly are motor and sensory dysfunctions of facial muscle.

   According to the motor dysfunction part of facial muscle, there are different clinical manifestations such as palpebral fissure enlargement, unable to frown or close eyes, forehead wrinkle disappearance, grinningly, agitating cheek and unable to whistle. There are also clinical manifestations such as forehead wrinkle disappearance, palpebral fissure enlargement, nasolabial groove becoming shallow, droop, stretching face to offside, lacrimation or salivation.

   The dysfunctions are different in different injured part of facial nerve. It can be summarized as follows:
   (a) Facial nerve branch below stylomastoid foramen is injured, which can induce peripheral facial paralysis. The main manifestations are forehead wrinkle disappearance in injured side, unable to crinkle forehead and frown, palpebral fissure enlargement, unable to close or close incompletely, Bell syndrome (eyeball rotate upward and outside when closing eyes and white sclera is exposed), nasolabial groove becoming shallow, corner of the mouth skews to uninjured side, corner of the mouth deviate to uninjured side when exposing teeth, air leakage in agitating cheek or whistle, food retention in teeth buccal space when eating.
   (b) Facial nerve branch above tympanic cord is injured. Besides peripheral facial paralysis, there is dysgeusia in two third front of tongue in the ipsilateral.
   (c) Facial nerve branch above stapedius is injured. Besides peripheral facial paralysis and dysgeusia in two third front of tongue in the ipsilateral, there is hyperakusis.
   (d) Geniculate ganglion is injured. Besides peripheral facial paralysis, dysgeusia in two third front of tongue in the ipsilateral and hyperakusis, there is pain in mastoidea, hypaesthesia of auricle and external auditory canal, herpes of external auditory canal or tympanic membrane, which is called Hunt syndrome [3].
4. Sequelae: Facial dysfunction still exists half a year after the disease.

   The main signs include no raising eyebrow movement or incomplete raising eyebrow movement, incomplete opening eyes, corner of the mouth going upward when raising eyebrow, stretching the corner of the mouth when closing eyes, eyes becoming small when agitating mouth (synkinetic movement of mouth and eye), shallow nasolabial groove, facial stiffness, food retention, tears, secondary prosopospasm and denervated muscle atrophy.

Sequelae are due to delay of the illness or improper therapy method. Some reports deem that half a day after attach is the best therapeutic opportunity. Nerve in injured side is not recovered timely, which lead to incomplete conduction of neural impulse or conduction generalization. In addition, some sequelae are due to irreversible injury of facial nerve.

11.1.2 Functional Assessment Method of Facial Paralysis

International functional assessment methods of facial paralysis are House-Brackmann assessment method and Portmann simple measuring scale.

1. House-Brackmann assessment method [4] is divided into six grades (Table 11.1).

   Assessment standard of therapeutic effect of House-Brackmann: six grades assessment standard of facial nerve of House-Brackmann facial nerve are as follows:

   - Grade I: Normal.
   - Grade II: There may be slight asymmetry in the facial movement functions and slight synkinetic movement.
   - Grade III: There is obvious asymmetry and secondary defect, but there is still movement in frontal part.
   - Grade IV: There is obvious asymmetry, but there is no movement in frontal part.
   - Grade V: There is merely slight movement in the face.
   - Grade VI: the paralysis is complete and there is no movement. The higher the grade of House-Brackmann is, the better the functional recovery of facial nerve is.
2. Portmann score: The full mark of this score is 20.
   (a) Specific assessment method: Simple assessment method of Portmann includes six autokinetic movements such as frown, closing eyes, moving wing of nose, smiling, whistle and blowing cheek. The scores of movement in injured side and uninjured side are 3. The score is 2, which stands for weak movement. The score is 1, which stands for slight movement. The score is 0, which stands for autokinetic movement inability. In addition, there are 2 score for impression. The score of completely normal is 20. Scoring scale refers to Table 11.2.
   (b) Portmann assessment standard.
   - Completely recovery (more than 17).
   - Partially recovery (16–14).
   - Just good (13–10).
   - Bad (less than 9).

The lower the score is, the more severe the disease is.

11.2 The Mechanism and Method of Rehabilitation Therapy of Facial Neuritis

11.2.1 The Mechanism of Rehabilitation Therapy of Facial Neuritis

Facial muscle includes orbicularis, masticatory muscle and mimetic muscle, which are the same as muscles of the trunk that are controlled by motor center of brain cortex. They can generate voluntary movement. Therefore, promotion of CNS plasticity [5] and functional recovery, activation of reserved conduction pathway are suitable for recovering lost motor functions after injuries of functional nucleus of facial nerve or facial nerve fiber.

In clinical therapy, there is usually of voluntary autonomous movement of facial muscle, which is neglected because they are not obvious as joint motion. The therapeutic methods usually are passive methods such as medicine, physiotherapy, acupuncture, massage, sunken cord and surgery in the late phase.

Although the potential ability of neural fiber (nerve trunk) is not so good as functional nucleus of central nerves, they also have reserved conduction pathway, because one nerve trunk includes many neural fibers. In addition, there is

Table 11.1 House-Brackmann functional assessment form of facial paralysis

Grade	Dysfunction degree	Percent of normal function (%)	Normal condition	Clinical symptoms		
				Rest	Movement	Secondary defect
I	None	100	The function of facial muscle is normal	The function of facial muscle is normal	The function of facial muscle is normal	The function of facial muscle is normal
II	Slightly	99–75	Mild myasthenia after close examination	normal Symmetry muscle tension	Forehead movement is partially normal or completely normal. Closing eyes is normal regardless of the force	There is slight facial synkinetic movement. There is no conbundleure or spasm of face in paralytic side
III	Slight and medium	75–50	There is significant but non-disfigured difference between two sides and there is no functional impairment. There is usually non-severe synkinetic movement, conbundleure and (or) spasm of face in paralytic side.	normal Symmetry muscle tension	There is slight or no forehead movement and there is asymmetry when closing eyes with force	There is obvious non-disfigured synkinetic movement. There is conbundleure or spasm in Grade III. There is voluntary movement in Grade II
IV	Medium and severe	50–25	There is obvious inability and (or) disfigured asymmetry	Normal Symmetry muscle tension	There is slight or no forehead movement. The patients cannot close eyes with force. There is symmetry movement in corner of the mouth	There are spasm and synkinetic movement in Grade IV regardless of severe impairment of autonomous movement
V	Severe	25–1	There is merely observed movement	There may be distortion of commissure, asymmetry in two sides. Nasolabial groove in one side become shallow or disappear	There is no movement in forehead. The patients cannot close eyes or can do slight eyelid movement with greatest force. There is slight movement in the corner of mouth	There is no synkinetic movement but there are conbundleure and spasm of facial muscle in paralytic side
VI	Completely paralyzed	0	There is no tension, movement, symmetry, synkinetic movement, conbundleure or spasm of face in paralytic side	Non	Non	Non

overlap domination phenomenon in the nerve. For example, fiber end of intercostal nerve in the third thoracic vertebra is involved in the domination of intercostal nerve in the fourth thoracic vertebra. Forepart of five pairs of intercostal nerves and subcostal nerves from the bottom, go forward into abdominal wall and distributes in the skin of abdominal muscle and abdominal wall. Therefore, if the lower intercostal nerves and subcostal nerves are stimulated, they can induce reflex tonus of muscles in abdominal wall and skin pain. In abdominal surgery, if too many

Table 11.2 Portmann simple scoring scale

Items	The same as uninjured side	Weaken	There is slight movement	There is no autonomous movement	Impression score	Normal
Scoring standard	3	2	2	0	2	20
Frown						
Closing eyes						
Moving wing of nose						
Smile						
Whistle						
Plumping cheek						

lower intercostal nerves are cut off, there will be paralysis of muscles in abdominal wall of dominated area, cutaneous sensation bluntness or disappearance. Therefore, peripheral nerves also have reserved functions and potential ability to be developed. In addition, peripheral nerves have strong regeneration ability.

Promotion of CNS plasticity and functional recovery, activation of reserved conduction pathway are suitable for recovering lost motor functions after injuries of functional nucleus of facial nerve or facial nerve fiber.

1. Musculus facialis is the muscle of voluntary movement. Musculus facialis can complete active movement under the domination of somatic nerve. Therefore, through the training of promoting the active movement of musculus facialis, the lost functions due to injuries of facial nucleus and other neural fibers can be recovered, which is in accordance with the mechanism of promoting CNS plasticity and functional reorganization.
2. Synkinetic movement of musculus facialis is abnormal motor pattern. Motor function nucleus of CNS can give out electrical signal to control voluntary conbundleion of muscle. The electrical signal is given out sequentially and orderly. The formation of synkinetic movement of musculus facialis is the same as synkinetic movement of limbs. The basis is disordered motor program in motor center. Therefore, it should be reestablished through motor program reestablishment technique. Through motor pattern remodeling technique, facial movement is coordinated and orderly. During this process, preventing or decreasing facial synkinetic movement is good for the rectification of synkinetic movement of musculus facialis. Therefore, recovery of coordinated movement of musculus facialis is suitable for three-stage rehabilitation method of "neural potential development, motor program reestablishment and motor pattern remodeling", which is called three-stage rehabilitation method of musculus facialis movement in order to be distinguished from three-stage method of motor pattern training of limbs.
3. The basis of developing facial nerve potential is reserved neural cells and nerve fiber bundles. Electrical signal from CNS to the dominated muscle is the most effective stimulus of activating neural reserved conduction pathway. As mentioned above, nerve trunk includes many nerve bundles and nerve bundles are composed of numerous neural fibers (Fig. 11.1).

The injury of nerve trunk doesn't mean all the nerve bundles are injured. Through training, incompletely injured nerve bundle can be recovered. In addition, human tissues have a great reservoir so that nerve bundle in nerve trunk is enough to recover functions. Under normal circumstances, because the motor degree and intensity are different, the number of activated nerve bundles is different. The rest are still in standby state. These reservations are the potential ability of nerve trunk. Therefore, when the nerve trunk in not injured completely, it is possible to be recovered and the reserved nerve bundle is

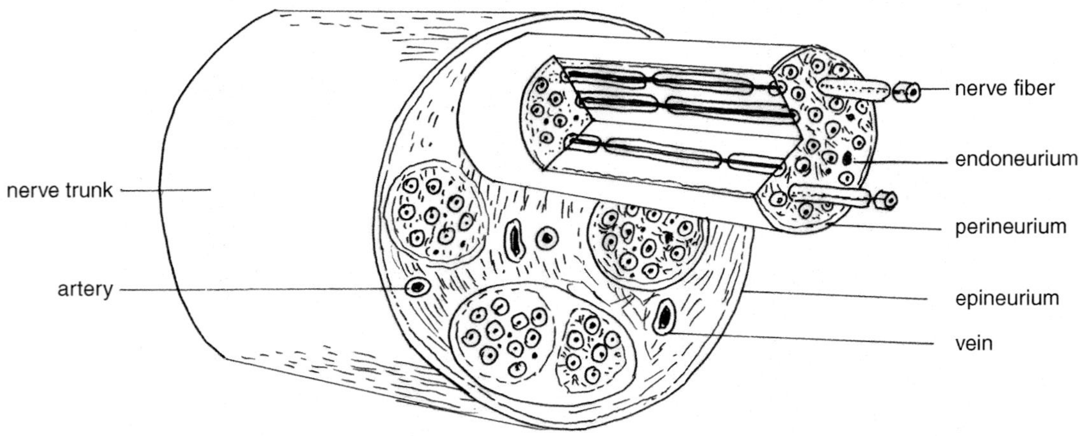

Fig. 11.1 Basic structure of nerve trunk

possible to be activated. Active movement is the effective method to recover and activate functions of nerve bundle. Daoyin technique is applied to encourage the patients to try to do anti-resistance in order to induce autonomous contraction of facial paralytic muscles. Musculus facialis contraction signals from brain cortex or facial nucleus are increased. The increase of this signal has the following effects: electrical signal from central nerves can promote the conduction functions of nerve trunk. Inherent muscle contraction driven electrical signal form neural nucleus is suitable for the current in nerve bundle. The current intensity and frequency can be accepted by nerve bundle and the orientation the current is from inward to outward to promote recanalization of injured part of nerve bundle. External stimulus such as acupuncture and electrical stimulus can generate impulse that is from outward to inward. It is not physiological signal so that it is not suitable for the conduction in nerve bundle. It not only can recover neural functions, but also emphasizes on the recovery of sensory function, which has no effect on the recovery of motor functions. In dangerous situation, nervous system may generate some kind of inducible factor to activate reserved nerve bundle in order to replace the injured nerve bundle. When the cells of neural nucleus generate electrical signal or give out electrical signal through residual nerve bundle, the intensity is not enough to induce muscle contraction needed for movement and bioactive substance (some kind of inducible factor) can be increased through feedback mechanism. The effect of this factor is to activate nerve bundle in dormant state to replace injured nerve bundle to play conduction functions and recover neural functions.

11.2.2 The Method of Rehabilitation Therapy of Facial Neuritis

Because central facial neuritis in the early phase requires management of neurology or neurosurgery, it is not discussed in this chapter. After therapy, remaining motor and sensory dysfunction refer to rehabilitation therapy of recovery period and chronic period of facial neuritis.

At present, there are many methods to treat facial paralysis such as hormone, neurotrophic medicine, physics, surgery, acupuncture, partial closure, sunken cord, passive massage of facial muscle. Among these methods, simple medicine therapy is not good and most patients reject hormone therapy. Operative therapies include facial nerve decompression, facial nerve transplantation and facial nerve anastomosis. Because the surgical trauma is severe and there is certain risk, it cannot be widely applied in clinic. In some reports, acupuncture and acusector have good therapeutic effects, but most scholars deem that the doctors should choose proper therapeutic opportunity. For example, in acute phase, acusector can lead to sequelae such as musculus facialis spasm [6]. In addition, there are 26 facial muscles. They interlap with each other with different functions. Acupuncture, acusector, partial closure, sunken cord or surgical therapy can easily damage facial muscle, even muscular hemorrhage, fibrosis and inflammation response. Some research indicate that it is impossible to recover active motor functions of musculus facialis through simple facial muscle massage.

11.2.2.1 Rehabilitation Therapy in Acute Phase

The clinical stages of facial neuritis are different. Generally, the acute phase is 2 weeks after facial neuritis. The recovery period is from 2 weeks to 1 month. The sequelae is more than 1 month. Someone think that half a year or more than 2 years is defined as the sequelae. The clinical stages are to instruct therapy and ascertain the therapeutic opportunity of facial nerve. The characteristics of acute phase are the progressive disease. Timely and effective therapy can increase cure rate and decrease disability rate.

1. Anti-inflammatory, detumescence and increasing local blood circulation: The therapeutic purpose in acute phase is to eliminate inflammation and alleviate mucosa edema of facial nerve canal in order to eliminate the injury of facial nerve from facial nerve and alleviate compression of facial nerve.

   For the early compression of facial nerve, medicine, acupuncture, ultrashort wave, far infrared rays and injection around stylomastoid foramen are used for the therapy.

   (a) Far infrared rays: Far infrared rays is used to improve local blood circulation, increase metabolism, increase immune function, enhance stability of cell membrane, promote elimination of toxic substance and metabolite, accelerate absorption of exudate, control inflammation, eliminate edema and accelerate tissue repair.

   Specific therapeutic method: The power of normal far infrared ray lamp is 250–300 W. The distance between injured musculus facialis and stylomastoid foramen is 30–50 cm. There is slight heat or warm heat. The frequency of musculus facialis is 15–20 min per time and the frequency of stylomastoid foramen is 10–15 min per time. There is 15 times in one therapy course (one time a day). It can be applied persistently.

   During therapy, the thermal insulation pad should be covered on the eyes in case of ocular damage.

   (b) Ultrashort wave: Ultrashort wave can ease pain, improve microcirculation, diminish inflammation, sterilize bacteria, promote wound healing, promote regeneration of incompletely injured neural fiber to eliminate inflammation of facial nerve canal and mucosa edema and promote recovery of neural functions and lost motor functions.

   Specific therapeutic method: Ultrashort wave of the five sense organs is used. The diameter of round capacitor electrode is 4–8 cm. Stylomastoid foramen in injured side is concatenated with eye part. Air distance space is 0.5–1.0 cm. There is no heat. The frequency is 6–10 min per time (one time a day) and there is 15 times in one therapy course. Through 3–5 days' rest, the second therapy course can be done.

   (c) Medium frequency electrotherapy modulated by low frequency (computerized modulated medium frequency): Medium frequency electrotherapy can ease pain, promote blood circulation, diminish inflammation, loosen adhesion and prevent scar formation. Medium frequency electrotherapy modulated by low frequency has the characteristics of low frequency and medium frequency and can stimulate skeletal muscle contraction. It has slight stimulation effect on cutaneous sensory nerve ending and there is no electrolytic action, which can be used for a long time. The current is deep, which is good for the therapy of deep lesion.

Specific therapeutic method: The diameter of round electrode is 2 × 5 cm (eye electrode). Stylomastoid foramen area is concatenated with the front of ear. Tolerance dose, bidirectional pulse and amplitude are increased and decreased gradually. The frequency is (modulated wave) is 100–150 time in 1 min. There is one time (10–20 min) a day and ten time in one therapy course.

(d) He-Ne Laser irradiation: In elementary beam irradiation, the distance between stylomastoid foramen and temple is 20–30 cm. The power is 10 mW. If the power is 3–6 mW, contaction irradiation can be used. The diameter of beam is 0.5 cm. There is one time (3–5 min) a day and 7–10 times in one therapy course.
   - Microwave therapy: round radiator is selected and the center points to the space between the front of ear and mastoid process. The distance is 10 cm. The dose is no heat or slight heat. There is one time (10–15 min) a day and ten times in one therapy course.

(e) Acupuncture therapy: Acupoints are Taiyang, Dicang, Yangbai, Yingxiang, Xiaguan, Jiache, Hegu and Lieque. The therapists select 3–4 acupoints every time with medium stimulation. The needle is kept for 10–20 min and is twiddled for 3–5 times. There is one time a day and 7–10 times in one therapy course. Electrical acupuncture can also be used.

(f) Massage therapy: Touching, pressing, pinching, rubbing, holding and trembling are used for paralytic muscle or selecting acupoint along channel. In early phase, the manipulation is slight in case of neural injury because of too great force. The patients can do massage by themselves. They use hand in the offside of facial paralysis, wash it clean, put thumb into mouth, use index finger and middle finger to pinch and rub outside. There is 1–2 times (10–15 min) a day and 10–20 times in one therapy course.

(g) Physiotherapy is the associated application method of rehabilitation technique of neurological training. Generally, far infrared rays, ultrashort wave, medium frequency and facial massage are used. In the early phase of the disease, acupuncture therapy should be used and the author thinks that there is a certain therapeutic effect. The times of therapy course should be observed, because too many acupuncture can induce muscle spasm, corners of the mouth deviating to injured side.

The therapists should ask the patients to keep the face warm and do standard therapy timely in case of sequelae because of incomplete therapy.

2. Recovering autokinetic movement of musculus facialis and preventing tissue adhesion and facial deformity: The best method of recovering autonomic nerve innervation of musculus facialis is to develop functional nucleus of facial nerve and potential ability of nerve bundle through active movement training. On the basis of regulation of mind and breathing, neurological training is active movement training with definite target and has good therapeutic effect, which is better than self-exercise and normal autonomous movement exercise or training.

Neurological training includes physical exercise therapy of neurological training (bare-handed operation method), neurological training (six-step Daoyin technique training under the detection of motor program signal) and training method of virtual reality. According to the actual situations that facial muscle is small and is distributed complicatedly, it is difficult to place signal acquisition electrode, pin electrode is not suitable to be used repeatedly and it is not easy to extract motor program signal of training muscle, during training, it is to detect the movement part of motor signal, place receiving electrode and set a surpassing goal associated with muscle movement.

The training of facial active movement includes raising eyebrow, wrinkling one's forehead, frowning, opening eyes, closing eyes, pulling up the corner of mouth, exposing teeth, pouting one's lips and sucking. Involved muscles include Occipitofrontalis muscle, orbicularis oculi muscle, zygomaticus major or minor, Albinus' muscle, orbicular muscle of mouth, nasalis, levator labii superioris, depressor labii inferioris and buccinators.

The starting and ending points, effect and innervation of facial muscle refer to Table 11.3 and Fig. 11.2.

(a) Physical exercise therapy of neurological training of musculus facialis is bare-handed manipulation method of six-step Daoyin technique in traditional Chinese medicine. The training is done according to start-stop and line feed of musculus facialis.

Operational approach: In supine position, the patients lie in therapy bed. In order to decrease the friction of face, the therapists can wear rubber gloves and smear a little cream or liquefied petrolatum on the gloves and face. On the basis of regulation of mind

Table 11.3 The starting and ending points, effect and innervation of facial muscle

Muscle group	Name	Starting point	ending points	Main effect	innervation
Facial muscle	Occipitofrontalis muscle	Frontal belly: galea aponeurotica	Frontal skin	Raise eyebrows and wrinkle forehead	Temporal branch (VII)
		Occipital belly: neck line of the occipital bone	Galea aponeurotica	Pull back scalp	Auricular branch (VII)
	Orbicularis oculi muscle	Face: around palpebral fissure Pars orbitalis: around orbit Lacrimal part: from lacrimal sac to face		Blink, close eyes, expand lacrimal sac to discharge tear	Temporal branch, zygomaticus (VII)
	Nasalis	Transverse part: canine teeth of upper jaw bone and teeth of second incisor Alar part of groove process: facies lateralis of nasal alar cartilage		Narrow nostril, expand nostril	Buccal branch (VII)
	Orbicular muscle of mouth	Around schistostoma		Close schistostoma	Buccal branch and marginal mandibular branch (VII)
	Levator labii superioris	The orientation of upper lip	The skin of the corner of mouth	Raise upper lip	Rami zygomatici and buccal branch (VII)
	Zygomaticus			Raise the corner of mouth	Rami zygomatici (VII)
	Albinus' muscle	Parotid masseter muscle fascia		Pull outside the corner of mouth	Buccal branch and marginal mandibular branch (VII)
	Depressor anguli oris	The orientation of lower lip		Lower the corner of mouth	Marginal mandibular branch (VII)
	Levator anguli oris	Below infraorbital foramen		Raise the corner of mouth	Buccal branch (VII)
	Depressor labii Inferioris	The orientation of lower lip		Lower the corner of mouth and lower lip	
	Buccinator	Deep part of cheek		Make lip and cheek close to teeth to chew and suck	
	Mentalis	Second incisor of lower jawbone and alveolar process of central incisor	Skin of mental region	Raise skin of mental region to put upper lip forward	Marginal mandibular branch (VII)

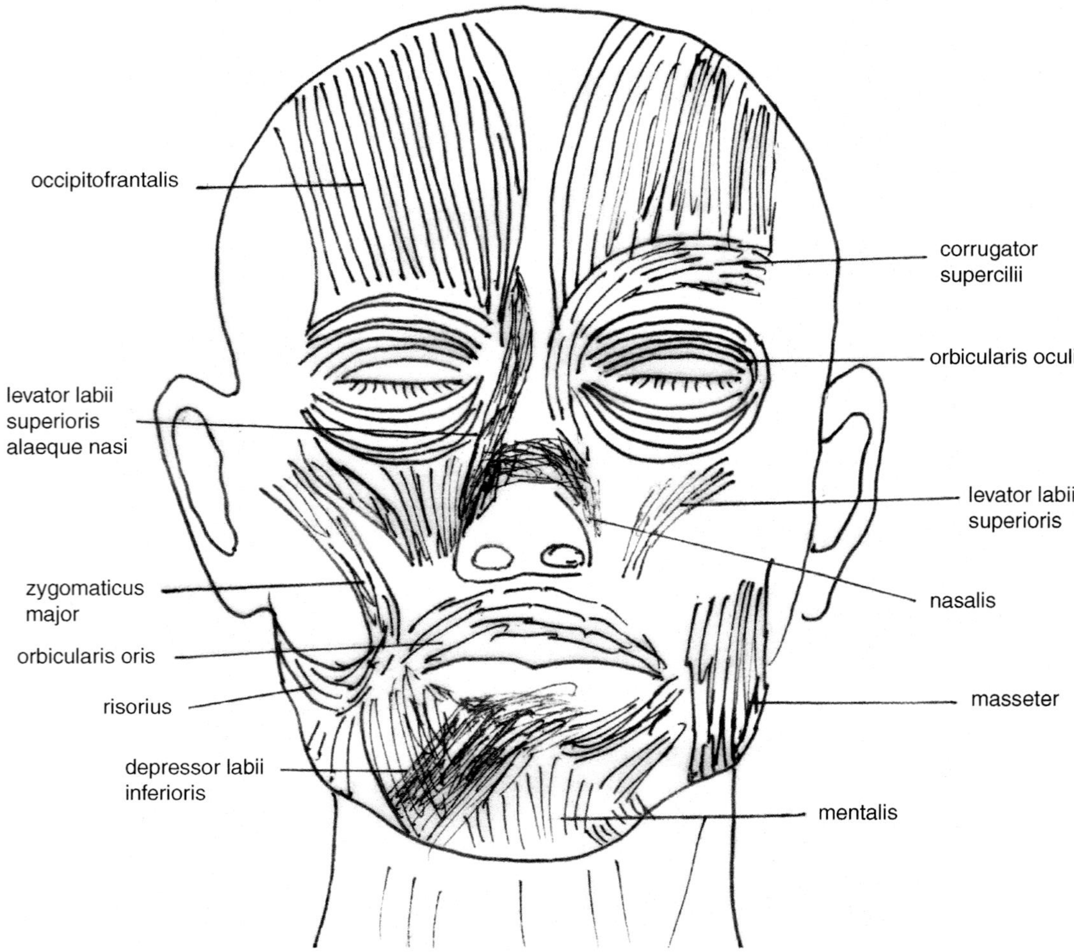

Fig. 11.2 The distribution of facial muscle

and breathing, the patients are guided to raise eyebrow, wrinkle forehead, open eyes, close eyes, pull outside the corner of mouth, close schistostoma, expose teeth, pout and suck. During the training, in the ending of training muscle, the therapists use finger belly to press the muscle and pull the muscle in the negative direction of muscle contraction to complete anti-resistance training. The patients are guided to persist for 6 s. After completing one movement, the therapists use palm or finger belly to do massage of training part in order to loosen tissue and increase blood circulation. The anti-resistance orientations of muscles are as follows:

The training of opening eyes and wrinkling forehead: The involved muscle is occipital frontalis. The press part of the finger is superior border of geisoma. The anti-resistance orientation is downward form eyelid (Fig. 11.3). The effect is to recover the functions of wrinkling forehead and opening eyes.

The training of closing eyes: The involved muscle is orbicularis oculi muscle. The press part of the finger is lower and upper orbit. The therapists use thumb and finger to enlarge eyelid from above and below to increase resistance (Fig. 11.4). The effect is to recover the functions of closing eyes.

The training of raising the corner of mouth: The involved muscle is levator anguli oris, zygomaticus major and minor and Albinus'muscle. The press part of the finger is outside and upward side of the corner of mouth. The therapists use finger to exert force inward and downward along the corner of mouth to increase resistance (Fig. 11.5). The effect is to recover the functions of raising the corner of mouth upward and outside to rectify distortion of commissure to uninjured side.

The training of exposing teeth: The involved muscle is levator labii superioris and depressor labii inferioris. The press part of the finger is upper and lower lip. The therapists use thumb and finger to exert force upward and downward of schistostoma to increase resistance (Fig. 11.6). The effect is to recover

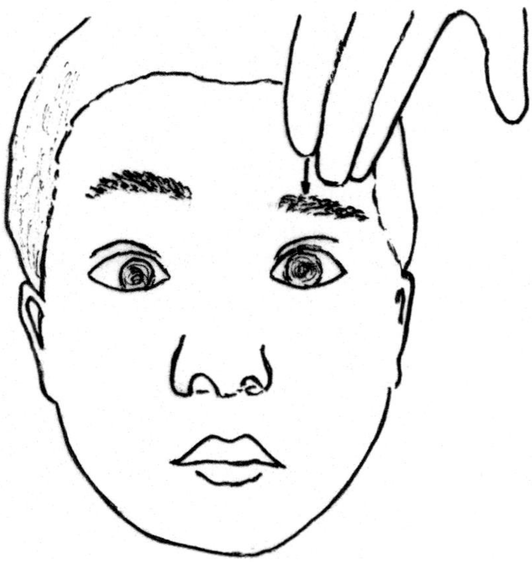

Fig. 11.3 The training of opening eyes and wrinkling forehead

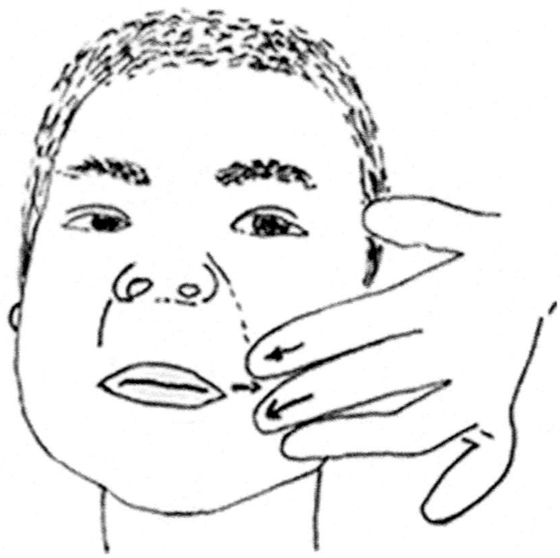

Fig. 11.5 The training of raising the corner of mouth

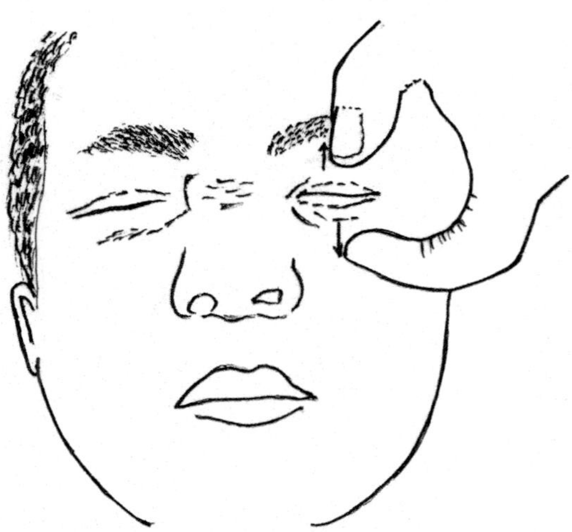

Fig. 11.4 The training of closing eyes

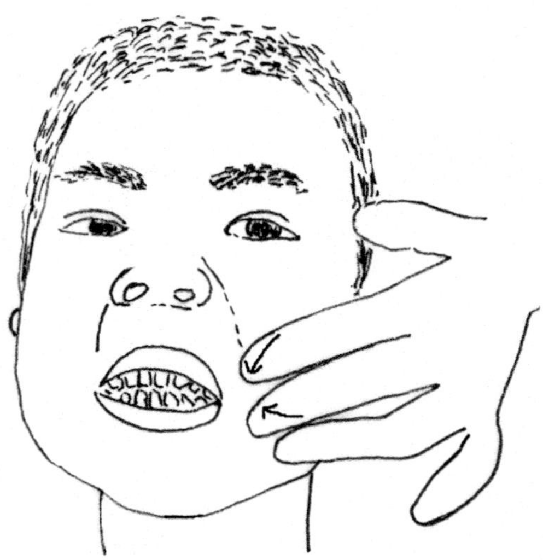

Fig. 11.6 The training of exposing teeth

the functions of moving the corner of mouth upward and downward.

The training of holding one's jaw: The involved muscle is orbicular muscle of mouth. The press part of the finger is the above and below of upper and lower lip. The therapists use thumb and finger to exert force upward and downward of schistostoma to increase resistance (Fig. 11.7). The effect is to recover the functions of holding one's jaw to prevent non-autonomous overflow of oral content such as salivation and rice grain falling.

The training of sucking: The involved muscle is buccinators. The press part of the finger is upper and lower lip. The therapists use thumb and finger to exert force upward and downward of schistostoma to increase resistance (Fig. 11.8). The effect is to make lip and cheek close to teeth to decrease oral cavity. The effect is to recover the functions of chewing and sucking.

The training of pouting: The involved muscle is mentalis. The press part of the finger is chin. The therapists use thumb and finger to exert force downward to increase resistance (Fig. 11.9). The effect is to close upper and lower lip further and pout forward.

The training of twitching one's nose: The involved muscle is nasalis. The press part of the finger is two side of the front of nose wing. The therapists use finger to increase resistance to the two sides of nose wing (Fig. 11.10). The effect is to recover the control ability of enlarging or narrow nostril.

In clinical application, according to the results of functional assessment, the therapists find out the main obstacles and use the trainings mentioned above. The patients can do the training of three parts every time alternatively (15 min for each part). There is one time a day (45 min) and there are 66–90 times in one therapy course.

(b) Neurological training: Six-step Daoyin technique training is under the detection of motor program signal.

According to the start-stop and line feed of musculus facialis, the therapist use fastener electrode or 3M electrode that is cut small and paste electrode according to the location demonstrated in Figs. 11.11, 11.12, 11.13, 11.14, 11.15, 11.16, 11.17, and 11.18. If it is not fastened stably, the therapists can use non-woven fabrics adhesive tape to fix it. Daoyin technique is used to encourage the

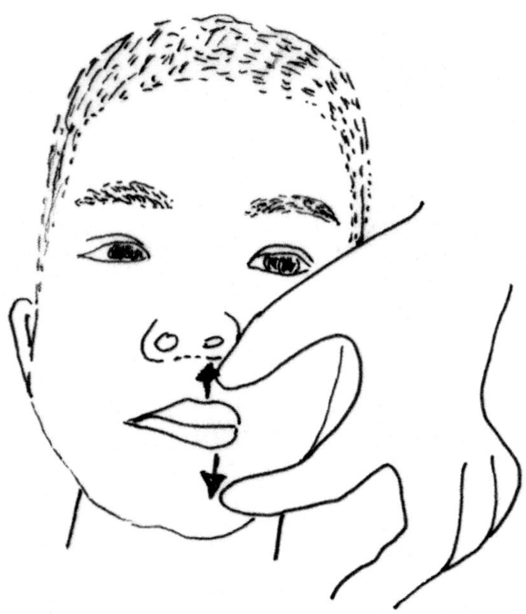

Fig. 11.7 The training of holding one's jaw

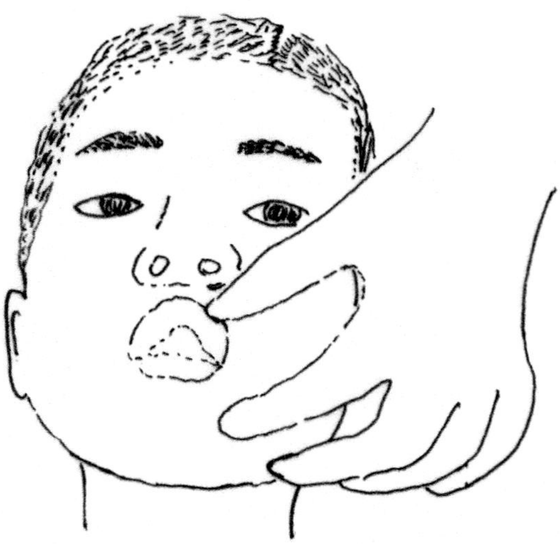

Fig. 11.8 The training of sucking

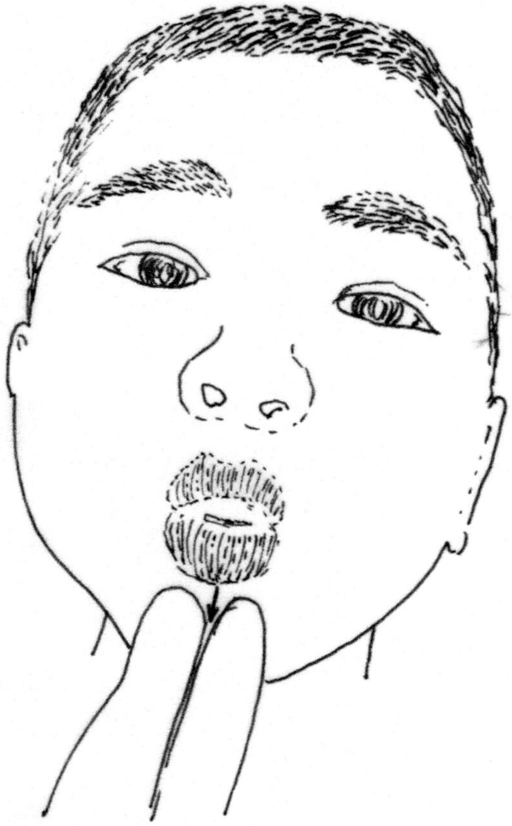

Fig. 11.9 The training of pouting

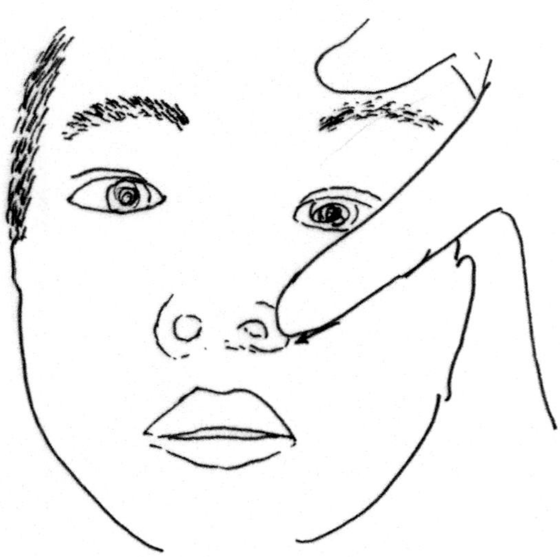

Fig. 11.10 The training of twitching one's nose

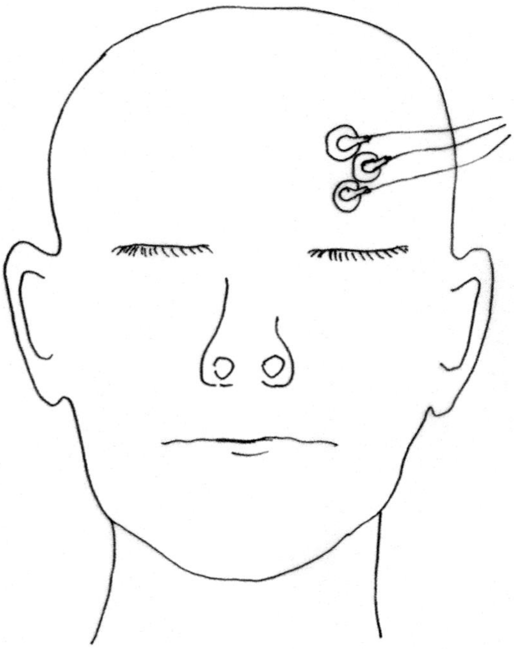

Fig. 11.11 The training of opening eyes and wrinkling forehead (occipitofrontalis muscle)

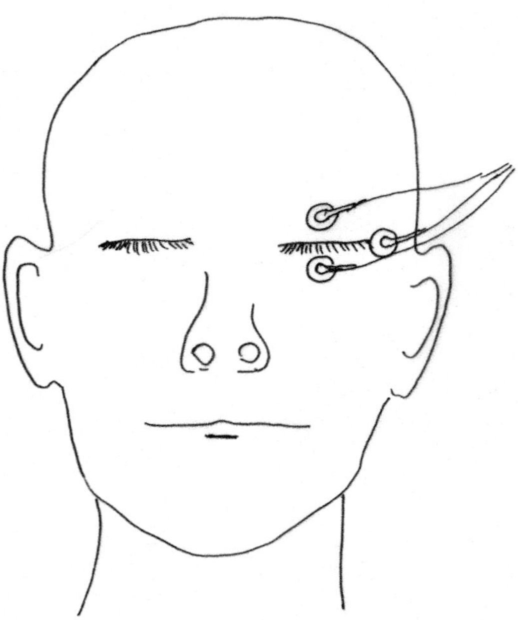

Fig. 11.12 The training of closing eyes (orbicularis oculi muscle)

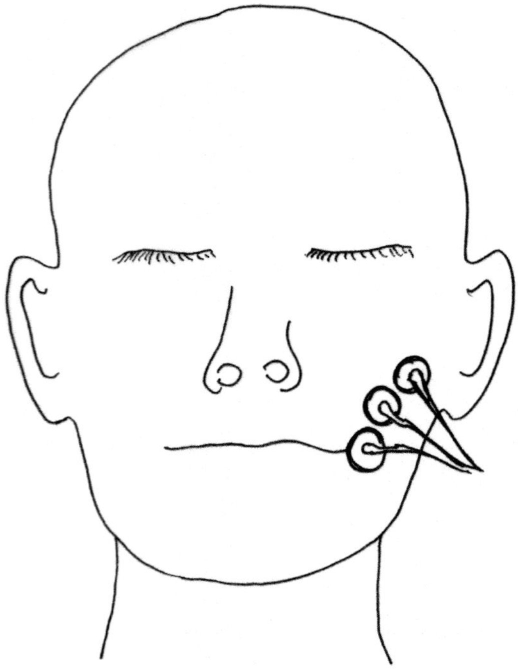

Fig. 11.13 The training of raising the corner of mouth (zygomaticus)

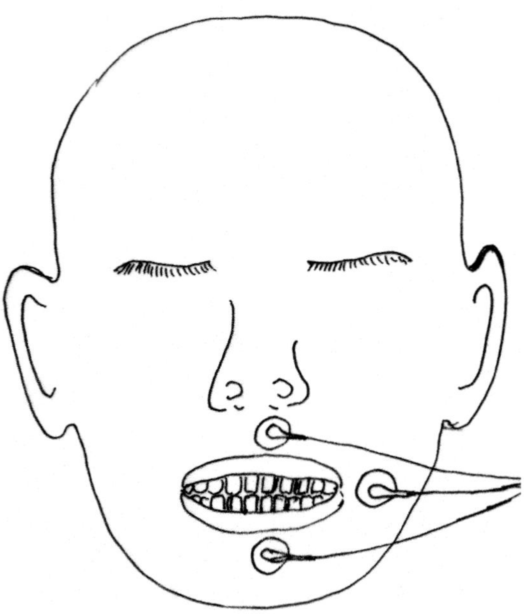

Fig. 11.14 The training of exposing teeth (levator anguli oris)

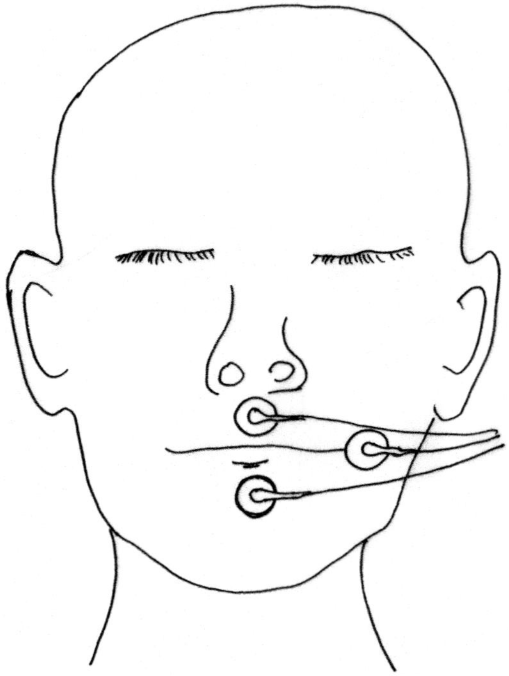

Fig. 11.15 The training of holding one's jaw (orbicular muscle of mouth)

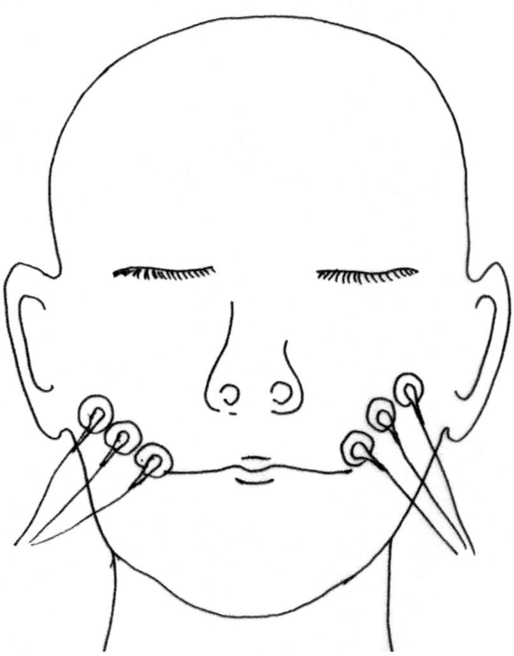

Fig. 11.16 The training of sucking (buccinator)

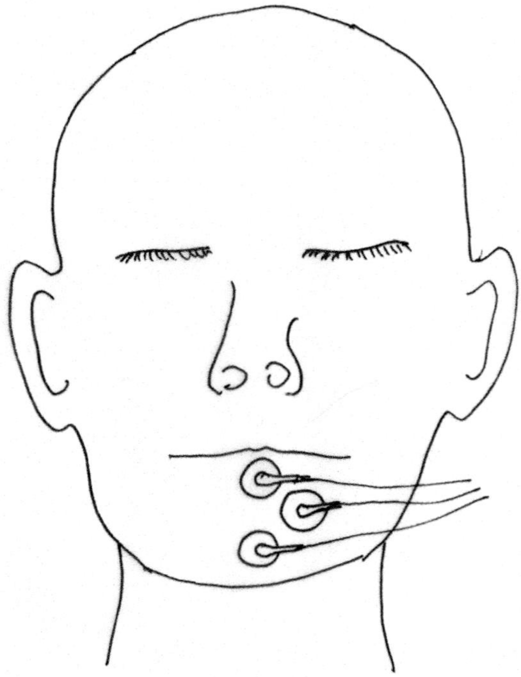

Fig. 11.17 The training of pouting (mentalis)

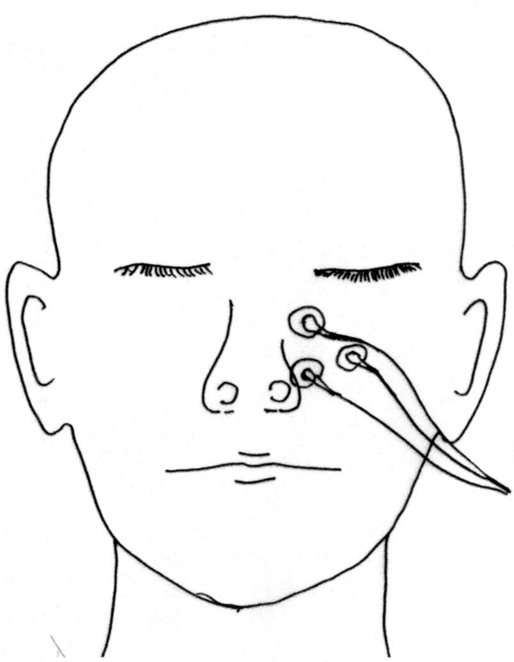

Fig. 11.18 The training of twitching one's nose (oculonasal muscle)

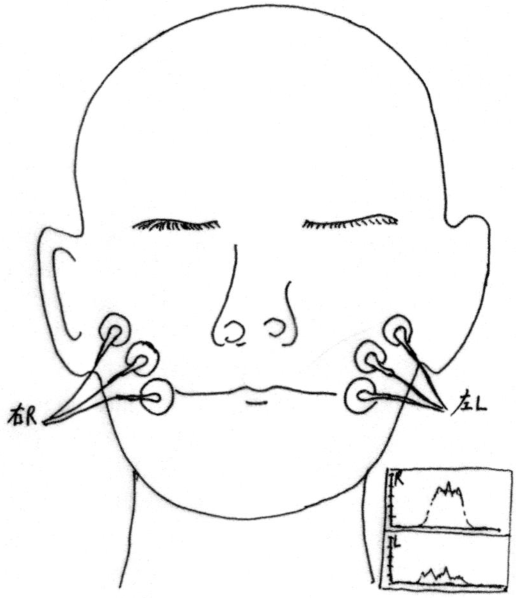

Fig. 11.19 Double screen training method

patients to complete designed contraction training of musculus facialis and neurological training equipment is used to receive and display motor program signal real-timely. Initial or last signal intensity baseline is regarded as the target line. Daoyin technique is used repeatedly to encourage the patients to surpass new goal and increase signal intensity of agonistic muscle. During the process of developing facial nerve potential and enhancing myodynamia, autonomous motor function of the muscle can be recovered gradually.

Double screen method can be used for neurological training therapy of musculus facialis. The motor program signals from injured and uninjured muscle are detected and the signal form uninjured muscle is used as target to guide the patients to do surpassing training of autonomous movement of injured muscle (Fig. 11.19).

(c) Virtual reality training of neurological training is that virtual reality training equipment of neurological training is used in this training.

Because there are many small pieces of musculus facialis, it is difficult to paste single muscle electrode. Moreover, face is not suitable to be pasted with electrode with binding agent repeatedly in case of skin injury. In addition, it is hard to do anti-resistance training of musculus facialis. The training progress takes a long time and the patients cannot see the increase of the signal for a long time, which can affect the confidence of therapy.

Virtual reality training can figure out these problems well. Virtual increased signal can make the patients see the progress of the therapy. Although the signal is virtual, it can develop neural potential because the patients actually do the anti-resistance and surpassing training with definite goal in the training process.

The virtual reality training and neurological training can be combined, which is one kind of good rehabilitation training. It can not only make the patients know the actual situation and change of motor program signal, which is good for the formulation of therapeutic schedule and training with a purpose, but also can compensate the defect that actual motor program signal cannot endure for a long time and may affect the therapeutic enthusiasm easily. The combined way is that the neurological training is once a week and virtual reality training is 4–5 times a week. There are 50 min per time and 66–90 times in one therapy course.

(d) Massage and loosening of musculus facialis can increase blood circulation of facial tissue in paralytic side, loosen tissue adhesion and alleviate facial distortion.

Paralysis of musculus facialis can lead to myodynamia asymmetry in two sides of facial muscle. Facial tissues are stretched by the muscles in uninjured side to uninjured side, which form facial distortion. At this time, the muscle in paralytic side is lengthened and the muscle in uninjured side is shortened. They all lose the proper initial length and affect diastolic and systolic function of facial muscle further in case of adhesion between muscle fibers or muscle fiber and peripheral tissue. They can further affect muscle contraction and rectification of facial demormity. Therefore, rehabilitation therapy of facial paralysis includes therapy of the injured side and therapy of the uninjured side.

In addition, because muscular movement is decreased, the local blood circulation is poor. Metabolite cannot be excluded timely and then are accumulated. Acid metabolite can stimulate local neural ending and induce soreness, numbness, dysesthesia and stiffness.

Manual massage can increase local tissue blood circulation, promote exclusion of metabolite, loosen adhesive tissue and extend contracture muscle in order to alleviate facial discomfort and distortion.

Because of the beauty of the face, facial massage and tissue loosening should be gentle and with proper force. The therapists can smear cream on the face such as paroline and facial cleanser to alleviate abrasion of facial skin.

Facial massage and tissue loosening are the common manipulations. On-the-point pressing includes finger on-the-point pressing and palm on-the-point pressing. Finger on-the-point pressing is that the therapists use thumb or finger prominence of index finger and middle finger to press the face or acupoint of the patients. Palm on-the-point pressing is that the therapists use palm or heel of hand to press the face of the patients. Touch method is that the therapists put finger or palm on face and do massage in straight line or in a loop, which includes finger touch method and palm touch method. Finger touch method is that the therapists adduct four fingers and use finger pulp of index finger, middle finger and ring finger to touch the patients. The movement should be gentle and rapid. The frequency is 120–160 times per min. Palm touch method is that the therapists use the center of the palm to touch the patients in a loop. The movement should be gentle and slow. The frequency is about 180 times per min. The speed of finger touch method is faster than that of palm touch method. The force of palm touch method is greater than that of finger touch method. Kneading is that the therapists use thenar eminence and heel of the hand to press the lesion part and knead the patients in a circle round gently and mildly with force, which includes finger kneading, thenar kneading and heel of hand kneading. Finger kneading is that the therapists use thumb (single finger kneading), index finger and middle finger (double-finger kneading) or index finger, middle finger and ring finger (three-finger kneading) to knead the patients to and fro. Thenar kneading is that the therapists use thenar eminenceto press on the face and knead it in a circle round. Heel of hand kneading is that the therapists use heel of hand to press on the face and knead it in a circle round. The frequency is 120 times per min. The force of heel of hand is great and is suitable for loosening of adhesive tissue and contracture muscle of the face in uninjured side.

The frequency of musculus facialis massage is 20 min per time. There is once a day and 30 times in one therapy course.

(e) Traction of musculus facialis: For the muscles that induce the corner of mouth deviate to the uninjured side and contracture in uninjured side, such as zygomaticus major and minor, although the cause of facial distortion is the paralysis of muscles in injured side, traction of muscles in uninjured side is one of the reasons that induce facial deformity such as facial distortion. It can affect the functional recovery of paralytic muscles.

The traction method is that the therapists wash the hands clean or wear sterile latex gloves and put index finger into oral cavity in uninjured side. At first, the therapists use index finger and thumb outside of oral cavity to do massage of oral cavity from outside to inside. After that, the therapists use thumb and finger pulp of index finger to pinch the corner of mouth slightly and exert force slowly to tract it to the injured side for several seconds. The therapists pull it repeatedly for 10–15 times and time of duration is 20 min. There is 1–2 times a day and 15–30 times in one therapy course. The effect of traction is better after local heating of far infrared rays.

(f) Self-exercise of musculus facialis includes facial massage, active muscle contraction and self-traction of musculus facialis. Facial massage is that the patients sit on the chair, twist two hands until they are warm, adduct five fingers, touch, knead and run on the face until the face is warm. The movement should be gentle. The face doesn't feel any discomfort. The patients use index finger, middle finger and ring finger or thenar eminence to do massage with big force. Active contraction exercise of musculus facialis is that the patients do active exercise of muscle contraction through facial movement. The patients sit before the mirror and use six-step Daoyin technique to raise forehead (occipital frontalis), frown, close eyes, smile, blow cheek, open mouth (zygomaticus) and pout (mentalis) after regulation of mind and breathing. The patients exert resistance using fingers in the negative orientation of muscle contraction for 6 s. if the patients use the uninjured side as the target for surpassing exercise, the effect is better.

The frequency of self-exercise is 10–15 min per time. There is 1–2 time a day and 15–30 times in one therapy course. Normal people who do this exercise can delay aging.

Self-traction of musculus facialis is the important content of self-exercise. Facial massage can loosen tissue, but cannot fully loosen zygomaticus in uninjured side with contracture that induce facial distortion. The patients should do self-traction. The patients use left hand to pull right cheek and use right hand to pull left cheek. The specific method is the same as that in the traction of musculus facialis.

11.2.2.2 Rehabilitation Therapy in Recovery Phase

Two weeks to 1 month after disease is the recovery phase of facial neuritis. During this phase, the progression of disease stops, edema of facial nerve fade away and incomplete injured neural functions are recovered.

The key point of this phase is to develop neural potential, further promote edema elimination, enrich blood circulation and loosen adhesive tissue. Rehabilitation method of neurological training is used to develop neural potential better, recover autonomous movement function of musculus facialis. Physical method is used to improve blood circulation of local tissue, alleviate facial numbness and stiffness, loosen tissue adhesion manually.

1. Physiotherapy mainly includes thermal therapy and medium frequency electrotherapy.
   (a) Facial irradiation of far infrared rays: the method is the same as the therapy in acute phase. There is once a day and ten times in one therapy course.

(b) Medium frequency electrotherapy modulated by low frequency (Computerized modulated medium frequency or low frequency): the method is the same as the therapy in acute phase. The diameter of round electrode is 2–5 cm (eye electrode). Stylomastoid foramen is juxtaposed with the front of the ear. Tolerance dose, bidirectional pulse and amplitude are increased and decreased gradually. The frequency is (modulated wave) is 100–150 times in 1 min. There is one time (10–20 min) a day and ten times in one therapy course.
(c) Microwave therapy: the therapists choose no-heat or slight heat and the frequency is 10–15 min per time. There is once a day and fifteen times in one therapy course.

2. Active movement training of musculus facialis: Development of neural potential and reestablishment of motor program are the key therapeutic measures of recovering autonomous movement of musculus facialis.
   (a) Physical exercise therapy of neurological training of musculus facialis: Bare-handed manipulation of six-step Daoyin technique in traditional Chinese medicine is used. In clinical application, according to the start-stop and line feed of musculus facialis and the results of functional assessment, the therapists find out the main obstacles and use the trainings mentioned above. The patients can do the training of three parts every time alternatively (15 min for each part). There is one time a day (45 min) and one therapy course takes 3 months.
   (b) Neurological training: Six-step Daoyin technique training under the detection of motor program signal is used alone or combined with virtual reality training method of neurological training. if it is used alone, there are 50 min per time and one therapy course takes 3 months. The combined way is that the neurological training is once a week and virtual reality training is 4–5 times a week. There are 50 min per time and one therapy course takes 3 months.
   (c) Massage of musculus facialis: the method is the same as the massage of musculus facialis in acute phase (20 min per time). There is once a day and thirty times in one therapy course.
   (d) Traction of musculus facialis: the method is the same as the traction of musculus facialis in acute phase (20 min per time). The traction time is 10–15 and 1–2 times a day. There are 15–30 times in one therapy course. The effect of traction is better after local heating.
   (e) Self-exercise of musculus facialis: the method is the same as that of self-exercise in acute phase. The frequency is 10–15 min per time and there is 1–2 times a day.

11.3 Rehabilitation therapy in sequelae phase.

One month after facial neuritis is called sequelae phase. Because some cases are not recovered completely, there are linked movement of mouth and eyes, ptosis, closing one's eyes incompletely, facial distortion, salivation, dysesthesia of face in injured side, numbness, stiffness and inarticulateness, which affect the life quality and beauty of the patients greatly. The occurrence rate is about 25%.

The key point of rehabilitation in this phase is symptomatic therapy such as the training of active movement of muscle, coordinated movement of musculus facialis, balanced capacity of myodynamia and speech and the therapy of facial paresthesia.

1. The mechanism of synkinetic movement of face: After facial paralysis, there are synkinetic movement (synkinesia) and musculus facialis spasm, which are all the complications of facioplegia. Synkinetic movement is that when closing eyes the corner of mouth moves to injured side or when moving the corner of mouth the patients close eyes, which is abnormal motor pattern of orbicularis oculi muscle and zygomaticus. The mechanism of synkinetic movement remains unclear until now and there are three hypotheses.

(a) Abnormal regeneration of degenerated nerve: Synkinetic movement is induced by malposition connection in the regeneration process of small neural fiber. Although is widely accepted, there is still controversy. Some researchers think that if synkinetic movement is induced by abnormal regeneration of nerve, there is synkinetic movement in the recovery of the nerve. However, in clinic, synkinetic movement and musculus facialis contracture appear 4 months after the disease. After injury, the nerve regenerates from 2 weeks after the disease.

The author thinks that the reason is not solid, because regeneration of neural fiber from 2 weeks of the disease is not equal to completion of regeneration and connection of targeted muscles. On the contrary, if the regeneration speed of nerve is 1 mm a day, the regeneration of facial nerve takes 4 months until the process is completed. The process is in accordance with the time of synkinetic movement in clinic. Therefore, dislocation signal conduction is one of the reasons that lead to synkinetic movement of musculus facialis.

(b) Potential abnormal propagation in injured part: In the injured part, the regenerated nerve fibers form potential and this potential can spread misdirected to other parts to induce synkinetic movement.

This hypothesis cannot explain why synkinetic movement doesn't happen in the injury of facial nerve, but after the recovery of facioplegia. Certainly, when facial nerves are not injured, it may be related to musculus facialis paralysis and motor inability, but there is evidence of abnormal potential and wrong conduction without regenerated neural fibers.

(c) Excitability increase of nerve nucleus: The formation of synkinetic movement may be induced by erethism of neural cells in intermediate group of facial nucleus, which is one kind of synkinetic effect.

Anatomic study of facial nucleus put forward questions to abnormal neural regeneration. Human facial nucleus includes four kinds of cell groups such as dorsomedial group, ventral medial group, intermediate group and lateral group. The cells in intermediate group project fibers to dominate frontal belly of occipitofrontalis, orbicularis oculi muscle, corrugator and zygomaticus that are related to synkinetic movement. Small cells in intermediate group dominate stapedius. Dorsomedial group cells project to nervus auricularis posterior to dominate auricularis muscle and occipital belly of frontal occipitalis. Ventral medial group cells project fibers to dominate platysma myoides through cervical branch. Lateral group cells project fibers to dominate buccinators and muscles in cheek and lip through cheek branch. Erethism of intermediate group cells that dominate orbicularis oculi muscle and zygomaticus may lead to synkinetic movement of mouth and eye.

Further peripheral nerve examination found that motor fibers of facial nerve are distributed in diffusivity around temporal part, which can easily induce synkinetic movement because of imprecise excitation transmission.

(d) Motor program disorder: the author think that synkinetic movement of musculus facialis is similar with abnormal motor pattern of limbs, which may be induced by abnormal motor program in facial nucleus or cortex motor center.

Facial muscle is the same as muscles in the whole body, which are all dominated by motor program signal in CNS. This dominance is sequential and orderly. When facial nucleus or facial nerve is partially injured, the ability of giving out or conduct motor program signal is affected, the associated muscles are paralyzed. During the process of functional recovery of paralyzed muscles, before paralytic muscles' functions are recovered, inappropriate facial movement can lead to abnormal motor pattern because of synkinetic movement through activating other muscles to replace the functions of the unrecovered muscles. Repeated compensation can lead to abnormal motor program in CNS so that synkinetic movement is more difficult to be rectified.

In clinical practice, this viewpoint is primarily verified in rehabilitation training. For the patients with synkinetic movement of musculus facialis, 3 months' motor program reestablishment training can alleviate synkinetic movement greatly, but the effect should be verified in multicenter and large sample size study.

2. Rehabilitation therapy of synkinetic movement includes the training to enhance flexibility of musculus facialis and reestablish motor program of musculus facialis.
   (a) Rehabilitation training of neurological training: The training includes flexibility training of single muscle with definite surpassing goal and motor program reestablishment and myodynamia coordination training of musculus facialis with a purpose. Flexibility training method is the flexibility training of aingle muscle according to different muscles of forming abnormal face. For example, zygomaticus should be mainly trained in distorted mouth, occipital frontalis should be trained in ptosis and orbicularis oculi muscle should be trained in incomplete closing one's eyes. Signal detection electrode should be placed in the same position where neurological training electrode of musculus facialis is placed. However, the difference between flexibility training of musculus facialis and reestablishment training of motor program is that motor program reestablishment training is to enhance signal intensity of agonistic muscle and decrease signal intensity of antagonistic muscle in order to recover the normal proportion, while flexibility training is to shorten muscle contraction time at first as soon as possible and then to enhance contraction signal intensity in order to relax the muscle and make the signal return to zero. The purpose of this training is to make the diastolic and systolic movement of musculus facialis in accordance with all or none law of neural signal conduction. Both contraction and relaxation are fast to recover the flexibility of autonomous nerve innervation (Fig. 11.20). Synkinetic movement rectification method: The most advanced motor pattern is separation movement. Synkinetic movement demonstrated that the injured nerves are not completely recovered. Through reestablishment of motor program of musculus facialis, it can be rectified. The muscles with synkinetic movement are regarded as agonistic muscle and antagonistic muscle in one movement for training. When in the training of closing eyes, orbicularis oculi muscle is agonistic muscle and zygomaticus is antagonistic muscle. Six-step Daoyin technique is used to guide the patients to increase signal intensity of orbicularis oculi muscle and decrease signal intensity of zygomaticus in order to eliminate synkinetic movement (Fig. 11.21). In the training of zygomaticus, zygomaticus is agonistic muscle.

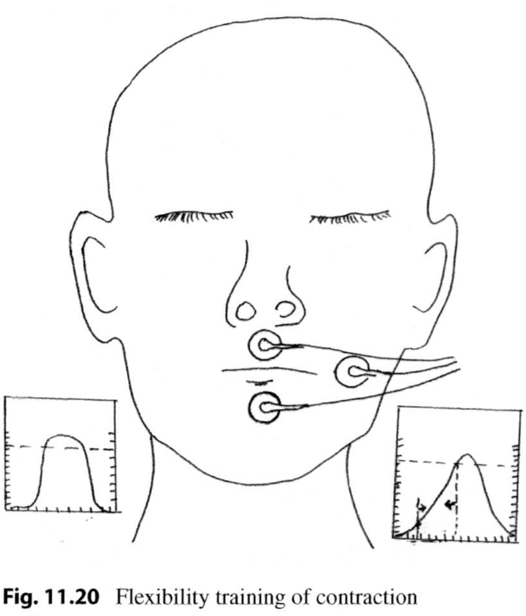

Fig. 11.20 Flexibility training of contraction

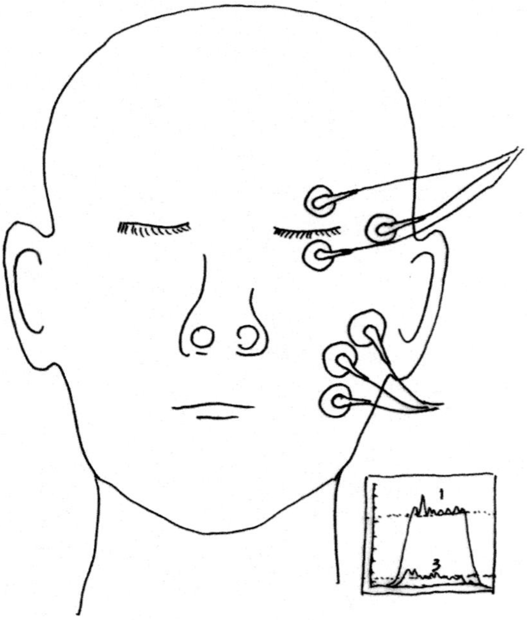

Fig. 11.21 Synkinetic movement rectification training

Six-step Daoyin technique is used to guide the patients to increase signal intensity of zygomaticus and decrease signal intensity of orbicularis oculi muscle in order to eliminate synkinetic movement. Bilateral comparison method: it is suitable for the patients with simple facial distortion, closing eyes inability and raising forehead inability. The first and the second channel of neurological training equipment are separately used to detect the motoe program signal of the same muscles in uninjured side and injured side and display them in double screens. The therapists use signal in uninjured side as the surpassing goal and use six-step Daoyin technique repeatedly to guide the patients to increase signal intensity in uninjured side to rectify the facial demormity.

(b) Increasing local blood circulation and promoting metabolism: Far infrared rays are used for therapy. Twenty centimeter away from aural skin in injured side, irradiation cover of far infrared rays is placed and the heat should be comfort and don't burn the skin. The frequency is once a day (15–20 min per time) and there are 15 times in one therapy course.

(c) Medium frequency electriotherapy to alleviate discomfort of face: The diameter of round electrode is 2 × 5 cm (eye electrode). Stylomastoid foramen area is concatenated with the front of ear. Tolerance dose, bidirectional pulse and amplitude are increased and decreased gradually. The frequency is (modulated wave) is 100–150 time in 1 min. The frequency is once a day (10–20 min per time) and there are 15 times in one therapy course.

After assessment, the patients can do the next therapy course. Once there is excitability increase or spasm of musculus facialis, the therapy should be stopped.

(d) Loosening tissue adhesion: The methods are introduced in the second part of this chapter such as on-the-point pressing, rubbing manipulation and kneading manipulation to do facial massage and tissue loosening. The frequency is 1–2 time a day (20 min per time) and there are 30 times in one therapy course. The effect is better after local heating.

(e) Traction of musculus facialis in uninjured side: the patients with facial distortion to uninjured side should receive traction therapy of musculus facialis in uninjured side. The traction method is that the therapists wash the hands clean or wear sterile latex gloves and put index finger into oral cavity in uninjured side. At first, the therapists use index finger and thumb outside of oral cavity to do massage of oral cavity from outside to inside. After that, the therapists use thumb and finger pulp of index finger to pinch the corner of mouth slightly and exert force slowly to tract it to the injured side for several seconds (10–15 times). The frequency is 1–2 time a day (20 min per time) and there are 15–30 times in one therapy course. The effect is better after local heating of far infrared rays.

(f) Self-exercise of musculus facialis: it is the same as that in acute phase. The frequency is 1–2 time a day (10–15 min per time).

3. Therapy of musculus facialis spasm: Musculus facialis spasm in the late phase of facial neuritis is common in the patients with central facial paralysis.

   Central facial paralysis is induced by injury of some part in the upstream pathway of facial nucleus, which is common in capsule interna. Internal carotid arterial system occlusion such as occlusion of trunk and branch of middle cerebral artery, hemangioma, intracranial hemorrhage and intracranial tumours due to hypertensive vasculopathy can lead to central facial paralysis.

   The mechanism of musculus facialis spasm may be that upper central nerves are injured and lose control of lower central nerves (facial nucleus). Cells of facial nucleus are disinhibited and cannot work coordinately. Therefore, recovering functions of upper central nerves is the important measure to alleviate musculus facialis spasm. Neural potential development and motor program reestablishment are the effective methods to recover functions of upper central nerves.

   (a) Physical exercise therapy of neurological training of musculus facialis: Bare-handed manipulation of six-step Daoyin technique is used for active contraction training of musculus facialis spasm. The frequency is once a day (30 min) and one therapy course takes 3 months.
   (b) Neurological training: According to the pathway of spasmodic facial muscle, signal reception electrode is placed. Six-step Daoyin technique is used for autonomous contraction and relaxation training of spasmodic muscle. Contraction training is to guide the patients increase the driven signal intensity from upper central nerves to spasmodic muscle to develop potential. Relaxation training guides the patients to control the intensity of spasmodic signal to let it weaken or disappear (Fig. 11.22), which is also a kind of way to develop potentials of central nerves. It is an effective measure for the therapy of spasmodic muscle. The signal is increased in muscle contraction, which demonstrated that the number and quality of central neural cells involved in spasmodic muscle are enhanced. The signal is decreased in spasm, which demonstrated that the control ability of upper central nerves to facial nucleus is increased.

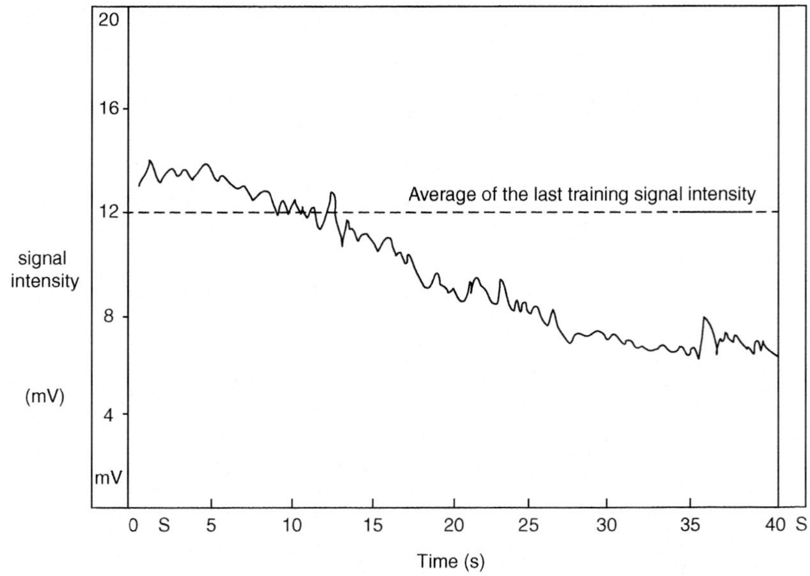

Fig. 11.22 Relaxation training of spasmodic facial muscle

The training time is 50 min. The contraction training takes 25 min and the relaxation training takes 25 min. One therapy course takes 3 months.

This training can be combined with virtual reality training of neurological training. The frequency of neurological training is once a week and the frequency of virtual reality training are 4–5 times a week (50 min per time). One therapy course takes 3 months.

In addition, it can cooperate with thermal therapy, massage, traction and self-exercise of musculus facialis. Spasmodic muscle and antagonistic muscle are stimulated in sequence. At first, spasmodic muscle contracts intensely and then antagonistic muscle contracts. Through reciprocal inhibition, spasmodic muscles are relieved (therapy equipment of muscle spasm). Because it is not in accordance with the mechanism of central nerve potential development, the effect is uncertain.

4. The prevention of facial neuritis includes invigorating health effectively, keep face and post aurem warm in cold weather, avoid sitting or sleeping in the wind blow to prevent attack or relapse.
   (a) Psychological counseling: The onset of facial neuritis is sudden. When getting up in the morning, the patients are in facial distortion and they feel nervous, anxious and terrified. They are anxious about facial sequelae after therapy and are ashamed of meeting other people. Therefore, during the therapy, the therapists should make explanations, comfort and ease the patients to relieve the nervous patients. The patients with stable mood can cooperate the training and therapeutic effect is increased.
   (b) Protecting eyes: because eyelid is not closed completely or cannot be closed, cornea is exposed and there is no blinking movement or corneal reflex. Intraocular infection is common. Therefore, protection of the eyes is very important. The patients can drip eyewash for lubrication, diminishing inflammation and nutrition in daytime. At night, the patients wear blinder or use saline gauze piece to cover the eyes. The patients should decrease using eyes and wear sunglasses in case of direct sunlight.
   (c) Facial partial nursing: hot compress to dispel the wind: fresh ginger residue is used on the face in paralytic side (half an hour a day). Moist heat: hot towel is used to cover the face (2–3 times a day). In addition, the patients should not wash face using cold water, take shelter from the wind, add clothes timely, do exercise and prevent from cold.
   (d) Persisted therapy and self-exercise: the rehabilitation of neural function injure takes a long time, 3 months or even longer. The patients and their family should know this and persist the therapy. In addition, whether the disease history is long or short, proper rehabilitation training can recover the functions further and the patients should not give up therapy because of long disease history.

Persisted self-exercise and health care of facial muscle has consolidated therapeutic effect, which can prevent relapse and facial neuritis.

11.3.1 Clinical Therapeutic Effect Observation of Peripheral Facial Paralysis Treated by Rehabilitation of Neurological Training

Facial neuritis is called Bell's Palsy, which belongs to peripheral facial paralysis and is usually induced by aseptic inflammation of facial nerve. The manifestations are special signs of facial mimetic muscle paralysis such as facial distortion, disappeared forehead wrinkle and incomplete closing eyes. It is usually accompanied with facial numbness, pain, dysgeusia and hyperakusis. If peripheral facial paralysis is not treated timely or properly, there are sequelae such as flaccidness of upper eyelid, no raising eyebrow movement, shallow nasolabial groove, facial distortion, facial stiffness, dyspepsia and water leakage when brushing the teeth. In severe patients, there are musculus facialis spasm, contracture and facial synkinetic movement. It can not only induce facial dysfunction to varying degrees, but also give mental stress to the patients because of affecting facial beauty, even affecting social contact and daily life.

At present, physiotherapies include hormone and nerve neurotrophic medicine, acupuncture, massage, sunken lead and electrical stimulus, but there are dysfunctions to varying degrees. The author use rehabilitation technique of neurological training to treat the patients and obtain good therapeutic effect.

11.3.1.1 Materials and Methods

1. Clinical materials: From August 2007 to August 2009, in rehabilitation center of neurological training of Capital Medical University affiliated Beijing Tongren Hospital, there are 30 inpatients and outpatients with peripheral facial paralysis. There are 18 males and 12 females. The age is 22–65 years old. The average age is 38.6 ± 12.5 years old. The shortest disease history is 3 months and the longest is 12 months. The average is 5.0 ± 9.5 months.
   Inclusion criteria:
   It is in accordance with diagnosis criteria of facioplegia.
   The lesion is unilateral in all patients.
   The disease history is 3–12 months.
   All the patients receive standard therapy such as hormone and nerve neurotrophic medicine, acupuncture and physiotherapy.
   The signs and symptoms of facial paralysis are still obvious such as numbness, facial distortion, air leakage when blowing mouth and shallow nasolabial groove in paralytic side.
   Exclusion criteria:
   Facial paralysis due to complete injury of facial nerve induced by trauma.
   Facial paralysis due to compression of tumor on facial nerve.
   Facial paralysis induced by central diseases.
2. Therapeutic method includes therapy of neurological training and physiotherapy.
   (a) Facial neurological training: in a warm, quiet, soundproof and lucifugl room, the patients sit in front of the display. Biofeedback equipment is used and 3 M Ag-AgCl surface electrode and reception electrode are separately placed in the two ends of the training muscle (the starting point and dead point). Reference electrode is pasted between the surface electrode and reception electrode or besides them. Under proper anti-resistance conditions, six-step Daoyin technique in traditional Chinese medicine is used to encourage the patients to do active contraction training of the muscle. Electrical signal from motor center to muscle is displayed on the fluorescent screen in a curve form and this curve is regarded as the baseline (transverse line). The therapists guided the patients to try to make the next signal intensity surpass the baseline. During therapy, when the signal intensity almost reaches the peak, the therapists exert resistance on the negative orientation of muscle contraction and use speeches to encourage the patients to surpass the baseline as much as possible such as "hold on, higher, higher, or you will bump!". After that, the therapists use new summit as the baseline and guide the patients to make new signal intensity surpass new baseline. The rest can be done in the same manner (Fig. 11.23, 11.24, and 11.25). The same method can be used for the training of frontalis, orbicularis oculi muscle, Albinus'muscle and orbicular muscle of mouth. The training time is 10 min for each muscle. The frequency is once a day (50 min) and there are 30 times.
   (b) Physical exercise therapy of facial neurological training: Six-step Daoyin technique in traditional Chinese medicine is used to do active movement training of facial muscle under anti-resistance training such as raising eyebrow, closing eyes,

exposing teeth, pouting, blowing mouth, smile and movement of upper and lower lips. Its purpose is to recover the innervation ability of facial nerve to dominate facial muscle, promote active movement of paralytic muscle and reestablish motor program of musculus facialis. During therapy, the environment should be kept quiet. The patients are in supine position and the therapists stand beside the head of the patients. The therapists wear gloves, smear adequate paroline or olive oil on the face in the paralytic side, make the face in uninjured side do the movement that the face in injured side will do, guide the patients to establish movement idea and target of facial muscle in injured side. The therapists ask the patients to take a deep breath, relax, concentrate on the brain and suddenly concentrate on the corresponding muscle of the face in injured side. The patients are guided to complete contraction movement of facial muscle. Meanwhile, the therapists exert opposite force and use speech to encourage the patients such as "1, 2, 3, go for it, 4, 5, hold on, fight!" the patients take deep breath and relax. Every facial movement should be trained for six times. In therapy interval, the therapists should do massage of facial muscle to relax muscle and alleviate spasm. If there is musculus facialis contracture in uninjured side, facial massage and manipulation traction in uninjured side are done to loosen adhesion.

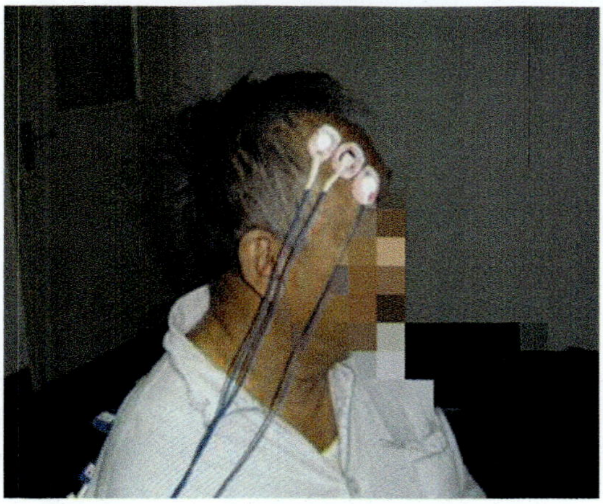

Fig. 11.23 Rehabilitation training of neurological training in the patients with obsolete facial paralysis

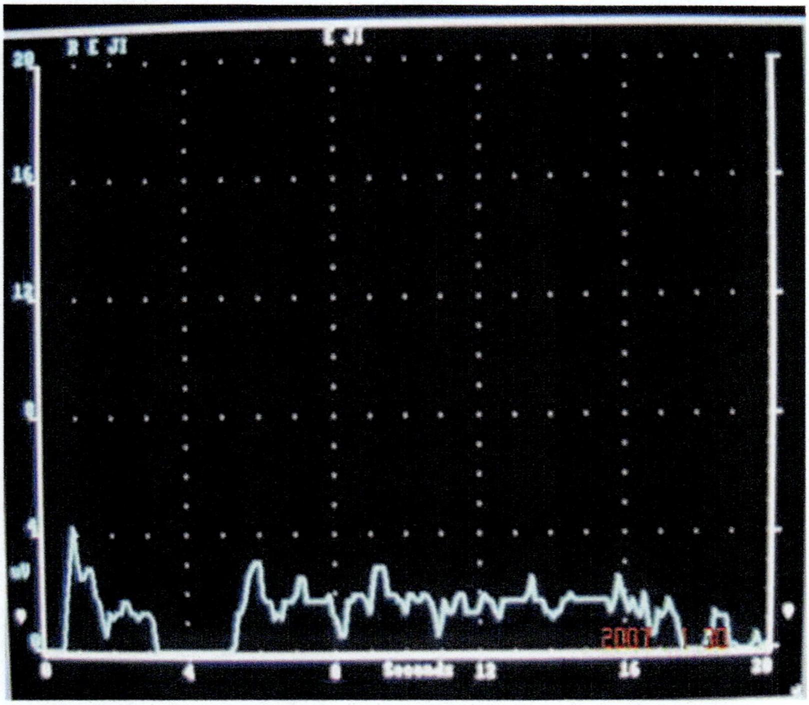

Fig. 11.24 Motor program signal at the beginning of the training

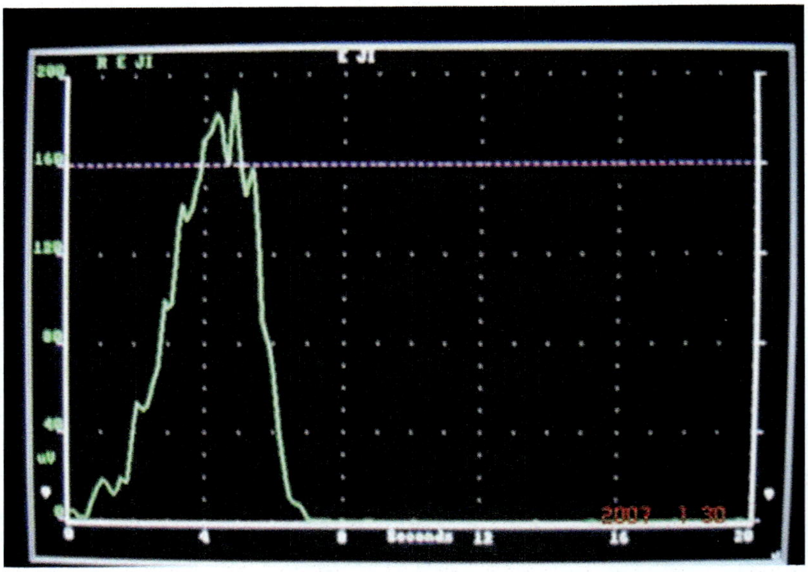

Fig. 11.25 After training, program signal is increased obviously and the functions are improved

There is one time a day (30 min per time) and there are 30 times in a therapy course.

(c) Medium frequency electrotherapy: Medium-frequency pulse therapeutic device with sinusoidal modulation is used. Two round electrodes are separately placed in frontalis and Albinus'muscle. The pulse frequency is 1–10 kHz. Medium frequency electrical stimulation can enhance excitability of muscle contraction to promote recovery of motor function, improve blood circulation, alleviate pain and numbness.

There is one time a day (20 min per time) and there are 30 times in a therapy course.

(d) Ultrashort wave: Two electrodes are separately placed in the front of ear and mastoid process. The micro-thermal (60–100 mA) is used to eliminate edema of facial nerve canal to relieve the compression of edema to facial nerve, recover functions of facial nerve and alleviate pain in mastoid process.

There is one time a day (20 min per time) and there are 30 times in a therapy course.

(e) Far infrared rays:20 cm away from aural skin in injured side, irradiation cover of far infrared rays is placed and the heat should be comfort and don't burn the skin. Its function is to improve local blood circulation, eliminate inflammation and edema.

There is one time a day (20 min per time) and there are 30 times in a therapy course.

(f) Self-facial muscle exercise: According to the training map of facial mimetic muscle, the patients do self-exercise of frown, closing eyes, smile, blow cheek and pouting. Compared with the uninjured side, the exercise effect is better.

There is two times a day (10 min per time) and there are 60 times in a therapy course.

3. Functional assessment: international general assessment method is used by special rehabilitation physician to do functional assessment at the beginning of the therapy and after the therapy. House-Brackmann and Portmann simple assessment methods are used for the intensity assessment of surface electromyogram signals of frontalis, orbicularis oculi muscle, Albinus'muscle and orbicular muscle of mouth. The data are recorded in database.

(a) Therapeutic effect assessment standard of House-Brackmann: House-Brackmann facial nerve classification standard is divided into six grades.

- Grade I: Normal.
- Grade II: There may be slight asymmetry in the facial movement functions and slight synkinetic movement.
- Grade III: There is obvious asymmetry and secondary defect, but there is still movement in frontal part.
- Grade IV: There is obvious asymmetry, but there is no movement in frontal part.
- Grade V: There is merely slight movement in the face.
- Grade VI: the paralysis is complete and there is no movement. The higher the grade of House-Brackmann is, the better the functional recovery of facial nerve is.

(b) Simple assessment method of Portmann includes six autokinetic movements such as frown, closing eyes, moving wing of nose, smiling, whistle and blowing cheek. The scores of movement in injured side and uninjured side are 3. The score is 2, which stands for weak movement. The score is 1, which stands for slight movement. The score is 0, which stands for autokinetic movement inability. In addition, there are 2 score for impression. The score of completely normal is 20.

- Portmann assessment standard.
- Completely recovery (more than 17).
- Partially recovery (16–14).
- Just good (13–10).
- Bad (less than 9).
- The lower the score is, the more severe the disease is.
- The higher Portmann score is, the stronger EMG signal is and the better the functional recovery of facial nerve is.

4. Statistical analysis: statistical software SPSS12.0 is used for statistical analysis. The data results are expressed as Mean ± SD ($\bar{X} \pm S$). T-test is used for the data comparison before and after therapy. $P < 0.05$ is regarded as significant difference.

11.3.1.2 Results

Assessment data analysis result of 30 before and after therapy patients refers to Table 11.4. There is significant difference of the data before and after therapy ($p < 0.01$), especially the therapy data of Albinus' muscle and orbicularis oculi muscle.

The comparison between Portmann scores and therapeutic effect refers to Table 11.5. There are 15 patients who are recovered completely in 30 patients. The Portmann scores is 17–20. There are two patients who are recovered poorly. The Portmann scores is less than 9 (Table 11.6).

Table 11.4 Statistical analysis data of facial muscle signal and Portmann scores before and after therapy ($\bar{X} \pm S$)

Assessment items	Before therapy	After therapy	t	p
Frontalis	13.93 ± 9.07	79.83 ± 42.80	9.17	<0.01
Albinus' muscle	22.76 ± 13.83	104.93 ± 41.35	13.76	<0.01
Orbicularis oris muscle	19.00 ± 20.71	81.40 ± 55.02	7.56	<0.01
Orbicularis oculi muscle	22.03 ± 12.44	109.17 ± 42.01	14.60	<0.01
Portmann scores	7.27 ± 2.20	16.20 ± 2.94	19.98	<0.01

Table 11.5 Recovery rate of therapeutic effect of Portmann scores before and after therapy

Therapeutic effect	Case number	Percentage
Completely recovery (more than 17)	15	50
Partially recovery (16–14)	10	33.33
Just good (13–10)	3	10
Bad (less than 9)	2	6.67

Table 11.6 The rate of therapeutic effect of House-Brackmann classification before and after therapy

Therapeutic effect	Before therapy		After therapy	
Grade	Case number	Percentage	Case number	Percentage
I	0	0	10	33.33
II	1	3.33	15	50
III	15	50	3	10
IV	10	33.33	2	6.67
V	2	6.67	0	0
VI	2	6.67	0	0

11.3.1.3 Discussion

There are many methods to treat peripheral facial paralysis such as medicine, acupuncture, physiotherapy, sunken cord and massage [7]. These methods have some therapeutic effects on the disease in the early phase, mainly through eliminating inflammation, alleviating edema, nurturing nerve and activating non-functional cells and neural fibers in shock state, but these methods usually have sequelae. They have no effect on the patients in recovery period or in obsolete cases. Because these methods all are passive measures, they are not in accordance with the mechanism of "skillful use and dependence" to promote neural plasticity.

Rehabilitation techniques of neurological training mainly are active movements, which are in accordance with the mechanism of promoting central neural plasticity and functional reorganization. Through neural potential development, motor program reestablishment and facial muscle motor pattern remodeling guided by Daoyin technique, the key point of therapy is put on recovery of neural functions to recover undead cells and conduction pathways and develop normal cells around injured area and conduction pathway so that they can play functions to replace the injured cells. On the basis of this, through motor program reestablishment technique, new activated neural cells can work coordinately and orderly. After that, through actual applied training, synkinetic movement of facial muscle is relieved. Meanwhile, cooperated with manual massage, facial muscle stretch and physiotherapy, adhesion and spasm of facial muscle and conbundleure of facial muscle in uninjured side are relieved effectively to recover autokinetic movement of facial muscle through neurological training method. Therefore, the comprehensive rehabilitation method of treating facial paralysis not only can recover autokinetic movement of facial muscle, but also relieve facial numbness, expression stiffness and unusual facies, which obtain good effect.

In short, this therapy not only includes the training of central facial nucleus to develop potential, enhance the control ability of brain to facial nerve and myodynamia of mimetic muscle, but also includes the training of peripheral facial nerve to promote its regeneration, activate reserved neural conduction pathway, recover autokinetic movement of paralytic facial muscle. With physical therapy, improvement of compression of facial nerve increases therapeutic effect, which is the new effective method to treat peripheral facioplegia. Long-term follow-up result of this method should be surveyed further. Coordination application of the method and formulation of therapy course require further exploration to rectify and improve this method in order to increase therapeutic effect.

References

1. Fishman Jonathan M. Corticosteroids effective in idiopathic facial nerve palsy (Bell's Palsy) but not necessarily in idiopathic acute vestibular dysfunction (Vestibular Neuritis). Laryngoscope. 2011;121(11):2494–5.
2. Jha AK, Nijhawan S, Nepalia S, Suchismita A. Association of Bell's Palsy with hepatitis E virus infection: a rare entity. J Clin Exp Hepatol. 2012;2(1):88–90.

3. Wackym PA. Molecular temporal bone pathology: II. Ramsay Hunt syndrome (herpeszoster oticus). Laryngoscope. 1997;107(9):1165–75.
4. Leal CL, Goffi GMVS, Ferreira BR, Roberto CL. Mime functional evaluation in facial paralysis following a stroke. Pró-Fono Rev Atual Cient. 2006;17(2):231–6.
5. Daniel A, Drubach MD, Michael Makley MD, Maryellen L, Dodd MD. Manipulation of central nervous system plasticity: a new dimension in the care of neurologically impaired patients. Mayo Clin Proc. 2004;79(6):796–800.
6. Fabrin S, Soares N, Regalo SCH, Verri ED. The effects of acupuncture on peripheral facial palsy sequelae after 20 years via electromyography. J Acupunct Meridian Stud. 2015;8(5):245–8.
7. Zhenzhen X. In recent years, clinical research progress in the treatment of facial paralysis. J Tradit Chin Med. 2010;25(05):1032–4.

12 Rehabilitation Therapy of Neurological Training of Cerebral Palsy in Children

12.1 The Characteristics of Cerebral Palsy

Cerebral palsy (CP) is short called brain paralysis [1]. From birth to 1 month after the birth, non-progressive brain injury syndrome is induced by some factors. The main manifestations are central movement dysfunction, muscle spasm, abnormal posture and bone and joint deformity accompanied with disorders of intelligence, speech, epilepsia, visual and auditory sense, behavior and perception.

12.1.1 Characteristics and Types of Cerebral Palsy in Children

The common causes of brain paralysis are maldevelopment, premature delivery, apnea, low body weight, craniocerebral injury and genetics [2]. The morbidity is 0.15–0.5% and is one of the main diseases that lead to disabilities in children, which affect the growth and development and self-care ability of children.

Clinical manifestations of movement dysfunction of cerebral palsy are various because of complicated pathological factors, injured parts and different degrees. The classification is according to the characteristic and degree of movement dysfunction and disease severity.

1. It can be divided into five types [3] according to the characteristic of movement dysfunction.
   (a) Spasmodic type is the most common type. The lesion is located in pyramidal tract system and the main manifestations are limbs movement restriction, increase of muscle tension, increase of passive movement resistance, clasp knife spasticity and tendon hyperreflexia.
   (b) Athetosic type is common. The lesion is located in basal ganglia and the main manifestations are uncertain muscle spasm, inconformity between movement will and movement results, involuntary movement, negative pathological reflex and dysarthria.
   (c) Ataxia type is rare. The lesion is located in epencephalon and the main manifestations are poor balance function, poor coordination of voluntary movement, volitional tremor and nystagmus.
   (d) Mixed type is common in clinic. It includes the characteristics of two or more types mentioned above, which is induced by injuries of pyramidal system and extrapyramidal system or epencephalon at the same time.
   (e) Other types are rare. The manifestation of relaxant type is low muscular tension. The manifestation of rigidity type is increase of motor resistance (lead-pipe rigidity).

W. Zhao, *Rehabilitation Therapeutics of the Neurological Training*,
https://doi.org/10.1007/978-981-13-0812-3_12

The manifestation of tremor type is static tremor of muscle.

2. According to the dysfunction degree of limb movement, it includes many types:
   (a) Paralysis of single limb: single limb is paralyzed, which is rare.
   (b) Hemiplegia: the limbs and trunk in one side are paralyzed, especially the upper limb.
   (c) Triplegia: the limbs and trunk in one side and one limb in offside are paralyzed.
   (d) Quadriplegia: all the limbs and trunk are paralyzed. The severity of upper limbs is the same as that of lower limbs.
   (e) Paraplegia: both lower limbs are severely paralyzed, but the trunk and upper limbs are normal.
   (f) Diplegia: all the limbs are paralyzed. The trunk and upper limbs are slight, but both lower limbs are severe.
   (g) Double hemipilegia: all the limbs are paralyzed. Both upper limbs are severe and sometimes the severity of left and right side may be different.
3. According to illness degree, it can be divided into three types.
   (a) Mild: the patients can look after themselves in their daily life.
   (b) Moderate: the patients can partially look after themselves in their daily life.
   (c) Severe: the patients cannot look after themselves in their daily life completely.
4. Cerebral palsy dysfunction in early phase [4]: The early phase is from birth to the ninth month after birth and the main manifestations are as follows:
   (a) General manifestations: the children patients have a short fuse, cry and scream persistently or are excessively quiet, have a weak sound of weeping, are difficult to be lactated or swallow, is easy to vomit and there is harmful weight gain.
   (b) Muscular tension and autokinetic movement: there are low muscular tension and decreased autokinetic movement.
   (c) Body posture and movement: the body becomes hand, the posture is abnormal and the movement is uncoordinated.
   (d) Cognitive state: the patients are slow in reacting, cannot recognize person and cry.
   (e) Motor development: big motor development fall behind such as unable to turnover, crawl, clench fist and grasp.
   (f) Myospasm: Convulsive seizure is usual.

The doctors know clinical manifestations of cerebral palsy in early phase and find out the dysfunction of cerebral palsy in early phase as soon as possible, which is the premise of realizing the basic rehabilitation principle of "early detection, early diagnosis and early therapy" of cerebral palsy.

12.1.2 Complications and Secondary Diseases

Except the main dysfunctions mentioned above, there are still complications and secondary diseases.

1. Complications: the common complications include dysgnosia (75% of all cerebral palsy), aphasis (30–70%), epilepsia (14–75%), hearing impairment (5–8%) and visual impairment (50–60%). In addition, there are dysfunctions of sensation and behavior.
2. Secondary diseases: it is induced by dysfunctions such as joint adhesion, deformity, tendon contracture, dislocation or subluxation of shoulder, hip and capitulum radii, osteoporosis, amyotrophy and scoliose.

12.2 Assessment Method of Cerebral Palsy in Children

There are many assessment methods of cerebral palsy, which are mostly used for effect assessment. There are few methods used for formulation of therapeutic schedule. Assessment method of children rehabilitation of neurological training includes myodynamia assessment, balance function assessment and myospasm assessment. This chapter only includes the assessment of motor function. Other functional assessment method of children cerebral palsy can refer to associated rehabilitation books or rehabilitation functional assessment monographs.

1. Comprehensive functional assessment of children cerebral palsy 4 (Tables 12.1 and 12.2).

Table 12.1 Comprehensive functional assessment table

Items	Scores		Items	Scores	
	Month day	Month day		Month day	Month day
I. Cognitive function			6. Stand		
1. Recognition of common shape			7.Walk		
2. Distinguishment of common concept			8. Walk up and down stairs		
3. Basic concept of space			9. Stretch out one's hand to fetch something		
4. Know four kinds of colors			10. Use thumb and index finger to fetch something		
5. Know something in the painting			Summation		
6. Be able to draw circle, vertical, transverse and oblique line			IV. Self-care movement		
7. Can concentrate on something instantly			1. Open bibcock		
8. Memory of the past			2. Wash face and hands		
9. Seek help and express ideas			3. Wash teeth		
10. Count, do addition and subtraction			4. Hold bowl		
Summation			5. Use hands or spoon to eat		
II. Speech functions			6. Put on or put off jacket		
1. Understand cold, heat and hunger			7. Put on or put off trousers		
2. Want to communicate with others			8. Put on or put off footgear		
3. Be able to understand others' expressions and behaviors			9. Untie and tie button		
4. Be able to express own needs			10. Can deal with is before or after using the toilet		
5. Be able to say sentence with 2–3 words			Summation		
6. Can simulate oral movement			V. Social adjustment		
7. Can pronunciate b, p, a, o and ao			1. Know family member		
8. Follow easy orders			2. Respect others and say hello to others		
9. Can repeat easy words			3. Take part in group game		
10. Can speak easy words according to pictures			4. Self-called and all relationship		
Summation			5. Can separate with mother		
III. Motor ability			6. Look out and know not to touch fire and electricity		
1. Head control			7. Know the environments		
2. Turn over			8. Are they familiar with family or not?		
3. Sit			9. Know health and disease		
4. Crawl			10. Can answer the social questions simply		
5. Kneel					
Total points: 1. _____ (2) _____ (3) _____					
General comments if functional status:					

Table 12.2 Evaluation standard of comprehensive function assessment (hundred-mark system)

Performance	Scores of each item	Total scores
All completed	2.0	100
Most completed	1.5	75
Half completed	1.0	50
Partially completed	0.5	25
Cannot complete	0.0	0

Table 12.3 Lovett myodynamia grading standard

Grade	Name	Standard	Percent of normal myodynamia
0	Zero	No detectable muscle contraction	0
1	Slightly	Slight contraction, but cannot induce joint motion	10
2	Bad	Can do full range of joint motion in weight support state	25
3	Just so	So can do full range of joint motion and do anti-weight movement, but cannot do anti-resistance movement	50
4	Good	Can do anti-weight movement and anti-certain-resistance full range of joint motion	75
5	Normal	Can do anti-weight movement and anti-sufficient-resistance full range of joint motion	100

2. Myodynamia assessment.

   Lovett manual muscle test Table 12.3.
3. Rehabilitation assessment of cerebral palsy spasm.
   (a) Improved Ashworth myospasm assessment method: in passive joint motion, according to range of joint motion with reflex muscular contraction force, myospasm can be classified into four grades (Table 12.4).

   Judgement of posture tension degree of lower limbs: The angle width of adductor and activities of children patients are used for the judgement of severity of lower limbs spasm.

   Severe: the angle of adductor is 0–30°. The patients cannot do exercise by themselves or are difficult to do exercise.

   Mild: the angle of adductor is 30–60°. The patients can do exercise with one pattern.

   Slight: the angle of adductor is 60–90°. The manifestations are poor motor coordination and tractability.

Table 12.4 Assessment of myospasm degree of cerebral palsy

Grade	Standard
0	Reflex muscular contractility is not increased and there is no resistance in the full range of passive limbs movement
1	Reflex muscular contractility is increased slightly and there is slight resistance when the limbs are moved passively to the terminals with slight resistance
1+	Reflex muscular contractility is increased slightly. In passive limbs movement, in the first half, there is sensation of slight locking and in the last half, there is slight resistance
2	Reflex muscular contractility is increased mildly. In passive limbs movement, there is resistance in the most range of limbs movement, but the limbs still can be moved
3	Reflex muscular contractility is increased moderately. In passive limbs movement, there is resistance in full range of limbs movement and limbs are hard to be moved
4	Reflex muscular contractility is increased highly. The limbs are stiff, the resistance is big and passive movements are difficult

4. Nervous reflex exam: Nervous reflex is the important index of CNS development and children movement development, which is significant for diagnosis of motor dysfunction.

During the process of assessment, the therapists should induce primitive reflex, correction response, balance response and protective extension response in every posture and observe the condition of response. If there is any abnormity, the therapists should find out the main reason that hinder the formation of response and observe the response of children patients with cerebral palsy to rehabilitation therapy of neurological training, which provides basis for formulation of therapeutic schedule. Specific assessment method should refer to rehabilitation medicine books about assessment of examination of the nervous system of children.

5. Development assessment of big motor function: Motor development of children patients with cerebral palsy is significantly lower than that of children in the same age. Motor functions and activities of daily life are required to be assessed.

   The degree of motor development retardation can be judged according to proverb such as raising head at second month, turning over at fourth month, sitting in sixth month, rolling at seventh month, creeping at eighth month and walking at ninth month. Motor development index of normal baby refer to Table 12.5.

6. Balance ability assessment [5]: It can be assessed by balance response.
   (a) Tilting reaction: The babies lie in their back or are in the prone position on the plate and they keep their head uptight when they are swayed left and right. There is equilibrium reaction to outside of the upper limbs and lower limbs in the upward side and protective extension of the upper limbs and lower limbs in the downward side.

       Tilting reaction appears in the sixth month after birth and lasts for lifelong, which is the basic element of standing balance and walking balance.
   (b) Sitting balance reaction includes balance reaction in the front, sideward and backward of sitting position. When the children patients are in sitting position and are pushed forward, sideward and backward, they extend upper limbs forward, sideward and backward to keep balance.

       Sitting balance reaction appears in the sixth–tenth month after birth and lasts for lifelong.
   (c) Standing balance reaction: when the babies are in standing position and incline to all around by external force. Under normal circumstance, when they incline forward and backward, they can step forward and backward actively. When they incline left and right, the lower limbs in one side stretches out to the other side to support the body weight, counteract external force and keep the body upright.

Table 12.5 Motor development index of normal baby

Month	Main motor development index
1	The baby can raise head in the prone position. Chin can be way from bed for 3 s. They can grasp pen with two hands. They can open month and simulate speaking
2	The baby can raise head for a while and turn it around in the prone position. They can extend fingers and play them in front of chest. They can suck thumb
3	The baby can raise half the chest in the prone position and can use elbow to support the upper body. The head can be straight and upright. The hands can grasp each other and can be used to grasp clothes
4	The baby can raise upper body until it is vertical to the bed. They can use leg to kick clothes, quilt or lifting toy
5	The baby can turn over, sit against cushion. When sitting, they can unbend waist. They can stand up when they are helped. They can put something into their mouth
6	The baby can use hand to hook the foot. They can extend the body in flat. They can hold one toy in each hand separately. They can take biscuit to eat
7	The baby can sit. They can creep with help. They can use hand to take toy. They can use voice and behavior to notice that they want to defecate
8	The baby can stand up with handrail. They can give the toy to specified people. They can use fingers to grasp something to eat
9	They baby can stand up with something. They can step crosswise with two feet. They can use thumb and index finger to pinch tiny thing. They can cooperate to wear clothes
10	The baby can stand for a while by themselves. The can creep quickly. They can walk hand in hand and get close to other children
11	The baby can walk when lead by one hand. They can point body part and can extend one finger to stand for 1-year-old
12	The baby can stand still and walk a few steps independently. They can complete simple requirements and are willing to play games with other children

7. The assessment of deformity: the common deformity includes hip flexion, adduction, intorsion, flexion of knee joint or genu recurvatum, talipes equinus, foot drop, dislocation or subluxation of hip joint, dislocation or subluxation of patella.

12.3 The Formulation of Therapeutic Schedule

Rehabilitation therapy of cerebral palsy is complicated and is a systemic large-scale project. It not only recovers autonomous contraction function of single muscle, but also establishes motor program of associated movement of single joint motion and multiple joints. On the basis of this, normal motor pattern is established, which is three-stage rehabilitation method. In addition, the therapy of intelligence speech, swallow and gatism and the rectification of bone and joint deformity are the important condition of motor function recovery. In most cases, medicine and surgery cannot solve these problems. Only rehabilitation training can achieve the anticipated goal. Therefore, the rehabilitation of cerebral palsy is challenging and it is a difficult and complicated disease so that rehabilitation is a great human building project.

However, on the other hand, because of the advantages of age and development, CNS plasticity [6] is good, only if we don't fear difficulty, treat it seriously, exam it carefully, analyze it in detail, use proper therapeutic method, implement therapy on the condition that the case is easy to obtain therapeutic effect. For decades, the author summarized a lot through clinical practice.

Through detailed functional assessment, we can find the main obstacles and do therapy according to order of priority, which is the key to recover main functions and increase daily life ability of children patients.

Because cerebral palsy is complicated and the age of the patients is different with different clinical manifestations, we should formulate individual therapeutic schedule, which includes baby and infant types. On the basis of three-stage rehabilitation training principle, individual therapeutic schedule is formulated.

12.3.1 Rehabilitation Therapy Principle of the Baby and Infant with Cerebral Palsy

The baby is the new born from birth to one full year of life, while the infant is the children from 1 year old to 3 years old, which is the important development stage of children. In this stage, nervous system and system of bone, joint and muscle of children patients are not developed completely. In addition, the baby cannot or just learn to walk and they cannot cooperate anti-resistance training of developing neural potential like older children patients and adult with cerebral palsy. However, cerebral palsy is due to injury of brain tissue induced by some factors. The basis of recovering injured brain tissue is CNS plasticity. When some methods are used to recover undead brain cells in injured area, normal cells around injured area play functions to replace the injured cells. However, the process that cells around injured area play functions to replace injured cells is different from the natural development of brain. On the basis of normal movement, the training should be intensified to promote CNS plasticity and functional reorganization.

Therefore, rehabilitation therapy method of cerebral palsy should meet the requirements of active movement and intensified active movement. In addition, because the patients with cerebral palsy are always accompanied with complications and secondary disease, the therapy of complications and secondary disease is necessary on the moment of developing neural potential. Therefore, children patients can be recovered comprehensively. This is the basic principle of rehabilitation therapy of baby and infant.

1. Induction training of active movement: Active movement is the effective method to recover and reestablish brain functions, but the baby and infant cannot cooperate with the training actively so that active movement rehabilitation training is difficulty. Rehabilitation method of neurological training can induce active movement of children patients with the help of posture change combined with game.

2. Rectification of limbs deformity: the patients with cerebral palsy are always with development impairments such as congenital dislocation of hip joint, patella instability, pointed foot and talipes equinovarus. Therefore, during the process of rehabilitation training, the therapists should observe the rectification therapy and prevention of bone and joint deformity, which can recover motor function of limbs on the basis of brain functions recovery.

12.3.2 Rehabilitation Therapy Schedule and Specific Method of the Baby and Infant with Cerebral Palsy

Because the baby cannot cooperate with rehabilitation training completely and the infant can cooperate with training to varying degrees, therapeutic schedules for the baby and infant are different.

1. Rehabilitation therapy schedule of babies with cerebral palsy.

   Induction training of active movement is used according to normal motor development.

   According to normal development law such as raising head at second month, turning over at fourth month, sitting in sixth month, rolling at seventh month, creeping at eighth month and walking at ninth month, the training method takes the body posture change as the principle thing and incudes active movement. Normal motor development law is that the baby in certain months can have the corresponding motor function. Therefore, motor induction training should be 1–2 weeks ahead of the normal development standard. For example, 3 weeks after birth, the baby starts the training of raising head. Three months after birth, the baby starts the induction training of turning over.

   (a) Induction training of raising head: 3 weeks after birth, the baby can start the training. Its purpose is to increase autonomous innervation of brain to musculi colli to make it control the head.

Specific method is as follows:

Support training of head forward: the therapists use upper limbs in one side to pick the baby up and make the baby standing upright with slightly incline backward. The therapists use the other hand to hold the head (Fig. 12.1), and hang or hand out a colorful toy in the front. The therapists loosen their hands and the baby heads backward. The therapists tell the baby "keep your head upright and touch the toy!" Meanwhile, the therapists waggle the toy and make it easy to see. If the baby cannot lift the limbs by himself, the therapists should help him to lift it up. Through several days' training, the support ability of the baby's head is strengthened and the support time can be lengthened to increase the angle of inclining backward. According to the specific condition of the baby, the therapists start to increase the resistance of inclining backward. The location of resistance is frons (Fig. 12.2).

Support training of head backward: the therapists use upper limbs in one side to

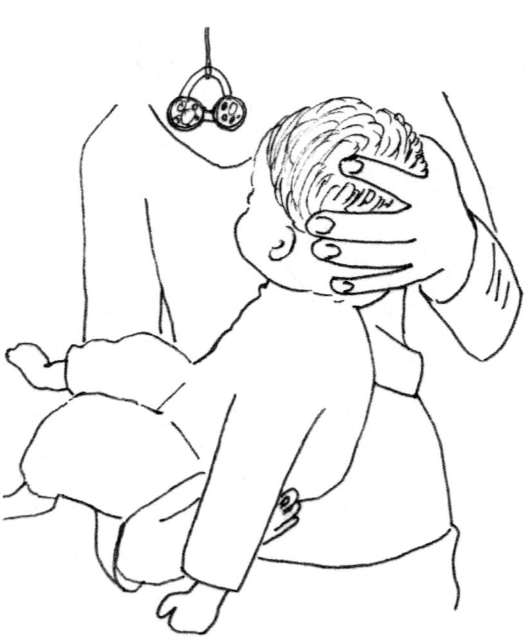

Fig. 12.1 Support training of head forward 1

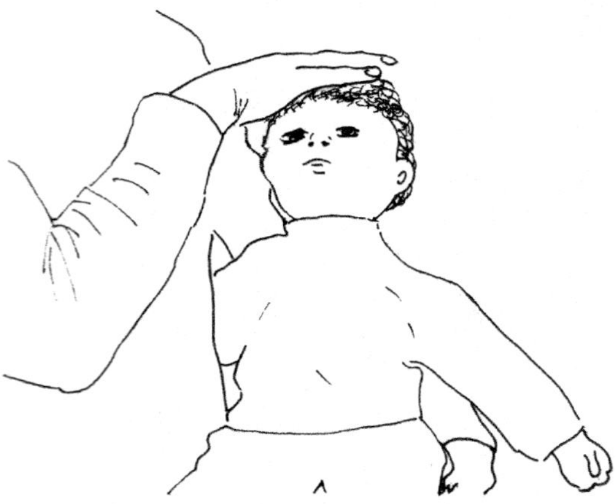

Fig. 12.2 Support training of head forward 2

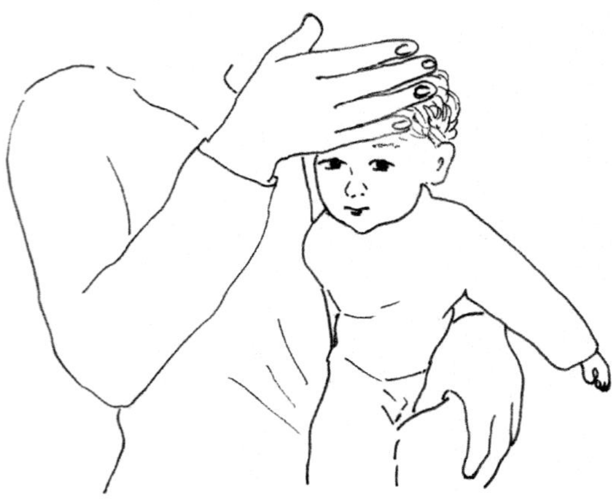

Fig. 12.3 Support training of head backward 1

pick the baby up and make the baby standing upright with slightly incline forward. The therapists use the other hand to hold the head (Fig. 12.3), and hang or hand out a small bell in the front. The therapists loosen their hands and the baby heads forward. The therapists tell the baby "keep your head upright and touch the bell". Meanwhile, the therapists waggle the bell to make noise. If the baby cannot protract backward, the therapists help children patients to restore the normal position of the head. Through several days' training, the support ability of the baby's head is strengthened and the support time can be lengthened to increase the angle of inclining forward. According

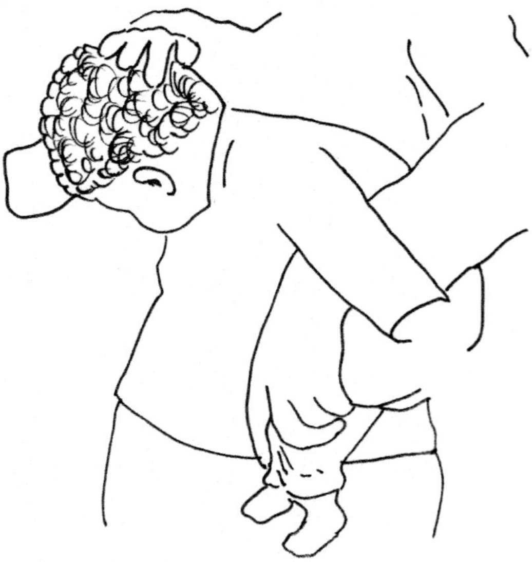

Fig. 12.4 Support training of head backward 2

to the specific condition of the baby, the therapists start to increase the resistance of inclining forward. The location of resistance is occipital region (Fig. 12.4).

The frequency is 1–2 times a day (30 min per time) and there are 30 times in one therapy course. The therapy course can be added according to the functional recovery.

(b) Induction training of turning over: 2.5–3 months after birth, the baby starts the ability training of turning over. Its purpose is to induce turning over ability of children patients.

The specific method is as follows:

Motor induction training of turning over to the right: in the training bed (3–5 m × 1 m) with adjustable inclining angle, the training bed is adjusted to 10–30°. The bed surface at the beginning terminal of the training is high and the bed surface at the ending terminal of the training is low. The bed is like a slope to decrease the difficulty of turning over, which is called downslope turning over training. Children patients recline on it and a colorful toy is hanged in the front of the right of the body. The therapists sway left lower limb of children patients

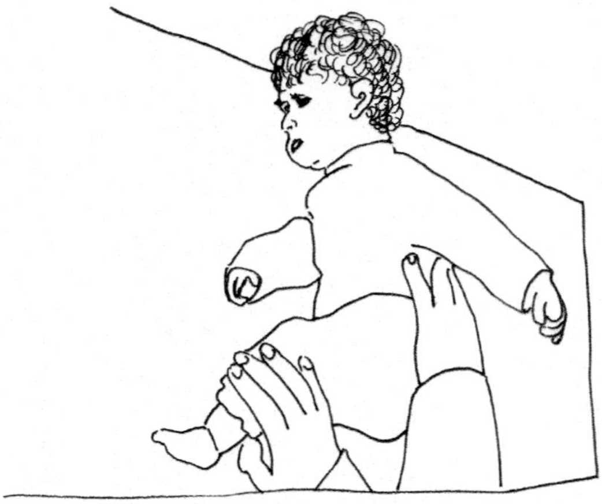

Fig. 12.5 Training of turning over to the right 1

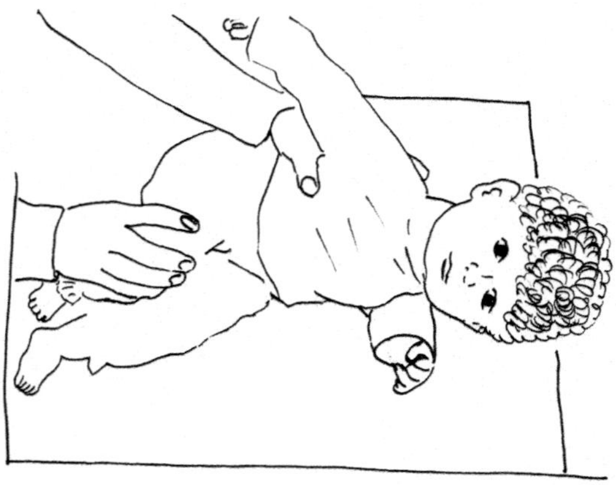

Fig. 12.6 Training of turning over to the right 2

to the right, make it cross over right lower limbs and put it on training bed. After that, the therapists use speech to tell children patients to get the toy through turning over to the right and help children patients to sway their upper part of the body and left upper limb to the right (Fig. 12.5). After completing turning over movement, the children patients are in ventral decubitus. The therapists sway right lower limb of children patients to right backward and make it cross over left limb until foot touch the bed surface. After that, the therapists use speech to tell children patients to get the toy through turning over to the right and help children patients to sway their upper part of the body and left upper limb to the right (Fig. 12.6). After completing turning over movement, the children patients are in supine position. The baby does the next training of turning over to the right until he gets the other end of the training bed. With the increase of turning over ability of children patients, the inclining angle of training bed is decreased gradually and is transmitted to upslope turning over training.

Motor induction training of turning over to the left: Children patients lie on the back in bed and a colorful toy is hanged in the front of the left of the body. From the downslope turning over training, the therapists sway right lower limb of children patients to the left, make it cross over left lower limbs and put it on training bed. After that, the therapists use speech to tell children patients to get the toy through turning over to the left and help children patients to sway their upper part of the body and right upper limb to the left (Fig. 12.7). After completing turning over movement, the children patients are in ventral decubitus. The therapists sway right lower limb of children patients to right backward and make it cross over left limb until foot touch the bed surface. After that, the therapists use speech to tell children patients to get the toy through turning over to the left and help children patients to sway their upper part of the body and right upper limb to the left (Fig. 12.8). After completing turning over movement, the children patients are in supine position. The baby does the next training of turning over to the left until he gets the other end of the training bed. With the increase of turning over ability of children patients, the inclining angle of training bed is decreased gradually and is transmitted to upslope turning over training.

The frequency is 1–2 times a day (30 min per time) and there are 30 times in one therapy course. The therapy

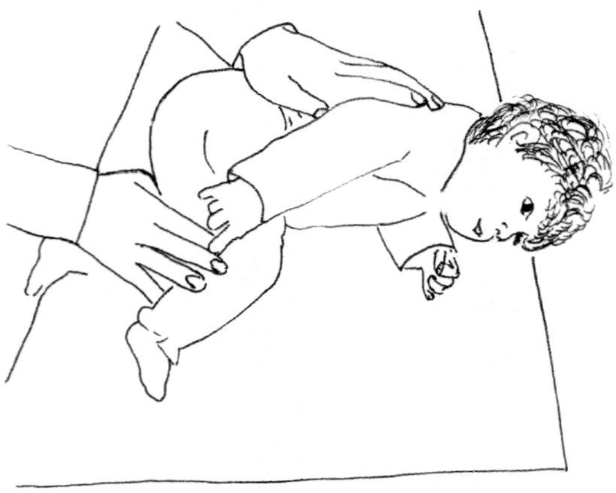

Fig. 12.7 Training of turning over to the left 1

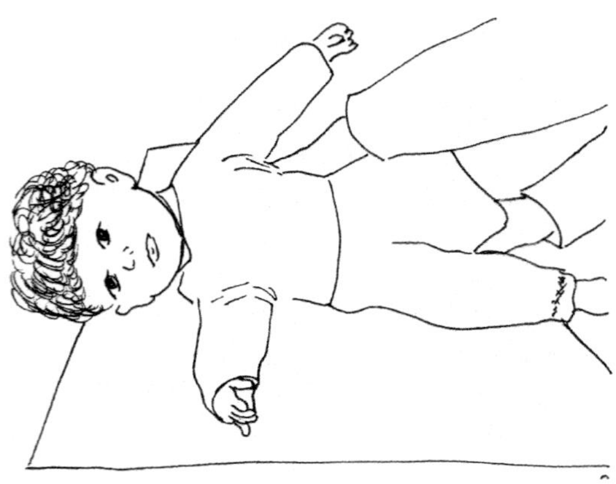

Fig. 12.8 Training of turning over to the left 2

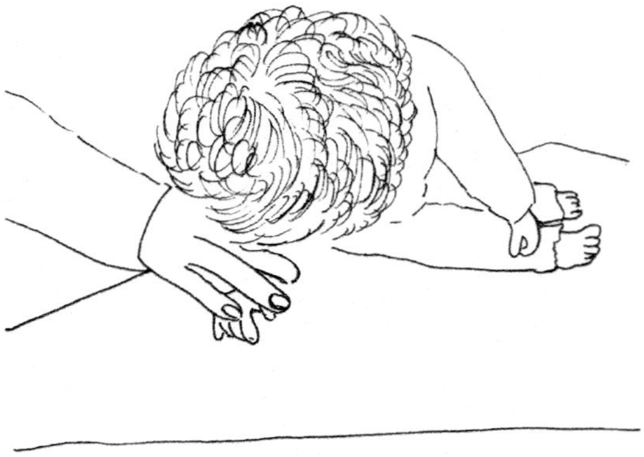

Fig. 12.9 Sitting up training in right side

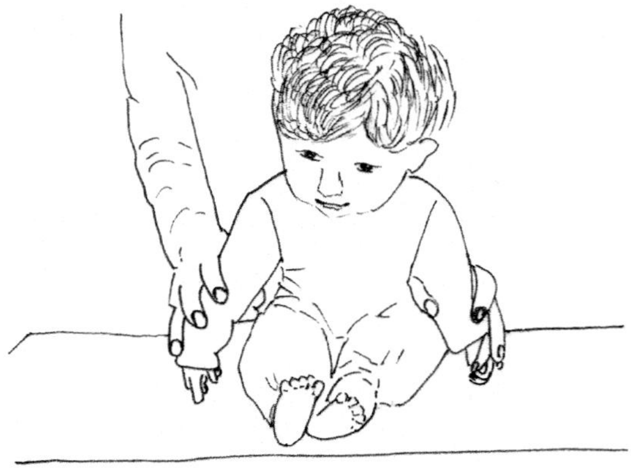

Fig. 12.10 Sitting up training in the center

course can be added according to the functional recovery.

(c) Induction training of sitting up: 4–5 months after birth, the baby starts the training of sitting up and balance ability in sitting position. Its purpose is to induce sitting up and balance ability in sitting position of children patients by themselves.

The specific method is as follows:

- Induction training of sitting up to the right: when children patients are in supine position, the therapists guide and help children patients to turn upper part of the body to the right. The therapists let children patients use elbow of right upper limb and left palm to support the body on bed surface and use upper limbs to make the trunk upright in sitting position. With the increase of the ability, the therapists reduce the support force and exert resistance from left back to forward in the process of sitting up to further increase strength of low back muscle (Fig. 12.9).
- Induction training of sitting up in the center: when children patients are in supine position, the therapists guide and help children patients to lift up the upper part of the body, use two hands to support the body on bed surface and use upper limbs to make the trunk upright in sitting position. With the increase of the ability, the therapists reduce the support force

and exert resistance from forward to backward in the process of sitting up to further increase strength of abdominal muscle (Fig. 12.10).

Induction training of sitting up to the left: when children patients are in supine position, the therapists guide and help children patients to turn upper part of the body to the left. The therapists let children patients use elbow of left upper limb and right palm to support the body on bed surface and use upper limbs to make the trunk upright in sitting position. With the increase of the ability, the therapists reduce the support force and exert resistance from right back to forward in the process of sitting up to further increase strength of low back muscle (Fig. 12.11).

Induction training of balance movement in sitting position: The therapists help children patients to sit upright and tell them "sit still and do not fall down". The therapists loosen their hands but still in protection and use counting method to encourage children patients to keep in sitting position for longer time. If children patients are going to fall down, the therapists help children patients to sit upright again. With the increase of the ability, the therapists reduce the support force and exert resistance from every direction to push children patients slightly in order to increase balance ability in sitting position (Fig. 12.12).

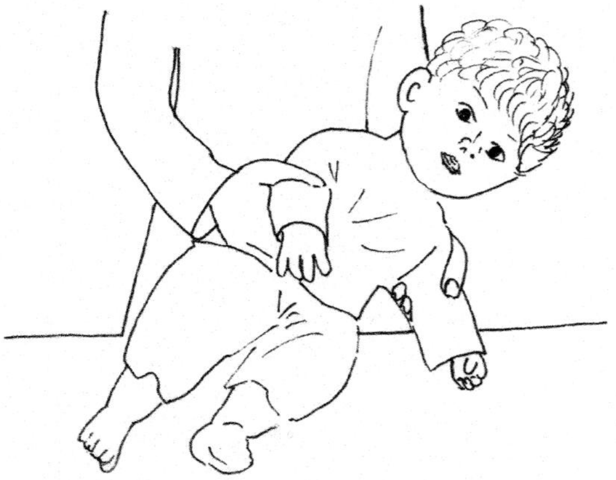

Fig. 12.11 Induction training of sitting up in the left side

The frequency is once a day (30 min per time) and there are 30 times in one therapy course. The therapy course can be added according to the functional recovery.

(d) Induction training of rolling movement: 5–6 months after birth, the baby starts the training of rolling ability. Its purpose is to induce continuous rolling ability of children patients.

The specific method is as follows:

- Induction training of rolling movement to the right: in the training bed (3–5 m × 1 m) with adjustable inclining angle, the training bed is adjusted to 45° downslope positions. Children patients recline on it and a colorful toy is hanged in the front of the right of the body. The therapists sway left lower limb of children patients to the right, make it cross over right lower limbs and put it on training bed. After that, the therapists use speech to tell children patients to get the toy through turning over to the right and help children patients to sway their upper part of the body and left upper limb to the right. After completing

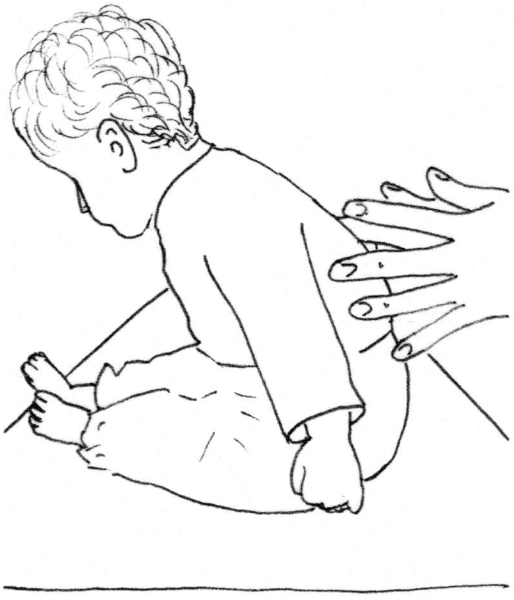

Fig. 12.12 Induction training of balance movement in sitting position

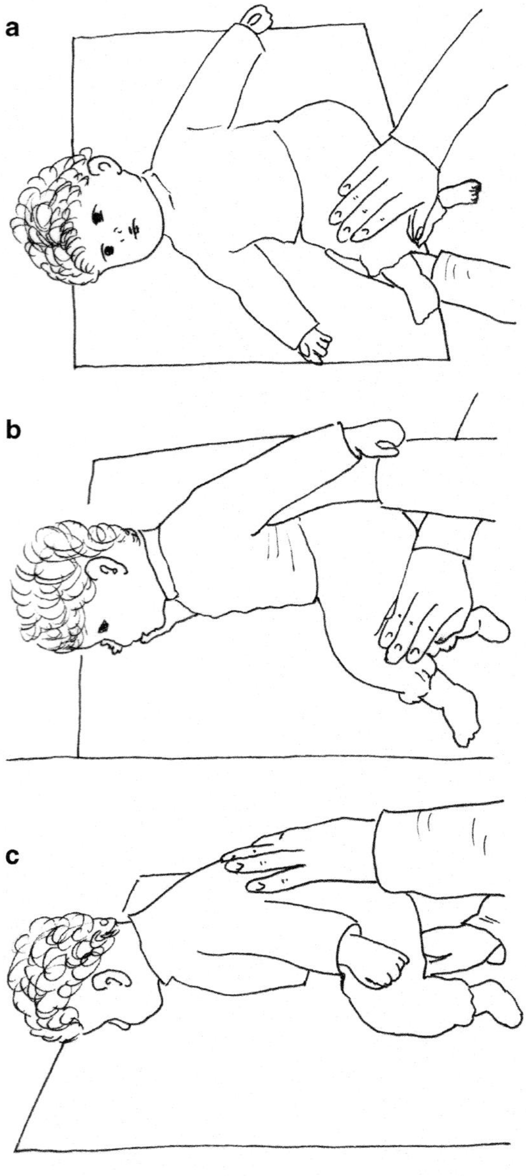

Fig. 12.13 (**a**) Induction training of rolling movement to the right. (**b**) Induction training of rolling movement to the right. (**c**) Induction training of rolling movement to the right

turning over movement, the children patients are in ventral decubitus. After that, the therapists guided children patients to toll the body to the right to complete continuous rolling movement (Fig. 12.13) until they get to the other end of the training bed. With the increase of rolling ability of children patients, inclining angle of training bed is decreased gradually until they start the rolling training of inclining upward to increase training difficulty and promote the rolling ability of children patients.

- Induction training of rolling movement to the left: in the training bed (3–5 m × 1 m) with adjustable inclining angle, the training bed is adjusted to 45° downslope positions. Children patients recline on it and a colorful toy is hanged in the front of the left of the body. The therapists sway right lower limb of children patients to the left, make it cross over left lower limbs and put it on training bed. After that, the therapists use speech to tell children patients to get the toy through turning over to the left and help children patients to sway their upper part of the body and right upper limb to the left. After completing turning over movement, the children patients are in ventral decubitus. After that, the therapists guided children patients to toll the body to the left to complete continuous rolling movement (Fig. 12.14) until they get to the other end of the training bed. With the increase of rolling ability of children patients, inclining angle of training bed is decreased gradually until they start the rolling training of inclining upward to increase training difficulty and promote the rolling ability of children patients.

The frequency is once a day (30 min per time) and there are 30 times in one therapy course. The therapy course can be added according to the functional recovery.

(e) Induction training of crawling movement: 6.5–7 months after birth, the baby starts the training of crawling ability. Its purpose is to induce autonomous crawling ability of children patients.

The specific method is as follows:

- Induction training of crawling movement in downslope: in the training bed of crawling movement, the baby is in prone position. The therapists wear thoracoabdominal weight support band for the baby. The purpose is to make the trunk of the baby 5 cm away from bed surface. The thera-

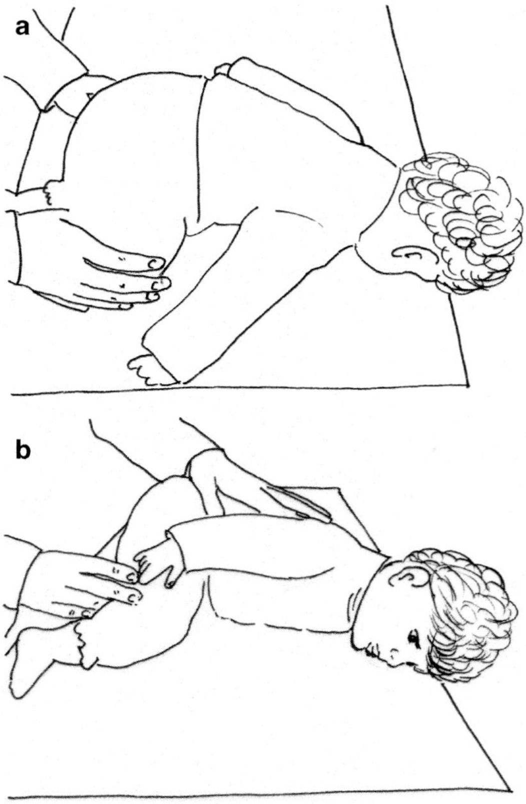

Fig. 12.14 (**a**) Induction training of rolling movement to the left. (**b**) Induction training of rolling movement to the left

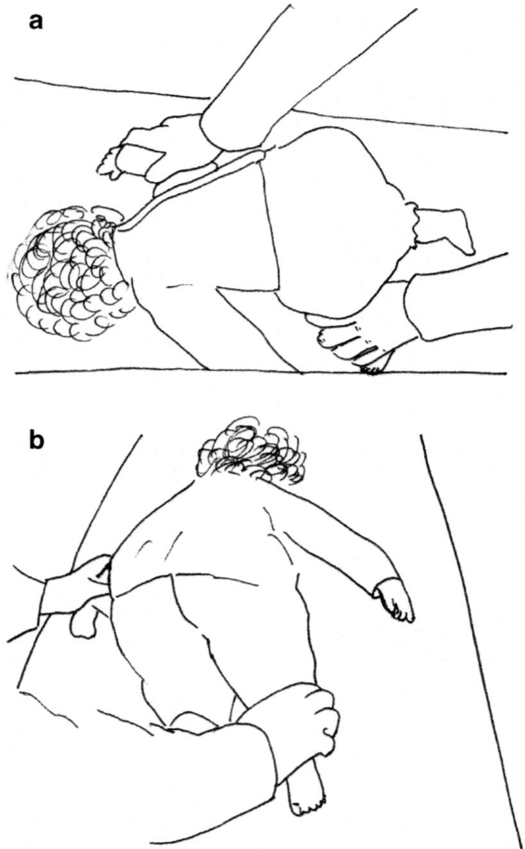

Fig. 12.15 (**a**) Induction training of crawling movement in downslope. (**b**) Induction training of crawling movement in downslope

pists adjust the angle of training bed to 30° Trendelenburg. The therapists help the baby and guide them repeatedly to complete crawling forward movement according to the sequence that right upper limb moves forward to make forearm and palm touch the bed, left lower limb moves forward to make knee joint and thigh touch the bed, the body moves forward, left upper limb moves forward to make forearm and palm touch the bed, right lower limb moves forward to make knee joint and thigh touch bed and the body moves forward (Fig. 12.15a, b). With the increase of crawling ability of children patients, inclining angle of bed surface is decreased gradually to the plane and the weight is gradually decreased.

- Induction training of crawling movement in upslope: preparation and training method are the same as induction training of crawling movement in downslope. With the protection of weight support system, the training should be started from small angle such as 10° and 15°. With the increase of ability, the difficulty is increased gradually (Fig. 12.16a, b).
- Induction training of retroaction crawling movement: in the training bed of crawling movement, the baby is in prone position. The therapists wear thoracoabdominal weight support band for the baby. The purpose is to make the trunk of the baby 5 cm away from bed surface. The therapists adjust the angle of training bed to 30° Trendelenburg. The therapists help the baby and guide them repeatedly to complete crawling backward movement according to the sequence that right lower

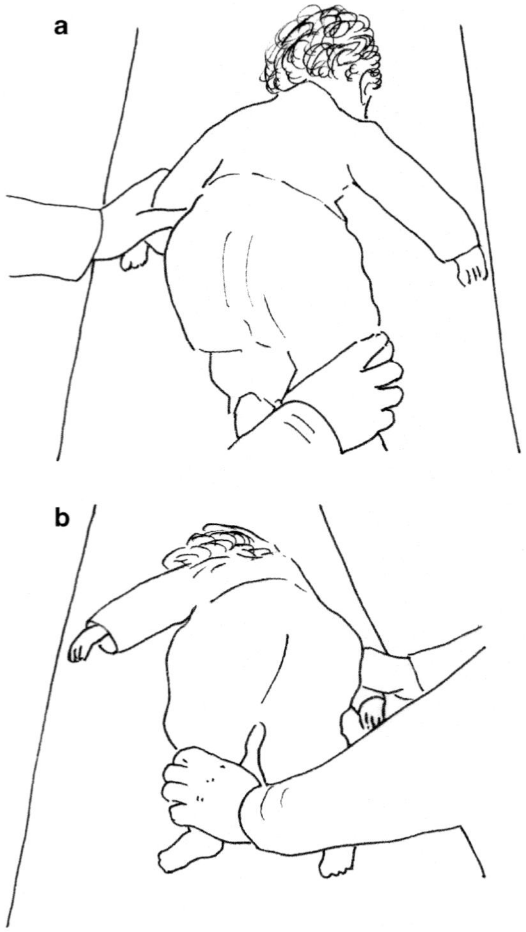

Fig. 12.16 (**a**) Induction training of crawling movement in downslope. (**b**) Induction training of crawling movement in downslope

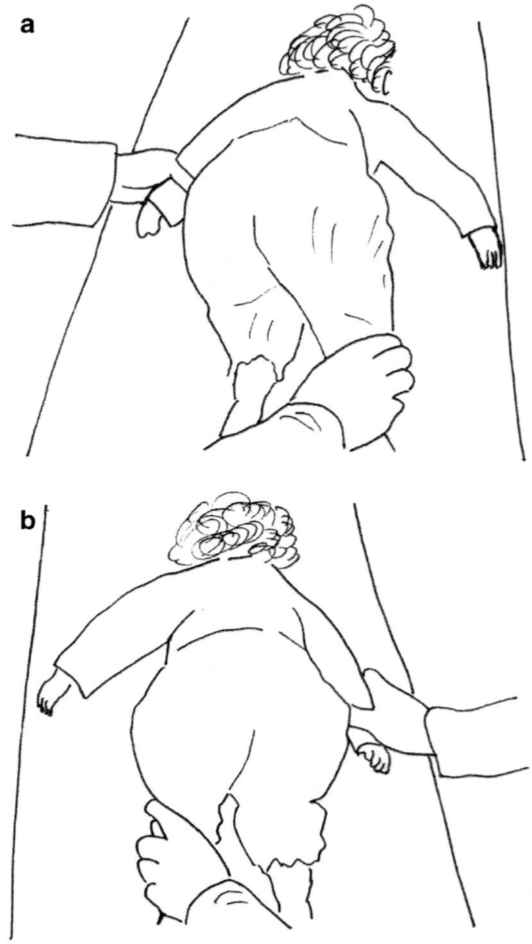

Fig. 12.17 (**a**) Induction training of retroaction crawling movement. (**b**) Induction training of retroaction crawling movement

limb moves forward to make knee joint and thigh touch the bed, left upper limb moves forward to make forearm and palm touch the bed, the body moves backward, left lower limb moves backward to make knee joint and thigh touch the bed, right upper limb moves forward to make forearm and palm touch bed and the body moves backward (Fig. 12.17a, b). With the increase of crawling ability of children patients, inclining angle of bed surface is decreased gradually to the plane and the weight is gradually decreased.

The frequency is once a day (30 min per time) and there are 30 times in one therapy course. The therapy course can be added according to the functional recovery.

(f) Induction training of walking movement: 9–11 months after birth, the baby starts the training of walking ability. Its purpose is to induce walking ability of children patients such as standing, stepping and gait training.

The specific method is as follows:

- The standing bed training: its purpose is to increase bearing ability of bony joint and spinal cord of children patients. Standing bed of children is applied from 45°. The frequency is two times a day (10 min per time). If children patients are not suitable for this training, the standing training can be done directly.

- Standing training: weight support balance training equipment is used for training. The therapists help children patients to stand in the middle of training equipment and wear weight support protection band. The weigh is from half of the body weight of children patients. Many colorful toys are hanged around the training equipment. The therapists distract children patients through game to make children patients in standing position (Fig. 12.18). The frequency is two times a day (10 min per time).
- Standing balance training: in the weight support standing balance training equipment, children patients fasten balance training belt and the therapists adjust the tension of elastic rope in the four corners of training equipment. When children patients swing to one orientation, the opposite elastic rope can keep the patients away from the arm of training equipment (Fig. 12.19). If lower limbs of children patients cannot support the body weight, weight support system can be used to decrease the bearing of lower limbs of children patients. The frequency is two times a day (15 min per time).
- Shifting of weight training of stride and gait: this is the basic training before walking training. It is the training of shifting of weight, weight bearing and stepping. Children Shifting of weight training equipment of stride and gait is used for the training. Abnormal gait rectification weight support walking training equipment is also used to do segment training of gait. In the

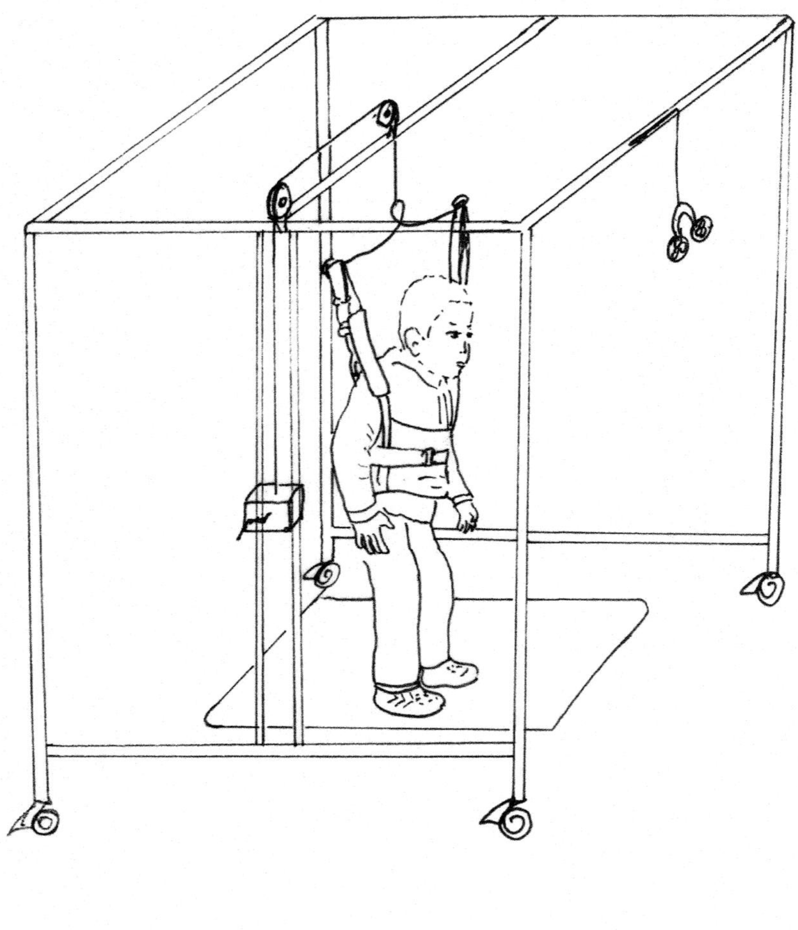

Fig. 12.18 Sketch map of standing training

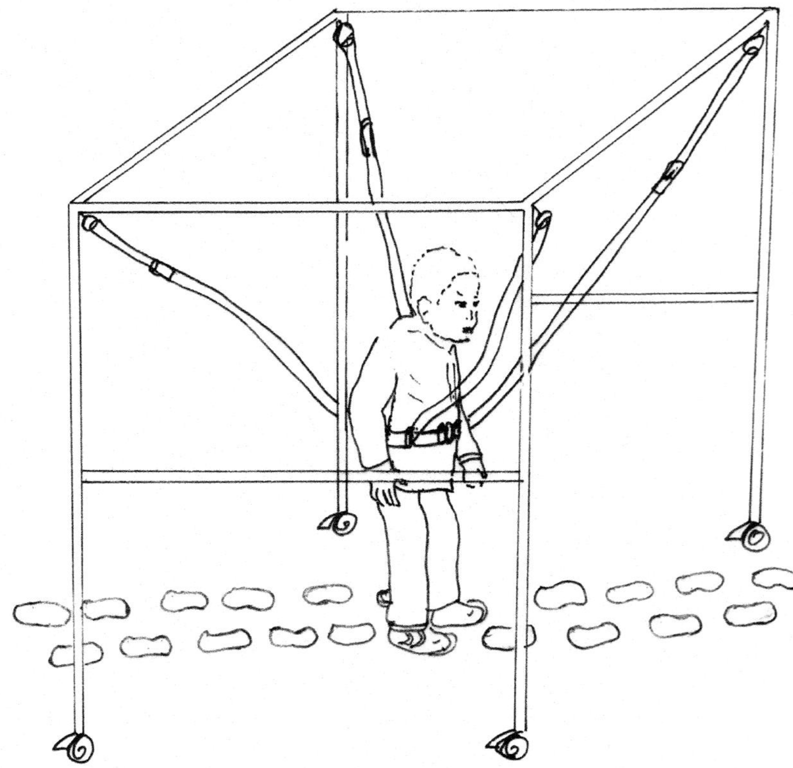

Fig. 12.19 Sketch map of standing balance training

weight support and secure protection, the therapists guide children patients to move the weight center to one side and life up lower limb in the other side to step forward. The heel firstly touches the ground, the foot lands on the footprint of footpath, the body moves forward, knee joint extend straightly to bear weight and weight center moves to this side. The patients lift up lower limb in the other side to step forward and do segment training repeatedly. With the increase of walking ability of children patients, the weight is decreased gradually to increase the walking speed (Fig. 12.20). The frequency is two times a day (15 min per time).

- Abnormal gait rectification weight support walking training: through induction training of walking ability mentioned above, children patients with certain walking ability can start this training. It is suitable for compulsive active walking training of children patients who cannot

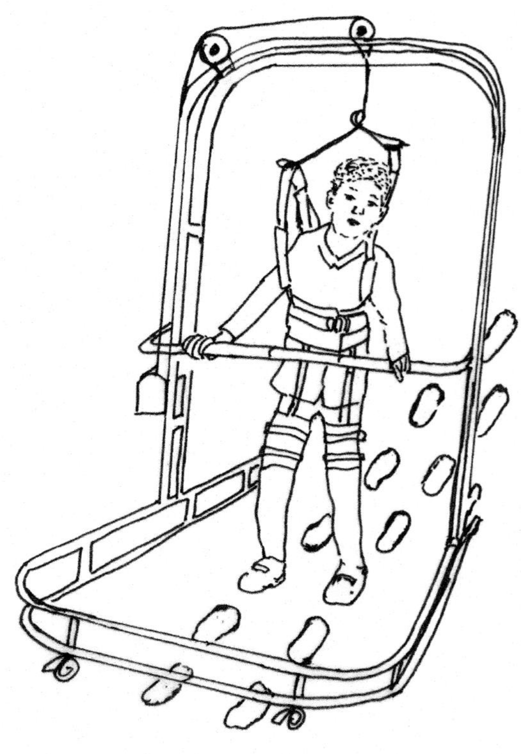

Fig. 12.20 Shifting of weight training of stride and gait

stand independently after therapy. The training is done in the abnormal gait rectification weight support walking training equipment. The therapists wear weight support pectoral girdle for children patients and adjust the weight loss on the standard that children patients can walk. If children patients are accompanied with adduction of lower limbs (scissors gait), circle gait (foot drop) and so on, rectification elastic band of adduction of lower limbs or foot drop is used. The tightness of elastic band can basically overcome adduction of lower limbs or foot drop. In the footprint training footpath, children patients are guided to land every foot on the footprint of footpath precisely (Fig. 12.21). With the increase of walking ability, the weight and strength of elastic band of adduction of lower limbs or foot drop are decreased gradually until the elastic band is removed completely.

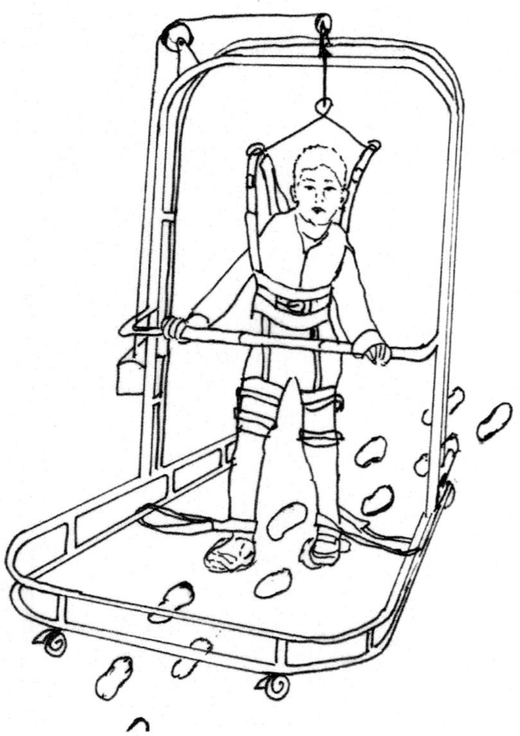

Fig. 12.21 Abnormal gait rectification weight support walking training

The frequency is once a day (15 min per time) and there are 30 times in one therapy course.

(g) Potential development training: Although induction training of movement has some effect on potential development, it is not enough. For the elder baby who can stand or cooperate with training, potential development training of lower limbs, trunk and upper limbs can be done. The frequency is once a day (15 min per time) and there are 30 times in one therapy course.

(h) Motor program reestablishment training: For children patients with basic understanding ability and cooperation ability, the therapists find out main obstacles through detailed functional assessment and do therapy in sequentially and orderly. Motor program of single joint is established at first and then motor program of associated movement with multiple joints is established. The therapy should be interesting and joyful. The children can receive therapy with game. The frequency is once a day (20 min per time).

(i) Motor pattern remodeling training: On the basis of potential development and motor program reestablishment, motor pattern remodeling training equipment is used and weight support equipment of abnormal gait rectification is applied. In the training footpath, gait modeling training is done and transmitted to walking without weight support gradually. The frequency is once a day (15 min per time).

(j) Rectification of limb deformity: because the baby's tissue is soft, if the therapists can find deformities of trunk, limbs or joints in the phase, the therapeutic effect is good after early rectification.

- Scoliosis deformity: Macromolecule fibrous materials are used to make back dry rack. The dome and the bottom of the curve are under pressure to rectify scoliosis. The materials are ventilated, absorbent, radioparent. The side effect is small. Back dry rack can be adjusted or changed with the increase of the height of the baby.
- Muscle spasm or contracture joint deformity: it is common in elbow joint, wrist

joint and knee joint, which is mostly induced by muscle spasm or tendon contracture and includes deformity in flexion or extension position. Traction and local thermal therapy should be done first to loosen adhesion of tissue and joint. Rectification splint is used to fix them in functional position, which can be adjusted or changed at any time.

Rectification of ankle deformity includes talipes equinovarus and foot drop, which is induced by development deformity and paralysis of tibialis anterior muscle or peroneus longus and brevis. On the basis of joint loosening by manipulation, foot tray is used to fix them in functional position. The materials of foot tray can be selected according to degree of deformity such as high temperature thermoplastic plate and slim thermoplastic materials. With the month of height, it should be adjusted or changed timely. The patients with severe deformity should consider surgical therapy.

(k) Passive exercise of children patients is suitable for children patients who cannot cooperate with active movement training. Proper passive movement can prevent adhesion of joint and muscle and promote development of children patients, but it has no effect on recovery of brain function. Passive exercise of children patients includes eight movements (four movements of upper limbs and four movements of lower limbs).

Upper limbs movement: Children patients are in supine position. The therapists use two hands to hold the wrist of children patients, put thumb into the palm of children patients, let children patients make a fist and put two hands beside children patients. Passive exercises are as follows:

Chest expanding exercises: the patients divide right and left hand, open and flat them, make them vertical to the body and the center of the palm goes up. Two hands cross before the chest. The patients divide right and left hands again and flat them outside. The patients restore the movement and repeat them for four times.

Elbow flexion movement: the patients flex bilateral elbow joints upward until the forearm is attached to upper arm, extend elbow joints straightly until they are parallel to the bed. The patients flex bilateral elbow joints upward until the forearm is attached to upper arm. The patients restore the movement and repeat them for four times.

Shoulder joint movement: the therapists hold the hands of the baby and rotate left shoulder joint in circle from inward to outward. The therapists hold the right hand of the baby and rotate right shoulder joint in circle from inward to outward. The patients restore the movement and repeat them for four times.

Upper limbs movement: the patients divide right and left hand, open and flat them and make them vertical to the body. The patients raise two hands to the front, make the centers of two palms face to face. The distance is as wide as the shoulder. Two hands cross before the chest. The patients lift two hands over the head and the center of the palm goes upward. The patients restore the movement and repeat them for four times.

Lower limbs movement: When the baby is in supine position, the therapists use left hand to hold left ankle of the baby and use right hand to hold half sole of left foot. Ankle joint movement: the therapists move the toe of the baby upward to flex ankle joint and move the toe of the baby downward to extend ankle joint. The baby does the same movements using right foot and repeats it for four times. Lower limbs extension and flexion movements: The therapists use two hands to hold two thighs of the baby and extend knee joint alternatively like pedaling a bike. The baby flexes left leg to touch the abdomen and then extend straightly downward. The baby flexes right leg to touch the abdomen and then extend straightly for four times. Leg raising movement: the baby extends straightly two lower limbs and flats them. The therapists pronate two palms and hold two knee joints of the baby. The baby extends two lower limbs straightly and lift up them in 90°. The baby restores the movement and repeats them for four times. Turning over movement: when the baby is in supine position, the therapists use one hand to support the chest and abdomen of the baby and use the other hand to support the back of the baby. The therapists help the baby turn over from supine position to lateral position, from lateral position to prone position and then from prone position to supine position. The baby repeats it for four times.

This exercise is suitable for the baby in the second month to sixth month after birth. The frequency is 1–2 times a day. When the baby is awake or after shower, the baby can do the exercise in good mood. The exercise should be orderly. During training, the baby wears soft and loose clothes. The operation should be soft and orderly with the music that the baby likes.

12.3.2.1 Cerebral Palsy

The schedule and specific method of rehabilitation therapy of neurological training of children patients with cerebral palsy who are older than 3 years old. These children are able to understand, describe the symptoms and cooperate with training. According to the condition of cognitive disorder and motor ability of the children, Rehabilitation therapy principles of neurological training are different.

1. There are three rehabilitation therapy principles:

   Three-stage rehabilitation therapy principle of atypical neurological training is suitable for children patients with single limb paralysis and slight double lower limbs paralysis.

   - The main purpose of three-stage rehabilitation method is to reestablish motor pattern of normal walking. Therefore, for children patients with slight limb paralysis in one side, on the basis of restriction of paralytic limbs in short time, according to the functional recovery condition, it can be transmitted to actual using training such as motor pattern remodeling training.
   - Neural potential development training: according to paralytic part, corresponding potential development training is done such potential development training of lower limbs. If the patients can cooperate with the training well, potential development method of guiding collaterals through meridians or normal potential development method is used. The frequency is 1–2 time (25 min per time) a day and there are 30 times in one therapy course.
   - Motor program reestablishment training: neurological training equipment is used to do the training of motor program reestablishment of single joint and associated movement with purpose. The frequency is 1–2 time (25 min per time) a day and there are 30 times in one therapy course.

2. Motor pattern remodeling training: during the reestablishment of motor program, motor pattern remodeling training can be started. The patients wear motor pattern remodeling training device and use abnormal gait rectification weight support walking training device to do the training in training footpath. Gradually, the patients do independent walking training without help. The frequency is 1–2 time (25 min per time) a day and there are 30 times in one therapy course.

   Three-stage rehabilitation principle of typical neurological training is suitable for the patients with a certain function with the help of rehabilitation method of neurological training and assistive device, which can improve abnormal motor pattern on the basis of recovering body motor function. Moreover, the trained children patients can cooperate with training.

   - The first phase is neural potential development phase. Children patients are required to sit in wheelchair and are forbidden to walk. According to the results of functional assessment, corresponding potential development training equipment is applied. Six-step Daoyin technique or six-step Daoyin technique of guiding collaterals through meridians is used to guide the patients to do the potential development training of upper limbs, trunk, lower limbs, tibialis anterior muscle, musculus gastrocnemius and hamstring muscles. The frequency is 1–2 time (25 min per time) a day and there are 30 times in one therapy course.

- The second phase is motor program reestablishment phase. Children patients are required to sit in wheelchair and are restricted to walk. According to the main obstacles after functional assessment, neurological training equipment and virtual reality training system are used to do motor program reestablishment training of single joint and associated movement with purpose and in order. The frequency is 1–2 time (25 min per time) a day and there are 30 times in one therapy course.
- The third phase is motor pattern remodeling phase. Children patients can walk with motor pattern remodeling training device and do a series of gait training. After that, they can do independent walking without help. The frequency is 1–2 time (25 min per time) a day and there are 30 times in one therapy course.

3. Rehabilitation principle of early standing and walking development is suitable for children patients with cerebral palsy who have severe motor dysfunction of limbs, lie in bed or sit in wheelchair for a long time, have cognitive disorder or joint deformity, cannot cooperate with the training and are difficult to stand up or walk even after rehabilitation method training of neurological training or application of assistive device.

For this kind of children patients, according to the procedure of three-stage rehabilitation method, the patients cannot meet the requirements of the third training phase, not to mention functional recovery of children patients. Therefore, the condition of motor pattern is not the key point. On the premise of reducing the assistance as much as possible, children patients are able to stand up and walk. Whether motor pattern is normal or abnormal, it can increase life quality of children patients and reduce life burden of children patients.

4. Preparations before walking training:
   - Rectification of limb deformity: standing is one of the basic elements and is the basic condition of extending double lower limbs and trunk to bear load. However, this kind of children patients belongs to mix type of cerebral palsy. Because muscle spasm can lead to joint flexion deformity, especially flexion deformity of double hips and knee joints, the basic condition of standing training is restoring double lower limbs to basic extension position through therapy. Traction: the patients can receive small dose continuous skin traction of lower limbs such as traction in extension position, abduction position and extorsion position. The weight is started from 1 kg and is increased gradually, but it doesn't exceed 3 kg. The traction is usually done at night. Thermal therapy: far infrared or kerotherapy is used to soften tissue adhesion or contracture to obtain better effect of loosening tissues by traction and manipulation. The frequency is 1–2 times a day (15 min per time) and one therapy course takes 3 months. The therapy course can be lengthened or the times can be increased. Manipulation: manipulation can be used to loosen adhesive joint and tissue to alleviate tendon contracture. The frequency is 1–2 times a day (15 min per time) and one therapy course takes 3 months. The therapy course can be lengthened or the times can be increased. Loosening method of trembling tissue: during the process of local thermal therapy and manipulation traction, hand massager is used to rub the muscle fiber to loosen adhesive tissue through tremble effect. The frequency is 1–2 times a day (15 min per time) and one therapy

course takes 3 months. The therapy course can be lengthened or the times can be increased. Orthopedic device fixation: in order to prevent second adhesion at night, adhesive joint is recovered to 15–30° through loosening and 6–8 layers of plaster support can be applied to fix adhesive joint in case of joint retraction and relapse of deformity. When the joint angle is hard to be recovered further, macromolecule fiber or thermoplastic orthopedic device is used to fix the joint. For the joint with fibrous and bony ankyloses, if the flexion angle affects the standing greatly, the therapists should ask for consultation of doctors and use surgery to rectify the deformity.

- Standing bed training: when the hip, knee and ankle joints are suitable for standing bed training, this training can be started. Its purpose is to increase bearing capacity of lower bony joint and cardiovascular stress capability. The training can be started from 45° to 90° in erect position. For long-term bed children patients, in the beginning phase, the training can be done under the monitor of Vital Signs Monitor. If there is any discomfort such as racing heart, palpitation or fall of blood pressure in children patients, the angle of standing should be adjusted or the training should be suspended. The frequency is 1–2 times a day (15 min per time) and one therapy course takes 1 month. The therapy course can be lengthened or the times can be increased.
- Walking training: abnormal gait rectification weight support walking training device and wearable children motor pattern remodeling device are used for the training. According to the degree and types of children patients' dysfunction, the tightness of lower limbs abduction and rectification elastic band of foot dorsiflexion are adjusted in case that foot touches the ground and lower limbs adduces. Children patients can keep in standing position and the weight can be adjusted. The training is implemented by 1–2 therapists. Weight support walking training device is moved forward. Meanwhile, children patients are guided to step forward. When children patients are not able to step forward, the therapists can help the patients to step forward through assistive band. The rest can be done in the same manner. With the increase of the ability of children patients, the weight, elastic force of rectification band and the help of the therapists can be decreased. The frequency is 1–2 times a day (25 min per time) and one therapy course takes 1 month. The therapy course can be lengthened or the times can be increased.
- Potential development training: according to the results of functional assessment, corresponding potential development training device can be used. Six-step Daoyin technique or six-step Daoyin technique of guiding collaterals through meridians is used to guide the patients to do the potential development training of upper limbs, trunk, lower limbs, tibialis anterior muscle, musculus gastrocnemius and hamstring muscles, but the walking of children patients is not restricted. The frequency is 1–2 times a day (25 min per time) and one therapy course takes 1 month. The therapy course can be lengthened or the times can be increased.
- Motor program reestablishment training: According to the main obstacles after functional assessment, neurological training equipment and virtual reality training system are used to do motor program reestablishment training of single joint and associated movement with purpose and in order. The frequency is 1–2 times a day (25 min per time) and one therapy course takes 1 month. The therapy course can be lengthened or the times can be increased.

5. The principle of proper application of assistive devices: assistive devices can compensate functions, prevent and rectify deformity. However, every assistive device has aide effect. For example, after the patients wear waistline band, the stability of lumbar vertebra is increased, which can alleviate pain of

waist in the patients with fibrositis of psoas. If the patients wear it for a longtime, because the waist muscles are used less, the myophagism and myodynamia decrease can be induced. For example, ankle-foot orthosis can rectify foot drop and strephenopodia to increase walking stability. If the patients wear it for a long time, it can induce myodynamia decrease of tibialis anterior muscle and musculus gastrocnemius, in addition, the purpose of babaka sold in the market is to rectify posture hunchback. The cause of posture hunchback is that low head position when people are watching book or working and the low myodynamia of back muscles. The fundamental measures of rectification are rectifying wrong posture and strengthen active movement exercise of back muscles. If people only wear babaka, but don't do functional exercise of back, not only bad posture cannot be rectified, but also the autonomous movement of back muscles can be restricted further. If people wear it for a long time, the myodynamia of back muscles can be decreased, which may aggravate the degree of humpback. Therefore, assistive devices are the measures by necessity but not the first choice. It cannot be overused for profit.

Through rehabilitation training, the active contraction of muscle that induces joint deformity cannot be recovered. The patients should wear orthotics to replace partial functions of paralytic muscles. Otherwise, it not only aggravates joint deformity, but also leads to abnormal motor pattern and affect movement quality. If autonomous contraction function of paralytic tibialis anterior muscle cannot be recovered in a short time, the patients can wear foot tray to rectify foot drop. Otherwise, foot drop can lead to abnormal motor pattern such as circle gait. Moreover, long-term foot drop can stretch tibialis anterior muscle further and make it lose the proper initial length, which cause difficulties to functional recovery.

Motor pattern remodeling training device developed by the author only restricts the unnecessary joint motion and doesn't restrict normal joint motion. Therefore, the patients can wear it for a long time. According to external normal motor pattern, abnormal motor program in motor center of cortex can be modified and can be transmitted to normal motor program. Motor pattern remodeling training device is good for the formation and solidification of normal motor pattern.

6. Assistive training induced by other autonomous movements:
   - Fine motor training mainly trains the fine motor ability of upper limbs and hand such as nutting, game of string beads and building blocks.
   - Divertive game training such as sensory integration training, combined ladder-climbing training and climbing sand dune training can increase the interests of children patients, induce autonomous movement and increase motor ability.
   - Hydrotherapy has thermal, mechanical and chemical stimulation effect. Through the mechanism of neurohumoral regulation, the functions of organs can be improved. With the help of hydrostatic pressure, water flow impact pressure and buoyancy, the therapists can induce water exercise of children patients and make them complete autonomous movements that cannot be completed in normal condition.

12.3.3 Amount of Training of Children with Cerebral Palsy

Because the baby and the infant cannot express their ability and feeling of amount of training and recovering dysfunction induced by CNS injury movement is recovering CNS function but not physical training to enhance myodynamia, the patients are required to keep vigorous physical power to do neural potential development training well. Therefore, proper amount of training is very important. The therapists can assess the feeling and degree of fatigue to adjust the training timely (Table 12.6).

Table 12.6 Proper amount of training assessment table in children with cerebral palsy

Items	0	1	2
Self-perception	A little tired	Tired	exhausted
Muscular soreness, low myodynamia and muscle hardness increase	Recovered after rest	Recovered in the second day	Cannot be recovered in the second day
The heart rate is increased ten times per minute	The heart rate is normal after rest for 5 min	The heart rate cannot be recovered after rest for 5 min	The heart rate cannot be recovered in the second day
Myocardial enzyme	Normal	Increase	Double

Criteria: the total score is less than 2, which means insufficient. The total score is 3–4, which means proper. The total score is more than 5, which means overdose.

12.3.4 Training and Therapy in Other Aspects

1. Daily life ability training: The purpose is to transform the training results into daily life self-care ability through life autonomous movement on the basis of trainings mentioned above.
   (a) Feeding training: When the children with cerebral palsy are eating, the training can be done according to recurring problems. Feeding position placement can help the patients to relax and alleviate spasm. Control of children patients' jaw can increase masticatory ability of children patients. The patients should choose plastic tableware with shallow surface and use skid resistance dish and bowl with handle. The therapists should be patient during training and split feeding movement into several coherent petty actions. With the increase of feeding ability, the therapists can combine several coherent petty actions. On the basis of keep the feeding amount of children patients, the training should be done three meals every day persistently.
   (b) Dressing and undressing training: According to individual condition of children patients with cerebral palsy, different training mode can be selected. The training can be started from dressing and undressing simple clothes. The therapists should let children patients know the sequence of dressing and undressing clothes. The children patients should undress the clothes in uninjured side and then in injured side. The children patients should dress the clothes in injured side and then in uninjured side. The therapists help children patients to dress and undress clothes at first. With the increase of ability of children patients, the help force can be decreased until the patients can dress themselves independently.
   (c) Defecation training: Defecation training should be started from 2 years old and is a comprehensive training includes dressing and undressing trousers, standing, sitting balance and squatting. Disposal after defecation is a process of hand functions training of children patients. The therapists use children bed pan with handle in the front or in two sides to provide stable sitting posture for children patients. The patients should concentrate on defecation process. They don't listen to the story or read books and only concentrate on defecation. The children patients defecate regularly and learn to control defecation. In every defecation, the children patients should train themselves.
   (d) Other life movements training such as cleaning (tooth brushing and washing hands), face-lifting, social contact and using appliances. According to the gender, age and disease severity of children patients, the therapists formulate actual individual plan and implement it.

   Daily life ability training mentioned above can increase daily life ability and social life ability of children patients, promote mental and physical development of children patients and make them do the movements independently in all aspects. For severe children patients, not only the functions should be improved, but also the life self-care ability should be increased through compensation according to the degree of dysfunction.

2. Speech training: Its purpose is to provide speech stimulation and to motivate the interest of children patients to use speech. It can help children patients to establish and increase applying ability of interpersonal skills to meet the requirements of daily life and learning.
   (a) The training of ability to accept language: attention training: under instructions, children patients stop what they are doing, listen to their own name and follow the order of the therapists to do one thing. Comprehension ability training of symbols includes comprehension ability of real object and toy. Comprehension ability training of speech includes environment comprehension, one character word or two characters word comprehension. The training associated with interpersonal skills includes the training of vision, auditory sense and other perceptions.
   (b) The training of expression ability: the training before spoken language includes the training of movements or gesture, environmental pronunciation and imitation ability. The training of expression ability includes the training of single words, two words and simple sentence. The training of non-verbal expression ability includes the common gesture or movements training and communication graph.
   (c) The training of dysarthria: Basic training includes improvement of control of lower jaw and upper lip, improvement of control of tongue, control of involuntary movements, promote coordinated movements and improvement of oral perception. The training of articulation: according to the examination results, the therapists give articulation training to children patients from simple sound such as bilabial sound to difficult sounds such as velar, dental and linguo-dental.

       In order to increase the effect and interest of speech training, pictures and slides can be used. Speech biological feedback therapy can also be used. Through speech biofeedback equipment, abnormal tone and sound are displayed in fluorescent screen in a wave form or curve form. The therapists can do pectorophony or sound attenuation training with a purpose.

3. Cognitive training: Cognitive training can be divided into three phases such as primary phase, middle phase and advanced phase.
   (a) The training content in primary phase: enlightenment training includes acquaintance of color, graph, digit, time, space and quantity of object. Basic cognitive ability training includes the training of attention, outsight and memory.
   (b) The training content in middle phase is information coding ability training, which includes the training of sequence inferential capability, analogic reasoning capability, transmissibility inferential capability and group ability.
   (c) The training content in advanced phase is organizational strategy training, which includes the training of information integration ability using linear structure, net structure, coordinate structure and comprehensive structure.

       The hypothesis of human brain memory gate: whether the memory in human brain is ring current or memory protein, they are all the process that something is known, understand and memory is formed, storage and retrieved. There is a memory channel or gate. If there is a problem in any gate, the memory is incomplete. The process of cognitive training is to use methodology to reestablish memory and open the memory gate. Through training, cognitive competence can be increased.

4. Physiotherapy.
   Physiotherapy includes medium-frequency electrical stimulation, ultrashort wave, far infrared and kerotherapy [7].
   Medium-frequency electrical stimulation is given to paralytic nerve and muscles to increase the excitability. Transcranial electromagnetic stimulation can promote the wake of undead brain cells. Far infrared and kerotherapy can promote local blood circulation, soften adhesive tissue or tendon contracture, which is good for strengthening the effect of manipulation loosening. Continuous Passive Motion (CPM) training device is used for continuous passive motion of the joint in the maximum range of motion after manipulation loosening to increase range of joint motion, prevent relapse of adhesion and not to affect the implement of rehabilitation therapy. CPM training can be done at night when children patients fall asleep.
5. The application of orthotics and walking aid.
   Orthotics is the appliance to prevent and rectify the deformity of body and trunk. Walking aid is assistive appliance to help the patients to walk. The therapists should select the appliance according to the actual requirements of children patients. The purpose of orthotics is to decrease load bearing of injured limbs, keep in good limb position, maintain local stability, prevent and rectify contracture of limbs, help the patients to complete necessary movements and control involuntary movement. Walking aid includes wheelchair, crutch and walker. They can enlarge the support surface of children patients, decrease swing of the center of weight, increase body stability and help the patients to stand and walk.
6. Psychotherapy and education rehabilitation.
   Child psychology [8] is a branch of psychology. It is a science to investigate children's law of psychological development and mental profile in every age stage of children.
   (a) Psychotherapy: because children patients with cerebral palsy have motor dysfunction, restricted movements, small motion range, mental retardation and abnormal psychological development. Abnormal mentality usually leads to abnormal behaviors and restrict the motor and speech ability development of children patients. The clinical manifestations are immoderate reliance and coward, extremely unstable emotion, low self-control, impulsion, sensitivity, intense self-respect, distracted attention, bad memory, loneliness, self-abasement, poor adaptation to environment, unstable characteristic, autolesion or injury by another.
   Psychotherapy, group therapy, behavior therapy, family therapy and other culture, sports or musicotherapy are used in therapy. The therapy should be patient and step by step. It can integrate learning and doing, has a positive education effect. It can encourage the patients and create normal mental environment. During the process of motor and intelligence, psychological rehabilitation is done.
   (b) Education rehabilitation: Education is the basis of human life. The earlier Children patients receive the education, the better the effect is, especially for the disabled infant. The education objects include children patients and their parents. The content includes instruction of spirits and thoughts and instructions of training methods. Rehabilitation staff should receive education and the level should be increased to achieve the effect of education rehabilitation.

The disabled children are restricted in motor and intelligence. The environment of general schools is not suitable for their teaching. According to their special ability and required equipment, special curriculum is formulated and special education is done using different teaching methods. Pavlov's classical conditioning theory indicated that learning any functional skill requires continuous practice entirely or partially. The therapists should combine therapy and education, combine therapy with prevention, combine persistence (lengthways) and continuity (crosswise). The therapists should integrate learning and training contents into the whole day's life of children patients, which is good for the rehabilitation of mind and body of children patients.

7. Surgical therapy: The main purpose is to rectify line of bearing load, rectify deformity, balance myodynamia, decrease muscle spasm and contracture.

   It is suitable for congenital bone and joint deformity, fibrous joint ankyloses, bony joint ankyloses and unrecovered paralytic muscles. Surgical therapy includes tenotomy, tendon lengthening, tendon loosening, tendon transfer, osteotomy, joint fusion.

   Neurosurgery: Partial neurotomy and selectivity or high selective posterior rhizotomy to alleviate spasm [9].

   It should be noticed that the cause of motor dysfunction of patients with cerebral palsy is brain dysfunction. Therefore, recovering brain function is the important measures of solving the problems. Before recovering brain functions, muscle tendon surgery may only improve the functions for a short time. It will relapse after a certain time. For example, denervation of tibialis anterior muscle leads to paralysis of the muscle and myodynamia imbalance between tibialis anterior muscle and musculus gastrocnemius, which induce over plantar flexion of the foot. The most effective method to treat foot drop is to recover the domination of brain to tibialis anterior muscle. If brain functions are not recovered, tendon lengthening can alleviate foot drop temporarily after surgery. However, the paralysis of tibialis anterior muscle is not recovered and the imbalance between tibialis anterior muscle and musculus gastrocnemius still exists. After a certain time, foot weight in walking and traction of musculus gastrocnemius can induce foot drop again.

   Therefore, for patients' interest, rehabilitation training should be done first. The functions can be recovered with proper methods. The patients who cannot be recovered completely use orthotics to rectify the dysfunction and then do rehabilitation training. If these methods mentioned above cannot recover functions, surgical therapy can be considered. It should be cautious to suggest the patients with cerebral palsy to receive surgical therapy.

12.4 Case Report: The Rehabilitation Process of an Elder Child with Cerebral Palsy

The child with cerebral palsy named YanYan (alias) who is 14 years old and never stand up, finally is able to stand up after half year's rehabilitation training. All the rehabilitation staff, wardmate and family members are excited and yell out "YanYan can stand up!" her mother has confidence in the rehabilitation and recognizes the importance of rehabilitation. Her mother said "we only know taking medicine before or did surgery. We think rehabilitation is moving arms and legs and it is dispensable. We then realize the importance of rehabilitation and we use western rehabilitation technique, but there is no effect after 1 year's western rehabilitation training of rehabilitation method. I realize that Daoyin technique in traditional Chinese medicine is good. Rehabilitation technique of neurological training developed from Daoyin technique in traditional Chinese medicine will contribute to human rehabilitation enterprise".

YanYan was born after 36 weeks' pregnancy (cesarean) and there is no abnormity during birth. After birth, growth and development of she is slower than the infant in the same age and there are involuntary movements of hand and foot, which is diagnosed with mixed type cerebral palsy in one hospital in Beijing. When she is 1 year old, she is able to raise head, turn over and sit up. She can speak but the speed is slow with expression retardation. There are many involuntary movements of upper limbs (chorea). She cannot use fingers to grasp and hold something. There are severe spasm and adduction of lower limbs. Maldevelopment of left acetabulum and caput femoris lead to congenital complete dislocation of left hip joint. All these with instability of double ankle joints make YanYan cannot stand up, even with the help of her family.

Her mother sees the doctors in many big hospitals after YanYan's birth. Once there is any therapy method, they will try it and never let off any chance. In 2007, she received standard rehabilitation training for almost 1 year in a well-known rehabilitation hospital and she can sit independently, but cannot sit upright. She cannot raise her head. Her fingers are twisted so she cannot eat food and comb by herself. When she tries to extend upper limbs, she will yell out and the speech is unclear. Increased muscle tension of lower limbs, adduction deformity, flat feet, unstable ankle joint, complete dislocation of left hip joint make her cannot stand up, not to mention walking.

She never goes to the kindergarten and read books when she is 14 years old. Her mother feels painful in heart. Her mother never stops seeking doctors for YanYan. Her mother is a great mum.

In the early of 2008, her mother realized rehabilitation therapy of neurological training in internet. Potential development and motor program reestablishment theory and method are used for the patients, which have good effects on the patients with cerebral palsy and are not restricted by therapy course. She took the child to Beijing as soon as possible. After detailed examination and assessment, although the state of disease is complicated and the disease history is long, it is possible to recover the functions of independent standing and assistive walking through rehabilitation method of neurological training. They rebuilt the hope of rehabilitation.

According to her dysfunctions, the therapists formulate specific therapeutic schedule and decide to give three-stage rehabilitation training of neural potential development, motor program reestablishment and motor pattern remodeling to her. The therapeutic goal is to recover the functions of independent standing and assistive walking.

Complete dislocation of left hip joint make her cannot stand up, which makes it difficult for potential development training of lower limbs. Six-step Daoyin technique in traditional Chinese medicine is used for her to do potential development training of upper limbs, lower limbs and trunk bedside, motor program reestablishment training. According to biofeedback mechanism that archery accuracy can be improved through target exercise, under the instruction of motor program signal, the patients are guided to do the training with a purpose. Through goal-motive mechanism, the patients are guided to enhance signal intensity of agonistic muscle, decrease signal intensity of antagonistic muscle, establish normal motor program and increase control ability of limbs movements.

After 2 months' motor program reestablishment training, she can raise her head and sit upright. The involuntary movements are decreased and she can eat food by herself. All the family is excited. Over the years, this is the first time to see the great effect of rehabilitation therapy. They have confidence in the rehabilitation with surprise and amaze.

Dislocated left hip joint and unstable double ankle joint are the important factors to influence standing, lower limbs training and functional recovery. The patient must bear load with left limb so that she can stand up. How to make the dislocated left hip joint and unstable double ankle joints bear load? In fact, the best method is hip joint moulding or artificial joint replacement of full hip and double ankle arthrodesis. She is young and the limbs function is poor. Therefore, hip replacement and double ankle arthrodesis may not be used for a long time. Because the child grows and the life of artificial joint is limited, it is not suitable for the child to do hip replacement and double ankle arthrodesis.

After repeated discussion, hip surgery is not suitable for her. The therapists decide to use orthotics to abduce hip joint to make undeveloped caput femoris bear load in acetabulum and use ankle joint molding brace to make double ankle joint bear load. During the process of establishing motor program, she can do standing and walking training. However, this is hypothesis. Moreover, bearing load of immature developed caput femoris may lead to femoral head necrosis. Undeveloped acetabulum may moves upward and damages peripheral tissues when caput femoris is bearing load. It is risky to use this kind of hip joint to stand up with the help of assistive device. It is no sense to give up training that can recover standing and walking functions in order to keep an undeveloped caput femoris. It is meaningful to recover standing and walking functions regardless of undeveloped caput femoris, because hip joint can be reestablished through hip replacement and hip replacement is meaningful after recovering standing and walking functions.

In order to cooperate with orthotics, basic training is given to her before the standing and walking training. Training intensity of lumbodorsal muscles, hip flexor, hip abductor and quadriceps femoris is increased because they are necessary for standing and walking.

When she wears orthotics to practice standing, everybody look forward to the amazing standing and watch the detailed of wearing orthotics with attention and caution. When she wears hip joint abduction orthotics and double ankle joint molding brace and walk with the help of the therapists and without pain, everybody is excited and cheer for the success. It is lucky that the caput femoris is not moved upward. There is no accident in the standing for a while, which not means there is no injury after long-term standing. She receives X-ray examination in the first month and third month after standing training and there is no injury.

After that, on the basis of motor program reestablishment and potential development training of upper limbs, the therapists add potential development training of lower limbs. When she is able to stand independently, according to the neurological training of early standing and walking development and rehabilitation principle of treating cerebral palsy, she starts walking training.

With the help of abnormal gait rectification weight support walking training device and the instruction of the therapists, she steps forward for the first time. Although the gait is not beautiful and is very slow, she feels excited, because this is the first step in her life.

Because severe adductor spasm of double lower limbs, although elastic band of walking device can prevent partially over adduction of lower limbs, there is still scissors gait in walking. Abduction supporter of lower limbs is used to make her do walking training successfully, which can effectively prevent scissors gait induced by adduction of double lower limbs. It is difficult to walk with several orthotics such as hip joint abduction orthotics, abduction supporter of lower limbs and rectification brace of double ankle joints, but she finally can step forward with these help. It is very important for her. Standing can make bone bear load, which is good for bone development. Walking can promote the increase of domination ability of brain to limbs and the establishment of walking center functions in spinal cord. Standing and walking can strengthen muscle and myodynamia. Standing and walking is the necessary training procedure to make her take care of herself.

Meanwhile, in order to increase her walking ability, therapists add the center of body weight training of stride and gait, balance training, hip abduction, coordinated motor program reestablishment training of hip flexion and knee extension and myodynamia enhancement training.

In a long period, she gets into a stable training program phase. In every day, the therapists use innovated six-step Daoyin technique in traditional Chinese medicine to do potential development training of upper limbs, lower limbs and trunk with the help of potential development equipment, to do gait training with the help of weight support stride and gait weight center shifting training device, to do motor program reestablishment training with the help of virtual reality of neurological training system, to do walking training with the help of abnormal gait rectification weight support walking trainer and motor pattern remodeling training device. The doctors and the therapists in rehabilitation center observe the change of her carefully and adjust therapeutic schedule timely.

In this way, 1 month later, 2 months later, there is no obvious progress. She feels frustrated and her mother feels confused. The therapists feel that she and her family lose confidence of rehabilitation. For this, the therapists explain the detail to her and her family and tell them functional recovery of central nervous system is a chronic process, which likes a man can walk 1 year after birth and is the necessary development process of central nervous system. Because she cannot stand and walk after birth, she loses the best development period of central nervous system. At present, motor program of standing and walking should be established in her brain, which takes longer time than that in the phase of the baby. If the patients can persist on it, there will be good results.

She and her family know the mechanism and receive the training happily. In the tenth month after training, the walking speed of her is increased and self-care ability is improved. She can wash her face, brush her tooth, eat and write. Slowly, she can bear load without double ankle joint molding. There is no abduction of lower limbs without abduction supporter of lower limbs. She can walk with the help of walking aid and without abnormal gait rectification weight support walking device.

After a period of time of rehabilitation training and schedule adjustment, she can walk with the help of walking aid and without others' help. She and her family have a higher goal. They believe family affection can conquer disease and YanYan can achieve it. They believe they find the effective method to treat the disease.

Family affection, tenacity and methods are three necessary factors in rehabilitation therapy, which are similar and essential. The patients who require rehabilitation are unable to move, need to be taken care of, are lack of finance resource and have no ability of choose and decision making. Therefore, they are the group who require family affection and care. Rehabilitation is a chronic process, even lifelong. The patients and their family should be decisive, willpower and tough. All of these are the basis of good effects of effective rehabilitation method.

Good method is the accumulation of experience. The process of her therapeutic process not only testifies the rationality and effectiveness of neural potential development, motor program reestablishment and motor pattern remodeling training, but also shows the great potential and plasticity of human body. In the training of standing and walking, through bearing load of limbs and innervation of brain to muscle, the joint motion is done. Unstable ankle joint is stable, muscle strength is increased and the movement is flexible. It indicates that proper therapeutic method can develop human potential. Whether the course of disease is long or not, the state of disease is complicated or not, it is possible to increase the functions. It is incorrect to give up the therapy and predicate that there is no improvement.

In the clinical practice year after year, the therapists can fully realize the importance of three elements of rehabilitation. They should tell the patients, patients' family and other medical staff timely and extensively and make the whole society realize the importance and particularity of rehabilitation. It is good for the increase of rehabilitation consciousness and progress of rehabilitation medicine.

References

1. Torres VM, Saddi VA. Systematic review: hereditary thrombophilia associated to pediatric strokes and cerebral palsy. J Pediatr. 2015;91(1):22–9.
2. Bearden DR, Monokwane B, Khurana E, Baier J, Baranov E, Westmoreland K, Mazhani L. Steenhoff AP pediatric cerebral palsy in botswana: etiology, outcomes, and comorbidities. Pediatr Neurol. 2016;59(6):23–7.
3. Södermark L, Sigurdsson V, Näs W, Wall P, Trollfors B. Neuroborreliosis in Swedish children: a population-based study on incidence and clinical characteristics. Pediatr Infect Dis J. 2017;36(11):1052–6.
4. Horan MP, Stuart Blankenship JS, Iwinski HJ. Recent developments in functional assessment tools for ambulatory cerebral palsy. Curr Orthop Pract. 2008;19(6):667–70.
5. Hamer Elisa G, Bos Arend F, Mijna H-A. Assessment of specific characteristics of abnormal general movements: does it enhance the prediction of cerebral palsy? Dev Med Child Neurol. 2011;53(8):751–6.
6. Martinuzzi A, De Polo G, Bortolot S, Brogå PMC. Pediatric neurorehabilitation and the ICF. NeuroRehabilitation. 2015;36(1):31–6.
7. Bailes Amy F, Paul S. Factors associated with physical therapy services received for individuals with cerebral palsy in an outpatient pediatric medical setting. Phys Ther. 2012;92(11):1411–8.
8. Lorenzee EJ, Cancro R. Role of nondirective play therapy as a technic of psychotherapy in cerebral palsy. Arch Phys Med Rehabil. 1955;36(8):523–36.
9. Becmeur F, Schneider A, Flaum V, Klipfel C, Pierrel C, Lacreuse I. Which surgery for drooling in patients with cerebral palsy? J Pediatr Surg. 2013;48(10):2171–4.

13 Rehabilitation Therapy of Neurological Training of Paraplegia

13.1 The Main Dysfunctions of Spinal Cord Injury

Spinal cord injury (SCI) [1] is injury of structure and function of spinal cord induced by various nosogenesis, which lead to dysfunctions of spinal cord under the injured level such as motor, sensation and reflex. It is severe disabled injury. It can induce paraplegia or quadriplegia to varying degrees and affect the self-care ability and social ability of the patients greatly. It is difficult in the therapy, especially complete spinal cord injury. Except for implantable functional electrical stimulation and compensation of assistive device, there are no other effective methods for the disease such as surgery, medicine and neural stem cells transplantation [2].

Up to this day, many patients, their family and clinical physicians still think that rehabilitation therapy can be considered only if other methods are hopeless. Dependence of surgery or aimless use of medicine and therapy method without clinical verification can affect effects of rehabilitation training because of delaying opportunity of rehabilitation therapy.

13.1.1 Classification and Diagnosis of Spinal Cord Injury

Spinal cord injury is transverse injury of spinal cord due to various pathogenic factors. It leads to dysfunctions of spinal cord after injured level such as motor, sensation, sphincter and autonomic nervous function. According to pathological factors and neural dysfunctions, spinal cord injury is classified, which is important for the diagnosis, rehabilitation therapy and prognosis of the patients.

13.1.1.1 Classification of Spinal Cord Injury

Many factors and diseases can lead to SCI. It can be divided into traumatic injury and non-traumatic injury.

1. Traumatic spinal cord injury: Traumatic injury is injury of structure and function of spinal cord induced by destruction of spinal cord stability due to mechanical action.
   - Direct external force: Blade puncture or penetrating injury of spinal cord by bullet, shrapnel can lead to open spinal cord injury. Stone or weight can hit the small of the back directly, which is the common cause of spinal cord fracture and spinal cord injury.
   - Indirect external force: In traffic accidents and fall accident from high place, external force acts on spine and spinal cord, but external force can lead to different spinal fractures and dislocations, which can induce spinal cord injury.

External force is the main cause of injury of spine and spinal cord. Some spinal cord injuries

W. Zhao, *Rehabilitation Therapeutics of the Neurological Training*,
https://doi.org/10.1007/978-981-13-0812-3_13

are not always accompanied with fractures and dislocations of spine, even there is no abnormal phenomenon in imaging changes, which are common in spinal cord injury of children and adult patients with degenerative spondylodynia and spinal canal stenosis. It can be misdiagnosed so that we should pay attention to it. MRI and electrophysiological examination have some effect on the diagnosis of spinal cord injury without fractures and dislocations.

2. Non-traumatic spinal cord injury: There are many causes of non-traumatic spinal cord injury. They can be divided into two classes.

Developmental pathogenesis includes congenital scoliosis, spina bifida and spondylolisthesis. Spina bifida can lead to tethered cord syndrome.

Acquired pathogenesis: Spinal cord injury due to non-spinal cause mainly includes:

Rehabilitation centre of first affiliated hospital of Henan College of Traditional Chinese Medicine: arteritis, thrombophlebitis of spinal cord, arteritis and phlebophlogosis.

Infection: Guillain-Barr syndrome, transverse myelitis, anterior poliomyelitis and spinal tuberculosis. Spinal tuberculosis was one of the important causes of spinal cord injury.

Degeneration: spinal amyotrophy, amyotrophic lateral sclerosis and syringomyelia.

Occupancy: various tumors, primary tumors such as meningioma (spinal meningioma), neuroglioma, neurofibroma and multiple myeloma, secondary tumors. Spine is the predilection site of metastatic tumor. There is spinal metastasis in pathological examination in 90% of cancer patients. In the patients with spinal metastasis, patients with spinal cord injury account for 20%.

Iatrogenic: accident injury of spinal surgery. We should master surgical indications and be familiar with surgical technic to prevent iatrogenic injury.

13.1.1.2 Diagnosis of Spinal Cord Injury

1. Qualitative diagnosis includes complete spinal cord injury and incomplete spinal cord injury.

Complete spinal cord injury: the functions of motor, sensation, physical reflex and sphincter below injured level are totally lost in spinal cord injury, especially the complete loss of motor and sensation functions of the lowest sacral segment below injured level. Sensation function of sacral segment is deep sensation of anal and sensation of the junction of skin and mucosa in anal. Motor function of sacral segment is the degree of autonomous contraction of musculus sphincter ani externus in digital rectal examination.

Incomplete spinal cord injury means that there is residual sensation and motor functions below injured level. There is motor or sensation function in the lowest sacral segment (S_{3-5}).

Spinal shock: After external force action (shock), the neural function of spinal cord are totally lost below injured level in a short time, but this is not definitely complete injury. It lasts several hours or weeks, even several months. In the period of spinal cord shock, the injured degree cannot be assessed correctly.

Quadriplegia: after cervical spinal cord injury, there is motor function lesion or loss of limbs and sensation lesion or loss below cervical injured level, which can lead to dysfunctions of trunk and pelvic organs.

Paraplegia means motor and sensation functions lesion or loss of chest, waist or sacrum of spinal cord. Paraplegia doesn't affect functions of upper limbs, but affect trunk, legs and pelvic organs, which includes injury of horsetail and conus medullaris.

Nerve root escape: after complete cervical cord or lumbar cord injury, spinal roots are recovered gradually above injured level and the neural injury level is decreased.

Qualitative diagnosis is very important for the degree of spinal cord injury and formulation of therapeutic schedule. Digital rectal examination, bulbocavernosus reflex and anal reflex are the essential items of qualitative diagnosis of the patients with spinal cord injury.

Digital rectal examination is the main indicator of complete injury. The procedure is that finger is used to be inserted into anal to exam the sensation and motor of anal. If there are still sensation and motor of anal, it is incomplete spinal cord injury. This exam can judge the completeness of injury.

Reflex examination includes bulbospongiosus-anal reflex and anal reflex. Bulbospongiosus reflex is the main indicator of spinal cord shock period. The procedure is that stimulation of glans penis or clitoris to see if there is reflex contraction of musculus sphincter ani externus. The reflex is negative in 15% of normal people. Therefore, except for bulbospongiosus reflex, muscle spasm below injure level is the indicator of disappearance of spinal shock period. Anal reflex: the procedure is that stimulation of anal to see if there is contraction of musculus sphincter ani externus.

If there is bulbospongiosus reflex, anal reflex and muscle spasm below injured level, it means the end of spinal shock period.

International Standards for Neurological Classification of Spinal Cord Injury (Table 13.1).

2. Localization diagnosis: According to sensory level and motor level, the injured level can be confirmed.

Segmental structure characteristics of spinal neurotomy determines the segmental manifestations of spinal cord injury. After spinal cord injury, the motor, sensation, reflex, sphincter and autonomous neural functions of spine are damaged to varying degrees below injured level. The relationship between injured level and sensory key point refer to Table 13.2.

3. Functional diagnosis: After spinal cord injury, the sensation, motor and daily life ability are assessed.

Inspection items and scoring methods of sensation and motor are used to assess sensory and motor functions to ascertain the sensory level, motor level and level of spinal cord injury and assess daily life ability of the patients.

The relationship between level of spinal cord injury and key muscle refer to Table 13.3. The level and severity of spinal cord injury are the main basis of determining the rehabilitation goal of the patients, which is important to rehabilitation therapeutic method selection, nursing schedule formulation, therapeutic effects evaluation and prognosis judgements.

13.1.2 The Common Clinical Syndrome After Spinal Cord Injury

Typical transverse spinal cord injury is divided into paraplegia and quadriplegia according to injure level. Some incomplete injuries have special manifestations, which is called clinical syndrome. Specific clinical manifestations and signs of these syndromes are good for understanding the parts of spinal cord injury, diagnosis and formulation of therapeutic schedule.

Central cord syndrome is commonly observed in the injury of spinal vessels. The injury may be started from the central of spinal cord to the peripheral. Because the motor nerve of upper limbs is close to the central of spinal cord and the motor nerve of lower limbs is close to the peripheral of spinal cord. The severity of nerves of upper limbs is more than that of lower limbs. The disorder of upper limbs is more severe than lower limbs. It is possible to walk for the patients, but the upper limbs may be partially or completely paralyzed.

Hemisection syndrome is common in blade injury or gun shot. It injures hemi-spinal cord. Because thermal sensory nerve and pain nerve cross over in spinal cord, proprioception and

Table 13.1 Grading table of international spinal function lesion (ASIA Impairment Scale)

Grade	Extent of injury	Sensory function	Motor function	Myodynamia of key muscle
A	Complete	None (sacral segment)	None	None
B	Incomplete	Have (sacral segment)	None	None
C	Incomplete	There is sensation below neurological level	There is motor function below neurological level	Less than Grade 3
D	Incomplete	There is sensation below neurological level	There is motor function below neurological level	No less than Grade 3
E	Normal	Sensation is normal	Motor is normal	Muscle tension is increased

Table 13.2 The relationship between injured level and sensory key point

Level	Parts	Level	Parts
C_2	Occipital tuberosity	T_8	The eighth intercostal (between T7 and T9)
C_3	Supraclavicular fossa	T_9	The ninth intercostal (between T8 and T10)
C_4	The top of acromioclavicular joint	T_{10}	The tenth intercostal (navel level)
C_5	Facies lateralis of antecubital fossa	T_{11}	The 11th intercostal (between T10 and T12)
C_6	Thumb	T_{12}	The middle part of inguinal ligament
C_7	Middle finger	L_1	Upper one-third of T_{12} and L_2
C_8	Little finger	L_2	Anterior middle part of thigh
T_1	Facies incisalis ulnaris of antecubital fossa	L_3	Medial femoral epicondyle
T_2	Armpit	L_4	Malleolus medialis
T_3	The third intercostal	L_5	The third metatarsophalangeal joint of acrotarsium
T_4	The fourth intercostal (milk line)	S_1	Lateral part of heel
T_5	The fifth intercostal (between T4 and T6)	S_2	Midpoint of popliteal space
T_6	The sixth intercostal (xiphoid level)	S_3	Ischial tuberosity
T_7	The seventh intercostal		

Table 13.3 The relationship between level and key motor muscles

Level	Key muscles	Level	Key muscles
C_5	Elbow flexor (musculus biceps brachii and pronator teres)	L_2	Hip flexor (iliopsoas)
C_6	Extensor carpi (extensor carpi radialis longus and brevis)	L_3	Knee extensor (quadriceps femoris)
C_7	Elbow extensor (musculus triceps brachii)	L_4	Ankle back extensor (tibialis anterior muscle)
C_8	Digital flexor of middle finger (flexor digitorum profundus)	L_5	Digital extensor (extensor digitorum longus)
T_1	Abductor of little finger	S_1	Ankle plantar flexor (musculus gastrocnemius and musculi soleus)

motor functions of ipsilateral limbs are lost in injured side and thermal sensation and pain sensation of offside limbs are lost.

Anterior cord syndrome: if the injury is located only in anterior spinal cord, because anterior horn motor cell is from higher motor information conduction bundle and thermal sensation and pain sensation are from anterior spinal cord, which can lead to loss of motor, thermal sensation and pain sensation below injured level, but the proprioception exists.

Posterior cord syndrome: The injury is located only in posterior spinal cord. Because slender fasciculus and fasciculus cuneatus of proprioception are located in posterior spinal cord, the proprioception below injured level is lost, but motor, thermal sensation and pain sensation still exist.

Conus medullaris syndrome: The injury is mainly located in conus medullaris in sacral segment of spinal cord, which induces areflexia of bladder, intestinal tract and lower limbs. The reflex is kept in sacral segment.

Cauda equine syndrome means the injury of nerve root in lumbosacral part of intraspine, which can induce areflexia of bladder, intestinal tract and lower limbs. Cauda equina belongs to peripheral nerve and is able to regenerate. The neural functions can be recovered and it takes a long time.

Spinal cord contusion means the temporary and reversible physiological function loss of spinal cord and cauda equine. It is only observed in simple compression fracture of centrum or short pressure wave of spinal cord. There is no mechanical compression in spinal cord and no organic injury. There are no positive results in radioactive rays. There is hyperreflexia in the patients without muscle spasm.

13.1.3 The Main Dysfunctions Induced by Spinal Cord Injury

Paralysis (motor dysfunction): Spinal cord injury in chest and lumbar segments lead to paralysis of lower limbs. Cervical spinal cord injury leads to quadriplegia.

Sensory disturbance: There are paresthesia, hyperesthesia, hypaesthesia, even sensory deprivation of paralytic limbs that are correspondence with injured level.

Gatism: After spinal cord injury, there is usually gatism or dysuresia and there is constipation or incontinence. Indwelling catheter term and residual urine volume can induce urinary system infection and stone, even renal dysfunction.

Pain: After spinal cord injury, there is usually pain below injured level and it is hard to cure.

Muscle spasm: There is usually muscle spasm after spinal cord injury above lumbar segments, which can not only affect limbs movements and nursing, but also induce pain.

Pressure sores: The most common spinal cord injury complications are infection and motor disorder.

Psychological disorder: After paraplegia, there are many problems. Most patients are with psychological disorders to varying degrees, which can aggravate the state of the disease, even suicide.

Others: Autonomic regulation disorder, heterotopic ossification and dyspnea because of respiratory muscle dysfunction.

13.1.4 Functional Assessment of Spinal Cord Injury

Rehabilitation assessment is the basis of formulation of rehabilitation therapy schedule. There are many methods that can be selected in the books of rehabilitation medicine and monograph of rehabilitation functional assessment. The following assessment methods are usually used in rehabilitation training of neurological training.

Functional assessment of spinal cord includes the level and severity of spinal cord injury.

Functional assessment of trunk includes assessments of range of joint motion, muscular strength, functional assessment of upper limbs and lower limbs, gait analysis, neural electrophysiology, spasm, sensory functional assessment, coordinated and balanced functional assessment.

Functional assessment of mentality includes assessments of psychological states, character and pain level.

Functional assessment of social ability includes assessments of life ability and independence ability.

Assessment of spinal stability: Because one of the conditions of the patients' rehabilitation training is the stability of spinal cord, or else it may aggravate or induce iatrogenic spinal cord injury. Therefore, the assessment of spinal stability is the essential assessment item before rehabilitation training.

If the spinal cord is in the physiological laden range, even if there is abnormal deformation, shifting and movement of spinal functional unit, the functions of spinal cord and nervous system cannot be injured. Unstable spinal cord is usually observed after the injury of functional unit or assistive structure of spinal cord. In the physiological laden condition, the functional units of spinal cord lose the ability of maintaining normal structure. Abnormal movements, shifting, deformity aggravation and functional impairments of spinal nerve are easy to occur. Diagnostic criteria of unstable spine from higher cervical spine to low lumbar spine refer to Table 13.4, 13.5, 13.6, and 13.7.

Under this circumstance, the patients with spinal cord injury receive rehabilitation are the patients who receive incision vertebrae reduction, spinal canal decompression and internal fixation. With the improvement of internal fixation devices and quality increase, internal fixation can meet the requirements of spinal cord stability. If it is not enough, the patients can wear orthopaedic assistive devices of back rack.

Functional assessments of spinal cord injury include injury degree, injured level, stability of spinal cord after surgery, range of joint motion,

Table 13.4 diagnostic criteria of unstable upper cervical spine (C_0–C_2)

Injured sites	Degree
Atlanto-occipital rotation	More than 8°
Atlanto-occipital shifting	More than 1 mm
Two sides shifting of atlanto-occipital lateral mass	More than 7 mm
Pre-gap sagittal odontoid	More than 4 mm
Unilateral rotation of atlanto-occipital vertebra	More than 45°
The space between posterior margin of epistropheus atlanto-occipital arcus posterior	No more than 13 mm

Table 13.5 Diagnostic criteria of unstable cervical vertebra (C_3–C_7)

Injured sites and degree	Score
Anterior column destruction and function loss	2
Posterior column destruction and function loss	2
The angle of sagittal surface rotation is more than 11°	2
Shifting distance of sagittal surface is more than 3.5 mm	2
Spinal cord injury	2
Cervical traction test is positive	2
Root injury	1
Spinal canal stenosis	1

Assessment criterion: the full score is 14. No less than 5 is defined as instability

Table 13.6 Diagnostic criteria of unstable thoracolumbar spine (T_{12}–L_1)

Injured sites and degree	Score
Anterior column destruction and function loss	2
Posterior column destruction and function loss	2
Shifting distance of sagittal surface is more than 2.5 mm	2
The angle of sagittal surface rotation is more than 5°	2
Spinal cord injury	2
Costovertebral joint rupture	1

Assessment criterion: the full score is 11. No less than 5 is defined as instability

myodynamis, spasm and balanced functional assessment, which are good for judgement of the patients' prognosis, formulation of rehabilitation therapy schedule, the design and application of assistive devices for walking.

Table 13.7 Diagnostic criteria of unstable lumbar segments (L_1–L_5)

Injured sites and degree	Score
Anterior column destruction and function loss	2
Posterior column destruction and function loss	2
The angle of sagittal surface rotation is more than 9%	2
Shifting distance of sagittal surface in flexion and extension position is more than 8–9%	2
Cauda equine injury	3

Assessment criterion: the full score is 11. No less than 5 is defined as instability

13.2 Spinal Cord Injury Rehabilitation Therapy of Neurological Training

13.2.1 Early Rehabilitation Therapy of Spinal Cord Injury

According to spinal function change and rehabilitation therapy method, spinal cord injury is divided into early phase of spinal cord injury and recovery phase of spinal cord injury.

The early phase of spinal cord injury includes the patients with unstable disease state within the 3 weeks after injury who receive incision vertebrae reduction, spinal canal decompression and internal fixation. Their wounds are just healed and the body reaches dynamic balance under new condition, which are not suitable for large dose motor function training such as off bed movements, standing and walking.

13.2.1.1 Rehabilitation Therapy Principle

Rehabilitation principle of this phase is to prevent complications and prepare for the preliminary training of off bed rehabilitation training.

13.2.1.2 Therapeutic Schedule and Method

After spinal cord injury, there are many complications. If they are not handled well, it is possible to induce secondary disease, which may affect functional recovery of the patients in the future greatly, even life danger.

1. Tertiary prevention to decrease disabled degree and secondary disease as much as possible.

Primary prevention is impairment prevention. After spinal cord injury, during the process of saving the patients, emergency treatment, immobilization fixation, drug therapy and correct surgery are adopted in the early phase to prevent secondary lesion and injury of spinal cord and the aggravation of spinal dysfunctions, which creates condition for the functional recovery of spinal cord. Clinical physicians should memorize that prevention of spinal cord injury is more important than therapy of spinal cord injury. Aggravation of spinal cord injury must be avoided in emergency. It must be pointed that correct surgical therapy is one part of therapy of spinal cord injury, while improper surgery may aggravate spinal cord injury.

Secondary prevention is disability prevention to prevent various kinds of complications, to carry out early rehabilitation training, to make full use of all residual functions to develop new functions, to reach self-care maximally, to prevent or decrease disability.

Tertiary prevention is handicap prevention. Spinal cord injury leads to spinal dysfunctions and rehabilitation measures (medicine, engineer and education) are used comprehensively to make full use of all residual functions and modify external conditions (barrier free accessibilities of house) to make the patients return to society in a short time.

2. Reflex bladder is established to prevent urinary system infection, promote functional recovery of defection and prevent constipation.

Prevention of urinary system infection and obstruction: urinary system infection and obstruction finally lead to renal failure, which is the main cause of death of the patients with neurogenic bladder and urethral dysfunction. Residual urine due to unable evacuation of bladder provide medium for growth and reproduction of bacteria and injure defense mechanism of bladder, which may induce urinary tract infection easily. If the kidney is infected, there is nephropyelitis.

The increase of residual urine can increase intravesical pressure, which increases the resistance of urine in ureter flowing into bladder, even regurgitation. High tension may lead to upper urinary tract dropsy and injure renal function, which finally induce renal failure. The main purpose of therapy is to recover balance function of bladder and urethra and prevent infection in order to protect renal function maximally. In clinic, preferred non-operation therapy method is intermittent catheterization and others include retention catheterization, bladder irrigation, bladder urination training, outer urine collection device and drug therapy.

Although retention catheterization can evacuate urine totally, avoid hyperinflation of bladder, improve blood circulation of bladder wall and promote functional recovery of bladder, indwelling catheter destroy germ free condition of bladder and urethra and germ can go into bladder through peripheral clearance of catheter and inner cavity, which can induce bacteriuria. If this is not handled properly, it will lead to urinary system infection. If the catheter is kept for 1 day, the incidence rate of bacteriuria is 50%. If the catheter is kept for 4 days, the incidence rate of bacteriuria is 98–100%. Therefore, it is used in the patients who are severe and feeble and cannot evacuate bladder, are with uroschesis or uroclepsia (female patients), are difficult to use intermittent catheterization or have upper urinary tract impairment and vesicoureteral regurgitation. Therefore, if possible, the long-term indwelling catheter should be avoided to prevent secondary disease such as urinary system infection and stone.

The preferred clean urethral catheterization technique is also called intermittent catheterization, which is the way of urethral catheterization without indwelling catheter by non-medical staffs such as patients, their family or caregivers to decrease the incidence of urinary system infection obviously.

If non-surgical therapy cannot figure out the problem, the patients can consider operation method therapy. Cystauchenotomy through urethra is suitable for the patients who with obstruction of export part of bladder, bladder contraction inability, but without external urethral sphincter dysfunction. Before surgery, phentolamine test can be sued to predict operation result. Transurethral sphincterotomy is suitable for the patients with spinal cord injury above sacral cord who have dysuresia due to hyper contraction of striated muscle of perineum and external urethral sphincter. Dysuresia can lead to increase of residual urine and this surgery can reduce urethral resistance effectively. External urethral sphincter incision is irreversible and there is uroclepsia to varying degrees after surgery. The surgery can be implemented 1 year after injury when the nervous system disease is stable and the functional recovery is finished. Suprapubic cystostomy is suitable for the patients who are with repeated severe urinary system infection, neurogenic bladder urethral dysfunction and urethral injury and it is temporary therapeutic measures. After surgery, fistula is adopted in scheduled time opening. When the bladder reaches certain filling volume, the patients evacuate it to avoid bladder contracture. When the disease is better, fistula should be removed as soon as possible to recover urination. Bladder augmentation is suitable for the patients who with increase of detrusor pressure and decrease of bladder volume due to bladder contracture. Terminal ileum is used to enlarge the volume of bladder in order to decrease intravesical pressure, alleviate and prevent hydronephrosis and hydroureter. Urinary diversion is only used for the patients with severe hydronephrosis and hydroureter and renal insufficiency. The most common used is napes fistulation of ileal loop replacing bladder. There are many secondary disease and it should be used with caution.

In some reports artificial urethral sphincter is used to reestablish the function of bladder urination. After surgery, the incidence rate of complications is high, which restricts the application of it. Implantation bladder stimulation device is used to stimulate detrusor of bladder directly to induce urination, but the effect is not satisfying. Electrode is implanted into conus medullaris or sacral nerve root directly, which is started to be used in clinic. The recent effect is satisfying and long-term effect remains to be observed.

Rectum training: After spinal cord injury, the problems of rectum include constipation. Enema, anus lubricating agent and laxative can be used. Diarrhea is rare and most are accompanied with intestinal infection. Antibacterial agents and intestinal astringents can be used for therapy. Functional training method of rectum active movement refers to the common complications disposition of spinal cord injury in the third section of this chapter.

3. Keeping joints in functional position to prevent amyotrophy, muscle tendon contracture and joint adhesion.
   - Application of retaining appliance of limbs functions position: Keeping joints in functional position or in good limbs position is the basis of motor functional recovery of limbs. After injury, without affecting first aid, it should be used as soon as possible.
   - Passive joint motion: After vital signs are stable, passive motion of all joints can be started. The times of movements in axial direction is 6–8 (1–2 times per day) to prevent muscle tendon contracture and tissue adhesion of joint and muscle.

The movement should be slow and reach the maximal physiological range to avoid straining a muscle or ligament. It should be operated according to regulations. For example, wrist and finger joints cannot be flexed at the same time in case of straining wrist and tendon of extensor digitorum muscle.

Continuous passive motion device of joints can be used such as CPM devices of ankle, knee, hip, finger, elbow and shoulder joint. The joints motion in maximal physiological range can be done in turns to eliminate joint adhesion without pain, improve the angle of joint motion, treat or prevent joint stiffness, amyotrophy, degenerative and traumatic arthritis. It can be used after traction of joint contracture and therapy of joint loosening to keep the therapeutic effect.

Massage of trunk and limbs can increase blood circulation of muscle, promote metabolism, prevent tissue adhesion and alleviate pain. Eight treating observances of massage is used for the massage of lower back and four limbs. The movement should be gentle and soft to avoid aggravating muscle spasm. The frequency is 1–2 times a day.

Active joint motion or induction training of active motion: For the patients with incomplete spinal cord injury, functional assessments are used to find out the main obstacles for physical training and occupational therapy of neurological training (six-step Daoyin technique). The patients are guided to do active joint motion and the therapists exert resistance in the orientation of movement to develop spinal potential and increase myodynamia in order to prevent amyotrophy and phlebothrombosis. Every time, the therapists choose three joints to do active flexion and extension motion training in turns. The training time is 45 min (1–2 times a day). For the patients with complete spinal cord injury, six-step Daoyin technique is used to do induction training. The patients should receive the therapy with patience. On the basis of regulation of mind and breathing, regulation of movement can induce the motor center in brain cortex to give out motor program signal to stimulate conduction bundle located in the part of spinal cord injury in order to recover the functions of incomplete injured conduction bundle and activate reserved conduction bundle around injure zone. In most cases, complete spinal cord injury in early diagnosis may be not the real complete injury and zero myodynamia from assessment may be not the real zero motor program signals. The functions are possible to be recovered. Medical staffs, the patients and their patients should have confidence and don't give up. The training of neurological training: In the early phase, rehabilitation training of neurological training can be done in the bedside. According to the actual situation of the patients, clinostatism, semireclining position or sitting position can be used. Neurological training device is used to monitor the motor program signal of agonistic muscle (single channel). Six-step method or six-step Daoyin technique of guiding collaterals through meridians is used to develop neural potential and recover lost motor function through setting surpassing goal. The training time is 45 min (one time a day).

Early sitting up and standing training: for the patients with stable spinal cord, the sitting training can be used in the early phase (after injury or 1 week after surgery). If the internal fixation is not stable, back rack can be used for protection. Sitting up training is started in 30° elevation from the head of the bed. If there is no adverse effect, the head of the bed can be increased 15° in every 3 days until the patient can sit upright and the duration is no less than 30 min. if there is any adverse effect in the training, the head of the bed should be decreased until the symptoms disappear. Under the guardianship of vital signs monitor such as electro cardio, the therapists can find the problem timely and keep the safety of the training. Standing bed training: after injury or 3 weeks after surgery, according to the specific condition of the patients, the training is done. If the patients can keep in sitting position (90°) for no less than 30 min and there is no adverse effect, the standing training can be started. Standing bed is used. The training can be started from 30° inclination and the angle can be increased gradually until the patients can stand upright for no less than 30 min and there is no adverse effect. In the training, the therapists should observe the change of the patients in case of postural hypotension. If there is any abnormity, the angle of standing bed should be decreased immediately and symptomatic treatment should be given to the patients timely. Vital signs monitor with alarm is used to monitor the patients continuously. If there is any abnormity of vital signs, the therapists can find out the problem and keep the safety of the training.

If the patients cannot stand upright for no less than 30 min, it means that the patient' injured level is higher and the cardiovascular stress response is poor. The following methods can be applied for therapy. Elastic bandage of lower limbs can be used with bellyband to increase returned blood volume. Pulse-activating injection is the Chinese materia medica preparation purified from red ginseng, Radix Ophiopogonis and Schisandra chinensis, which can regulate the flow of vital energy and remove obstruction toit, tonify qi and strengthen heart, promote the secretion of saliva or body fluid and restore the pulse, rescue from collapse by restoring Yang, strengthen the body resistance to eliminate pathogenic factors, promote blood circulation to remove blood stasis and anticoagulated.

Intramuscular injection: the injection dose is 2–4 ml every time (1–2 times per day). Intravenous drip: the dose is 20–60 ml every time. It should be diluted with 250–500 ml 5% dextrose injection (once a day).

4. Breathing and sputum excretion training to keep the airway open and prevent pulmonary infection.

Dyspnea due to spinal cord injury is rarely observed in high level injury, especially the patients with cervical spinal injury. Because paralysis of respiratory muscle and abdominal muscle, atelectasis can induce dyspnea and expectoration inability, which may easily induce pulmonary infection. The prevention methods are as follows: The therapists help the patients to turn over and slap back to excrete sputum. If possible, the patients should be in semireclining position to increase thorax volume through moving down visceral organs. If there is sticky sputum, aerosol inhalation is used to dilute sputum. Vibration sputum elimination apparatus is used to excrete sputum and the airway should be open. Active movement training of respiratory muscle: deep and slow abdominal breathing is the effective breathing form to increase tidal volume. Third-fourth gas is inhaled because of increase of thorax volume induced by moving down of diaphragm. For the patients with spinal cord injury and without diaphragmatic paralysis, pulmonary functional training device can be used to drill diaphragm to increase its contraction ability, which can form deep and slow abdominal breathing in order to prevent pulmonary infection.

5. Timely turning over and active and passive movements of lower limbs to prevent pressure sores and deep venous thrombosis effectively because of paraplegia, especially complete paraplegia, the patients lose sensation and motor function below paraplegic level, which easily induce pressure sores and deep venous thrombosis. When it does happen, it is difficult to be handled so that we should prevent them effectively.
6. Transfer training includes independent transfer training and transfer training with help. After injury, if the disease state is stable, the patients can start transfer training from bed to wheelchair and from wheelchair to toilet. Transfer training can be completed independently or with the help of others such as one person or two persons. Independent transfer is the transfer movement that the patients can complete by themselves. It is one kind of life stand-alone capability training, which includes transfer from clinostatism to sitting position, crosswise and vertical transfer on bed or cushion, transfer from bed to wheelchair, transfer from wheelchair to bed, transfer from wheelchair to stool, transfer from stool to wheelchair, transfer from wheelchair to the ground, transfer from the ground to wheelchair, transfer from wheelchair to pedestal pan and transfer from wheelchair to vehicle. In the transfer training, some assistive devices can be used such as sliding plate.

Assistive transfer training: the therapists face to the patients, use double knees to support the knee of the patients, use two hands to support the hip of the patients and lift up the patients. The patients use one hand to support the shoulder of the therapists and the other hand falls naturally. The patients are transferred to bed slowly.

Transfer forward training: Wheelchair faces to bedside and it is braked. The patients are transferred to bed slowly. The patients use two hands to hold the handrail of wheelchair to support the body in order to move to the bed from the front of wheelchair.

Transfer lateral training: the angle between wheelchair and bed is 45° and the wheelchair is braked. The patients put two legs on the bed, use one hand to support the bed and use the other hand to hold the handrail of wheelchair in order to move the hip out of bed.

In short, in the early rehabilitation phase of the patients with spinal cord injury, vasomotion training such as training from supine position to sitting position, form sitting in bedside to sitting in wheelchair, tilt bed transition, balance function training such as balance function training in sitting position, on cushion and in wheelchair, transfer training, wheelchair operation training, passive joint motion, muscle stretching, myodynamia training of residual muscles in the trunk and double upper limbs, breathing training are mainly used. In the late phase of rehabilitation, except for myodynamia training, balance function training and transfer training, standing training with the help of assistive device or the therapists, walking training with the help of body weight center shifting walking orthotics, knee-ankle-foot KAFO or ankle-foot orthotics are mainly used. Once the endurance is strengthened, overcoming obstacles, climbing stairs, standing up after falling are mainly used.

7. Physiotherapy can improve blood circulation of paralytic part and increase excitability of paralytic muscle. There are many physiotherapy methods. Nerve And Muscle Electrical Stimulation (NMES) can be used to treat disuse muscle atrophy to increase excitability of paralytic muscle, improve blood circulation, increase or maintain range of joint motion, promote muscle relearning and facilitate it. During therapy, electrode is placed on the muscle belly and symmetry bi-directional square wave (1–100 Hz) is used. Break-make ratio is from 1–1 to 1–15. Motor threshold is chosen in electricity and the time is 10–20 min (1–4 times a day). Transcutaneous Electrical Nerve Stimulation (TENS) is used to treat various acute and chronic pains to improve blood circulation. During therapy, the electrode is placed in the pain point and asymmetry bi-directional square wave (1–150 Hz) is used. Pulse width is 0.04–0.3 ms. The electricity is from sensation threshold to maximal bearing range. The time is 10–20 min (1–2 times a day). Vapor-pressure type limbs blood circulation drive device is used to accelerate return blood flow velocity from the distal to the proximal in order to eliminate edema, improve blood circulation of limbs, promote metabolism and prevent thrombogenesis. Therapeutic method is that the patients wear and regulate inflated bag of upper and lower limbs. The pressure is 20–220 mmHg, which can be adjusted according to the heart rate and pulse of the patients. Inflation and evacuation time is 5–10 s and the therapy time is 30 min (1–2 times a day). Medium-frequency electrical current, ultrashort wave, far infrared and interference current can eliminate inflammation, alleviate pain, promote blood circulation and recover neural functions. They can be selected according to the specific condition of the patients.
8. Psychotherapy: Psychotherapy is the only good medicine to encourage the patients to go out of the difficulty and fight with the disease. The patients with spinal cord injury become the person who lose functions from the person who are healthy. Because of function loss, the patients know nothing about their future. After injury, most patients have severe psychological disorder includes severe repression or depression, dysphoria, even mental symptoms. Therefore, psychotherapists must explain the psychotherapy to the patients with patience. They help the patients to analyze and know the three stages of the disease. Period of deny: the patients are thick suddenly and are lack of psychological preparation for this great fall. They don't think they are ill and they feel contradicted, anxious, hesitated and unwilling to cooperate with therapy. In allusion to this condition, on the basis of fact, psychotherapists explain to the patients that the law of birth, death, illness and old age is irresistible. The patients gradually recognize that they are the same as other people and they can be thick. If these laws can be preached in the normal population, it is good for increasing the consciousness of disease prevention and decreasing the morbidity. Period of sad: after a period of time, the patients recognize that they are the same as other people and they can be thick. They will wonder their illnesses are healed or not, there is sequela or not, they

can return to society and work or not and the family is worried or not. They may be caught in sorrow and then in sadness. They may have no appetite for food and drinks, insomnia, anxiety, and look extremely worried, which affect greatly physical and psychological health of the patients. Psychotherapists should do psychotherapy on time and help the patients to analyze the disease. They should ask the patients with the similar disease or with good therapeutic effect to introduce the experience and let the patients recognize that the disease cannot be defeated by pain and the patients should get up steam, face to the reality with courage, adjust psychology, cooperate with therapy and do hard-training. And then they can obtain good results. Period of positive in treatment: through the two stages, most patients finally recognize that only facing to the reality can figure out all the difficulties and cooperating with the therapists is the only way to functional recovery. The patients have faith and take part in rehabilitation training.

The mission of psychotherapy is to help the patients to realize the fact, get rid of the first two stages, transit to the third stage to alleviate extent of injury to mind and body of the patients and fight for best therapeutic effect.

13.2.2 Rehabilitation Therapy of Neurological Training of the Patients with Spinal Cord Injury in Convalescence

The convalescence of spinal cord injury means the period after acute phase. The undead cells or cells in shock in injured zone are already recovered through therapy. The compensation mechanism is activated to promote reserved conduction pathway and spinal nerve cells around injured zone to replace the injured cells. This compensation can be accumulated with time, which is good for the improvement and recovery of spinal functions. Therefore, spinal cord injury is in convalescence after acute phase. Although the recovery time is prolonged after injury, injured spinal cord can be further recovered and the patients should not give up.

13.2.2.1 Rehabilitation Therapy of Neurological Training Principle of the Patients with Spinal Cord Injury in Convalescence

Rehabilitation principle of this phase is to recover normal motor pattern, cooperate with assistive device, recover standing and walking functions, establish neural reflex bladder, control complications such as urinary system infection and stone effectively. Through vocational ability training, the patients have the ability of returning to the society and self-care.

The types of spinal cord injury include injury of central nerve (above sacrococcyx (sacral end)) and injury of peripheral nerve (below sacrococcyx). It also involves the abnormal motor pattern of peripheral nerve. Because traditional rehabilitation medicine thinks that central paralysis is qualitative change and peripheral paralysis is quantitative change [3]. After peripheral paralysis, there is no abnormal motor pattern and only the change of extent such as myodynamia. Central paralysis is changed with the extent of voluntary movements. Abnormal motor pattern is the main manifestation of qualitative change of central paralysis. The disability induced by peripheral nerve injury is amyotrophy, myodynamia decrease, muscle tension and tendon reflex decrease, while there is no abnormal motor pattern. The chief measure of recovering functions is the training of strengthening myodynamia.

This is because people don't recognize that human motor pattern is dominated and controlled by motor program in motor center of brain cortex and the formation of abnormal motor pattern is due to the appearance, completion and attenuation of associated response and associated movement.

However, it is not the case. Nervus peroneus communis injury and paralysis of tibialis anterior muscle and peroneus longus and brevis can lead to foot drop and strephenopodia, there is usually abnormal walking motor pattern such as circle gait ot drag gait. According to the theory of neurological training motor program, motor program decides motor pattern and motor pattern is the manifestation of motor program. Abnormal motor program leads to abnormal motor pattern and exterior abnormal motor pattern can modify the normal motor program in motor center of cortex. The abnormal motor program can be solidified with the application time. The exterior abnormal motor pattern is hard to be rectified. Therefore, there is abnormal motor pattern in peripheral nerve injury. The main purpose of rehabilitation is to recover lost neural function but not only strengthen myodynamia.

The final purpose of rehabilitation is to recover the normal motor pattern that is good for body functions. Therefore, recovering motor function of spinal cord injury is the basis of recovering normal motor pattern. For the patients with complete or incomplete function loss, the purpose of rehabilitation is to develop neural potential and residual functions maximally through training to make the patients use assistive device independently and recover standing, walking and daily self-care abilities.

13.2.2.2 Therapeutic Schedule and Method

1. The goal of rehabilitation training of neurological training of incomplete spinal cord injury to recover normal motor pattern, develop potential functions maximally and apply replacement function of assistive device in order to recover the standing, walking and self-care ability of the patients.

   According to detailed functional assessments and different degrees of paralysis, the training principles are as follows:

   Three-stage rehabilitation principle is suitable for the patients with more residual functions or slight dysfunction who can recover motor pattern through training.

   Three-stage rehabilitation principle with the functional compensation of assistive device is suitable for the patients with local dysfunctions such as strephenopodia and foot drop who can recover motor function through training and assistive device in spite the dysfunction is severe.

   Rehabilitation principle of early standing and walking recovery is suitable for the patients with severe functional injuries in multiple parts or cognitive dysfunction who are difficulty to recover functions because they are reluctant to cooperate with the training. Three-stage rehabilitation schedule cannot meet the requirements of the third stage training. At this time, recovering walking ability of the patients with partial help is the ideal result. If the therapists still use three stages therapy method, walking ability of the patients with partial help may not be recovered.

   Adoptive specific rehabilitation methods are as follows:

   - Neural potential development is suitable for central and peripheral nerve injuries. Normal method or six-step Daoyin technique in traditional Chinese medicine of guiding collaterals through meridians is used. According to the part of potential development, the corresponding training equipment is selected such as potential development training device or apparatus of upper limbs, lower limbs, trunk, tibialis anterior muscle, musculus gastrocnemius and hamstring muscles. They can be done gradually according to the difficulties. The training time is 30 (1–2 times a day) and there are 30 times in one therapy course. The patients can receive multiple therapy courses.
   - Physical therapy and occupational therapy of neurological training (six-step Daoyin technique bare-handed operation method): Normal method or six-step Daoyin technique in traditional Chinese medicine of guiding collaterals through meridians is used for active movement training of every joint. The therapists exert resistance in the orientation of movement to develop spinal potential functions fully. It is suitable for the functional training of upper limbs, lower limbs, trunk, neck and hand. The training time is 45 (1–2 times a day) and there are 30 times in one therapy course. The patients can receive multiple therapy courses.

- Neurological training: neurological training apparatus is used to monitor the motor program signal of agonistic muscle and antagonistic muscle continuously and the signal is displayed in real-time. Through setting surpassing goal, six-step method or six-step Daoyin technique of guiding collaterals through meridians is used to increase the signal intensity of agonistic muscle and decrease signal intensity of antagonistic muscle. Motor program of single joint is established at first and on the basis of that, motor program of associated movement is established gradually. The training time is 50 (once a day) and there are 30 times in one therapy course. The patients can receive multiple therapy courses. There is no side effect.

  Virtual reality training of neurological training: normal method or virtual reality training system of guiding collaterals through meridians is used for the training. The specific method is the same as the method of neurological training. The training time is 50 (once a day) and there are 30 times in one therapy course. The patients can receive multiple therapy courses.

  Motor pattern remodeling training: On the basis of potential development and motor program reestablishment, when the patients are able to stand up, flex hip and bear load with one leg independently or with the help of assistive device, the training of motor program remodeling can be started.

  The training of motor pattern remodeling after spinal cord injury is as follows:

  Balance training: under the weight support protection of balance training device, balance plate is used for balance training. The inclination angle is from small to big gradually.

  Shifting of weight training of stride and gait: Training device of stride and gait is used. Stride is divided into five grades according to the stride length. The lower the grade is, the shorter the stride is. The longer the stride is, the bigger the difficulty is. The sequence is from lower to higher and the difficulty is increased gradually. During training, the patients are guided to pay attention to correct shifting of body center and observe the balance in body shifting, which provides basis for walking training.

  Rectification weight support walking training of abnormal gait: Rectification weight support walking training device of abnormal gait is used. The patients wear motor pattern remodeling instrument for training. The weight depends on the specific condition of the patients. The weight usually is one fifth to one eighth of body weight. The patients do the walking training in the footpath marked by gait. The specific goal of stride and stride width is set in the walking training on the footpath.

  Walking balance training: Walking balance training device is used. The patients wear motor pattern remodeling instrument and lose weight. The patients do the training in the footpath marked by gait. In the first several trainings, except for weight support by suspension, there is no other helps, just like independent walking. During walking, swing of the body can make the patients feel nervous. The therapists should stand beside the patients, protect and guide the patients to alleviate psychological burden of the patients.

  Weight support walking training: Weight support walking training device is used for the training. According to the specific condition of the patients' motor pattern, the patients wear (abnormal motor pattern) or don't wear (normal motor pattern) motor pattern remodeling instrument. The weight usually is one fifth to one eighth of body weight. Rotational speed of track is from 0.22 m/s. With the increase of walking ability, the speed is increased gradually. The patients are guided to do the training according to the marked gait in the track of walking machine.

  Footpath training marked by gait includes balance bar footpath training marked by gait or walking aid footpath training marked by gait, the training of ascending and descending the stairs and the training of Footpath training marked by gait (Fig. 13.1). During the training, the patients wear or don't wear motor pattern remodeling instrument and gradually transited to independent walking without help and motor pattern remodeling instrument.

The patients can receive 4–6 therapy items every day. The therapy time is 30–50 min and there are 30 times in one therapy course. The patients can receive multiple therapy courses.

The application of assistive device: the functional recovery of the patients with incomplete paraplegia is usually slow and incomplete. Some patients have autonomous movements, but there are spasm or pain to varying degrees. Complete independent motor function is difficult to be recovered and the functional defects should be compensated by orthotics and support device. Therefore, the standing and walking abilities of the patients can be recovered. There are many kinds of orthotics and support assistive device including ankle-foot orthotics, knee-ankle orthotics, wheelchair, walking aid, interactive walking orthotics and intelligent standing and walking system.

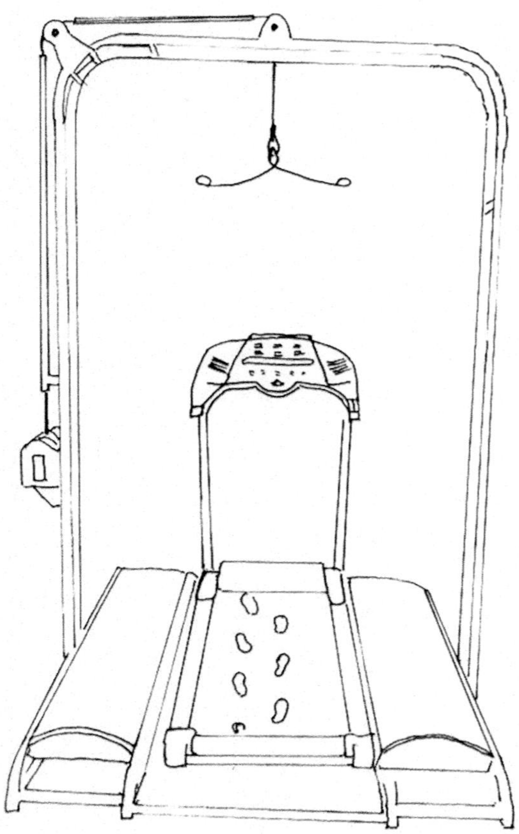

Fig. 13.1 The training of footpath training marked by gait

It would be specially mentioned that application of any assistive device is the unavoidable replacement measure and it should not be abused, especially for profit. Any replacement measure may lead to the disuse of the replaced part including muscle and bone, which affects the functional recovery of injured parts to varying degrees in the future.

For the patients with incomplete spinal cord injury, in order to make the patients stand up and walk in the early phase, the patients can wear walking assistive device. With the progress of training, the patients can remove some part of the assistive device gradually and stand up and walk independently on the basis of functional recovery.

The therapy of muscle spasm: for incomplete spinal cord injury, spinal cord below injured level loses the control of higher neural center. Its excitability can lead to muscle spasm. At present, the common therapy method of muscle spasm at home and abroad are as follows. Rehabilitation methods include prevention of harmful stimulation, motortherapy training such as extension, rectal probe electrical stimulation, other physical therapy such as stimulating antagonistic muscle and acupuncture and moxibustion therapy. Drug therapies includebaclofen, dantrolene and diazepam. Nerve block methods include motor spot block of phenol and Clostridium botulinum (creotoxin), paravertebral or nerve block of phenol and subarachnoid space block of phenol. Nerve damage methods include high selective posterior rhizotomy, selective posterior rhizotomy, rhizotomy, neurotomy, myotomy, myotenotomy, spinal tractotomy and myelotomy. The methods are not specific for etiological treatment (recover higher central neural functions) and there are some shortcomings.

Rehabilitation method of neurological training: Neural potential development training and motor program reestablishment training of spasmodic muscle are used for the therapy and there are some preliminary clinical effects such as disappearance of pathological reflex of the patients (ankle clonus) and obvious improvement of autonomous motor function. For example, a 9 years old Taipei child had paralysis of left limbs due to right cerebral infarction 2 years ago in America. After rehabilitation training in America and Taipei University affiliated children's hospital, there are still poor fine movement of left hand and left foot drop, circle gait in walking, strong positive of left ankle clonus, grade three of musculus gastrocnemius spasm, grade two of myodynamia of tibialis anterior muscle and no autonomous foot dorsiflexion. In Jan 22, 2013, the patient entered into national research center for rehabilitation technical aid affiliated hospital and receive the training of three-stage rehabilitation method of neurological training. During the process of neural potential development of upper and lower limbs, the patient received neural potential development training of musculus gastrocnemius and motor program reestablishment training of foot dorsiflexion. After 4 weeks' training, left foot dorsiflexion function is recovered with slight strephenopodia and ankle clonus disappears. Fine movements of every finger in left hand such as separating fingers, closing fingers, grasping and thumb opposing functions are recovered obviously. The long-term effect and therapeutic effect of muscle spasm after spinal cord injury need further clinical verification.

Physiotherapy is the same as rehabilitation therapy in the early phase after spinal cord injury.

Wheelchair use training: 2–3 months after injury, if the spinal cord of the patients is stable and the patients can sit independently for more than 15 min, the patients can start wheelchair use training if the patients cannot recover standing and walking ability in a short time. Upper body strength and endurance are the premise of wheelchair manipulation. Wheelchair use training includes forward drive. Backward drive, left and right turning, moving with tilting front wheel, rotation training, climbing slope and crossing barrier, up and down stairs, crossing curb kerb, going through narrow door, falling safely and sit up upright.

In every 20 min sitting, the patients should use upper limbs to support trunk or tilt the trunk to make hip away from seat in order to reduce pressure for 20–30 s, which can excrete local metabolism and guarantee blood supply in case that compression of tuber ischiadicum for a long time can lead to pressure sores.

Activities of daily living training: For the patients with paraplegia, especially self-care activities such as eating, combing and dressing in upper limbs. In addition, daily life ability training should be done after motor program reestablishment of hand through neurological training. it can be combined with traditional hand function training such as grasping ability of fingers, flexibility training, artware fabrication using plasticine, drawing, clipping clip, turning the screw, nut and tying knots.

2. Complete spinal cord injury: Prevention of complications effectively and recovery of functions with the help of assistive device are the rehabilitation training principle of complete spinal cord injury.

At present, for the patients with complete spinal injury, the functional recovery is impossible. Complete spinal cord injury in clinic is not always pathological complete spinal cord injury. Of the patients with spinal cord injury treated by the author, some are told by the surgical doctors that complete spinal cord injury is impossible to be recovered and they may spend all their life in wheelchair. After verification, it is not complete spinal cord injury and the functions are recovered partially through rehabilitation training, even independent walking ability. Therefore, for complete spinal cord injury in clinic, rehabilitation physicians should be cautious with it.

Prevention of complications: Effective prevention of complications such as urinary system infection, pressure sores, musculoskeletal disuse, joint adhesion and muscle tendon contracture is the premise to guarantee the life of the patients with paraplegia and functional recovery. It is the basis of recover functions using better therapeutic methods in the future.

Rehabilitation training of neurological training: although the patients are diagnosed with complete spinal cord injury, they should receive rehabilitation training. Its meaningfulness is as follows: There may be functional recovery. After spinal cord injury, through therapy or with time, the functions of undead cells and conduction pathways may be recovered. At this time, proper rehabilitation training can facilitate functional recovery. In addition, there are normal cells and conduction pathways around injure area. Neural potential development training is activated for functional recovery. The required conditions of using assistive device: rehabilitation training of neurological training, especially potential development training, can effectively prevent disuse atrophy of muscle to keep a certain muscle tension and prevent joint and soft tissue adhesion to keep a certain range of joint motion. These all the conditions required for the application of assistive device, walking aid or walking orthotics. Prevention of complications: motor function training of body can effectively promote blood circulation of limbs and trunk, promote metabolism of tissue, enhance body resistance, decrease long-term compression of local tissue. Therefore, it can improve body condition, prevent urinary system infection, pressure sores and organ function disease and make the patients' body keep in a basic good condition to prolong life, return to the society and create condition for waiting for the effective therapeutic method.

Specific therapeutic methods: the training of increasing cardiovascular stress response ability includes standing bed training and blood circulation drive training. on the moment increasing bearing load ability of bone and preventing osteoporosis, it can promote blood circulation of limbs and systolic and diastolic function of heart and vessels. Compulsive active movement training: Potential development training device is applied. On the premise of weight support and protection, six-step Daoyin technique is used to do autonomous movement induction training through changing body position. During therapy, the patients should be patient. On the basis of regulation of mind and breathing, regulation of movement can induce motor program signal of motor center of brain cortex to stimulate the conduction bundle in spinal cord injury part in order to recover the functions of incomplete injured conduction bundle and activate reserved conduction bundle around injure area. Abnormal gait rectification weight support walking training: with weight support and protection of abnormal gait rectification weight support walking training device, the patients wear motor pattern remodeling training aid or shoulder power walking assistive device and do walking training with the instruction and help of the therapists.

For the patients with higher paraplegia who are difficult to walk, they can wear walking aid pulley to do walking training. The shoe sole is equipped with four spring pulley. When the patients start to move the body center to offside, because the spring is compressed by the body weight, the shoe sole touches the ground and cannot move. The spring upspring without the compression of body weight in the stepping side, and the pulley touches the ground to make lower limb in stepping side slip forward. The movements are repeated alternatively, which forms stepping movement.

For the patients with complete paraplegia, the training should be progressive and from easy to difficult. The training time is 30 min. There are two breaks in the training. The frequency is once a day and one therapy course takes three months.

The application of walking orthotics: one of the main functions of orthotics associated with walking is to compensate lost muscle functions of lower limbs in order to increase standing and walking ability and improve gait.

Paraplegia orthotics for standing and walking assistive device includes hip-knee-ankle-foot orthosis (HKAFO) and alternate paraplegia orthotics (RGO). Its design principle is that through specific mechanical structure, the shifting of body weight center and the body are translated into impetus that can drives lower limbs forward, which realizes the stepping forward movement of lower limbs. Hip joint of orthotics, side lattice framing of the trunk and pelvis hipline guarantee the stability of the trunk to broaden the application of walking orthotics.

RGO is suitable for the patients with complete paraplegia below T_6. The patients with paraplegia below waist surface have normal functions of upper trunk. Therefore, the standing and walking ability can be recovered. The patients with lumbar cord level injury have unstable ankle joint, but have normal functions of lumbar and abdominal muscle. The patients who can control pelvis can use KAFO. For the patients with injury of lower thoracic cord level, when lumbar and abdominal muscles are injured, the patients can use HKAFO with pelvic support. The ankle joints of KAFO and HKAFO should be fixed on the dorsiflexion position. In standing, the lower limbs tilt forward to keep hip stable and balanced using hyperextension position of hip. Every segment of orthotics should be fixed on the limbs to disperse stress and prevent crush.

When wearing walking aid to walk, the users should use armpit crutch or elbow crutch. At first, the patients move the center of the body to one side and then tilt pelvis backward. Lower limb in this side is stretched by tightwire to step forward. The other leg can step forward with the same method. The movements mentioned above can be repeated continuously to realize functional walking of the patients with paraplegia.

The development of shoulder power walking assistive device: Walking orthotics mentioned above use passive walking. The author found that spinal cord injury includes cervical spinal cord injury but accessory nerve (the 11th cranial nerve) that dominates trapezius is not injured in most cases. Accessory nerve is motor nerve, which is composed of cranial nerve root and spinal nerve root. Cranial nerve root protrudes from medulla oblongata below vagus nerve root to dominate skeletal muscle of throat. Spinal root arises from cell population of grey matter parastyle in superior cervical spinal cord to dominate trapezius and sternocleidomastoid. These fibers go up from spinal cord and combine with cranial nerve into truncus nervi accessorii through foramen magnum.

Trapezius is located in the superficial layer of cervical part and the front of back (Fig. 13.2). It arises from superior nuchal line, external occipital protuberance, ligamentum nuchae and all spi-

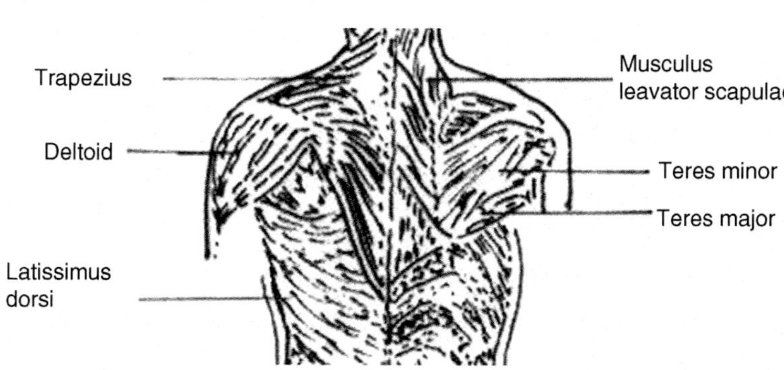

Fig. 13.2 An anatomy charting of the trapezius muscle, it is guided by cranial nerve (N XI), it's function can be reserved in high level spinal cord injures

nous processes of thoracic vertebra. Muscle fibers centralize to outside and end in outside one third of clavicle, acromion and mesoscapula. Its role is to shrug, elevating two shoulders to two ears. Contraction of this muscle can make scapula close to spinal column. Upper muscle bundle lifts scapula up and lower muscle bundle decreases scapula, which completes the shrug movement.

According to this function, the author designed shoulder power walking assistive device, which can use shrug as the power to complete hip and knee joint flexion in order to lift lower limbs. Through joint self-lock system, in the falling of lower limbs, hip and knee joints are locked in extension state. Through firm lattice framing of assistive device, the body weight can be supported and the standing position is kept. The movements can be done alternatively in two sides, which can complete stepping forward and independent walking.

The comprehensive effects make the patients walk independently. Through the force of shrugging, lower limb can be lifted and the patients can step forward, which is very close to the process and posture of normal walking. The patients can walk in asperous ground. In traditional walking, assistive device is use to move the center of the body and the other lower limb is passively waggled forward to complete functional walking.

For the patients with higher paraplegia whose upper limbs functions are not good, the author designed foldable individual weight support walking device (Fig. 13.3) to cooperate with the application of shoulder power walking assistive device in order to realize standing and walking of the patients.

The training before returning to home and society: through rehabilitation training in hospital, except for some patients, most patients should return to home, society, even work. Therefore, the special training should be done before to make the patients adapt to new environment or work. It includes several aspects of training: changing concept and conquering oneself: many patients think that they are with paraplegia and lose motor function, becoming the disabled. They cannot contribute to society and home. They usually are demoralized, depressed and are reluctant to contribute to the society and home even they can face the disease. In allusion to this condition, rehabilitation therapists should explain to the patients and help them to broaden their mind. The therapists should use fact to analyze the condition for the patients to make them know what is devotion. The author thinks that the disabled includes limbs disabled and spiritual or moral disabled. With the development of science and technology, limbs disabled can be replaced by many types such as assistive device, artificial limb and walking aid. The patients with limbs disabled have the functions of intelligence and speech. The patients can do manageable work with the help of modern facility. For example, through special technique training, the patients can complete associated

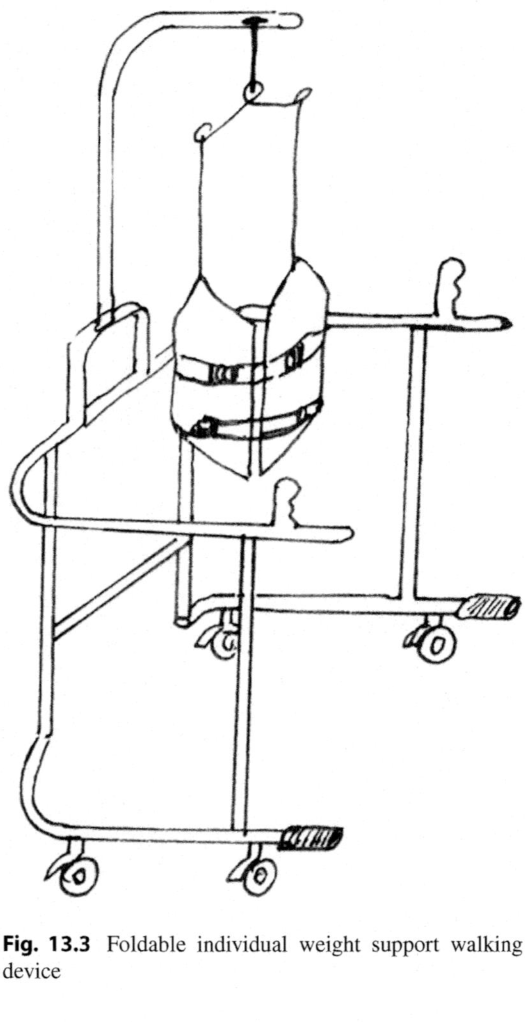

Fig. 13.3 Foldable individual weight support walking device

work through computer such as website establishment, internet marketing, drawing and finance and accounting. Stephen Hawking, a physicist in England, was diagnosed with Lou Gehrig's disease (Amyotrophic lateral sclerosis) who are totally paralyzed and can only live for 2 years. He cannot speak and only can communicate with others using dialog phone and voice operation demonstrator. He can read books with a machine to flip pages. However, his research achievement "black hole evaporation and quantum universe" shocks natural science and has a far-reaching influence on philosophy and religion. He becomes the recognized giant in Gravity physical science. In western world, if you don't read *A Brief History of Time*, you will be despised. The reason why he has a feather in one's cap is that he has strong sense of mission and tough will. His story is the maximum of human willpower and the miracle of scientific spirit. He is an integral person in spirit. The criminals are with four healthy limbs, but they do great harm to people's life and society. The criminals are the real disabled in spirits and morality. In all, the therapists guide the patients to exert subjective initiative to get a job and contribute to the society. Persisting on self-exercise and preventing functional decay: the rehabilitation of spinal cord injury is lifelong. Comparatively, rehabilitation therapy time in hospital is short and the therapists are responsible for figuring out the difficult and complicated diseases. Active self-exercise of the patients can induce slow functional recovery and prevent function decrease or loss. Persistence of self-exercise can induce stable functional recovery. If possible, the patients can do further consultation to the rehabilitation department of the hospital and receive standard rehabilitation training for a while. Tiny functional recoveries are accumulated to form meaningful functions. Modifying environment and adapting to the life of the disabled: according to functional recovery of the patients, family environment should be modified and the public environment should be presided by the government. In recent years, with the rapid development of technique and economy in our country, many communities are modified and there are many barrier-free facilities, which is convenient for the disabled. Rehabilitation medical staffs and the patients' family should cooperate with each other to provide support and help to the patients. The patients can rebuild their own life target and find proper life position under new condition.

13.3 The Prevention and Treatment of Common Complications of Paraplegia

13.3.1 Dysfunction of Urine and Stool and Rehabilitation Therapy

Dysfunction of urine and stool is the common complications of the patients with paraplegia. Urination dysfunction belongs to neurogenic bladder, which includes dysfunctions of sphincter vesicae and urethral sphincter, the early manifestation is uroschesis. The final manifestation is uroclepsia urinary retention with overflow incontinence.

Neurogenic bowel is the rectum dysfunction induced by injury of CNS or peripheral nerve that control rectum. The main manifestation is constipation. The fecal incontinence is rare.

The detailed rehabilitation therapy refers to the second section of this chapter.

13.3.2 Treatment of Pressure Sores

13.3.2.1 The Formation of Pressure Sores

Pressure sores is the necrosis and ulcer of skin and subcutaneous tissue induced by long-term local pressure and compression of human body.

Pressure sores is usually observed in the patients who are in wheelchair or bed for a long time, especially old people. The main external cause of pressure sores is mechanical factor. When the direct pressure exceeds normal capillary pressure (4.27 kPa) for a long time, the pressure sores is formed. In addition, shear force and friction force [4, 5] are the important factors that induce pressure sores. On the other hand, other external factors include medical factors such as various braking, improper nursing, therapy and medicine and internal factors include malnutrition, hypotension and poor tissue metabolism. They are the factors that include pressure sores.

13.3.2.2 Treatment of Pressure Sores

The treatment of pressure sores is prevention and there are many therapeutic methods.

- The prevention of pressure sores: The patients should select proper air bed and cushion. The patients should keep the skin and bed dry and clean. For the patients who cannot move their body, the posture should be changed in every two hours to avoid dragging the patients in turning over and prevent shear force injury of the tissue. In wheelchair, the patients need to extend double upper limbs in every 20 min and support the trunk to make the hip away from cushion to prevent the long-term pressure in ischial tuberosity. The support time should be prolonged 20–30 s every time. The patients should improve the nutrition status of the body and intake protein, vitamin and microelement. The therapists should improve the appetite of the patients and give fat emulsion, albumin, amino acid or whole blood into vein. Excessive body weight is one of the cause to induce pressure sores. Obese patients should lose fat and control the body weight. Convenient turning over device to prevent pressure sores: the author use macromolecule glass fiber material with good air-permeability to make tough support surface with arc bottom according to the shape of the trunk. It can reduce the pressure of the support from the body and the anti-acting force. It can enlarge the contact surface between skin and support surface to lower the pressure in skin. Through processing forming technique, the apophysis is suspended to avoid pressure, which is good for the prevention of pressure sores. The back of arc body is attached with four arc hollow strips made of macromolecule glass fiber material. The arc body is attached to the bed with four arc hollow strips. The inner face of arc body is attached with thin layer sponge with air-permeability and the two side in outside are fixed with fixing band. The therapists use terminal nylon thread gluing to fix it, which is convenient for dressing. The patients lie inside and one therapist push the device to make the patient turn over and change the pressure part of the body. The therapists use cuniform pad or thin pillow to fix the body of the patients. There is herringbone nursing opening of urine and stool in hip for turning over, which can prevent pressure sores effectively.
- The therapy of pressure sores includes physiotherapy, changing a medical prescription and surgical therapy. Physiotherapy can alleviate inflammation response and improve neural functions. Ultraviolet light therapy is suitable for the patients with skin injury but not muscle injury. Grade II–III erythema dose is used for the patients. The frequency is once every other day and there are 4–6 times in one therapy course. If the patients with muscle and bone injuries, grade III–IV erythema dose is used for the patients. The frequency is one time in every 1 or 2 days. Center overlap radiation method is used. If the granulation is fresh in the wound, in order to promote wound healing, the dose should be small, usually less than grade I erythema dose. Before therapy, the wound should be cleaned and should not be smeared with any medicine to facilitate the absorption of ultraviolet. Infrared therapy is suitable for the ulcer wound in every stage that the infection is controlled, granulation tissue is fresh and there is no purulent secretion. The usage is that the frequency is 1–2 time a day (20–25 min per time) and there are 15–20 times in one therapy course. Ultrashort wave therapy: if the skin injury cannot influence muscle, non-heating or micro-heating ultrashort wave is used. The frequency is 1–2 time a day (10–15 min per time) and there are 10–15 times in one therapy course. If the skin injury influences muscle, micro-heating ultrashort wave is used. The frequency is 1–2 time a day (10–15 min per time) and there are 10–15 times in one therapy course. Millimeter wave therapy: the secretions of wound should

be eliminated first and the radiator is placed above the wound. The therapy time is 20–30 min (once a day) and there are 10–20 times in one therapy course. Wound treatment: for the ulceration, saline is used to wash the wound and then it is covered with wet saline dressing. The dressing should be changed timely to promote the expel of secretions. Pressure sores paste can be used to change the medicine. Ulcer wound: necrosis tissue of the wound should be eliminated. Anti-infection: according to the whole symptoms and the results of bacterial culture, sensitive antibiotics are used. For the patients with pressure sores who has no constitutional symptoms and don't need antibiotics. The nursing of pressure sores: the clean of the wound and peripheral skin should be kept, especially pressure sores of hip and pars sacralis. The nursing of urine and stool should be paid attention to in order to prevent the contamination of excrement. Once contaminated, the wound should be cleaned immediately and the dressing should be changed. Surgical disposition: for the patients whose wound cannot be healed after long-term expectant treatment, the granulation of a wound is aged, the maiginal scar tissue is formed, the pressure sores reaches muscle, the bony joint is infected or deep sinus tract is formed, operation method therapy is used. The common surgical methods include skin transplantation, skin flap transplantation, muscular flap transplantation, neuromuscular flap transplantation and free skin transplantation. The pressure part should be avoided after surgery. Good pad is required to prevent new pressure sores. The diet and nursing of urine and stool should be enchanced.

13.3.3 The Common Cardiovascular Problem and Rehabilitation After Spinal Cord Injury

- The relationship between the level of spinal cord injury and cardiovascular function disorder.

The injury above thoracic cord level can lead to cardiovascular function disorder. The main manifestation is out of control of sympathetic modulation and the change of parasympathetic nerve. Spinal cord injury above T_6 level leads to out of control of sympathetic nerve and then the stress capability and vasomotoricity are abnormal. Thoracic cord injury below T6 leads to out of control of sympathetic nerve partially. Spinal cord injury in the level of lumbosacral spine not only influence the functions of sympathetic nervous system, but also damage the control ability of lower limbs' vessels.

The common abnormal manifestations of the patients with higher paraplegia or quadriplegia are hypotension, bradycardia and decrease of cardiac output. Generally, decrease of cardic sympathetic nerve tension is related to contractile mechanism disorder of vessels that make the blood stagnate in abdomen and lower limbs.

After spinal shock, segmental sympathetic nerve function is recovered gradually and cardiovascular function is improved, which form a new stable dynamic equilibrium state. Aged cardiac hypofunction can be aggravated after spinal cord injury, which can induce coronary heart disease, hypertension and heart failure.

- The common disposition of cardiovascular complication of spinal cord injury.

Just like the cases mentioned above, after spinal cord injury, the types of cardiovascular complications are related to the injured level. The common complications are as follows:

1. Arrhythmia usually includes bradycardia, supraventricular arrhythmia and primary cardiac arrest.
   - Prevention measures: maintenance of proper breathing is to keep oxygen content of blood and avoid hyoxemia. Alleviating heart load includes psychotherapy, relieving pain and reducing stimulation. Rating of perceived exertion during defecation should be noticed to save energy and reduce cardiac muscle load. Maintenance

of internal environment is to keep sufficient blood volume, water and electrolyte balance. Intake and output volume of liquid is measured timely to keep the organ perfusion and cardiac function. Avoiding stimulating vagus nerve: the movement should be gentle in sputum suction or trachea cannula. Before sputum suction, the patients can take in oxygen to prevent bradycardia induced by stimulation of vagus nerve. Reserved medicine: the reserved medicine includes atropine for bradycardia and drugs for arrhythmia.

- Rehabilitation training: In physical exercise therapy of neurological training, six-step Daoyin technique is used for rehabilitation training of autonomous movements of non-paralytic limbs in the early phase. For the paralytic limbs, induction training of autonomous movements is done. Passive movements of limbs and blood circulation drive can increase blood speed of paralytic limbs and cardiopulmonary function and alleviate hypotension and bradycardia.

2. Edema is usually observed in lower limbs. Lower limbs should be elevated in clinostatism and sitting position. For the patients with spinal cord injury below cervical level, the bed foot can be elevated 10–15°. Stretch socks or elastic bandage is used. Massage of injured limbs can promote blood circulation of muscle and lymphatic return. In the early phase after injury, active and passive movements of limbs are good for blood circulation of lower limbs and edema prevention.
3. Postural hypotension is usually observed in early phase of movements' recovery after injury. Through elevating the head of a bed gradually, prolonging sitting time and pressure dressing with abdominal elastic belly-band, all these can decrease blood stagnation in abdominal cavity. Standing bed is used for stand upright of the patients gradually. In order to prevent anxiety of the patients, in wheelchair, the patients can antevert waist to alleviate postural hypotension. If necessary, medicine such as dopamine can be used to keep the cardiac contractility and vascular tension.
4. Abnormal autonomic nervous reflex is usually observed in the patients with spinal cord injury above T_6.
   - The mechanism: Abnormal autonomic nervous reflex can be observed shortly after spinal shock. The main pathophysiological mechanism is out of control of sympathetic nerve excitability below injured level. The induction factors include filling of bladder, rectal stimulation, constipation, infection, spasm, stone and apparatus manipulation.
   - Clinical symptoms include hypertension (300/160 mmHg), headache, sweating, flushing, nausea, dermohemia and bradycardia.
   - Therapy: Through examination, the induction factors should be removed timely and the patients should be moved to the bed in sitting position. Drug therapy: For the slight patients, they can take calcium antagonists orally such as amlodipine (amlodipine besylate tablet), verapamil and diltiazem. For the severe patients, blocking agent of sympathetic nerve or nitroglycerin can be injected intravenously to dilate blood vessel. Rebound phenomenon of blood pressure should be noticed. If the patients want to stop taking the medicine, the dose should be decreased gradually to prevent rebound phenomenon. When the blood pressure is no less than 200/130 mmHg and the therapeutic effect is not good, epidural anesthesia can be used to block sympathetic ganglion to control blood pressure.

13.3.4 Deep Vein Thrombosis of Lower Limbs

Deep vein thrombosis (DVT) is one of the complications of circulatory system in the patients of long-term in bed. Blood clot in venous system of lower limbs leads to blood vessel stagnation. The main cause is the functional decrease of muscular contractility of lower limbs after long-term in bed and blood dilation and blood accumulation in venous system due to loss of sympathetic innervation. In addition, hypercoagulability of the blood is related to the trauma.

13.3.4.1 Occurrence Rate and Clinical Manifestation of Deep Vein Thrombosis

In the patients with spinal cord injury, occurrence rate of deep vein thrombosis is 40–100%. Occurrence rate of the patients with complete quadriplegia is higher than that of the patients with deep vein thrombosis. The patients with swell of thigh and shank, rise in body temperature and in local body temperature account for 15%. If the patients with deep vein thrombosis cannot be observed timely and treated, dropped embolism can induce pulmonary embolism and sudden death. Therefore, early diagnosis and therapy are very important. Color Doppler ultrasound examination contribute to early diagnosis.

13.3.4.2 The Therapy of Deep Vein Thrombosis Includes Rehabilitation, Medicine and Surgical Therapy

- Rehabilitation therapy: Elevation of injured limbs: the patients lie in bed and the injured limbs are elevated 20–30 cm higher than heart. The angle between elevated injured limbs and bed surface is 30°, which is good for blood backflow in lower limbs veins. Ten days after therapy, the patients can do exercise off bed and control the movement amount until the patients feel not tired or a little tired. If there is no effective anticoagulant therapy, it is forbidden to do passive joint movements. Supporting treatment is the common method of symptomatic treatment. Elastic bandage is used to bind up injured limbs or the patients wear stretch socks to eliminate edema. Physiotherapy: faradization is used to stimulate musculus gastrocnemius. Modulated low frequency electric stimulation: the wave width is 15 ms and the frequency is 20 Hz. The electricity with modulated frequency (10–30 Hz per min) is used to stimulate musculus gastrocnemius directly to induce intense muscle contraction. The effect is better than elastic sockings or elevating limbs. Functional electrical stimulation (FES): the frequency is 30 Hz and the wave width is 0.25 ms, the electrodes are placed in inward and outward heads of musculus gastrocnemius to induce intense muscle contraction. Blood circulation drive: trouser legs-like gasbag is used for air inflation and deflation in continuous cycle, which can give pulse mechanical pressure to all the lower limbs to accelerate backflow of venous blood of lower limbs. This method cannot be used in the early phase of thrombogenesis in case of falling off. This therapy can be used when thrombus is activated and becomes fiber.

The therapy frequency is once a day (10–15 min) and there are 15–20 times in one therapy course.

- Anticoagulant therapy: Heparin is the most definite and effective drug. After the diagnosis of deep vein thrombosis, heparin is given to the patients routinely overseas. It is rarely used in our country. Dextranum 40 and urokinase are usually used in our country, which are more convenient than heparin. The dose of dextranum 40 is 500 ml intravenously (drip, qd). The dose of urokinase is 1000 U/kg intravenously (drip) every day for 2 weeks. The patients can do exercise after reduction of swelling. Oral medicine includes warfarin sodium tablets that are suitable for the patients who need long-term anticoagulant. This drug is used for the therapy of thromboembolic disease to prevent the formation and development of thrombus. It can treat the venous thrombus formation after surgery or trauma and is the adjuvant drug of myocardial infarction. For the patients who had thromboembolic disease and are possible to have thrombus after surgery, it can be used for prevention.

The oral usual dose is 3–4 mg in the first to the third day to prevent impact therapy. The dose of older people, weak patients or the patients with diabetes should be cut half. Three days later, 2.5–5 mg can be given to the patients every day for maintenance. According to blood clotting time, the dose is adjusted until the INR is 2–3. This medicine is slow to take effect. There is transient hypercoagulability because anticoagulant protein in plasma is inhibited in the first 3 days. If anticoagulation is required immediately, the patients can take heparin meanwhile they start to take warfarin sodium tablets. The patients can stop heparin when the warfarin takes effect.

- Surgical therapy: The clinical application is rare, only in the patients with big or severe thrombus. Through surgery, the doctors can take out thrombus in deep vein of lower limbs. If there is stenosis or blocking in deep veins of lower limb, these problems can be treated together in surgery.

Thermal therapy is avoided during the treatment in case of infarction due to thrombus.

13.3.5 Rehabilitation of Thermoregulation Disorder

Heat-regulating center is located in hypothalamus. Through autonomous nerve conduction, after spinal cord injury, heat-regulating center loses control of body temperature to varying degrees and there is poikilothermia, which means body temperature is influenced by environment temperature. Hypothermia is common in the early phase after injury, which can lead to decrease of body function, especially in old patients. Because basal body temperature is low, sometimes 35 °C and the body temperature of the patients reaches 37.5 °C, it can be defined as high fever. Therefore, the body temperature should be measured at regular intervals. In addition, in the hot season, function disorder of sweat gland can induce high fever of the patients with spinal cord injury.

13.3.5.1 Prevention Measures Include Careful Observation, Early Detection of Induction Factor and Paying Attention to the Body Temperature Changes

- Keeping warm: According to temperature change, the patients can dress or undress clothes. When the temperature is 21 °C, if there is no proper clothes to keep warm, the body temperature of the patients with quadriplegia is possible to drop to about 35 °C. On the outside, the patients with paraplegia should keep warm in case of inducing thermoregulation disorder and influencing normal functions of tissues and organs.
- Keeping skin dry: The paralytic limbs are with heat dissipation disorder, which may induce sweating above paralytic level. There is no sweating below the paralytic level. The sweat should be wiped to keep the skin dry in case of catching cold.
- Eliminating induction factors: Overfilling bladder and rectum can stimulate sympathetic nerve system and induce damage autonomic hyperreflexia. The clinical manifestation includes excessive sweating that can induce hypothermia. The doctors should observe it timely and the patients should evacuate bladder and rectum.

13.3.5.2 Therapy Includes Cooling and Anti-infection

- Physical cooling is mainly used such as ice bag and lukewarm bath. In hot weather, heat dissipation should be noticed.
- Drug cooling: When the patients are with high fever, the effect of drug therapy is poor. Indometacin suppositories can be used in rectum. The hands and anus can be washed clean. Conical head of the drug points to the anus and is pushed by the index finger until it enters into anus. The space between the tail and anus is about 2 cm. The dose is 50–100 mg per time (half or one tablet, once a day). The dose of every day cannot exceed 200 mg and the effect is good.

- Anti-infection: For fever of undetermined origin, infection is the first factor that should be considered. Because there is sensory disorder in the patients, fever is the earliest or the only manifestation of infection. The doctors should find the source of infection as soon as possible and do bacterial culture test and drug sensitivity test. In allusion to infection source, the doctors adopt sensitive antibiotics for the therapy.

13.3.6 Tardive Neurological Deterioration

Several years after spinal cord injury, there may be neurological deterioration. Some reports showed that the patients with neurological deterioration account for 12.1% 3–5 years after injury. There are changes in sensation, motor or both, which affects self-care ability of the patients greatly.

Therefore, examination and assessment of the entire sensation and motor function of the patients should be done periodically. Compared with the last assessment results, the results are good for the early detection of neurological deterioration.

The cause of tardive neurological deterioration is unknown at present. It may be the result of degeneration or disuse. However, someone think that it is related to overuse. The author thinks that it may be related to disuse.

13.4 Clinical Application of Neurological Training for Paraplegia

13.4.1 Observation of Therapeutic Effects of Chronic Cervical Cord Injury

In the past, 1 year after spinal cord injury, the patients lost the hope of further functional recovery. In recent years, some literatures [6–8] showed that the patients with obsolete spinal cord injury had the potential to be recovered further. Biological feedback is an operant conditioning technique that can establish autonomous control training technique of specific physiological reflex. The effect is verified preliminarily [9]. Biological feedback technique has been applied for clinical rehabilitation therapy for more than 20 years [10]. Rehabilitation therapy of spinal cord injury is very limited and the results are various [11]. The author observes the therapeutic effect of biological feedback on spinal cord injury. The author wants to verify whether this therapy can increase autonomous electromyographic signal and myodynamia of all muscles in upper limbs of the patients with obsolete spinal cord injury above C_6 on the basis of various original electromyographic signal and myodynamia.

13.4.1.1 Materials and Methods

1. Subjects: There are 139 patients with spinal cord injury. There are 108 males and 31 females. Male female ratio is 3.5 versus 1. The age range is from 8 to 68 years old. The average age is 32.8 (*SD* is ±11.12). Injured segments are from C_1 to C_6. There are 59 patients with spinal cord injury at C_5, which accounts for 42.45% of all the patients. There are 32 patients with spinal cord injury at C_4, which accounts for 23.02% of all the patients. There are 28 patients with spinal cord injury at C_6, which accounts for 20.14% of all the patients. There are ten patients with spinal cord injury at C_3, which accounts for 7.19% of all the patients. There are six patients with spinal cord injury at C_2, which accounts for 4.32% of all the patients. There are four patients with spinal cord injury at C_1, which accounts for 2.88% of all the patients. There are 111 patients due to motor traffic accidents (79.86%), 15 patients due to sport injury (10.79%), four patients due to gunshot wound (2.88%), nine patients due to other causes (6.47%). The disease history is 0.5–20 years and the average is 4.07 years (*SD* is ±4.02). There are 57 patients (41%) whose disease history is from 0.5 to 1 year, 37 patients (26.6%) whose disease history is from 1 to 5 years, 32 patients (23%) whose disease history is from 5 to 10 years, 13 patients (9.4%) whose disease history is more than 10 years.

The longest disease history is 23 years. All the cases have no further functional recovery after various kinds of rehabilitation method therapy. All the patients in this group complete one therapy course of biological feedback therapy with EMG. The therapy time is 50 min and there are 15 times in a day.

2. Instruments: Four-lead Neuroeducator II and 3M Ag-AgCl surface electrode are produced by Therapeutic Alliances in America. Neuroeducator II is used to analyze EMG signal and provides EMG signal for feedback. This signal is analyzed from analysis of EMG signal that is the square root of mean value of potential whose noise level is lower than 0.2 μV. The bandwidth is from 10 to 1000 Hz and the noise is less than 140 dB. If the combination time of EMG signal exceeds 0.1 s, it can be standardized into μVs. The data in one tenth second is displayed in color screen in a continuous curve form. The scan time limit in every screen is 20 s and the data can be stored in soft disk.
3. Therapeutic method: In a quiet and lucifugal therapy room, the patients sit in the front of the display. Two 3 M surface electrode are attached on the skin surface of the two terminals of muscle belly separately. Ground surface is placed between the two electrodes. Surface electrode is connected to the corresponding lead of Neuroeducator II through wire. This method can be used to treat one group (agonistic muscle and antagonistic muscle) or two groups of muscles. The patients are guided to observe the change of EMG signal in display. Meanwhile, the patients try to do shoulder abduction, elbow flexion and extension, wrist flexion and extension, finger flexion and extension actively. The highest EMG signal collected from this movement is the primary data and is recorded. The highest EMG signal is marked as a baseline and the patients are asked to make EMG signal surpass the baseline. The patients are asked not to concentrate on joint motion and muscle contraction, but should observe the change of EMG signal curve in display. If EMG signal surpasses baseline, the new highest point is defined as the new baseline. The patients are asked to make new EMG signal surpass this baseline in next movement. The rest can be done in the same manner until the EMG signal cannot surpass the baseline. Usually, the process requires 6–8 movements, which is defined as one therapy. There are 15 times in one therapy course. The data of the highest EMG signal is recorded.

13.4.1.2 Observational Index

- Myodynamia assessment: According to improved Lovett myodynamia assessment method, myodynamis of all muscles can be assessed and graded before therapy.
- EMG data collection: The highest EMG signal data of all muscles are collected before therapy and are used for statistical analysis. These standard EMG data can be converted according to conversion that the percentage of Brucker in normal electromyographic signal (Table 13.8).

13.4.1.3 Results

According to injured segments, injured degree and clinical manifestations, there are 108 deltoids, 89 bicipital muscles of arm, 220 triceps muscles of arm, 194 wrist extensors, 234 wrist flexors, 234 finger extensors and 205 finger flexors in 139 patients who receive therapy. The statistical results of electromyographic signal and myodynamia of all muscles refer to Table 13.9 before therapy. T-test showed that after therapy there are significant difference of electromyo-

Table 13.8 The percentage of standard electromyographic signal in normal electromyographic signal

Electromyographic signal (μV)	The percentage of normal electromyographic signal
0	0
1	1
3	2
10	5
80	15
160	25
320	50
480	75
640	100

Table 13.9 Statistical analysis results of EMG and myodynamia before and after therapy ($\overline{X} \pm S$)

Name	Number		Electromyographic signal (μV)	Myodynamia (0–5)
Middle deltoid	108	Before therapy	233.95 ± 221.33	2.48 ± 1.51
		After therapy	464.44 ± 264.77[a]	2.96 ± 1.53[a]
Bicipital muscle of arm	89	Before therapy	173.25 ± 192.38	2.42 ± 1.65
		After therapy	396.64 ± 284.59[a]	3.01 ± 1.68[a]
Triceps muscle of arm	220	Before therapy	119.07 ± 142.52	1.96 ± 1.16
		After therapy	356.47 ± 218.11[a]	2.49 ± 1.19[a]
Wrist extensor	194	Before therapy	171.44 ± 179.75	2.65 ± 1.51
		After therapy	419.70 ± 256.87[a]	3.13 ± 1.58[a]
Wrist flexor	234	Before therapy	113.01 ± 164.66	1.60 ± 1.35
		After therapy	289.41 ± 231.78[a]	2.04 ± 1.40[a]
Finger extensor	234	Before therapy	56.78 ± 100.06	1.12 ± 1.26
		After therapy	162.16 ± 162.26[a]	1.41 ± 1.40[a]
Finger flexor	205	Before therapy	52.33 ± 73.34	1.07 ± 1.22
		After therapy	153.54 ± 165.44[a]	1.43 ± 1.41[a]

[a]$P < 0.01$. The comparison before and after therapy

graphic signal and myodynamia ($P < 0.001$). EMG of deltoid after therapy is increased 36% than that before therapy EMG and myodynamia is increased 12%. EMG of bicipital muscle of arm is increased 36.5% and myodynamia is increased 20.1%. EMG of triceps muscle of arm is increased 37.1% and myodynamia is increased 11.5%. EMG of wrist extensor is increased 38.5% and myodynamia is increased 20.4%. EMG of wrist flexor is increased 27.6% and myodynamia is increased 5.5%. EMG of finger extensor is increased 16.5% and myodynamia is increased 2.9%. EMG of finger flexor is increased 15.8% and myodynamia is increased 3.6%. Compared with before therapy, EMG of all the muscles are increased 29.8% averagely after therapy and myodynamia is increased 10.9% averagely.

13.4.1.4 Discussion

In the past, they think that central nervous system has no regeneration capacity. Therefore, there is no further functional recovery in 1 year after central nervous system injury [12]. Recently some research showed that human central nervous system has compensation and regeneration capability [13], even in adult. In addition, undead cells in injured area (penumbra cells) [14], are able to recover functions through improving local condition. The more important is that the connection between human central nervous cells, the conduction pathway of information, is changed and perfected in lifetime. After the death of central nervous cells, the axon is not dead. The undead axon can regenerate central nervous cells when the condition is complete. Just like a dead tree, the undead bud grows up and becomes a tree. All these showed that central nervous system has compensation ability and can recover or improve functions through proper therapy and training.

Therapeutic mechanism of biological feedback of EMG is that through observation of autonomous signal displayed in display in a smooth curve by the patients and central nervous system integration of this signal through visual afferent pathway feedback, it can be overlapped in the next efferent autonomous electromyographic signal and the signal intensity is increased [15]. Therefore, the patients are asked to increase autonomous electromyographic signal and concentrate on the changed curve in monitor. The patients are asked to forget joint motion and muscle contraction and concentrate on increasing autonomous electromyographic signal in monitor. The subjects in this group require 6–8 blocks to reach the highest point of this training. After that, the patients can train other muscles. In next therapy, autonomous electromyographic signal of this muscle can still be increased.

The average history of the patients is 4.07 years and disease history of some patients is more than 10 years. The longest disease history is 23 years. All the cases have no further functional recovery through other therapeutic methods. After therapy, the results showed that biological feedback therapy of EMG can obviously increase autonomous electromyographic signal and myodynamia obsolete cervical cord injury. The recovery has no relation with the disease history after injury. The recovery is related to the position of upper limbs' muscle. The functional recovery of muscles of hand is lower than that of muscles of upper arm. The author thinks that the recovery of autonomous electromyographic signal is more than that of myodynamia and it is related to biological feedback therapy of EMG. The increase of autonomous electromyographic signal is dependent on functional recovery of central nervous cells and reestablishment and improvement of conduction pathway between central nervous cells, which is not proportional to the intensity of muscle contraction. This was verified in the therapy. Biological feedback therapy technique is to recover functions of central nervous cells to establish and improve the conduction pathway between central nervous cells, but not to recover myodynamia. Therefore, the recovery of autonomous electromyographic signal is earlier and more than that of myodynamia. The recovery of myodynamia can be increased in the training of myodynamia through biological feedback of EMG after therapy.

The results of this research are the same as some other reports [16]. It indicated that chronic central nervous system injury is possible to be recovered further. In addition, understanding and use of biological feedback therapy of EMG is important and its purpose is to use modulated conditional feedback technique to establish and consolidate specific physiological reflex of autonomous signal. It usually is mistaken that biological feedback is a simple visual and audio physiological reflex phenomenon for the patients. Without using actual feedback technique, the effect of biological feedback therapy may be influenced. This is why the effect is not good in some reports [11]. In short, there is further functional recovery in long-term spinal cord injury. If it is used properly, biological feedback is an effective method to treat spinal cord injury and recover functions.

13.4.2 Multiple-Course Observation of Curative Effect of Treating Obsolete Cervical Cord Injury

The good functional recovery of long-term spinal cord injury is proved preliminarily [17, 18]. However, the patients are the first time to receive this therapy and just one therapy course. The effects of multiple-course of biological feedback therapy require further verification.

The purpose of this study is to observe the effect of four coursed of biological feedback therapy. On the basis of electromyographic signal and myodynamia in the previous therapy course, autonomous electromyographic signal and myodynamia of all muscles in upper limbs are increased obviously further in the patients with obsolete spinal cord injury above C_6.

13.4.2.1 Materials and Methods

Subjects: There are 39 patients with cervical cord injury who come from orthopedics or rehabilitation department of Miami University in America. There are 31 males and 318 females. Male female ratio is 3.9 versus 1. The age range is from 11 to 62 years old. The average age is 33.1 (SD is ±11.8). Injured segments are from C_1 to C_6. There are 14 patients with cervical cord injury at C_4, which accounts for 35.9% of all the patients. There are 11 patients with cervical cord injury at C_5, which accounts for 28.2% of all the patients. There are nine patients with cervical cord injury at C_6, which accounts for 23.1% of all the patients. There are two patients with cervical cord injury at C_3. There is one patient with spinal cord injury at C_2. There are two patients with cervical cord injury at C_1. There are 31 patients due to motor traffic accidents (79.5%), eight patients due to sport injury (20.5%). The disease history is 0.5–19 years and the average is 4.5 years (SD is ±4.5). All the cases have no further functional recovery after various kinds of rehabilitation method therapy.

Therapeutic method: In a quiet and lucifugal therapy room, the patients sit in the front of the display. Two 3M surface electrode are attached on the skin surface of the two terminals of muscle belly separately. Ground surface is placed between the two electrodes. Surface electrode is connected to the corresponding lead of Neuroeducator II through wire. The patients are guided to observe the change of EMG signal in display. Meanwhile, the patients try to do shoulder abduction, elbow flexion and extension, wrist flexion and extension, finger flexion and extension actively. The highest EMG signal collected from this movement is the primary data and is recorded. The highest EMG signal is marked as a baseline and the patients are asked to make EMG signal surpass the baseline. The patients are asked not to concentrate on joint motion and muscle contraction, but should observe the change of EMG signal curve in display. If EMG signal surpasses baseline, the new highest point is defined as the new baseline. The patients are asked to make new EMG signal surpass this baseline in next movement. The rest can be done in the same manner until the EMG signal cannot surpass the baseline. Usually, the process requires 6–8 movements, which is defined as one therapy. The therapy time is 50 min and there are 15 times in one therapy course. The data of the highest EMG signal is recorded. All the patients in this group complete four therapy courses in 4 years.

13.4.2.2 Observation Indicators

- Myodynamia assessment: According to improved Lovett myodynamia assessment method [19]· myodynamis of all muscles can be assessed and graded before therapy.
- EMG data collection: The highest EMG signal data of all muscles are collected before therapy and are used for statistical analysis. The comparison is done between the data of the first therapy course after therapy and raw data before therapy. The comparison is done between the data of every therapy course after therapy and the highest data of previous therapy course after therapy.

13.4.2.3 Statistical Analysis

T-test is done using SPSS 6.0.

13.4.2.4 Results

According to injured segments, injured degree and clinical manifestations, there are 12 deltoids, 10 bicipital muscles of arm, 18 triceps muscles of arm, 17 wrist extensors, 17 wrist flexors, 20 finger extensors and 21 finger flexors in 39 patients who receive therapy.

The data of electromyographic signal and myodynamia data of all muscles before therapy refer to Table 13.10 and statistical analysis results refer to Tables 13.10, 13.11, and 13.12.

Table 13.10 Mean value and standard deviation of raw EMG signal data and EMG signal data of every therapy course after therapy

Name	Number[a]		Raw	1	2	3	4
Middle deltoid	12	Mean value	290.17	472.42	501.25	511.92	516.75
		Standard deviation	246.83	246.83	251.01	276.48	289.17
Bicipital muscle of arm	10	Mean value	87.90	333.40	428.70	455.90	430.61
		Standard deviation	115.96	274.75	346.36	329.53	342.51
Triceps muscle of arm	18	Mean value	106.17	315.39	434.56	451.28	431.61
		Standard deviation	167.16	215.13	281.54	289.07	306.63
Wrist extensor	17	Mean value	172.25	381.76	516.94	570.65	552.47
		Standard deviation	213.22	219.96	204.57	220.31	239.36
wrist flexor	17	Mean value	159.47	277.88	364.24	374.88	373.94
		Standard deviation	244.61	279.10	292.74	298.58	299.57
finger extensor	20	Mean value	88.22	195.90	236.00	297.41	361.23
		Standard deviation	126.21	165.17	201.14	263.43	273.53
finger flexor	21	Mean value	74.71	213.76	236.95	339.67	376.38
		Standard deviation	61.78	183.94	216.50	254.98	253.56

[a]Number of muscles

Table 13.11 Mean value and standard deviation of raw myodynamia data and myodynamia data of every therapy course

Name	Number[a]		Raw	1	2	3	4
middle deltoid	12	Mean value	2.86	3.08	3.12	3.22	3.29
		Standard deviation	1.50	1.52	1.51	1.61	1.62
bicipital muscle of arm	10	Mean value	2.00	2.43	2.80	2.86	3.23
		Standard deviation	1.56	1.59	1.54	1.61	1.75
triceps muscle of arm	18	Mean value	1.87	2.33	2.52	2.54	2.85
		Standard deviation	1.23	1.29	1.32	1.41	1.44
wrist extensor	17	Mean value	3.13	3.69	4.07	4.04	4.13
		Standard deviation	1.14	1.29	1.38	1.36	1.34
wrist flexor	17	Mean value	1.04	1.68	1.76	1.59	1.88
		Standard deviation	1.38	1.92	1.19	1.31	1.18
finger extensor	20	Mean value	1.67	1.80	1.73	1.95	2.22
		Standard deviation	1.47	1.60	1.52	1.54	1.54
finger flexor	21	Mean value	1.62	1.97	2.00	2.09	2.40
		Standard deviation	1.36	1.60	1.58	1.63	1.64

[a]Number of muscles

1. Comparison with raw data: After every therapy course, electromyographic signal and myodynamia are compared with raw electromyographic signal and myodynamia of the first therapy before therapy. There is significant difference between electromyographic signal data from the first to the fourth therapy course and raw electromyographic signal date ($P < 0.05$ or $P < 0.001$). In the grading scores of myodynamia, there is no significant difference of deltoid between the end of the fore three therapy courses and raw data, but there is significant difference of deltoid between the end of the fore four therapy courses and raw data ($P < 0.05$). There is no significant difference of bicipital muscle of arm between the end of the first therapy and raw data, but there is significant difference of bicipital muscle of arm between the end of the second therapy and raw data ($P < 0.01$). There is no significant difference of finger extensor myodynamia between the end of the fore two therapy courses and raw data, but there is significant difference of finger extensor myodynamia between the beginning of the third therapy course and raw data ($P < 0.05$ in the third therapy course and $P < 0.001$ in the fourth therapy course). There is significant difference of raw grading score of myodynamia in the beginning of the first therapy ($P < 0.05$ or 0.01). At the end of the fourth therapy, there is significant difference between electromyographic signal and myodynamia and raw grading score of electromyographic signal and myodynamia ($P < 0.001$).
2. Comparison with the first therapy course: The comparison between the end of the first therapy course and the end of the second, the third or the fourth therapy course. Except for electromyographic signal of finger extensor, finger flexor of the second therapy course, middle deltoid of the first or the third therapy course, there is significant difference of all the other muscles between the end of every courses and the first therapy course after therapy ($P < 0.05$ or 0.01). There is significant difference of triceps muscle of arm between the end of the

Table 13.12 T-test results of electromyographic signal and myodynamia data between raw and every therapy course using biological feedback after therapy

Name	Classes	0–1	0–2	0–3	0–4	1–2	1–3	1–4	2–3	2–4	3–4
Middle deltoid	Myoelectricity	3.90^{**}	4.59^{***}	4.50^{***}	4.17^{**}	1.66^{ns}	2.36^{*}	1.49^{ns}	0.60^{ns}	0.59^{ns}	0.29^{ns}
12	Myodynamia	1.80^{ns}	1.94^{ns}	2.04^{ns}	2.54^{*}	0.47^{ns}	0.83^{ns}	1.62^{ns}	0.72^{ns}	1.89^{ns}	0.70^{ns}
Bicipital muscle of arm	Myoelectricity	3.45^{**}	3.44^{**}	3.90^{**}	3.49^{**}	2.62*	3.22^{**}	2.72^{*}	1.56^{ns}	0.55^{ns}	1.36^{ns}
10	Myodynamia	1.85^{ns}	3.77^{**}	4.46^{**}	6.20^{**}	2.90^{*}	3.54^{**}	4.27^{**}	1.00^{ns}	3.88^{**}	3.98^{**}
Bicipital muscle of arm	Myoelectricity	5.84^{***}	5.61^{***}	5.60^{***}	5.03^{***}	3.10^{*}	3.41^{**}	2.73^{*}	1.25^{ns}	0.17^{ns}	1.88^{ns}
18	Myodynamia	2.53^{*}	3.98^{**}	3.86^{*}	6.29^{***}	1.61^{ns}	1.83^{ns}	3.44^{**}	0.15^{ns}	2.63	3.45^{**}
Wrist extensor	Myoelectricity	7.88^{***}	8.44^{***}	7.54^{***}	6.92^{***}	4.51^{**}	4.51^{**}	4.10^{**}	1.64^{ns}	1.04^{ns}	1.01^{ns}
17	Myodynamia	5.36^{**}	6.36^{***}	5.28^{***}	5.62^{***}	3.32^{**}	2.40^{*}	2.98^{**}	0.42^{ns}	0.68^{ns}	1.63^{*}
Wrist flexor	Myoelectricity	4.31^{***}	5.04^{***}	4.85^{***}	4.81^{***}	3.68^{**}	3.67^{**}	3.35^{**}	0.81^{ns}	0.62^{ns}	0.08^{ns}
17	Myodynamia	4.10^{***}	4.05^{***}	3.12^{**}	5.29^{***}	1.17^{ns}	0.81^{ns}	1.54^{ns}	1.53^{ns}	0.81^{ns}	2.43
Finger extensor	Myoelectricity	5.64^{***}	7.41^{***}	4.72^{***}	5.99^{***}	1.88^{ns}	2.29^{*}	3.51^{**}	1.60^{ns}	2.87^{**}	2.21^{*}
20	Myodynamia	1.14^{ns}	0.63^{ns}	2.55^{*}	4.01^{***}	1.28^{ns}	1.38^{ns}	3.20^{**}	2.46^{*}	4.04^{**}	2.32^{*}
Finger flexor	Myoelectricity	3.76^{**}	3.86^{**}	5.31^{***}	6.17^{***}	1.01^{ns}	3.38^{**}	3.73^{**}	2.67^{*}	3.39^{**}	2.07^{ns}
21	Myodynamia	2.80^{*}	2.75^{*}	2.91^{*}	3.97^{***}	0.46^{ns}	1.40^{ns}	3.34^{**}	1.82^{ns}	4.11^{**}	3.80^{**}

*p < 0.05; **p < 0.01; ***p < 0.001; Ns: no significant difference

second or the third therapy course and the end of the first therapy course ($P < 0.01$).

3. Comparison with the second therapy course: The comparison between the end of the second therapy course and the end of the third or the fourth therapy course. Except for electromyographic signal of finger extensor of the fourth therapy course, and finger flexor of the third or the fourth therapy course ($P < 0.05$ or 0.01), there is no significant difference of all other muscles between the end of every course and the end of the second course ($P > 0.05$). There is significant difference of the grading score of myodynamia of bicipital muscle of arm, triceps muscle of arm and finger extensor between the fourth therapy course and the end of the second therapy course. There is significant difference of the grading score of myodynamia of finger extensor between the end of the third or the fourth therapy course and the end of the second therapy course ($P < 0.05$ or 0.01). There is no significant difference of myodynamia of the other muscles between the end of the second therapy courses and other therapy courses ($P > 0.05$).
4. Comparison with the third therapy course: There is significant difference of electromyographic signal of finger extensor between the end of the fourth therapy course and the end of the third therapy course ($P < 0.05$). There is no significant difference of electromyographic signal of all other muscles between the end of the fourth therapy course and the end of the third therapy course ($P > 0.05$). Except for myodynamia grading of deltoid, there is significant difference of the value of electromyographic signal of all other muscles between the end of the fourth therapy course and the end of the third therapy course ($P < 0.05$ or 0.01).

13.4.2.5 Discussion

There are many latent neural conduction pathways and synapses in human body. Proper training method can activate them and make them play functions to compensate injured conduction pathways and synapses [20]. The damage can destroy the soma of neurons or proximal synapse and leads to the death of neural cells. Uninjured nerve cell axon can protrude from the branch and establish axon connection with neural tissue in target area to replace the neural axon that loses functions. Rehabilitation training can change gene expression of some proteins in central nervous system, promote axon budding, synaptic reestablishment and repair or compensation of tissue in necrosis area. The peripheral tissue around injured area can replace the functions of offside brain cortex and promote motor function recovery [21]. These functions are called the neural plasticity of central nervous system, which is proved in anatomy [22]. In addition, undead cells in injured area (penumbra cells), are able to recover functions through improving local condition. The more important is that the connection between human central nervous cells, the conduction pathway of information, is changed and perfected in lifetime. All these demonstrated that central nervous system has regeneration ability and the functions of injured central nervous system can be improved or recovered through proper therapy and training. In-depth exploration should be done for the better method that can promote plasticity of central nervous system and recover injured central nerves.

The exercise method of functional rehabilitation includes active method and passive method. Passive functional exercise can move joints and prevent adhesion through passive movements. Active functional exercise not only can move joints and enhance myodynamia, but also can promote functional recovery of nervous system. The author think that active functional exercise method is better for brain functions and functional recovery of brain cells, which can activate reserved conduction pathway and synapse.

The therapeutic mechanism of biological feedback therapy of operant conditioning EMG designed by the author is different from biological feedback therapy of EMG at home at present. Biological feedback therapy at home at present is one kind of electrical stimulation without feedback of bio-electricity signal. EMG biological feedback therapy of operant conditioning EMG is a new technique of modern physiotherapy, which is related to many subjects such as physical medicine, Contrology and Physiology. In this sense, it is a new technique that is related to comprehensive application of multiple subjects. Feedback is a word that is created by Norner Winner (an American mathematician). Feedback is that efferent signal of control system return to control system through some way in order to control control system. Biofeedback means the subjective initiative of the patients. When the patients do autonomous movements, skin surface electrode of the contracted muscle can receive this kind of voluntary slight electrical signal. Through a series of overlay treatment, the signal is displayed in monitor in a smooth curve form. The patients observe this smooth curve. The signal gives feedback to central nervous system through visual afferent pathway and is integrated. The next efferent autonomous electromyographic signal is modulated and the accuracy and intensity is increased. The generation of this kind of electromyographic signal is dependent on the functional state of central nervous cells and the soundness of neural conduction pathway from nerve cells to motor end plate. Therefore, this kind of electrical signal received from tissue surface actually reflects electroencephalogram of motor neuron in brain cortex. This kind of signal can be strengthened quickly and continuously in the therapy, because this method can activate functional recovery of injured neural cells, potential conduction pathway and synapse.

The average disease history of the patients in this group receive biological feedback before therapy is 4.5 years. There are 13 patients whose disease history is more than 5 years. The longest disease history is 19 years. All the patients have no further functional recovery using other therapeutic methods. Comprehensive results of electromyographic signal and myodynamia before and after four-course therapy refer to Fig. 13.4.

From the therapeutic results, we can conclude the following key points: Recovery speed and degree of electromyographic signal and myodynamia of all muscle of upper limbs are related to the nerve innervation level. Electromyographic signal and myodynamia of muscles dominated by higher nerve segment can be recovered faster and better. For example, the functions of deltoid dominated by C_4 and finger flexor and extensor dominated by C_6 can be recovered faster and better. The intensity of electromyographic signal is related to the strength of myodynamia. For central nervous injury, myodynamia is stronger than electromyographic signal. For peripheral nerve injury, electromyographic signal is stronger, but myodynamia is very weak. Electromyographic

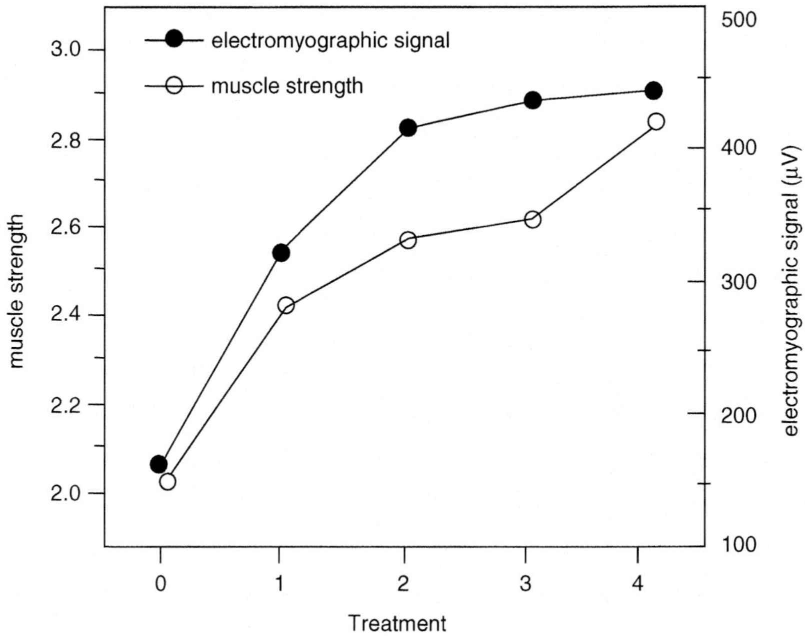

Fig. 13.4 Comparison sketch map of electromyographic signal and myodynamia before and after four-course therapy

signal is mainly recovered in the fore three biological feedback therapy courses and myodynamia is mainly recovered in the fourth therapy course. Electromyographic signal is recovered faster than myodynamia recovery. For highly paralytic muscles, there is no significant difference between the results of single therapy course and raw electromyographic signal and myodynamia. There is significant difference between the results at the end of the second therapy course or the third therapy course and raw electromyographic signal and myodynamia. If the therapeutic effect of single therapy course is not obvious, the patients should not give up therapy. Accumulated therapeutic effect can induce meaningful functional recovery.

13.4.3 Therapeutic Effect Analysis of Muscles with Zero Myodynamia in the Patients with Obsolete Cervical Cord Injury

For biological feedback therapy of long-term spinal cord injury, multiple therapy courses can promote further functional recovery on the basis of therapeutic effect of previous therapy course, which is proved. For the muscles with zero myodynamia, whether biological feedback therapy can recover autonomous signal and myodynamia and whether zero myodynamia equals to zero electromyographic signal, all these require confirmation.

The author do biological feedback therapy of 343 muscles with zero myodynamia of upper limbs in the patients with obsolete spinal cord injury above C_5, observe the relationship between muscles with zero myodynamia and autonomous electromyographic signal, analyze therapeutic effect and find out the therapy experience of muscles with zero myodynamia.

13.4.3.1 Materials and Methods

1. Subjects: There are 77 patients with spinal cord injury. There are 62 males and 15 females. Male female ratio is 4 versus 1. The age range is from 11 to 64 years old. The average age is 31.7 (SD is ±9). Injured segments are from C_1 to C_5. There are 40 patients with spinal cord injury at C_5, which accounts for 51.9% of all the patients. There are 19 patients with cervical cord injury at C_5, which accounts for 24.7% of all the patients. There are 60 patients due to motor traffic accidents (77.9%), eight patients due to sport injury (10.4%). The disease history is 0.5–20 years and the average is 4.2 years (SD is ±4.3). All the cases have no further functional recovery after various kinds of rehabilitation method therapy. All patients in this group complete biological feedback therapy of EMG in one therapy course. The therapy time is 50 min and there are 15 times in one therapy course.
2. Instruments: Four-lead Neuroeducator II and 3 M Ag-AgCl surface electrode are produced by Therapeutic Alliances in America. Neuroeducator II is used to analyze EMG signal and provides EMG signal for feedback. This signal is analyzed from analysis of EMG signal that is the square root of mean value of potential whose noise level is lower than 0.2 μV. The bandwidth is from 10 to 1000 Hz and the noise is less than 140 dB. If the combination time of EMG signal exceeds 0.1 s, it can be standardized into μVs. The data in one tenth second is displayed in color screen in a continuous curve form. The scan time limit in every screen is 20 s and the data can be stored in soft disk.
3. Therapeutic method: In a quiet and lucifugal therapy room, the patients sit in the front of the display. Two 3M surface electrode are attached on the skin surface of the two terminals of muscle belly separately. Ground surface is placed between the two electrodes. Surface electrode is connected to the corresponding lead of Neuroeducator II through wire. The patients are guided to observe the change of EMG signal in display. Meanwhile, the patients try to do shoulder abduction, elbow flexion and extension, wrist flexion and extension, finger flexion and extension actively. The highest EMG signal collected from this movement is the primary data and is recorded. The highest EMG signal is marked as a baseline

and the patients are asked to make EMG signal surpass the baseline. The patients are asked not to concentrate on joint motion and muscle contraction, but should observe the change of EMG signal curve in display. If EMG signal surpasses baseline, the new highest point is defined as the new baseline. The patients are asked to make new EMG signal surpass this baseline in next movement. The rest can be done in the same manner until the EMG signal cannot surpass the baseline. Usually, the process requires 6–8 movements, which is defined as one therapy. The therapy time is 50 min and there are 15 times in one therapy course. The data of the highest EMG signal is recorded.

13.4.3.2 Observational Index

- Myodynamia assessment: According to improved Lovett myodynamia assessment method, myodynamis of all muscles can be assessed and graded before therapy.
- EMG data collection: The highest EMG signal data of all muscles are collected before therapy or at the end of the therapy and are used for comparison and statistical analysis.

13.4.3.3 Results

There are 16 middle deltoids, 21 bicipital muscles of arm, 28 triceps muscles of arm, 31 wrist extensors, 61 wrist flexors, 97 finger extensors and 89 finger flexors of 343 muscles with zero myodynamia of 77 patients. Analysis results of electromyographic signal and myodynamiastatistical of all muscles before and after therapy refers to Table 13.13.

Statistical analysis of electromyographic signal and myodynamia of 343 muscles with zero myodynamia before and after therapy is done. Electromyographic signal: t = 14.17, myodynamia: t = 13.52. There are significant differences of electromyographic signal and myodynamia before and after therapy ($P < 0.001$).

In 343 muscles with zero myodynamia, there are only 11 muscles with zero myoelectricity. At the end of one therapy course, the myodynamia of 11 muscles with zero myodynamia is recovered to 0.15, but there is no significant difference before and after therapy ($P > 0.05$). The myoelectricity is increased to 8.01 μV and there is significant difference before therapy and after therapy ($P < 0.05$). In 343 muscles with zero myodynamia, there are 121 muscles whose myoelectricity is lower than 10 μV. At the end of one therapy course, the myodynamia of is recovered to 0.32 and there is significant difference before and after therapy ($P < 0.01$). The myoelectricity is increased to 45.34 μV and there is significant difference before therapy and after therapy myoelectricity ($P < 0.001$, Fig. 13.5).

Table 13.13 Mean value of EMG signal after therapy in every therapy course and raw data

Name	Number[a]		Electromyographic signal (μV)		Myodynamia	
			Before therapy	After therapy	Before therapy	After therapy
Middle deltoid	16	Mean value	27.69	134.81[a]	0.00	0.67[a]
		Standard deviation	28.72	69.95	0.00	0.54
Bicipital muscle of arm	21	Mean value	26.10	105.76[a]	0.00	0.74[a]
		Standard deviation	41.08	124.79	0.00	0.58
Triceps muscle of arm	28	Mean value	21.39	165.21[a]	0.00	0.92[a]
		Standard deviation	33.14	188.18	0.00	0.84
Wrist extensor	31	Mean value	24.19	120.45[a]	0.00	0.46[a]
		Standard deviation	21.84	124.80	0.00	0.64
Wrist flexor	61	Mean value	34.59	95.69[a]	0.00	0.75[a]
		Standard deviation	137.73	153.97	0.00	0.81
Finger extensor	97	Mean value	16.89	78.96[a]	0.00	0.27[a]
		Standard deviation	32.89	97.65	0.00	0.46
Finger flexor	89	Mean value	24.75	70.04[a]	0.00	0.39[a]
		Standard deviation	44.92	95.51	0.00	0.82

[a] $p < 0.01$

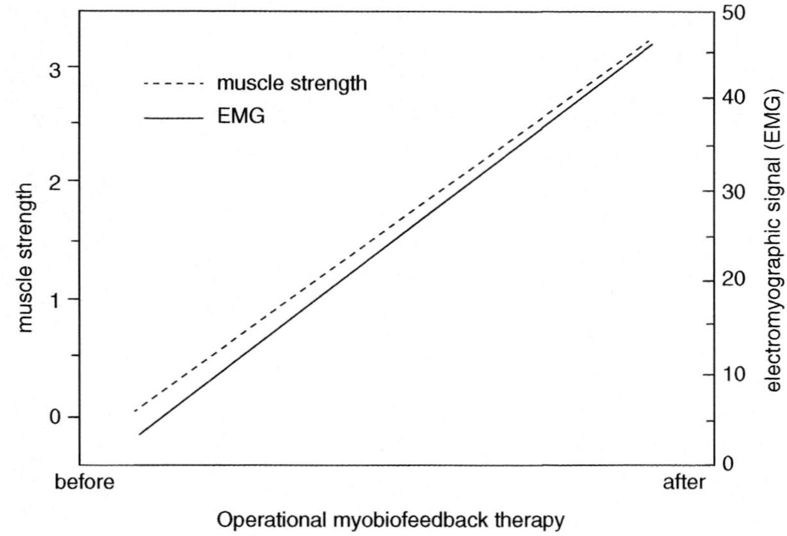

Fig. 13.5 Comparison of 343 muscles with zero myodynmaia before and after therapy

13.4.3.4 Discussion

According to manual muscle test, zero myodynamia means the patients are required to contract certain muscle and the examiner cannot feel muscle contraction on skin surface of this muscle using hands, which indicates that this muscle is completely paralytic without denervation. Under this circumstance, except for the muscles with zero myodynamia due to spinal shock in acute phase that can be recovered after shock phase, for the patients in chronic phase, it is impossible to recover autonomous muscle contraction and the patients may give up therapy and functional exercise, especially for the muscles with zero myodynamia due to obsolete nerve injury in the patients whose disease history is more than 1 year. It is impossible to recover autonomous innervation and the patients lose functional recovery and improvement of life quality ability. The disease history in this group is 0.5–20 years after injury and the average is 4.2 years. After therapy, there are significant increases of electromyographic signal and myodynamia, which is related to the following factors.

1. MMT is not sensitive. MMT is an essential assessment method for diagnosis, therapeutic schedule formulation and therapeutic effect assessment. MMT is widely used [23] in clinic because of obvious distinctive symptoms between different myodynamia grades, better quantification, strong comparability and repeatability. No specific equipment is required and the method is easy to memorize and master. MMT is one of the most credible and subjective methods for assessment of motor function loss due to pain in lower limbs and waist. MMT is usually used in rehabilitation area. Bohannon [24] deemed that myodynamia grades of lower limbs are consistent with the range of joint motion. Some reports point out that MMT is less sensitive in the myodynamia assessment below grade four than myodynamometer. In the assessment of myodynamia that is no less than grade four, MMT is better than myodynamometer. In the myodynamia comparison after spinal cord injury through isokinetic myodynamia assessment, MMT is not sensitive for myodynamia assessment. MMT is less sensitive than isokinetic myodynamia assessment method [25]. Operant biological feedback of myoelectricity is analyzed from analysis of EMG signal that is the square root of mean value of potential whose noise level is lower than 0.2 μV. The bandwidth is from 10 to 1000 Hz and the noise is less than 140 dB. It is highly sensitive. In 343 muscles with zero myodynamia through clinical assessment, there are only 11 muscles with zero myoelectricity. Coincidence

rate is 3‰. It proved that MMT is less sensitive than biological feedback signal reception equipment of myoelectricity. If the muscle can receive autonomous electromyographic signal, the functions of this muscle can be recovered to varying degrees.

2. The effect of weak electrical signal. The disabled patients are usually pessimistic and with severe mental disorder, especially the patients who are not recovered after rehabilitation therapy or who are impossible to be recovered. Therefore, if the patients can see the progress of the therapy timely, their rehabilitation desire and confidence can be further activated. The effective method of autonomous muscle contraction and joint motion is to induce the appearance or enhancement of autonomous nerve signal through active movements. The autonomous contraction and joint motion of muscles with zero myodynamia cannot be observed. The patients try their best, but cannot see the progress. They may lose confidence and feel absent. They may give up the therapy. Under the monitor of operant biological feedback equipment of bioelectricity, when the patients actively do autonomous contraction and joint motion of muscles with zero myodynamia, weak electromyographic signal can be received. Through amplification and computer processing, the signal can be displayed in monitor in a smooth curve. At this time, the therapists must explain the origin and meaning of this curve to the patients. Some researchers found that the intensity of electromyographic signal is not proportional to the strength of myodynamia. The received electromyographic signal is a mixed signal that is mainly electroencephalogram. This curve means the functional level of the muscle dominated by brain. The therapists tell the patients to observe the change of the curve and increase the height. The patients are asked not to concentrate on contracted muscle and moved joint. Therefore, it is easy to induce innervation signal of autonomous nerve. The patients and the therapists can see the therapeutic progress at any time and the rehabilitation confidence is further increased.

3. Providing objective target for learning and functional training. Objective indicator is essential for learning and functional training. In daily life, there is a truth that archery athlete aims at arrow target to practice archery so that degree of accuracy in archery can be increased. Otherwise, the degree of accuracy in archery cannot be increased without target. This is because archery is a motor program that is constructed in cortex motor center. Through repeated practice, the archery skill will be promoted continuously. When archery athlete aims at arrow target to practice archery, the first arrow may be shoot in the above of the bull's-eye. The archery result is sent to the brain and the brain will analyze numerous factors (altitude of arrow target, distance, wind direction, bow weight, arrow weight, arm strength and emotion) comprehensively. After calculation, the gesture of the second arrow can be decided such as lowering the arrowhead. The second arrow may be shoot in the below of the bull's-eye. The archery result is sent to the brain and the brain will know the arrowhead is too low. The gesture of the third arrow can be decided such as raising the arrowhead. The third arrow is shoot in the bull's-eye. After repeated training, the speed and accuracy of the movements are controlled precisely by the brain so that the speed and accuracy of the movements will be increased. During this process, arrow target is the subjective indicator for illustration and feedback, which make the brain know the mistake, rectify it timely and set clear objective. Therefore, arrow target is essential external conditions for increasing the degree of accuracy in archery and constructing archery motor program. After repeated training, the motor program is consolidated.

4. There is residual partial neural conduction pathway. Some reports demonstrated that the occurrence rate of complete spinal cord injury, which is related to the anatomy of spinal cord. Generally, after spinal cord injury, if there is one third of normal spinal tissue left, the spinal cord can have normal func-

tions. If the original conduction pathway is injured, potential conduction pathway can be activated through proper training method. For example, scientific training can improve the performance of the athletes. The muscles with zero myodynamia and non-zero potential can receive autonomous signal through active movements and the potential conduction pathway can be activated. The muscles with zero myodynamia and zero potential cannot receive autonomous signal through active movements and the potential conduction pathway cannot be activated. At this time, the therapists should have confidence and ask the patients to try their best to give out signal to the muscles. Semi-active method is used to induce autonomous signal. For example, bicipital muscle of arm can induce autonomous signal and activate conduction pathway through pull-up with help and quadriceps femoris can induce autonomous signal and activate conduction pathway through standing up from semi-kneeling-squatting position. The author found that if there is autonomous signal, it can be increased quickly and cannot be lost. Reflex signal from spinal cord can induce autonomous signal.

References

1. Garrido AG, Espitia AML, Magraner LM, et al. Validación española del cuestionario International Spinal Cord Injury Pulmonary Function Basic Data Set para valorar la repercusión de la lesión medular en el sistema respiratorio. Med Clin. 2015;145(11):477–81.
2. Mothe AJ, Tator CH. Review of transplantation of neural stem/progenitor cells for spinal cord injury. Int J Dev Neurosci. 2013;31(7):701–13.
3. Zeuke W, Heidrich R. Late paralysis of the peripheral nerves from the neurologic viewpoint. Zentr Neurochir. 1983;44(1):53–5.
4. Lahmann NA, Tannen A, Dassen T, Kottner J. Friction and shear highly associated with pressure ulcers of residents in long-term care-classification tree analysis (CHAID) of Braden items. J Eval Clin Pract. 2011;17(1):168–73.
5. Ohura N, Ichioka S, Nakatsuka T, Shibata M. Evaluating dressing materials for the prevention of shear force in the treatment of pressure ulcers. J Wound Care. 2005;14(9):401–4.
6. Newstead AH, Dragotta NJ, Wood P. Prevention of spinal cord and head injury. J Neurol Phys Ther. 1994;18(2):21–8.
7. Yarkony GM, Roth EJ, Heinemann AW. Functional skills after spinal cord injury rehabilitation:three-year longitudinal follow-up. Arch Phys Med Rehabil. 1988;69(2):111–1114.
8. Kolse KJ, Schmidt DL, Needham BM. Rehabilitation therapy for patients with long-term spinal cord injuries. Arch Phys Med Rehabil. 1990;71(9):659–62.
9. Brucker BS. Biofeedback and rehabilitation. In: Ince LP, editor. Behavioral psychology in rehabilitation medicine: clinical application. New York, NY: Williams & Wilkins Co; 1980. p. 188–217.
10. Brucker BS. Biofeedback and rehabilitation. In: Golden R, editor. Current rehabilitation psychology. San Diege, CA: Grune and Ttratton; 1984. p. 173–99.
11. Brucker BS, Bulaeva NV. Biofeedback effect on electromyography responses in patients with spinal cord injury. Arch Phys Med Rehabil. 1996;77(2):133–7.
12. Vogel G. New brain cells prompt theory of depression. Science. 2000;290(590):258–9.
13. Wenru Z, Qiqiu Q, Bing Q. Exploration of pedicled epicardial spinal cord in the treatment of paraplegia. Chin J Orthop. 1994;9(14):561–5.
14. Mulholland TB. Biofeedback as scientific method. In: Schwarta GE, editor. Biofeedback: theory and research. New York, NY: Academic; 1977.
15. Stein RB, Brucker BS, Ayyar DR. Motor units in incomplete spinal cord injury: electrical activity contractile properties and the effects of biofeedback. J Neurol Neurosurg Psychiatry. 1990;53(10):880.
16. Klose KJ, Needham BM, Schmidt D. An assessment of the contri bution of electromyographic biofeedback as an adjunct therapy in the physical training of spinal cord injured persons. Arch Phys Med Rehabil. 1993;74(5):453–6.
17. Wenru Z, Brucker BS, Xiuru W, et al. Application of myobiofeedback in the injury of old cervical spinal cord. J Chin Rehabil Med. 2003;18(2):91–3.
18. Yulong W. Rehabilitation evaluation, vol. 88. Beijing: People's Health Publishing House; 2000.
19. Delisa JA. Rehabilitation medicine: principles and practice. Philadelphia, PA: Lippincott Williams & Wilkins Inc.; 1998.
20. Li X, Ling L, Zhiren R, et al. Effect of rehabilitation training on the expression of GAP-43 in brain of cerebral infarction rats. The Fourth Military Medical University. Neurosci Res. 2001;22(16):1469–72.
21. Shifang Z. Research and rehabilitation of brain plasticity after cerebral apoplexy. Chin J Phys Med Rehabil. 2002;14(7):437–9.
22. Bohannon RW, Corrigan D. A broad range of force is encompassed by the maximum manual muscle test grade of five. Percept Motor Skills. 2000;90(1):747–50.
23. Yasuoka M, Yoneda H, Hasegawa N. Application of the treadmill test for estimation of motor due to pain

in lumber region and lower extremities. Masui Jpn J Anesthesiol. 1991;40(03):367.

24. Bohannon RW. Internal consistency of manual muscle testing scores. Percept Motor Skills. 1997;85(2):736–8.
25. Schwartz S, Cohen ME, Herbison GJ. Relationship between two measures of upper extremity strength:manual muscle test compared to hand-held myometry. Arch Phys Med Rehabil. 1992;73(11):1063–8.

14 Rehabilitation Therapy of Neurological Training of Pulmonary Dysfunction

14.1 Respiratory Movement and Pulmonary Function

There are many types of pulmonary dysfunction. In this chapter, we mainly introduce voluntary movement dysfunction of breathing [1] and its rehabilitation therapy of neurological training.

In the entire life course, gas exchange between human body and environment is required to maintain relative stability of O_2 and CO_2. Therefore, the metabolism and physiological functions of tissue and cells can be maintained. The process of gas exchange is called respiration.

The entire process of respiration includes three stages.

External respiration is the process of gas exchange between environment and pulmonary blood, which includes pulmonary ventilation and pulmonary gas exchange.

The transportation of gas in blood includes the O_2 transportation from lung to tissue and CO_2 transportation from tissue to lung.

Internal respiration is the gas exchange process between blood in capillary and tissue cells.

If there is respiration disorder, there are histanoxia and carbon dioxide retention, which can influence metabolism of tissue cells to varying degrees, even endanger vital movements.

14.1.1 Pulmonary Ventilation Function

Pulmonary ventilation is the gas exchange process [2] between pulmonary alveoli and environment. The structures of pulmonary ventilation include respiratory tract, pulmonary alveoli, thoracic cage and pleural cavity.

14.1.1.1 Gas Exchange and Power of Pulmonary Ventilation

Gas exchange includes pulmonary gas exchange and gas exchange in tissues through diffusion. Gas molecule always moves from high pressure to low pressure. When intrapulmonic pressure is lower than barometric pressure, gas enter into pulmonary alveoli. Conversely, when intrapulmonic pressure is higher than barometric pressure, gas flows from pulmonary alveoli to external atmosphere until the pressure is equal. Barometric pressure is relatively constant, but intrapulmonic pressure fluctuates with the changes of pulmonary volume. The volume change is induced by dilation and shrink of thoracic cage that is due to contraction and relaxation of respiratory muscle. Therefore, contraction and relaxation of respiratory muscle is the source power of pulmonary ventilation.

W. Zhao, *Rehabilitation Therapeutics of the Neurological Training*,
https://doi.org/10.1007/978-981-13-0812-3_14

14.1.1.2 Respiratory Movement and Modulation

Respiratory movement is rhythmic dilation and shrink of thoracic cage that is due to contraction and relaxation of respiratory muscle, which includes inspiratory movement and expiratory movement.

1. Muscles involved in breathing include respiratory muscle and auxiliary respiratory muscle [3]. These muscles are the same as muscles that drive joint motion, which belong to voluntary skeletal muscle.
   - Respiratory muscle includes diaphragm and external intercostal muscles. Diaphragm: when the person inhale gas, diaphragm contracts, diaphragmatic dome decreases, abdominal organs decline, thoracic cage enlarges, pulmonary volume increases, pulmonary negative pressure increases and gas flow into lung. When the person exhale gas, diaphragm relaxes, diaphragmatic dome increases, abdominal organs move up, thoracic cage shrinks, pulmonary volume decreases, intrapleural pressure increases and gas flow out of lung. External intercostal muscles: when the people inhale gas, external intercostal muscles contract, rib moves upward and outward, pulmonary volume increases, gas flow into lung. When the people exhale gas, external intercostal muscles relaxes, rib moves downward and inward, pulmonary volume decreases, gas flow out of lung.

     In this process, inspiratory movement is active movement and expiratory movement is passive movement.
   - Auxiliary respiratory muscle is the muscles that are involved in respiratory movements except diaphragm and external intercostal muscles in forced respiration.

Auxiliary respiratory muscles include internal intercostal muscles, muscles of the back, muscles of chest and abdominal muscle. When the patients put forth their strength to inhale gas, except the contraction of diaphragm and external intercostal muscles, Auxiliary respiratory muscles such as sternocleidomastoid and pectoralis major constrict to further enlarge thoracic cage and pulmonary volume in order to inhale more gas. When the patients put forth their strength to exhale gas, except relaxation of inspiratory muscles, expiratory muscles such as internal intercostal muscles and abdominal muscles are relaxed to further reduce thoracic cage and pulmonary volume in order to exhale more gas.

In the process of forced respiration, both respiration and expiration are active movements.

2. Respiratory movements include abdominal respiration, thoracic respiration and combined respiration.

   Abdominal respiration is a respiration process completed by diaphragm movement. Diaphragm contraction makes abdominal organs move downward. The external manifestation is apophysis of abdomen in inspiration and return of abdomen in expiration. Therefore, respiration process mainly completed by diaphragm movement is called abdominal respiration [4].

   Thoracic respiration is a respiration process completed by external intercostal muscles. When people inhale gas, external intercostal muscles contract, rib moves upward and outward, thoracic volume enlarges. The external manifestation is that thoracic cage enlarges and returns to home position in respiration. The manifestation is fluctuation of chest? Respiration process mainly completed by external intercostal muscles is called thoracic respiration.

   Combined respiration: Generally, the manifestation of respiratory movement in normal person is thoraco-abdominal combined respiration. Abdominal respiration is mainly observed in infants because the thoracic cage is not developed. When the patients with pleuritic or pleural effusion, thoracic cage movement is limited so that abdominal respiration is the main respiration process. For the pregnant women in the late phase, or the patients with huge abdominal mass or ascites, the respiration movement mainly is thoracic respiration because abdominal movement is limited.

Human thoracic cage is flat cone with short anteroposterior diameter, long right and left diameter, small top and big bottom. The displacement induced by upward and outward movement of rib is limited. The enlargement of thoracic cage volume is small. Diaphragm at the bottom of thoracic cage contract and viscera decline. Slight displacement can induce big change of thoracic volume. Therefore, abdominal respiration is a more effective respiration form. If there is eupnea, diaphragm contraction can increase thoracic volume, which equals to fourth fifth of total lung ventilation. Diaphragm contraction plays an important role in pulmonary ventilation.

3. Regulation of respiratory movement: According to different regulation mode, respiratory movement includes rhythmic respiration and voluntary respiration. Rhythmic respiration is the main regulation way [5].
   - Rhythmic respiration is non-voluntary respiration, which is respiratory movement completed by rhythmic excitability of respiratory center located in pons and medulla oblongata. The depth and frequency can change with the change of internal and external environments in order to adapt to the requirements of body metabolism. Peripheral chemoreceptor located in carotid body and aortic body and central chemoreceptor located in ventrolateral superficial part of medulla oblongata can detect the change of oxygen partial pressure and partial pressure of carbon dioxide in blood and regulate respiration rhythm through feedback mechanism in order to maintain physiological dynamic balance.
   - Voluntary respiration: respiratory movement is controlled by brain consciousness. For example, people can hold their breath in swallowing, speaking, defecation and diving. Strenuous exercise requires deep and fast respiration to ensure the normal process of these movements.

   In short, respiratory movement is completed through interaction of various grades of respiratory centers and regulation of peripheral afferent impulse.

14.1.1.3 Potential Capacity of Respiratory Function

Potential capability of respiratory system and respiratory function is the key for pulmonary function rehabilitation training and functional improvement through training.

In fact, pulmonary function is the same as the functions of other tissues and organs. They all have great functional potential. The main manifestations are as follows:

1. Tissue reservation is the histological basis of potential capability. There are 300 million [6] Alveoli in the two lungs. The total diffusion area is about 70 square meter. In resting state, the number of alveoli of gas diffusion is about 180 million. Respiratory membrane area is about 40 square meters. Therefore, reserved area of respiratory membrane is huge. Moreover, when in movements, open number and open degree of pulmonary blood capillary are increased and effective diffusion area is greatly increased.
2. Respiratory muscle of voluntary movement can increase respiratory function through developing neural potential and enhancing myodynamia. Respiratory muscle and auxiliary respiratory muscle are skeletal muscle at will. Through training, on the basis of developing neural potential of dominated muscle, muscle contraction ability is increased and pulmonary respiratory function is improved. Through training, respiratory function of athletes can meet the requirements of oxygen supply in strenuous exercise.
3. We can increase pulmonary function through changing respiratory form. Of the entire gas, partial gas in respiratory tract, weasand and pulmonary alveoli that cannot be used for gas exchange is called dead space. The more functions Dead space plays, the less oxygen content in blood is. According the part of dead space, it divided into three parts. Anatomical dead space: in every respiration, gas in upper respiratory tract to respiratory bronchiole cannot be used for gas exchange between pulmonary alveoli and blood. The space is about 150 mL in adult. Dead space of pulmonary

alveoli: the gas flows into pulmonary alveoli but not used for gas exchange. Physiological dead space: in every respiration, gas in physiological dead space cannot be used for gas exchange, which includes anatomical dead space and dead space of pulmonary alveoli. For healthy people, physiological dead space is equal to anatomical dead space, which means the gas that flows into pulmonary alveoli can be used for gas exchange entirely.

The volume of valid gas exchange in every minute is alveolar ventilation volume. The formulation is:

$$\text{Alveolar ventilation volume} = (\text{tidal volume} - \text{dead space volume}) \times \text{respiratory frequency}.$$

Under normal circumstances, minute ventilation volume is 8 L. Tidal volume is0.5 L (inhaled or exhaled gas every respiration). The relationship between respiration frequency and alveolar ventilation volume refers to Table 14.1.

Therefore, deep and slow abdominal respiration can obviously improve alveolar ventilation volume, increase volume of gas exchange. Shallow and fast respiration can decrease ventilatory efficiency of pulmonary alveoli.

4. Improving compliance of pulmonary tissue and reducing respiratory resistance Exercise can improve suppleness of elastic fiber in pulmonary tissue. In a certain range, the more the lung expands, the stronger the lung elastic recoil is, the stronger the inspiratory resistance is.

Elastic resistance can confront shape change, which is the elastic recoil. Its intensity can be manifested by elasticity. Elasticity is the dilation difficulty of elastic tissue under the influence of external force. Big Elasticity means the tissue is easy to dilate and small elasticity means the tissue is difficult to dilate. Small elastic resistance makes it easy to dilate and big elastic resistance makes it difficult to dilate.

Table 14.1 The effect of different respiration form on ventilation volume (L/min)

Breathing form	Minute ventilation volume	Alveolar ventilation volume
Eupnea	0.80 (0.50 × 16)	0.56 [(0.50 – 0.15) × 16]
Shallow and fast respiration	0.80 (0.25 × 32)	0.32 [(0.25 – 0.15) × 32]
Deep and slow respiration	0.80 (1.00 × 8)	0.68 [(1.00 – 0.15) × 8]

Through deep and slow abdominal respiration training, pulmonary tissue can be dilated fully and relaxed fully. Therefore, suppleness of elastic fiber in pulmonary tissue is increased gradually to increase elasticity of pulmonary tissue and improve respiration quality.

14.1.2 Evaluation of Pulmonary Ventilation Function

Pulmonary ventilation is an important link for gas circulation between pulmonary alveoli and environment, which can refresh gas in pulmonary alveoli. The change of lung volume and pulmonary ventilation volume are the indicators of assessing pulmonary ventilation function.

1. Lung volume: lung volume is the gas volume in lung. The change of lung volume is closely related to the depth of respiration.
   - Tidal volume: If there is eupnea, gas volume that is inhaled or exhaled is called tidal volume. Tidal volume of normal people is 0.4–0.6 L and the average is about 0.5 L.
   - Inspiratory reserve volume: At the end of inspiration, people try their best to inhale gas, which is called inspiratory reserve volume. Inspiratory reserve volume of normal people is 1.5–2.0 L and it is the reserved capacity of inspiration.

- Inspiratory capacity: The sum of inspiratory reserve volume and tidal volume is inspiratory capacity, which is an important indicator to assess potential ability of maximal ventilation.
- Expiratory reserve volume: At the end of expiration, people try their best to exhale gas, which is called expiratory reserve volume. Expiratory reserve volume of normal people is 0.9–2.0 L and it is the reserved capacity of expiration.
- Vital capacity: After maximal inspiration, people try their best to exhale gas and the exhaled gas volume is called vital capacity. The sum of tidal volume, inspiratory reserve volume and expiratory reserve volume is vital capacity. The vital capacity in male adult is about 3.5 L and in female adult is about 2.5 L.
- Forced expiratory volume: at the end of forced inspiration, when people try their best to exhale gas as soon as possible, the gas volume exhaled in the first several seconds is called forced vital capacity, which is manifested by the percent of vital capacity in forced expiration. At the end of the first second, forced expiratory volume accounts for 83% of FVC. Forced expiratory volume reflects the fluency of air tract and elasticity of pulmonary tissue in respiratory process, which is a good indicator of pulmonary ventilation function.
- Residual volume and Functional residual volume: at the end of maximal expiration, the gas volume in lung that cannot be exhaled is called residual volume. Residual volume of normal person is 1.0–1.5 L. Poor pulmonary ventilation function can attenuate pulmonary elasticity and increase residual volume. Functional residual volume is the gas volume in lung at the end of respiration. It is the sum of expiratory reserve volume and residual volume. Functional residual volume of normal person is about 2.5 L.

  Functional residual volume can buffer the change of oxygen partial pressure in pulmonary alveoli in expiration process, which is good for pulmonary gas exchange.
- Total lung capacity is the most gas volume in lung. It is the sum of vital capacity and residual volume. Total lung capacity of male adult is about 5.0 L and of female adult is about 3.5 L.

2. Pulmonary ventilation volume.
   - Minute ventilation volume is the gas that flow in or out of lung in every minute. It is the tidal volume plus respiration frequency. If there is eupnea in adult, minute ventilation is 6–9 L.
   - Alveolar ventilation volume: during respiratory movement, the gas volume into pulmonary alveoli in every minute is called alveolar ventilation volume.

14.2 Pulmonary Motor Dysfunction and Rehabilitation Therapy of Neurological Training

14.2.1 Assessment of Pulmonary Motor Dysfunction

Motor dysfunction of lung is mainly due to paralysis of respiratory muscle, which is commonly observed in injuries of central nervous system such as brain trauma, brain infarction and spinal injuries. It is also observed in neural diseases such as myasthenia gravis and motor neuron degeneration that affect respiratory muscle in one side or two sides, paralysis and brain damages that usually affect respiratory muscle in one side, neurological disease and paraplegia that affect respiratory muscle in two sides.

In clinic, international general assessment method is usually used to assess pulmonary function and dysfunction degree.

1. Exercise test is used to assess cardiopulmonary function and motor capacity of the patients with pulmonary disease.

   Because of dyspnea, cardiopulmonary function is weakened to varying degrees and maximal oxygen consumption is decreased, which restricts endurance and motor ability. Exercise test is one of the important methods to assess the disability of the patients with pulmonary disease. Heart and lung are one functional unit. The following materials can be obtained through exercise test.

- Maximal oxygen uptake (VO_{2max}) is the important indicator to reflex physical activity ability and cardiopulmonary function. The specific method can be referred in rehabilitation evaluation books.
- Oxygen consumption of quantitative movement: in resting state, after quantitative exercise and in the middle of recovery, oxygen consumption can be tested and heart rate and minute ventilation volume are recorded. Because the motor intensity is small, it is easily accepted by the patients. It is safe and convenient.
- O_2 pulse: the ration of V O_2 to HR can be used to assess the entire pulmonary function.
- Anaerobic threshold: when energy requirement exceeds oxygen supply, ATP can be generated by anaerobic metabolism to meet energy requirements. However, this cannot last long. At this time, acid metabolite such as lactate is increased, which is the beginning of anaerobic metabolism (anaerobic threshold).

2. The assessment of dyspnea: according to the third edition of permanent injury evaluation guideline amended by American Medical Association in 1990, the dyspnea is divided into three degrees (Table 14.2).

Table 14.2 Assessment of dyspnea

Degrees	Characteristics
Slight	It may appear when the patients are walking in the flat ground or climbing gentle slope. If the patients walk in the flat ground, walking speed is the same as healthy people of the same age and physique, but they may fall behind when climbing gentle slope or stairs
Moderate	When the patients walk in flat ground or climb stairs with the healthy people of the same age and physique, there will be dyspnea
Severe	In flat ground, the patients walk 4–5 min using their own speed, there is dyspnea. If the patients put forth their strength slightly, there is dyspnea, even in rest

14.2.2 Rehabilitation Therapy of Neurological Training

Both respiratory muscles and auxiliary respiratory muscles are skeletal muscles involved in voluntary movements, which are dominated by central nervous system and can be used for rehabilitation training of neurological training.

In addition, respiratory function is the basis to work on productive labor and competitive sports. However, respiratory function training is accompanied with productive labor or physical exercise. Special respiratory function training is not universal. The effects of special training and accompanied training are different.

1. Signal enhancement training of neurological training: Its purpose is to develop neural potential and recover motor function of respiratory muscle.
   - Rehabilitation training of neurological training of diaphragm: diaphragm is the main muscle to complete abdominal respiration. Fourth fifth of gas is inhaled through diaphragm movements. Therefore, diaphragm is the important inspiratory muscle for training.

   Diaphragm is dominated by nervus phrenicus that is composed of C_4 nerve root. Only C_4 and spinal nerve above it can lead to paralysis of diaphragm. Spinal cord injury below C_4 usually doesn't influence the function of this muscle. In the patients with hemiplegia induced by cerebral hemorrhage, cerebral infarction and cerebral trauma, it usually induces paralysis of diaphragm to varying degrees in one side.

   Neurological training technique is applied for rehabilitation training of diaphragm. According to the attachment point of diaphragm in the inner surface of thoracic cage, surface electrode is pasted in the corresponding part of thoracic cage. Two groups of electrodes (three electrodes in each group, Fig. 14.1) are pasted in two sides of sixth intercostal space in midclavicular line, 8th intercostal space in midaxillary line and tenth intercostal space in

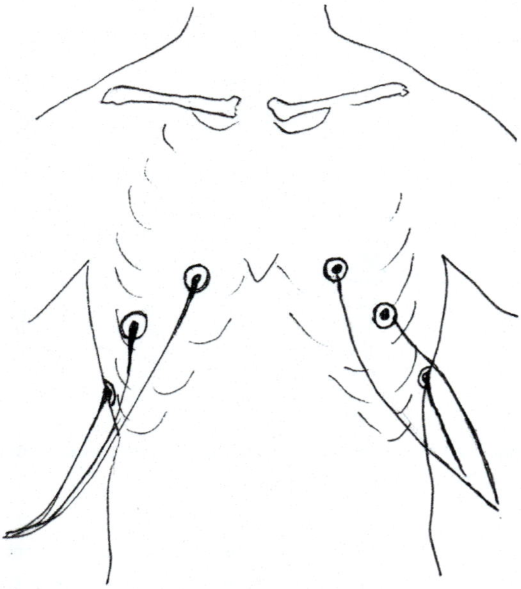

Fig. 14.1 Training electrode placement sketch map of diaphragm

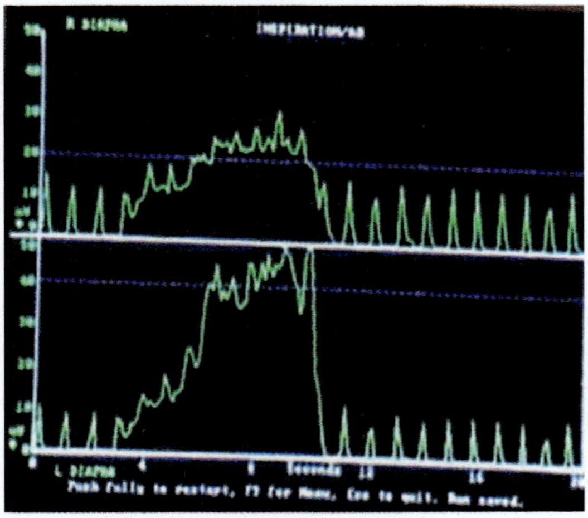

Fig. 14.2 Control display of diaphragm signal in two sides

linea scapularis or posterior axillary line. Two groups of electrodes are connected to the first and the third lead of neurological training equipment. One screen is used to display diaphragm signal in two sides (Fig. 14.2). Control training of diaphragm in two sides is done to provide visual surpassing goal (the healthy side) for the patients.

Specific method: normal Daoyin technique or six-step Daoyin technique of guiding collaterals through meridians in traditional Chinese medicine is used. Main and collateral channels are operated by guiding collaterals through meridians. Stomach meridian of foot-yangming: wing of nose (Yingxiang), inner canthus (Jingming), upper teeth and ring lip (philtrum), supraclavicular fossa (Quepen), 2 in. besides xiphoid (Burong). On the basis of regulation of mind and breathing, the patients are required to inhale gas with force using abdominal respiration. The therapists put palm on the upper abdomen and increase resistance according to the patients' condition (Fig. 14.3). The therapists encourage the patients to try their best to increase signal intensity of diaphragm. The patients insist for 6 s and enter into the process of guiding collaterals. After diaphragm contraction, the patients are guided to relax. The mind goes downward along 2 in. besides midline of abdomen (Guanmen), inguen (Qichong), hip joint (Biguan), outside of tibia (Zusanli), the anterior of thigh (tibialis anterior muscle), acrotarsium (Chongyang), inside of middle toe (Neiting) and finally arrives at outside of the second toe (Lidui).

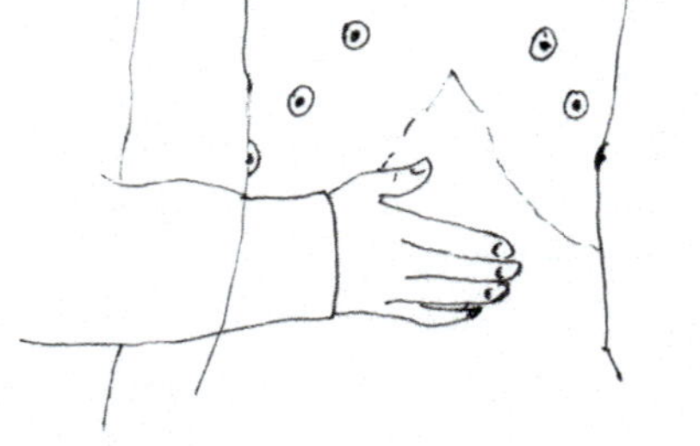

Fig. 14.3 Anti-resistance training of neurological training of diaphragm

After that, the patients relax, take a deep inspiration and exhale it slowly.

In the second training, signal intensity induced in the first training is used to make an elevation line, which is the surpass goal of the second training. The patients are guided to make signal intensity surpass the elevation line. The rest can be done in the same manner. Signal intensity of diaphragm dominated by central nervous system is increased gradually to recover motor function of diaphragm.

The training time is 25 min (once a day) and there are 30 time in one therapy course.

- Rehabilitation training of neurological training of external intercostal muscles: External intercostal muscles are the main inspiratory muscles, which is dominated by intercostal nerve. There is cross dominance phenomenon in intercostal nerve. For example, the fourth external intercostal muscles not only dominated by the fourth intercostal nerve, but also innervated by the branches of the third and fifth intercostal nerve. Therefore, the training of external intercostal muscles can be done separately. The fourth, sixth, eighth and tenth external intercostal muscles can be trained.

There are two groups of surface electrode that receive signal in left and right sides. There are three electrodes in each group. The paste parts of fourth external intercostal muscles are as follows: the first electrode is placed in intercostal space of midclavicular line. The second electrode is placed in intercostal space of anterior axillary line. The third electrode is placed in intercostal space of posterior axillary line (Fig. 14.4). The rest can be done in the same manner.

Specific method: the normal Daoyin technique or six-step Daoyin technique of guiding collaterals through meridians in traditional Chinese medicine is used for training. When the training of guiding collaterals through meridians is used for the fourth, sixth and eighth external intercostal muscles, Qi is guided to Wuyi, Ruzhong and Burong to activate contraction movements of external intercostal muscles. The therapists put one hand on the corresponding part of thoracic wall, exert resistance inward and upward properly use count method to encourage the patients to enhance continuous contraction intensity of external intercostal muscles. The specific method is the same as diaphragm training. The training time is 25 min (once a day) and there are 30 time in one therapy course.

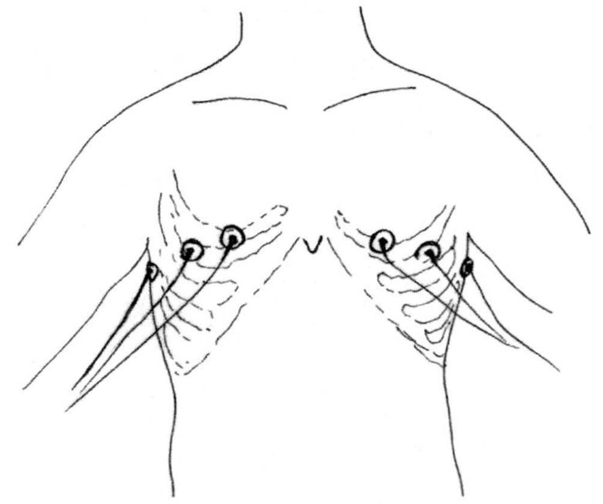

Fig. 14.4 Sketch map of paste part of surface electrode on external intercostal muscles

- Rehabilitation therapy of neurological training of auxiliary inspiratory muscles: when the patients inhale gas, pectoralis major contraction enlarges thoracic cage and pulmonary volume to inhale more gas.

Rehabilitation training of neurological training of pectoralis major: pectoralis major is from inside of clavicle, the anterior of sternum, the first to the sixth costicartilages and the upper of the anterior wall of vagina musculi recti abdominis to spine of greater tubercle of humerus. The function of pectoralis major is to adduct and intort shoulder joint in proximal fixation. In distal fixation, the trunk is stretched to upper arm and the rib is elevated for inspiration.

The paste part of received electrode: surface electrodes are placed in two fingers in the level of anterior axillary line in infraclavicula, four fingers below midclavicular line, six fingers in infraclavicula and two fingers besides sternum. Reference electrode are between upper and lower electrodes (Fig. 14.5).

Upper arm adduction induces autonomous motor program signal of pectoralis major and anti-resistance enhances the signal intensity (Fig. 14.6). Other trainings are the same as the methods mentioned above. The training time is 25 min (once a day) and there are 30 time in one therapy course.

- Rehabilitation training of neurological training of auxiliary expiratory muscles: when the patients put up their forth to exhale gas, except the dilation of inspiratory muscles, contraction of expiration muscles of internal intercostal muscles and abdominal muscles shrink thoracic cage and pulmonary volume to exhale more gas and decrease residual gas volume in pulmonary alveoli.

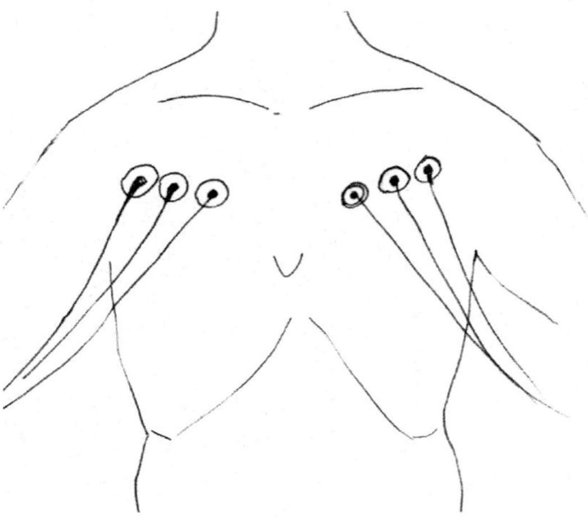

Fig. 14.5 Sketch map of paste part of surface electrode on pectoralis major

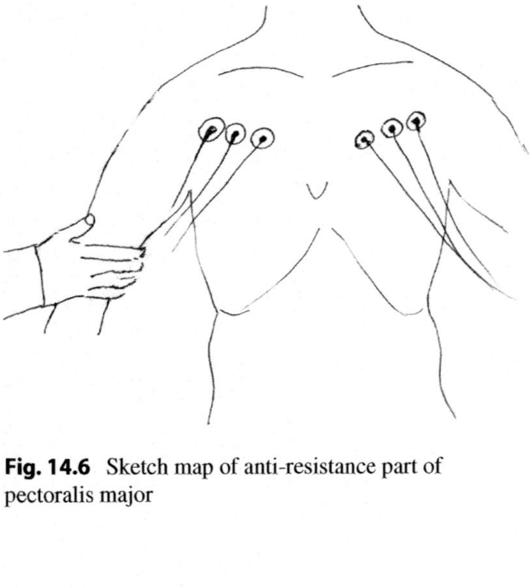

Fig. 14.6 Sketch map of anti-resistance part of pectoralis major

Rehabilitation training of neurological training of internal intercostal muscles: internal intercostal muscles are in intercostal space and in deep layer. The direction of diagonal muscle fibers is contrary to that of external intercostal muscles. Muscle fiber is from the upper rib besides sternum to the lower rib besides spinal cord. The contraction of internal intercostal muscles decrease sternum. The rib inclines downward and rotates inside to shorten the anteroposterior and left and right diameter of thoracic cage to generate expiration effect.

Electrode paste place and training method of rehabilitation training of neurological training of internal intercostal muscles are the same as these of external intercostal muscles training (Fig. 14.7). During the anti-resistance of internal intercostal muscles, the therapists use palm to exert resistance inward and downward from costal margin to resist the shortening of anteroposterior diameter of thoracic cage. The training of internal intercostal muscles refers to Fig. 14.8. The training time is 25 min (once a day) and there are 30 time in one therapy course.

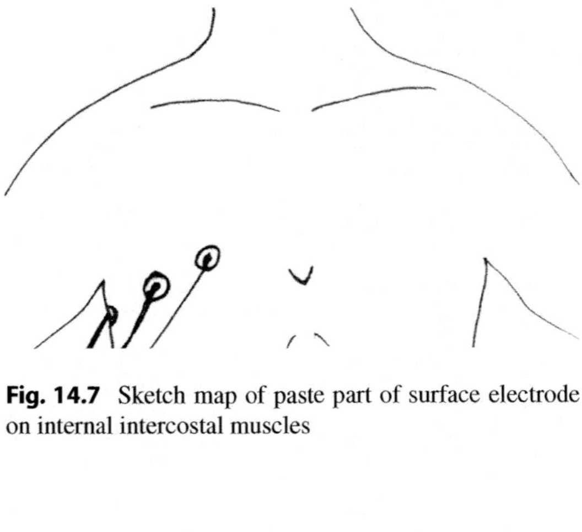

Fig. 14.7 Sketch map of paste part of surface electrode on internal intercostal muscles

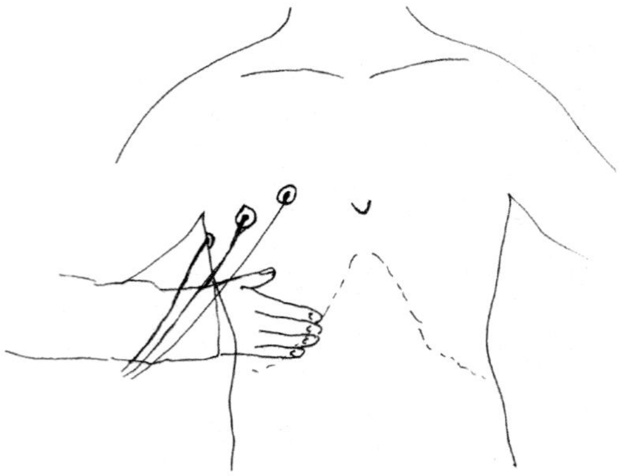

Fig. 14.8 Sketch map of anti-resistance part of internal intercostal muscles

2. Potential development training of neurological training: Auxiliary respiratory muscles can be used for potential development training.
   - Potential development training of pectoralis major: With the help of potential development training equipment of upper limbs, the patients knee in training equipment and wear weight support band. According to the condition of the patients, the weight can be decreased. Six-step Daoyin technique is used to guide the patients to do pushing up and down of upper limbs. During pushing up and down with upper limbs, fluctuation of the trunk requires pectoralis major and latissimus dorsi. Through decreasing weight support or increasing resistance gradually, the patients can recover neural functions and strengthen the muscles. The training time is 25 min (once a day) and there are 30 time in one therapy course.
   - Rectus abdominis training: sit-up is used to train rectus abdominis. With the help of potential development training equipment of upper limbs, the patients knee in training equipment and wear weight support band. According to the condition of the patients, the weight can be decreased and lower limbs are fixed. Six-step Daoyin technique is used to guide the patients to sit up and lie down. Through decreasing weight support or increasing resistance gradually, the patients can develop neural potential and enhance the strength of rectus abdominis. The training time is 25 min (once a day) and there are 30 time in one therapy course.
3. Abdominal respiration training: the patients can train diaphragm and breathe in a deep and slow way to increase vital capacity. There are many ways of respiration exercises, such as diaphragm respiration, anti-resistance respiration, segmentation respiration, deep and slow respiration, and retraction lip respiration. They have certain therapeutic effects, but there is no special equipment for respiration training and there is no visual real-time objective indicator of inspiratory capacity. In some hospitals, home-made paper bag is the tool for respiration training, but the patients cannot insist on it, which can influence exercise effect.

   Pulmonary function exercise device developed by the author is a kind of exercise device of active movements of inspiratory muscles (Fig. 14.9). It is made from non-toxic medical plastics. It is equipped with main measurement barrel to measure inspiratory capacity and flow measurement barrel to measure gas volume in unit interval. The main measurement barrel is equipped with scale and float. The float can fluctuate flexibly. Therefore, the users can know their progress of exercise and get inspired. Flow measurement barrel is marked with three gears that include good, better and best. When the floater in flow measurement barrel is on good gear, the gas volume in unit time is big and the inspiratory time is short, which belongs to shallow and fast respiration mode. When the floater in flow measurement barrel is on best gear, the gas volume in unit time is small and the inspiratory time is long, which belongs to deep and slow respiration mode. The users observe the inspiratory capacity and flow volume in the process of exercise. Through biofeedback mechanism, they can keep gas flow at minimum and inspiratory capacity at maximum and the deep and slow abdominal respiration mode is formed gradually.

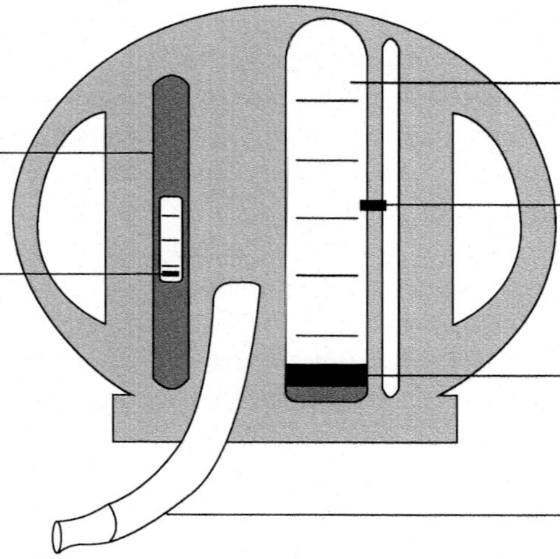

Fig. 14.9 Sketch map of pulmonary function exercise device

- Pulmonary function exercise device: through objective and motive mechanism, the users can strengthen diaphragm and turn the breathing to deep and slow abdominal respiration mode to increase alveolar ventilation volume, increase oxyhemoglobin saturation, prevent pulmonary alveoli collapse and re-inflate the collapsed pulmonary alveoli.
- Application methods and therapy course: application methods: the patients usually are in sitting position or lying position. The patients in sitting position should keep their heads up. The patients lying in bed should be in semireclining position. At first, they should do deep inspiratory practice for several times and then use pulmonary function exercise device. The patients should concentrate when in exercise. According to individual physical truth, they adjust scale Vernier of inspiratory capacity. At the time of inspiration, the patients observe the vernier change in flow measurement barrel and keep the floater in flow measurement barrel at best gear. In the next exercise, on the basis of keep the floater in flow measurement barrel at best gear, the patients try to make the inspiratory capacity surpass it. The new capacity is marked by floater and the rest may be deduced by analogy. The inspiratory capacity is increased gradually. The therapy time is 20 min (2–3 time a day) and there are 30 times in one therapy course. It can be used for a long time as health care.
- Indications: pulmonary function exercise device is widely used to replace traditional respiration exercise modes such as blowing paper bag and retraction lip respiration. It can be used for prevent or treat pulmonary atelectasis, obstructive emphysema and chronic bronchitis. It can be used for the old weak patients, the patients with lung and heart disease, chest trauma, respiratory muscle paralysis, various kinds of surgery especially thoracotomy and respiration that is influenced to varying degrees. It can be used for the patients lying in bed for a long time, the patients with stroke, spinal injury, myodystrophy and abdominal wall relaxation after birth. All the patients have pulmonary alveoli collapse. Rehabilitation of respiratory function disorder is significantly meaningful to respiratory diseases. Arthritis and Ankylosing Spondylitis can affect breathing to varying degrees so that these are the indication of pulmonary function exercise device.
- Contraindications: There is no obvious contraindication. It should be used under the instructions of the doctors in the patients with severe cardiopulmonary dysfunction, ascites and late pregnancy.

- Cautions: in order to get better training effect, there are some announcements. The expiratory speed should be slow. The ration of inspiration and expiration is one to two. The patients should bulge abdomen in exercise to guarantee the exercise of diaphragm. The exercise should be step by step. The patients should be preserved to obtain good therapy and prevention effect. Pulmonary function exercise device is the equipment for inspiratory training. It is forbidden to blow it. The water in expiratory gas can make floater in measure barrel get wet and lose flexibility. Under this circumstance, pulmonary function exercise can be placed in shade until the water in measurement barrel evaporates completely.

14.3 Rehabilitation Methods of Keeping Fluency of Respiratory Tract

The premise of normal ventilation is the fluency of respiration tract. Elimination of secreta timely and effective in trachea is an important method to keep the fluency of respiration tract, prevent and decrease respiratory system infection.

14.3.1 The Control and Adjustment of Cough

Shallow and frequent cough and fulminant cough must be controlled timely. The control method is that the patients should relax fully, sit comfortably, incline their body and inhale gas deeply using abdominal respiration. Inhaled gas can reach deep part through trachea with secreta. After holding breath for a while, the patients shrink abdominal muscles and cough for 2–3 times. There is usually sputum. If there is still difficulty, the patients can use two hands to compress the lower part of chest and upper abdomen to cough forcedly in order to excrete sputum.

14.3.2 Postural Drainage

According to different anatomical position in lung, the patients are in proper position and use fluid mechanics to make sputum flow from higher position to lower position and decrease energy consumption [7].

1. Position and procedure: Pillow, elevating bed or tailor-made therapy bed is used to place the patients. There are five basic positions.
   - The position of inclined prone position and lowering head at 45° is suitable for drainage of rear back area in lobus inferior pulmonis.
   - The position of inclined lying on one side and lowering head at 45° is suitable for drainage of outer back area in lobus inferior pulmonis.
   - The position of inclined supine position and lowering head at 45° is suitable for drainage of forward back area.
   - The position of inclined semi-lateral position and lowering head at 30° is suitable for ligule drainage of middle lobe of right lung and superior lobe of left lung.
   - The position of semi-lateral position and backward position is suitable for drainage of superior lobes of two lungs. Inclining forward position is suitable for drainage of apex pulmonis of two lungs and extensive lung diseases.
2. Drainage procedure and time: Postural drainage should be done before meal to prevent gastric reflux. The drainage time of each part is 5–10 min and the total time cannot exceed 45 min (2–4 times a day).
3. Indications and contraindications.
   - Indications: The sputum is more than 30 mL a day or the sputum is medium, and other methods cannot excrete sputum.
   - Contraindications: Postural drainage is forbidden in the patients with myocardial infarction, cardiac insufficiency, pulmonary edema, pulmonary embolism, pleural exudation, acute chest trauma and hemorrhagic disorders.

During postural drainage, if there is cyanosis, dyspnea exacerbation, oxygen partial pressure that is less than 6.6 kPa (50 mmHg), partial pressure of carbon dioxide that is more than 8 kPa (60 mmHg), the drainage should be stopped and handled.

14.3.3 Patting and Chattering to Excrete Sputum

The therapists grasp hollow arc and use finger pulp or palm side to pat the dorsal part of chest, or use one hand to press the other hand to vibrate the dorsal part of chest. Secreta in trachea may fall off to big trachea and is easy to be excreted. During this process, the patients are asked to do slow abdominal respiration and the therapists use hand to pat and vibrate the dorsal part of chest from lower to upper in expiration for several times. Patting and vibrating should be gentle to avoid pain. The therapists should keep away from regio scapularis and upper abdomen. Sputum excretion vibrator can be used to excrete sputum and the effect is better.

14.3.4 Aerosol Inhalation Therapy

Aerosol inhalation can make 90% medicine particles whose diameter is less than 3 pm disperse in bronchus and bronchiole. The water in aerosol gas whose dose is more than 50 mL/L can wet respiration tract and are good for liquidation and excretion of secreta. Antibiotics and mucus lytic agent can be added to aerosol to liquidate sputum and prevent infection or resist infection.

During aerosol inhalation, the patients do deep and slow abdominal respiration to make aerosol reach the bottom of the lung extensively and deeply. Several minutes after inhalation, it contributes to sputum excretion with the help of cough. Aerosol inhalation therapy is given to the patients before postural drainage to increase the effect of sputum excretion.

Inhaled particles can stimulate respiration tract and may induce bronchospasm. For the patients who are tendentious to bronchospasm, in aerosol inhalation, bronchodilators can be added to prevent bronchospasm.

Aerosol inhalation therapy: the therapy time is 20 min (3–4 times a day). It can be done after getting up and before going to sleep.

14.3.5 Mucus Lytic Agent

Mucolytic medicine is a kind of medicine that can change viscous ingredient in sputum, decrease viscosity of sputum, reduce cough frequency, relieve thoracic discomfort, excrete sputum and improve general body state. It is applied in bronchial or lung diseases such as cough, expectoration and sticky sputum. It includes bromhexine, acetylcysteine and chymotrypsin. Mucolytic medicine can destroy gastric mucosal barrier. It should be used with caution in the patients with medical history of gastric ulcer.

In addition, in the health care of respiratory system, the patients should keep away from stimulation substance of respiration tract such as toxic gas, dust fog, lampblack in kitchen and smog in smoking.

14.4 Development and Clinical Application of Pulmonary Function Exercise Device

14.4.1 Design Principle of FG-01 Pulmonary Function Exercise Device

Oxygen is required for human life. Human body acquires oxygen through gas exchange. Through respiration, inhaled oxygen required for human physiological activities. The exhaled metabolite is carbon dioxide. Respiration is one of the basic life processes to maintain body metabolism. Respiratory arrest means death. The patients who stay in a position for a long time, especially in an inhibitory state because of disease, are easy to catch pneumonia. For the patients who lie in bed for a long time, the old weak patients, the patients with lung and heart disease, chest trauma, respiratory muscle paralysis, various kinds of surgery especially thoracotomy and respiration that is influenced to varying degrees, oxygen saturation in blood is decreased, tissue oxygen supply is poor, the energy is insufficient, functions are decreased due to lack of required energy. Mechanical movement of chest and lung is decreased, which can affect returned blood volume, decrease ejection blood volume and block the excretion of secreta that induce pulmonary atelectasis. Secreta retention can make the bacteria grow in lung, which can lead to pulmonary infection, increase resistance of pulmonary ventilation, decrease gas diffusion speed, further influence ventilation and gas exchange volume. It forms a vicious circle. It can delay the cure of the disease and rehabilitation time, even endanger life.

Rehabilitation of pulmonary function is important for preventing pulmonary complications and increasing visceral functions. Western developed country attaches great importance to pulmonary function rehabilitation and accumulates enriched experience. Special equipment of pulmonary function training is used. In our country, some medical books introduce rehabilitation knowledge of pulmonary function, but clinical application is rare. There is no specialized rehabilitation training equipment and apparatus of pulmonary function. Development of rehabilitation training equipment of pulmonary function with special proprietary intellectual property rights is good for promotion and popularization of rehabilitation work of pulmonary function in China.

14.4.1.1 Design Principle

Pulmonary function exercise device is designed according to human respiratory physiology function.

1. The mechanism of formation of respiratory movement: respiratory movement is formed by dilation and shrink of thoracic cage induced by respiratory muscle contraction and relaxation.

   When there is eupnea, inspiratory movement is completed by contraction of inspiratory muscles. Expiratory movement is induced by relaxation of inspiratory muscles. Inspiration is active movement and expiration is passive movement. Thoracic cage is bid in the bottom and small in the upper part. Minor diaphragm movement can induce large volume change of thoracic volume. In a resting state, fourth fifth of inhaled gas is completed by diaphragm movement. Therefore, the key point of pulmonary function exercise is to enhance diaphragm function, which is exercise of inspiratory muscles.
2. Gas volume contained in lung is the basis of capacity of pulmonary function exercise device. Lung volume can be measured by vital capacity.

   Vital capacity is the maximal volume that people can exhale after forced inspiration. It is the sum of tidal volume, inspiratory reserve volume and expiratory reserve volume. There is individual difference in vital capacity that is related to stature, gender, age, position and strength of respiratory muscle. Generally, vital capacity of male adult is 3500 mL and vital capacity of female adult is 2500 mL. Therefore, the volume of pulmonary function exercise device should be considered by the patients to meet the requirements of different crowds. It can be divided into different types according to the difficulty and volume.
3. Deep and slow respiration can reduce dead space effectively.

   The inhaled gas into lung is not all used for gas exchange between pulmonary alveoli and blood. There are 150 mL gas left from respiration tract to respiratory bronchiole, which is called anatomical dead space. Only the gas that flow into pulmonary alveoli can be used for gas exchange. Only deep and slow respiration can decrease dead space and increase alveolar ventilation volume. Shallow and rapid respiration is on the contrary.

   The design of pulmonary function exercise device must contribute to the formation of deep and slow abdominal respiration.

14.4.1.2 Main Structure

In order to meet the physiological requirements, FG-01 pulmonary function exercise device is equipped with exercise devices to measure inspiratory capacity and inspiratory flow measurement. The users can use them to train diaphragm, form deep and slow abdominal respiration and increase alveolar ventilation volume.

1. Inspiratory capacity measurement system is equipped with measurement barrel. The volume is 2500 and 3500 mL separately. There is surpassing goal.

   In order to measure the inhaled gas volume, the barrel is equipped with floater that can fluctuate with inhaled gas volume. The outside of measurement barrel is equipped with movable Vernier. The users can set the gas volume at the first time according to their own conditions and increase it with the increase of gas volume. The merit of it is that the users can see their own progress of inspiratory capacity at any time and there is always a new surpassing goal for the users. Through objective and motive mechanism, it has a feedback role that contribute to enhancement of rehabilitation confidence of pulmonary function and acceleration of rehabilitation process.
2. Gas flow measurement system: Flow measurement barrel is equipped with floater. Flow measurement barrel is marked with three gears that include good, better and best.

   This barrel can help the users to control the gas volume in unit time. When the floater is at good gear, gas volume in unit time is huge, inspiration time is short and respiration process is easy to be completed. When the floater is at better gear, gas volume in unit time is small, inspiration time is long, respiration process is difficult to be completed, but alveolar ventilation volume can be increased and diaphragm may be trained well. When the floater is at best gear, gas volume in unit time is minimum, inspiration time is the longest and respiration process is the most difficult to be completed. At this time, deep and slow respiration can make the alveolar ventilation volume reach the maximum. Diaphragm may be trained best. The users can have deep and slow respiration using abdominal respiration.
3. Performance index.
   - The materials of pulmonary function exercise device are made from qualified medical plastics. This medical plastic is in accordance with medical standard and non-toxic. There is no radioactive substance, non-carcinogenic and no sensitization.
   - Floater in measurement barrel is flexible and can reflect minor gas volume change.
   - It is equipped with gas infiltration device that can prevent dust effectively.
4. Functions.

   FG-01 respiratory function exercise device is an active inspiratory muscles exercise device. Inspiratory muscles can get better exercise and functional recovery. The respiration form is transformed to deep and slow abdominal respiration to increase alveolar ventilation volume, increase oxyhemoglobin saturation, prevent pulmonary alveoli collapse and re-expand collapsed pulmonary alveoli.
5. Discussion.

   Rehabilitation consciousness of medical staffs and the patients is increased, but the development of rehabilitation work of pulmonary function is limited. Except some professional departments such as respiration medicine and chest surgery, other departments seldom notice the rehabilitation of pulmonary function, even in department of rehabilitation medicine. For the patients with poor pulmonary function, most physicians use oxygen uptake to deal with pulmonary ventilation insufficiency and hyoxemia. Oxygen uptake is an emergent measure, but is not the common measure to deal with chronic pulmonary ventilation insufficiency and hyoxemia. The physician may ignore rehabilitation exercise of pulmonary function of the patients. Hyperoxia environment is artificial and can inhibit respiratory center. Long-term hyperoxia environment can injure pulmonary function. The people who live in hyperoxia environment don't adapt to plateau section with low oxygen content. Insufficiency of pulmonary function can lead to severe hyoxemia. Therefore, it is very important to pay attention to rehabilitation training of pulmonary function of the patients.

Pulmonary alveoli collapse and hypostatic pneumonia are the common complications of the old weak patients, the patients who lie in bed for a long time, the patients with lung diseases or after thoracotomy. The early phase after surgery, vital capacity of the patients is decreased 50–60% and ventilatory capacity in one time is decreased 25% [8]. These problems cannot be solved by oxygen uptake. Oxygen uptake cannot increase ventilation capacity, but may decrease ventilation capacity because of high oxygen content. Insufficiency of ventilation capacity cannot prevent pulmonary alveoli collapse and cannot re-expand collapsed pulmonary alveoli. Only active pulmonary function exercise can increase pulmonary ventilation volume to prevent and treat pulmonary complications.

The rehabilitation of respiratory dysfunction is meaningful to many diseases. Many diseases can lead to pulmonary dysfunction. Poor pulmonary function is an important factor to induce and aggravate many diseases. Tockman [9] and his colleagues found that the decreased percentage of forced inspiratory volume to predicted value is one of the risk factors of coronary heart diseases. Singh [10] and his colleagues found that there is restricted ventilatory dysfunction in the patients with type 2 diabetes mellitus. Lung is one of the most common involved organs in uremia. Pulmonary dysfunction may be induced by direct or indirect factors of uremia [11]. Arthritis, ankylosing spondylitis, myodystrophy, weak, stroke and spinal cord injury can lead to ventilation insufficiency. The pulmonary complication is the main reason of death, especially in the patients with quadriplegia. In addition, pulmonary function in healthy people may be changed greatly with age. Human pulmonary function reaches the peak at the age of 25. There is regeneration change at the age of 30 and there is obvious regeneration change at the age of 60. The degeneration changes include diaphragm hypomotility, increase of airway resistance and decrease of alveoli number [12]. From this, we can see the close relationship between pulmonary dysfunction and other diseases and the meaningfulness of respiratory function exercise [13, 14].

Increasing alveolar ventilation volume is the key to increase gas exchange, expand pulmonary alveoli and prevent pulmonary complications. In order to increase alveolar ventilation volume, the training of deep and slow respiration form is required. Tidal volume and respiration frequency have different impacts on pulmonary ventilation capacity and alveolar ventilation volume. When tidal volume is reduced by half and respiration frequency is doubled, alveolar ventilation volume is decreased obviously. When tidal volume is double and respiration frequency is reduced by half, alveolar ventilation volume is increased obviously [15] in spite that pulmonary ventilation volume is constant. The key point of pulmonary function exercise is active diaphragm exercise and training of deep and slow respiration mode.

FG-01 pulmonary function exercise device is an active inspiratory muscles exercise device that is equipped with inspiratory capacity and gas flow measurement device. The users can learn deep and slow abdominal respiration form to increase alveolar ventilation volume [16], activate reserved respiratory membrane area, expand pulmonary alveoli, promote gas exchange and prevent lung complications. In addition, deep inspiration training can contribute to negative pressure increase in pleural cavity, which can promote backflow of venous blood and lymph and increase blood circulation volume.

It is needed to be mentioned that rehabilitation methods of pulmonary function in some hospitals are home-made simple expiration practice device. Some reports found that expiration exercise method cannot prevent or treat pulmonary atelectasis, but can aggravate pulmonary atelectasis [17]. Only inspiration practice can prevent or treat pulmonary atelectasis. The effect of it on the sober patients is better than interval positive-pressure respiration method.

14.4.2 The Therapeutic Effect of FG-01 Pulmonary Function Exercise Device on Pulmonary Function Rehabilitation of the Patients with Pulmonary Fibrosis

The main pathological features of severe acute respiratory syndrome are hypoimmunity and pulmonary fibrosis, which greatly affect pulmonary function. In order to explore rehabilitation methods of pulmonary function damage after SARS, the author developed pulmonary function exercise device according to respiration physiology. Approved by the state administration of traditional Chinese medicine, the author chooses the patients with coalworker pneumoconiosis whose manifestation is pulmonary fibrosis as subjects. The manifestation of coalworker pneumoconiosis is similar with SARS. Pulmonary function exercise device is used for the patients to do inspiration function training to observe its effect on vital capacity and daily life of the patients.

14.4.2.1 General Conditions

Seventy-two patients with coalworker pneumoconiosis are all from pneumoconiosis and tuberculosis department of Beijing Jingmei group general hospital from August 2003 to December 2003. All the patients are diagnosed of coalworker pneumoconiosis complicated with tuberculosis by diagnosis group of occupational disease in Beijing Jingmei group. The pulmonary fibrosis is diagnosed in antituberculosis therapy. All the patients are male. The age is from 51 to 81 years old. The average is 69.9 years old. They are diagnosed in I–II phase of tuberculopneumoconiosis. The disease state is stable and there is no severe complication. The patients don't need continuous oxygen uptake. The patients are randomly divided into training group and control group. There are 36 patients in each group. There are 19 patients in I phase of tuberculopneumoconiosis and 14 patients in II phase of tuberculopneumoconiosis in training group. There are 20 patients in I phase of tuberculopneumoconiosis and 12 patients in II phase of tuberculopneumoconiosis in control group. The patients in two groups all receive antituberculosis therapy. There is no significant difference of general condition between two groups (Table 14.3).

14.4.2.2 Exercise Method

According to application method and announcements introduced in the second section is this chapter, the patients in training group use FG-01 pulmonary function exercise device to do active inspiration training. The training time is 20 min (twice a day) and therapy course can last 4 months.

At first, rehabilitation physicians give training to physicians in ward about application method and assessment method of pulmonary function exercise device. After that, physicians explain the importance of pulmonary function exercise and application method and assessment method of pulmonary function exercise device to the patients. The key point of explanation is to teach the patients to learn to observe the floater in measurement barrel, data reading method in inspiration, the effect of gas measurement floater on deep and slow abdominal respiration. The patients master it and can do exercise by themselves. The patients should try to increase inspiratory capacity in each time and record it. The patients in control group not only receive antituberculosis therapy, but also do exercise by themselves. The physicians should explain the importance of pulmonary function exercise and deep and slow abdominal respiration to the patients.

14.4.2.3 Assessment Criteria

1. Pulmonary function measurement: CHESTGRAPH HI-101 portable pulmonary function apparatus made in Japan is used. Orifice plate flowmeter is used for flow measurement. Flow integral method is used for volume assessment. Volume accuracy is ±3% or ±50 mL. Flow range is 0.05 ± 14 L/s. Volume range is 10 L. The functions are measured at the

Table 14.3 Comparison of general condition in two groups

Group	Stages of pneumoconiosis			Vital capacity breathe hard					Breathlessness activity grade of daily living					
	I	II	(L)	I	II	III	IV	V	0	I	II	III	IV	V
Training group	19	14	2.24 ± 0.64	0	18	11	3	1	0	2	12	18	1	0
Control group	20	12	1.97 ± 0.74	0	14	12	6	0	0	0	17	14	1	0

beginning of the experiment, 1 month after the experiment and at the end of the experiment.

2. Grading assessment of self-awareness of short of breath and breathlessness. According to the methods provided by Diagnosis and Treatment norms of Chinese rehabilitation medicine [18] grading assessment of self-awareness of short of breath and breathlessness is done (Table 14.4).
3. Assessment of daily life ability: According to the methods provided by Diagnosis and Treatment norms of Chinese rehabilitation medicine, daily life ability is assessed (Table 14.5).
4. Blood gas analysis: The blood are draw from the patients in training group and control group at the beginning and the end of the experiment. The blood is used to assess arterial partial pressure of oxygen, partial pressure of carbon dioxide in artery and arterial oxygen saturation.
5. Statistical analysis: Experiment data is analyzed by SPSS6.0 software. T-test is used for comparison between groups and within group.

Table 14.4 Grading standard of self-awareness of short of breath and breathless

Grade	Grading standard
I	No short of breath and breathlessness
II	Slight short of breath and breathlessness
III	Mild short of breath and breathlessness
IV	Obvious short of breath and breathlessness
V	Severe short of breath and breathlessness, Cannot endure

Table 14.5 Assessment standard of daily life assessment

Grade	Grading standard
0	The patients are with lung diseases to varying degrees, but their movements are the same as normal people. It has no effect on daily life and there is no short of breath
I	There is short of breath in labor
II	There is no short of breath in walking in flat ground. When the walking speed is fast or climbing stairs or uphill, the healthy people with the same age cannot feel short of breath, but the patients feel short of breath
III	There is short of breath within one hundred steps
IV	There is short of breath when the patients do minor movements such as speaking or dressing

14.4.2.4 Results

Vital capacity in different stages of experiment includes self-awareness of short of breath and breathlessness, blood gas analysis and daily life ability assessment.

In the 4-months experiment, there are three patients in training group and four patients in control group who quit the experiment because of economic condition. There are 33 patients in training group and 32 patients in control group who complete the experiment.

The results demonstrated that there is significant difference of vital capacity between training group and control group 1 month after experiment and at the end of the experiment ($P < 0.05$). There is significant difference of self-awareness of short of breath and breathlessness between training group and control group ($P < 0.05$). There is no significant difference of daily life ability between two groups.

14.4.2.5 Discussion

Pulmonary interstitial fibrosis can influence pulmonary gas exchange and decrease oxyhemoglobin saturation, reduce metabolic rate, affect functions of various organs and lead to disease [19, 20] It can decrease movement ability and life quality of the patients. There is pulmonary alveoli collapse in obstructive pulmonary disease such as chronic bronchitis, the patients who are long-term in bed or after thoracotomy.

Increasing alveolar ventilation volume, functional residual capacity and replacement rate of functional residual capacity can increase gas exchange rate and oxyhemoglobin saturation. There are several methods to increase these.

1. Decreasing dead space: The anatomical space in respiratory system that cannot be used for gas exchange is about 150 mL. In every respiration, dead space can play function once. The change of tidal volume and respiration frequency have different effects on pulmonary ventilation volume and alveolar ventilation volume.

   Tidal volume and respiration frequency have different impacts on pulmonary ventilation capacity and alveolar ventilation volume. When tidal volume is reduced by half and respiration frequency is doubled, alveolar ventilation volume is decreased obviously. When tidal volume is double and respiration frequency is reduced by half, alveolar ventilation volume is increased obviously in spite that pulmonary ventilation volume is constant. Diaphragm movement can induce big change of thoracic volume. In resting state, fourth fifth of inhaled gas is completed by diaphragm movement. Therefore, the key point of respiratory function exercise is on diaphragm, which means the exercise of inspiratory muscles. The manifestation of diaphragm movement is abdominal respiration mode.

2. Activating reserved lung volume: Human respiratory membrane area is the important factor to influence gas exchange.

   Under normal circumstance, there are 300 million Alveoli in the two lungs. The total diffusion area is about 70 m^2. In resting state, the number of alveoli of gas diffusion is about 180 million. Respiratory membrane area is about 40 m^2. Therefore, reserved area of respiratory membrane is huge. When there is pulmonary atelectasis, lung consolidation, pulmonary emphysema or pulmonary capillary close or obstruction, diffusion area of respiratory membrane is decreased. Through training, reserved lung capacity is activated to compensate the functions.

3. Prevention of pulmonary alveoli collapse to promote re-expand of pulmonary alveoli and alleviate pulmonary fibrosis.

   In the process of formation of pulmonary fibrosis, through respiratory function training, the increase of alveolar ventilation volume not only can prevent pulmonary alveoli collapse and promote re-expand of collapsed pulmonary alveoli, but also can interfere the process that fibrinogen in pulmonary alveoli wall forms fibrin because the increase of alveolar ventilation volume can increase the dilation degree of pulmonary alveoli, which can alleviate the effect of fibrosis on the dilation degree of pulmonary alveoli.

In short, diaphragm exercise can increase thoracic capacity and promote the formation of deep and slow abdominal respiration pattern, which can increase alveolar ventilation volume, increase oxyhemoglobin saturation and prevent lung complications.

FG-01 pulmonary function exercise device is a portable active inspiratory muscles exercise device. Inspiration volume measurement barrel can make the patients see their own progress of inspiration volume in exercise. The progress can be marked with Vernier. The patients can encourage themselves to increase inspiration volume. Gas flow limited device can help the patients to form deep and slow respiration. Long-term exercise can increase alveolar ventilation volume and oxyhemoglobin saturation. Overseas, in clinic, there is an equipment called pulmometer that is used for respiratory function rehabilitation of the patients in preoperative preparation and postoperative rehabilitation of surgeries [21] in heart, lung, abdominal cavity or thoracoabdominal combined surgery and the patients with neuromuscular diseases.

Researches show that inhaled gas volume displayed in exercise device in inspiration exercise is significantly correlated [22] two with vital capacity and inspiratory reserve volume measured by pulmonary function apparatus. Through exercise, myodynamia and endurance of inspiratory muscles can compensate the defect of inspiratory function restriction induced by pulmonary interstitial fibrosis. In recent years, pulmonary quantifier is used for inspiration practice, which is important for prevention or treatment of pulmonary atelectasis. Its effect is better than intermittent positive pressure ventilation and other obsolete methods such as blowing bottle that may aggravate pulmonary atelectasis. From the weak patients or the patients who lie in bed for a long time to the patients with stroke, spinal cord injury or myodystrophy, they all can obtain support from these devices, because all the patients have pulmonary alveoli collapse. In the early phase after surgery, pulmonary function of the patients is injured obviously and vital capacity is decreased greatly. Respiratory dysfunction rehabilitation is meaningful for respiration tract diseases. Arthritis, ankylosing spondylitis, myodystrophy, weak, stroke and spinal cord injury can lead to ventilation insufficiency. The pulmonary complication is the main reason of death. Therefore, respiratory function exercise has preventive and therapeutic effect on lung complications of the patients.

References

1. Minyaev VI. Temporal and spatial parameters of voluntary (assigned) human respiratory movements during various types of chemoreceptor stimulation. Bull Exp Biol Med. 1977;83(1):1–3.
2. Rossi N, Kolobow T, Aprigliano M, Tsuno K, Giacomini M. Intratracheal pulmonary ventilation at low airway pressures in a ventilator-induced model of acute respiratory failure improves lung function and survival. Chest. 1998;114(4):97–9.
3. Menezes KKP, Nascimento LR, Ada L, Polese JC, Avelino PR, Teixeira-Salmela LF. Respiratory muscle training increases respiratory muscle strength and reduces respiratory complications after stroke: a systematic review. J Physiother. 2016;62(3):138–44.
4. Costa D, Sampaio LM, de Lorenzzo VA, Jamami M, Damaso AR. Evaluation of respiratory muscle strength and thoracic and abdominal amplitudes after a functional reeducation of breathing program for obese individuals. Rev Lat Am Enfermagem. 2003;11(2):156–60.
5. Gaspari RJ, Paydarfar D. Respiratory recovery following organophosphate poisoning in a rat model is suppressed by isolated hypoxia at the point of apnea. Toxicology. 2012;302(2-3):242–6.
6. Smith U, Ryan JW. Pinocytotic vesicles of the pulmonary endothelial cell. Chest. 1971;59(5):12–5.
7. Toyama H, Hoshi K, Kobayashi T, Hashimoto K, Suzuki H, Matsukawa S, Hashimoto Y. The efficacy of postural drainage in a case of pulmonary edema following cholecystectomy. Masui. 1997;46(11):1503–7.
8. Jie C, Zhan H, Changying L, et al. Pulmonary function training in elderly patients with pulmonary insufficiency after pulmonary complications and course of disease. Chin Clin Rehabil. 2004;8(5):842–3.
9. Tockman MS, Pearson JD, Curb JD. Rapid cliclin in FEM:a new risk factor for coronary heart disease mortality. Int J Hypertens. 1995;151(02):121–6.
10. Singh S, Sircar SS, Singh KP. Are ventilatory impriements related to early onset and long history of diabetes? Int J Hypertens. 1995;93(12):7–10.
11. Guorong L. Study on the relationship between pulmonary function and extrapulmonary disease. Med Rev. 2002;8(7):400–1.
12. Nianqiu H, Shan L. Modern elderly respiratory disease. Beijing: People's Military Medical Publishing House; 1998. p. 109–12.
13. Yongxing W, yanfeng Y. Chronic obstructive pulmonary disease in patients with stable quality of life and pulmonary function relationship. J Chin Clin Rehabil. 2002;6(19):2851–2.
14. Xianqiao J, Lishuang H, Wenhua C. Respiratory rehabilitation treatment of patients with chronic obstructive pulmonary disease dyspnea, pulmonary function and exercise capacity. Journal of Chinese Clinical Rehabilitation. 2002;6(5):662–3.
15. Jingru Z. Physiology. Beijing: People's Medical Publishing House; 1998. p. 178–9.
16. Cahalin LP ue, Braga M, Matsuo Y, et al. Efficacy of diaphragmatic breathing in persons with chronic obstructive pulmonary disease: a review of the literature. J Cardiopulm Rehabil Prev. 2002;1(1):7–21.
17. Dengkun N. Rehabilitation medicine. 2nd ed. Beijing: People's Health Press; 2001. p. 10.
18. The Medical Department of Ministry of Health of the People's Republic of China. The Medical Department of Ministry of Health of the People's Republic of China. First volume. Beijing: Huaxia Press; 1998. p. 1–2.
19. De Vries J, Seebregts A, Drent M. Assessing health status and quality of life in idiopathic pulmonary fibrosis: which measure should be used? Respir Med. 2000;94(03):273–8.
20. De Vries J, Kessels BL, Drent M. Quality of life of idiopathic pulmonary fibrosis patients. Eur Respir J. 2001;17(05):954–61.
21. Bastin R, Moraine JJ, Bardocsky G. Incentive spirometry performance. A reliable indicator of pulmonary function in the early postoperative period after lobectomy? Chest. 1997;111(3):559–63.
22. Huijun Z, Yadong L. Coal workers pneumoconiosis with pulmonary infection on lung function. Chin Occup Med. 2002;(5):39–40.

Rehabilitation Therapy of Neurological Training of Cognitive Disorder

15

15.1 The Concept of Cognitive Disorder and the Mechanism of Memory Formation

The basis of cognition is one of the normal functions of brains. Any factor that can induce abnormity of cortex function and structure can lead to cognitive dysfunction. For example, after brain disease or brain injury, except motor and sensation dysfunctions, there is cognitive dysfunction to varying degrees, which can affect self-care ability, life quality and self-security [1] directly. The structure and function of brain are complicated and there is relationship among different cognitive disorders. Therefore, cognitive disorder is one of the most difficult clinical problems. At present, there is no effective therapy method and rehabilitation measure.

15.1.1 Basic Concept of Cognitive Disorder

15.1.1.1 Concept

Cognition is the process that human brain acquires information from the outside world and forms functions such as understanding, memory, speech and execution to acquire knowledge and apply them through processing such as acquisition, code, manipulation, extraction and use [2]. Cognitive disorder means there are one or several functions that are injured. If there two or more functions that are injured, it may influence daily movement or social ability, which is called dementia.

There are many types of cognitive disorders, including disorders of attention, memory and problem handling. There are subtypes in each type. The type of cognitive disorder is closely related to the part of cerebral injury. Right prefrontal lobe injury can lead to difficulties in attention, short-term memory and plan, indifference and lags in response. Injuries of left parietal lobe association area and callosum can lead to apraxia in different areas. Right parietal lobe injury can lead to spatial relationship disorder. Injuries in junctional zone among parietal lobe, temporal lobe and occipital lobe can lead to various kinds of agnosia.

15.1.1.2 The Common Types of Cognitive Disorder

1. Aphasia: if there are no visual and auditory defects and no muscles paralysis of vocal organs such as mouth, pharynx and throat and ataxia, the patients cannot understand the speech of others and themselves. They cannot declare the meanings. They don't understand or write the sentence they mastered before.
2. Agnosia: after brain injury, if there is no visual, auditory and touch defects, intelligence or consciousness disorder, they cannot recognize the objects that they are familiar before, but they can recognize them through

W. Zhao, *Rehabilitation Therapeutics of the Neurological Training*,
https://doi.org/10.1007/978-981-13-0812-3_15

other senses. For example, the patients see the glasses, but they don't know it is glasses. Only if they touch the glasses or they use it to watch books, they know it is a glasses.

3. Apraxia: after brain diseases, if there is no motor and sensation dysfunction, intelligence or consciousness disorder, the patients cannot complete the movements they do before through habitual movements. For example, they cannot blink, bulge cheek, dress and drink water, but they can complete these movements carelessly.
4. Dementia: This is the most severe type of cognitive disorder. It is an acquired and continuous disturbance of intelligence syndrome induced by chronic brain function deficiency.

Cognitive disorder has an effect on ability of daily life of the patients to varying degrees. Because understanding and memory ability decline, the patients require other people or special care to live [3]. Sometimes, the influence of cognitive disorder is bigger than the influence of physical dysfunction on the patients [4]. If the cognition function is normal, the patients with motor dysfunction can figure out problems with the help of assistive device, but they don't lose the abilities of communication and brainwork. On the other hand, cognition function has an effect on the rehabilitation effect of motor function, because the patients with cognitive dysfunction are hard to cooperate with rehabilitation training that are mainly active movements and are hard to promote plasticity and functional reorganization of central nerves. The effects are not ideal.

Therefore, early prevention, early detection and early therapy are meaningful for promotion of rehabilitation effect of cognitive dysfunction, enhancement of rehabilitation of motor dysfunction of limbs and improvement of life quality.

There are many types of cognitive disorder. In this chapter, we only discuss the mechanism of memory and understanding ability disorder and rehabilitation training method of neurological training.

15.1.2 The Mechanism of Memory Formation

Memory is the basic physiological function, including memorization, storage, recognition and reminiscence. If any part of the four processes is damaged, or they are all damaged at the same time, there is memory impairment.

15.1.2.1 The Definition of Memory

Memory is the process that the objects that are storage by the brain through perception, analysis, understanding and handling can be retrieved when required.

15.1.2.2 The Process of Memory Formation

The process of memory formation can be divided into several stages.

1. Registration is the process that the objects are marked in the brain through perception and learning.
2. Storage and consolidation is the memory that is transformed from short-term and unstable state to long-term stable state.
3. Recognition is the process that the perceived and experienced objects are recognized when they are perceived or experienced again.
4. Retrieval is the process that the trace in the brain reappear.

15.1.2.3 The Types of Memory

According to the duration time, memory is divided into three types.

1. Sensory memory is also called instant memory, which is formed with instant impression.
2. Short-term memory is also called short-term storage or the first memory, which is formed with experienced events with some mild stimulation.
3. Long-term memory is also called long-term storage or the secondary memory, which is formed with experienced events with some strong stimulation. There are two types of long-term memory.

- Declarative memory is the memory of fact, pilot and materials that are related to specific time, location.
- Nondeclarative memory is also called program memory that is related to actual operation or practice. It includes episodic memory and semantic memory. Episodic memory is individual experience associated with time and location. Semantic memory is the memory of organized knowledge such as concept, formula, semantics and grammar.

15.1.2.4 Amnesia

The patients are completely or partially unable to retrieve the objects in brain, which is called amnesia.

1. Anterograde amnesia is that the memory after attack cannot be formed.
2. Retrograde amnesia is that the patients cannot recall the experience in previous period.
3. Post-traumatic amnesia (PTA) is that the memory from cerebral injury to recovered continuous memory are totally lost.

15.1.2.5 Brain Functional Orientation of Memory

There are many areas in brain associated with memory.

1. Association cortex is the cortex that doesn't include sensation and motor areas.
   (a) Frontal cortex is associated with short-term memory.
   (b) Parietal lobe is associated with location memory.
   (c) The bottom of groove temporalis superior is associated with face memory.
   (d) Lateral surface of temporal cortex is associated with history memory.
   (e) Gyrus temporalis superior is associated with music memory.
   (f) Amygdaloid nucleus is associated with expression memory.
2. Hippocampus: Hippocampus is an important structure associated with memory such as long-term and short-term memory, declarative memory, and semantic memory.
3. Neural circuits of memory
   (a) Inside limbic system: areas parolfactoria and gyrus subcallosus—cingulate gyrus—hippocampus—fornix—corpus albicans of hypothalamus—tractus mamillothalamicus—nucleus anterior thalami—cingulate gyrus
   (b) Basolateral limbic system: pars orbitalis cortex of frontal lobe—prefrontal cortex—amygdaloid nucleus—dorsal medial nucleus of thalamus—pars orbitalis cortex of frontal lobe

   The first loop is associated with spatial memory and the second is associated with emotional memory. Both are associated with declarative memory. The loop of non-declarative memory includes the loop of extrapyramidal system between brainstem and cerebellum including epencephalon.
4. Memory characteristic of left and right cerebral hemisphere: Generally, left hemisphere process language, concept, symbol, time and conceptual work such as calculation and inference. Left hemisphere is usually associated with semantic memory. Right hemisphere is associated with spatial discrimination, music understanding and imaginal thinking. Right hemisphere is associated with episodic memory.

15.1.2.6 The Mechanism of Memory

The mechanism of memory is closely associated with neurotomy, neurophysiology and neurophysics.

1. Neurotomy: some research found that the neural basis of memory is mainly local neuronal circuit formed by loop structure of short axon neurons. It is associated with learning and memory. Mental retardation may be induced by the abnormity of these structures.
2. Neurophysiological mechanism: the plasticity of neurons or synapses.

(a) Neural circuit of memory is neural cells connected by synapses. Under certain circumstance, the transmission efficiency of synapse can be changed or the new synapse can be formed, which is plasticity of neurons or synapses. The synaptic plasticity usually exists in chemical synapses and is the potential basis of information storage.
(b) The types of synaptic plasticity: combination plasticity includes synaptic morphological change, formation of new synapses and establishment of conduction function. It is associated with long-term memory. Transmission plasticity is the change of transmission efficiency. It is associated with memory process that lasts several hours or several weeks.
(c) Establishment of conditioned reflex: Ivan Petrovich thought that conditioned reflex is the results of connection of two stimulus in brain. It is one of the basis of neurophysiology of memory.

3. Physical mechanism includes bionic memory and submolecule mechanism of memory.

Some physicists deemed that computers use ferromagnetic material to store information and its common physical features are many kinds of oscillation with the same oscillation frequency. Ferromagnetic material and DNA macromolecule have this nature. Therefore, DNA is the memory molecule and it can storage and playback information.

In addition, memory is related to neurobiochemistry mechanism. For example, in learning and memory, RNA synthesis is increased. Inhibition of RNA synthesis has an inhibitory effect on memory.

15.2 Rehabilitation Therapy of Neurological Training of Cognitive Disorder

Most cognition rehabilitation training methods are used for cognitive impairment in one aspect. Before training, according to the results of cognitive assessment, the degrees of cognitive disorder are analyzed and classified. Specific rehabilitation schedule is designed to highlight the purposiveness and interest.

In the process of rehabilitation training, according to the progress of the patients with cognitive impairments and the principle of step by step, rehabilitation physicians adjust training difficulties and content repeatedly to get satisfying clinical effect.

15.2.1 Assessment of Cognitive Disorder

There are four kinds of neuropsychology examination to assess cognitive disorder such as screening method, special inspection method, test of battery and functional examination method. All these are introduced in associated books of rehabilitation assessment. We only introduce screening method and behavioral memory examination in this chapter.

15.2.1.1 Screening Method

Screening method is a rapid examination method of neural comprehensive functions. Generally, screening method can detect whether there is cognitive disorder or not in the patients, but the results cannot be the basis of specific diagnosis. Clinical rehabilitation physicians cannot diagnose the patients with certain type of cognitive disorder through screening method or merely using the results of screening. Through screening, we can find out whether there are organic pathologic changes of brain or not, which can provide basis for further examination.

The common cognitive function screening scale includes mini mental state examination (Table 15.1) and cognition capacity screening examination.

1. Mini mental state examination is suitable for simple screening of cognitive disorder, which is the diagnosis basis of cognitive function impairment. There are 30 questions in MMSE [5] includes orientation, short-term memory, instant memory, attention, calculation, language and

Table 15.1 Mini mental state examination (MMSE)

Number	Question	Right	Wrong	Number	Question	Right	Wrong
1.	What year is this?	1	0	16.	86—7 (79)	1	0
2.	What season is this?	1	0	17.	79—7 (72)	1	0
3.	What's the date today?	1	0	18.	73—7 (66)	1	0
4.	What day is today?	1	0	19.	Recall: ball	1	0
5.	What month is this	1	0	20.	Recall: national flag	1	0
6.	Province (city)	1	0	21.	Recall: trees	1	0
7.	County (district)	1	0	22.	Identification: watch	1	0
8.	Village and town (street)	1	0	23.	Identification: pencil	1	0
9.	Which floor are we at?	1	0	24.	Repeat: 44 Chinese guardian lions	1	0
10.	What is here?	1	0	25.	Close eyes according to card	1	0
11.	Repeat: ball	1	0	26.	Hold the paper using right hand 1	0	
12.	Repeat: national flag	1	0	27.	Fold the paper	1	0
13.	Repeat: trees	1	0	28.	Put on the thigh	1	0
14.	100–7 (93)	1	0	29.	Say a complete sentence	1	0
15.	93–7 (86)	1	0	30.	Picture making	1	0

operation. Each examination takes 5–8 min. The patients get one mark through one right answer and the total scores are 0–30 marks.

Assessment standard: The patients with the mark that is less than 17 are in illiteracy level. The patients with the mark that is 17–20 are primary school level and the patients with the mark that is 20–24 are in middle school level.

Announcements: there are some key points in assessment. Year, month and season: the solar or lunar chronology are all right. Continuous subtrahend: if the previous answer is wrong and the next answer is right, the answer is right. When the subjects repeat the words such as balls, national flag and trees, the examiners only say it once and the subjects repeat them out of order. Under this circumstance, the answer is right. When repeating 44 Chinese guardian lions, the examiners only say it once and the subjects repeat the words clearly. Under this circumstance, the answer is right. In the 25th item, the card is given to the subjects and the subjects are asked to do movements according to the card. In order to avoid someone's taboo, the movement "please raise your left leg" can be changed to "please open your month". If the subjects answer that they won't do it, the answer is wrong. If the subjects are illiterates, the score of 25th item is zero.

2. Cognitive capacity screening examination (CCSE) is a new examination. Because cognition includes consciousness, attention, presentation, memory, language and thinking, and cognitive disorder is usually the disorders in these aspects, CCSE [6] can be used for the assessment of cognitive disorder. The specific contents refer to Table 15.2.

Assessment standard: one score for one right answer. The total score is 30. The score that is no more than 20 is defined as abnormity.

15.2.1.2 Behavioral Memory Test

Rivermead behavioral memory test (RBMT [7]) is used to assess memory ability of daily life with higher reliability and validity. There are eleven practical tests.

1. Remember the surname and given name: the examiners let the patients see a picture and tell them the surname and given name on this picture. A moment later, the examiners ask them the surname and given name on this picture. During this process, the examiners let the patients see other things to distract them.

   Score: if the patients answer the right surname and given name, they can get two scores. If they only answer surname or given

Table 15.2 Cognitive capacity screening examination (CCSE)

Serial number	Content	Serial number	Content
1	What day is today?	16	What is the opposite of big? What is the opposite of hard?
2	WHAT month is now?	17	If orange and banana belong to fruit, what red and blue belong to?
3	WHAT'S the date today?	18	What is five scores and two scores?
4	WHAT year is this?	19	What is the first word I want you to remember just now?
5	Where is this place?	20	What is the second word?
6	Please say 872	21	What is the third word?
7	Please say the three numbers reversely	21	What is the fourth word?
8	Please say 6371	23	110 Minus 7 equals?
9	Please listen to 694, please count the numbers from one to ten and repeat 694	24	Then minus 7 equals?
10	Please listen to 8143, please count the numbers from one to ten and repeat 8143	25	Then minus 7 equals?
11	Count from Sunday to Monday	26	Then minus 7 equals?
12	9 Plus 3 equals?	27	Then minus 7 equals?
13	Plus 6 equals?	28	Then minus 7 equals?
14	18 Minus 5 equals? Please remember these words "cap, car, tree and 26" and I will ask you a moment later	29	Then minus 7 equals?
15	If the opposite of quick is slow, what is the opposite of upper?	30	Then minus 7 equals?

name, they will get one score. Otherwise, they only get zero.

2. Remember the hidden objects: the examiners lend personal tissue, key chain, teacup and therapy card to the patients, hide them into drawer or therapy car and do some movements to distract the patients. A moment later, the examiners ask the patients where these objects are.

   Score: if the patients can point out the right location, they can get one score. Otherwise, they only get zero.

3. Remember the appointed application: The examiners tell the patients the appointment time is 20 min before see the doctor. The examiners set the alarm clock 20 min later. Twenty minutes later, when they hear the alarm, the patients make an appointment. The doctors can say "could you tell me when you can come to see me from now on?"

   Score: if the patients answer correctly when the bell rings, they can get one score. Otherwise, they only get zero.

4. Remember a short path: under direct vision of the patients, the examiners take an envelope, walk a path that can be divided into five segments such as chair-door-before the window-therapy desk-book table, and put the envelop on the book table. The examiners take the envelop from the table, put it in front of the patients and ask them to do it.

   Score: if the patients can do it in the same way, they can get one score. Otherwise, they only get zero.

5. A moment later, remember a short path: The method is the same as the fourth. A moment later, the patients are asked to repeat the path. During this process, the examiners talk with the patients to distract them.

   Score: if the patients can memorize all of these, they can get one score. Otherwise, they only get zero.

6. Remember one mission: the patients are asked to observe the right place of the envelop.

   Score: whether the patients answer the question immediately or later, they can get one score. Otherwise, they only get zero.

7. Learn a new skill: the examiners use calculator or electronic watch that can be set with time and date for the patients to learn the method of ascertaining month, day and hour. The procedures are as follows: pressing the setting button, inputing month, inputing day, pressing the date button, inputing time, pressing the time button, pressing time button, and press reset button to eliminate all inputs. The patients can try three times.

   Score: if the patients can succeed once in three times, they can get one score. Otherwise, they only get zero.
8. Orientation: the examiners ask the patients the following questions: What year is this? What month is this? What day (of the week) is it today? What's the date today? Where are we now? Which city are we in? How old are you? When is your birthday? Who is the prime minister? Who is the state president now?

   Score: if the patients can answer all the questions correctly, they can get one score. Otherwise, they only get zero.
9. Date: the examiners ask the patients the fourth question in the eighth item and write down whether the answer is right or wrong.

   Score: if the answer is right, the patients get one score. Otherwise, they only get zero.
10. Face discrimination: The examiners let the patients to see five pictures of face (5 s for one picture). After that, the examiners asked the patients questions. What is the gender of the face? What is the age of the face, more than 40 years old or less than 40 years old? The examiners show the patients ten pictures of face and there are five picture that the patients watched before. The patients are asked to pick the five out.

    Score: if the patients answer all the questions correctly, they can get one score. Otherwise, they only get zero.
11. Picture recognition: The examiners let the patients to see ten object drawings of bar (5 s for one drawing). After that, the examiners asked the patients to say the name of the object in each drawing. A moment later, the examiners ask the patients to pick out ten drawings that them watched before from all the twenty drawings.

    Score: If the patients answer all the questions correctly, they can get one score. Otherwise, they only get zero.

Except the maximal score is two in the first item, the maximal score of other items is one. The total score is 12.

For normal people, the total score is 9–12. The average is 10–12. The up-down error is 1.16.

The patients with brain injury cannot complete at least three items. The total score is 0–9. The average is 3.76. The up-down error is 2.84.

15.2.2 Rehabilitation Therapy of Cognitive Disorder

Rehabilitation therapy of cognitive disorder is difficult and the therapeutic effect is not ideal, but there are many therapeutic methods. In the clinical practice for more than 10 years, the author use rehabilitation therapy in three aspects and obtain some experience. The author introduced these experiences to everyone to start a discussion.

15.2.2.1 The Mechanism of Rehabilitation of Neurological Training of Cognition

There are three aspects in the mechanism of rehabilitation of neurological training of cognition.

1. Development of neurons and synapses potential to recover memory capacity.

   Neurons and synapses involved in memory have plasticity ability. Reinforced memory training induced by Daoyin technique can promote neurons and synapses around injured area to play functions in order to replace the functions of injured cells and recover lost memory.
2. Open the gate of memory and unblock memory loop.

   There are many links such as memorization, storage, recognition and reminiscence to form memory, especially the neural circuit of memory such as inside limbic system: areas parolfactoria and gyrus subcallosus—cingulate gyrus—hippocampus—fornix—corpus albicans of hypothalamus—tractus mamillothalamicus—nucleus anterior thalami—cingulate gyrus. If there is any loop is in disorder, there will be memory loss or memory function disorder to varying degrees. Therefore, the author think that if we take memory loop as memory electricity, memory electricity flows through every part, which can be defined as gate. When the gate is with pathological lesion, the gate closes and memory electricity cannot flow through it, which can induce memory impairments to varying degrees. Potential development and functional recovery to promote incomplete injured cells can re-open the gate to make memory electricity flow again. After that, memory can be recovered to varying degrees.

Not only cognition reinforcement training of neurological training can open memory gate, but also active movement to develop central neural potential may promote the open of memory gate and recover memory function, because there is positive correlation relationship between motor function and memory capacity.

3. The physical and biochemical mechanisms to recover ionic balance inside and outside memory cells and maintain permeability and electric activity of cell membrane.

   Memory cells are DNA macromolecules with magnetism that can be used for memorization, storage, recognition and reminiscence. In addition, functions of central nervous cells can be achieved by electrical activity. Under some pathological circumstances, the functions of proton pump are injured and the permeability of cell membrane is changed. Potassium ion overflows and sodium, chloridion and calcium flow into the cells, which can induce cell injury.

According to physical and biochemical characteristics of memory cells, electricity and magnetic wave interference can change permeability of cell membrane to promote the recovery of intracellular physiological status.

15.2.2.2 Rehabilitation Method of Neurological Training of Cognition

It includes reinforced memory training, motor potential development training, physical therapy and acupuncture.

1. Reinforced memory training: The mechanism of memory includes neural circuits and DNA memory protein theory. The memory is formed with some kind of matter. Easy for discussion, we called the matter that can store memory "memory matter." The cells that can produce memory matter are called memory cells. The formation and the quantity of memory are closely related to the stimulation degree of event on memory cells. The stronger the stimulation is, the longer the memory lasts.

   Reinforced memory training can reinforce the steps in the memory process such as memorization, storage, recognition and reminiscence through reinforcing the training of intended memory in order to promote undead central neural memory cells to recover functions and promote normal memory cells around injured area to play functions to replace the functions of injured cells.

   The memory formed by brain cells is the same as joint motion formed by muscles dominated by brain. They are one kind of efficiency. Six-step Daoyin technique can be used to promote brain potential development and recover lost motor function. Therefore, on the basis of regulation of mind and breathing, memory training can recover memory functions.

   Six-step Daoyin technique combined with biological feedback technique achieved objective indicator display of the effects of Daoyin technique. Therefore, the patients can do the training with purpose and the patients can see their training progress. Through setting surpassing goal, training interest can be increased and the training effects are enhanced.

   On the basis of this ultimate principle, cognition training system of neurological training is developed, which is called cognition training equipment for short. This system is equipped with automatic and manual memory training and can store plenty of pictures such as scenery, objects and person. It can be used for the training of reinforced instant memory, short-term memory, sequential memory, attention, figure, relative figure, memory game, reading, restatement and commander execution. Moreover, the system with self-comparison can display the results on the fluorescent screen in twinkled curve real-timely.

The specific training method: in a quiet and lucifugal warm room, the patients sit in front of cognition training equipment (Fig. 15.1). The therapists choose the content and music in the operation screen (three pictures in one group). For example, the therapists choose the great wall picture and light music. The therapists guide the patients to regulate mind and breathing to eliminate distracting thoughts. The therapists concentrate on the great wall picture on the screen and tell the patients this is great wall. The therapists guide the patients to notice the characteristics of the picture such as serpentine wall, tower, crenel and the surrounding mountains. The patients are asked to keep their eyes away from the picture twice, then regulate mind and breathing and stare at the panorama and characteristics of pictures for 1 min. The therapists use the same method to train the patients in the next two pictures. After completing all the three pictures such as great wall, Mount Huang and the Imperial Palace. There are three selection boxes under the picture. There are three words such as tower, great wall and the top of the wall under the picture. The patients click the box and choose the word. The selection system can be compared in the system. If the result is right, it is displayed in twinkled curve. Exploded fireworks are showed in the screen and the voice "congratulations, you are right" is played to the patients. If the result is wrong, the voice "never mind, try again" is played to the patients. The patients get 33.3 scores for each right answer. The total score of three right answers is 100. In the second training, on the basis of the first training, a baseline is displayed in one side of fluorescent screen and the other side of fluorescent screen show the pictures in the second training that are totally different from these in the previous group. The curve will increase one third after answering one question. If all the questions are answered correctly, or the curve surpasses the baseline, exploded fireworks are showed in the screen and the voice "congratulations, you are right" is played to the patients.

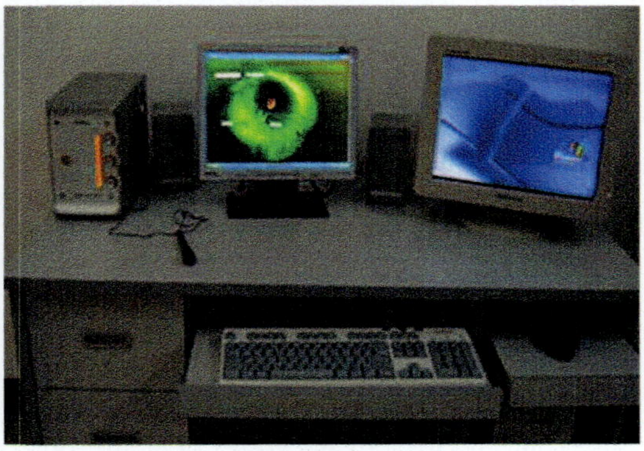

Fig. 15.1 Independently developed cognition training equipment

The training time is 30 min (once a day) and there are 30 times in one therapy course. The patients can do multiple courses of therapy.

2. Reinforcing autonomous movement training: Exercise can improve functions of nervous system, make the brain clear and make the action smart. Exercise can enhance the functions of various systems such as digestion, circulation and respiration. Exercise can meet the oxygen requirements of the body, promote tissue metabolism, and supply sufficient nutrition for all the parts including nervous system. Meanwhile, the brain needs the stimulation of movements to enhance reaction and judgement and increase memory and intelligence. Therefore, exercise can build the body and enhance intelligence.

Psychologists deemed that intelligence is developed with body movements. There is close relationship between exercise and intelligence. Generally, the movement is normal in the children with normal intelligence or more. If the body movements of children are later than the children in the same age, the children have the danger of mental retardation.

In fact, almost all rehabilitation methods of neurological training are based on the recovery of central nervous system to recover lost motor function. In the actual work of clinical rehabilitation, we noticed that there is position correlation between rehabilitation effect and the understanding of the patients and there is positive correlation between learning ability and memory capacity. Rehabilitation training of active movements not only can recover lost motor function, but also can improve cognitive status.

(a) Potential development training: Potential development training devices of upper limbs, lower limbs, the trunk, balance, tibialis anterior muscle, hamstring muscles and walking balance are used. On the basis of regulation of mind and breathing, six-step Daoyin technique is used to do neural potential development training of the corresponding parts (the second section of the third chapter). When the patients are guided to surpass the designed goal, the training not only promote plasticity of motor center in brain cortex, and also promote memory cells in these areas, because the patients use willpower and intelligence to overcome difficulties.

The training time is 25 min (once a day) and there are 30 times in one therapy course. The patients can do multiple courses of therapy.

(b) Motor program reestablishment training: Neurological training equipment is applied and normal method or Daoyin technique of guiding collaterals through meridians in traditional Chinese medicine is used to do motor program reestablishment training of all joints and associated movements. In the process of establishing single joint motor program training, the time limit of every screen is 40 s. The baseline of agonistic muscle and antagonistic muscle is set at the level that the patients are easy to reach. For example, in the training of wrist extension, the baseline of wrist extensor is set at 60 μV and that of wrist flexor is at 20 μV. The patients are guided to make the curve of wrist extensor surpass 60 μV and make the curve of wrist flexor under 20 μV. The patients are encouraged to maintain in this level for 25–30 s. During the training process, the patients are asked to use brain to control wrist extension, analyze the process and find the way to meet the training requirements in order to develop intelligence and recover memory.

After completing joint motion training, the patients are guided to watch the altitude and duration time of agonistic muscles and antagonistic muscles curves. After completing the next training of joint motion, the patients are helped to recall altitude and duration time of signal curve to enhance memory effect.

The training time is 50 min (once a day) and there are 30 times in one therapy course. The patients can do multiple courses of therapy.

3. Transcranial magnetic stimulation and electrical therapy: cell functions are that cell membrane permeability and change of ion concentration inside and outside cell membrane can maintain normal membrane potential through polarization, depolarization and repolarization. External electrical field and magnetic field can recover cell functions through recovering normal permeability and polarization of cell membrane.

The frequently used magnetic stimulation methods for brain in clinic are as follows:

(a) Transcranial magnetic stimulation (TMS): In recent years, the physiological effect of TMS on brain functions is highly focused. TMS can change physiological process in brain through generating painless induced current to activate cortex. On the other hand, TMS can treat nervous system diseases through changing the excitability of local cortex, cortex metabolism and blood flow. In clinic, it is used to treat motor disorder diseases, Parkinson's disease, myodystony, epilepsia, aphasia, cognitive disorder and depression. TMS has positive effect on peripheral nerve disease. In addition, it is suitable for the treatment of uroclepsia, uroschesis and frequent micturition.

With proper stimulation, transcranial magnetic stimulation is safe. Frameless stereo positioning and navigation transcranial magnetic stimulation can increase accuracy of stimulation part, which is good for increase of therapeutic effect. This research is done by Wangyong in Integrated Traditional and Western Medicine Department of Jinan Military General Hospital.

The action principle of transcranial magnetic stimulation is that rapid pulse current that is generated by induced electric field due to time varying magnetic field can stimulate coil to generate instant high-intensity magnetic field that can penetrate skull and induce secondary current in peripheral neural tissue. The intensity of magnetic field depends on stimulation frequency, the intensity, coil shape and coil orientation. Spatial resolution of TMS is 1 cm and depth of penetration is about 2 cm. Repeated TMS (rTMS) generates different effects because of different stimulation frequencies, even opposite effect. Low frequency rTMS (less than 1 Hz) stimulation can inhibit excitability of neural cells and cortex activities. High frequency rTMS (5–25 Hz) stimulation can increase cell excitability and cortex activities.

At present, the maximal side effect of TMS is epileptic seizure. Potential long-term safety problem requires further investigation. The therapeutic effect of cognitive disorder, especially long-term effect requires further observation.

The therapy time is 20–40 min (five times a week) and one therapy course takes 2 weeks.

(b) Cranial electrotherapy stimulation (CES): Low intensity minor electricity is used to stimulate brain through temporal skull. Research indicated that positive pole stimulation can excite brain cortex and negative pole stimulation can decrease the excitability of brain cortex. Both positive pole stimulation and negative pole stimulation contribute to functional recovery of the patients with stroke. It can be used to treat anxiety, depression, insomnia and children disease. There is no side effect.

Some reports demonstrated that CES can promote secretion of acetyl choline and 5-hydroxytryptamin. Acetyl choline can promote conduction speed of central nerves, enhance memory ability and improve brain functions. 5-Hydroxytryptamin is involved in many physiological functions and pathological states.

The therapy time is 20–60 min (once a day) and one therapy course takes 4 weeks.

4. Acupuncture therapy to restore consciousness, regulate mind, and promote blood circulation to remove meridian obstruction.
   (a) Basic therapy takes governor meridian, Foot shaoyang and Foot shaoyin. The main major acupuncture points are ophryon, Baihui acupoint with Sishengcong, Shangxing with Shenting, Fengchi, Taixi, Xuanzhong, Hegu and Taichong. Adjunct acupuncture points are Neiguan and Keshu in the patients with collateral obstruction by blood stasis syndrome. Acupuncture manipulation: Catharsis is used in Hegu and Taichong. Tonifying method is used in Taixi and Xuanzhong. mild Reinforcing-reducing method is used in other acupuncture points. Interval entwisting needle or acusector is used in acupuncture points of head.

The mechanism: Governor meridian lead Luonao, Baihui, Shenting, Sahngxing and ophryon to restore consciousness and regulate mind. Fengchi regulates Qi and blood in head. Taixi and Xuanzhong can benefit brain. Hegu and Taichong promote blood circulation to remove meridian obstruction. Sishencong is the acupuncture point to strengthen brain and benefit intelligence.

(b) Other therapies: head needle method: the therapists choose the top middle line, anterior oblique line of vertex-temporal, the oblique line of vertex-temporal and use two inches acupuncture needle to penetrate into galea aponeurotica. The therapists manipulate the needle quickly to make the point warm. Electroacupuncture stimulation can also be used. The needle is retained for 40 min. Auricular needle method: the therapists choose subcortex, forehead, occipital part, temporal part, heart, liver, kidney, endocrine and Shenmen and use acupuncture needle to stimulate 2–4 acupuncture points. Hvacupoint-injection therapy: the therapists choose Fengfu, Fengchi, Shenshu, Foot Three Li, Sanyinjiao and use compound angelic powder for injection, Danshen injection, citicoline or aceglutamide for injection. Every acupuncture point is injected 0.5–1.0 mL (once on alternate days).

15.2.2.3 Other Training Methods of Rehabilitation of Cognitive Disorder

The patients with cognitive disorder should do comprehensive rehabilitation training as soon as possible to alleviate symptoms and postpone progress of symptom. It includes memory training, thinking training, attention training and perceptive training. According to the damage condition of the patients, proper individual training schedule is designed, which can be applied with rehabilitation training of neurological training of cognitive disorder to obtain better effect.

Memory impairment is the prominent clinical manifestation. There is short-term memory impairment in the early phase. There is long-term memory impairment in the middle phase. There is memory loss in late phase. Memory training can maintain original memory or alleviate the decrease of memory.

Memory training is the movement exercise of brain cells. This kind of exercise can prevent brain aging. Epidemiological investigation found that occurrence rate of cognitive disorder in old patients with high standard of culture is higher than that in old patients with low standard of culture. For the old patients with cognitive disorder, memory training should emphasize on training process. The key point is the training process of thinking and memory, but not the content. The common training methods are as follows:

1. Maintain or repeat: Memory method of reading, memorization and rehearsal.

   The therapists read the content aloud, read it silently, analyze and memorize it. The therapists ask the patients to retell the content. Rehearsal enhance his attention, which is good to keep the information in short-term memory and promote short-term memory to long-term memory. For example, if the patients hear a car marker, they can memorize it through recitation or rehearsal. The more frequently the patients retell the content, the shorter the time spent in rehearsal is, the better the effect is. In every rehearsal, the patients can understand the content deeper and the memory is further consolidated. If the time spent in rehearsal is shorter, it demonstrates that the patients are more familiar with the content and it cannot induce fatigue. The maintain or rehearsal memory method requires the patients' cooperation, or else the therapeutic effect is poor. If the memory information is less, the effect is better.

2. Recall is reminiscence of events that happened to the patients before.

   The patients are asked to try to recover the events that happened to themselves before including environment, motion and physical state in order to obtain reminder and promote memory. This method is applied to train the patients with poor comprehending capacity after cerebral injury. The patients are guided to find the hint or the therapists give the hint to the patients to help the patients to recall the happened event.

3. Internal law or internal strategies: if there are obvious defects in the patients, they can use normal or less injured functions to memorize new information. If the linguistic memory of the patients is poor, they are encouraged to use visual memory, and vice versa.
   (a) General requirement: Potential development: The patients use the good functions to replace injured functions. The rate of progress is slow. The mission is divided into several segments and then linked gradually. If the therapists ask the patients, the patients are asked to answer a moment later. The difficulty can be increased gradually. The patients are asked to establish the increasing goal. Self-suggestion and instruction: the therapists ask the patients to ask themselves. Do I remember? What is the meaning? Do I need to ask again? How can I link this to the events I know? What should I do? Do I stray from the point? What am I going to do? The questions can be written in card so that the patients can refer to it frequently. The therapists communicate with the patients frequently. Every once in a while, the therapists and the patients analyze the condition together to find out the gap, clarify misunderstanding and rectify mistakes. The therapists should pay attention to reward. If the patients succeed, they should be rewarded or get oral commendations.
   (b) Specific methods include verbal mnemonics and visual imagery techniques.

   Verbal mnemonics is suitable for the patients with poor imaginal memory or right hemisphere. The first word memory method: the patients are asked to remember the first word of the information and compile it into phrase or sentence. Memory chunking: the information should be adapted to memory span of the patients. For example, if memory span of the patients is two items, the memory chunking is two items. When the patients do the training of verbal memory chunking, the information groups with the similar meaning are in union. Association: the patients associate semantics, voice and word with similar image to enhance memory. For example, semantic association is from walking stick to crutch. Auditory association is from fragrance to sound (the two words are similar pronunciation in Chinese). Visual association is from Shen to Jia (the two words are similar image in Chinese). Sequence of Time and Space: the patients used events that happen with the information to recall the memory. Causal relationship: the patients use causal relationship between the event and information to recall memory. Significance and recency: the important and new events are easier to recall than the unimportant and obsolete event. The patients use this characteristic to recall the memory. Elaborate processing: the patients are asked to memorize the information, analyze it, find out the characteristic and detail, and link it to the given information. Compatibility: the patients are asked to form a concept that can be compatible with their given information and link them together. Self-control: the patients are asked to analyze the relationship between the given information and themselves. Making up stories: the patients are asked to make up a familiar story using the given information according to their habit and hobby. Sunlight graphical method of new information classification: the patients are asked to compare the given information to the sun and ask six questions such as what, who or whose, how, where, when and why. This way can promote information encode and resurgence.

   Visual imagery techniques is suitable for the patients with poor verbal memory capacity and left hemisphere injury. The interaction of image logic is used to promote the memory effect. Verbal memory method: the chunking and association methods in visual image memory are used to promote recovery of verbal memory.

Place location method: the patients link new information to geometric position with permanent order. The patients can recall objects in order, which is suitable for the patients can memorize building or geometric position in permanent order. The connection or chained method: it is similar with association. The patients are asked to link the given information to associated image. Classification: the patients should classify the information for recall.

4. External strategy is that external adminicle or hint is used to recover memory.
   (a) Information storage: The calendar is the method to memorize time. For example, if the patients will do something in the future, the patients can tear one corner or fold one corner in the calendar to remind themselves. Big calendar with large grid has the similar effect. The patients can use pencil to mark the event on small calendar, but the effect is poor. Notebook can help the patients to memorize the past. If the page is large enough, the patients can write down all the details. The patients are asked to write page number on the diary and make an index on the last page. The place of the diary should be fixed. Memorandum: every week, the patients write a book and look up the memorandum every day. Schedule: the patients should design an organized schedule including therapy and rest. The patients use movable target to move along the orientation or use pencil to cross off the finished thing. The patients wear electronic watch that can give out signal and are asked to look for the unfinished thing in the schedule when the watch rings. The watch should be big and marked. Obvious sign: large map, big number, big arrow and obvious sign are used to instruct the patients to the common place. Picture: name, event and date are written on the back of the picture. Because there are imagery and verbal tips, the information is plenty and easy to recall.
   (b) Environment modification: The environment should be arranged to eliminate the factors to distract the patients' attention. Concentration training is the basic condition to obtain good effect. The amount of information and condition of the environment should be controlled properly. The amount of information should be minimized and the information should be presently as frequently as possible. The interval between the information presentation should be long. The stability of the internal environment should be maintained to keep constant repeated convention and environment for the functional recovery of the patients' memory. The external environment should be changed for environment recovery of the patients. For example, the door should be pasted with bright-coloured label and the event needed to be remembered. Tips: the verbal and visual tips associated with memory can be provided. For example, when the patients memorize one thing, the therapists ask the patients questions and let them see the associated picture to recover memory.

   Various memory aids used in external measures are compensatory measures to figure out permanent memory disorder and increase the patients' memory capacity.
5. Psychotherapy to eliminate psychological disorder of the patients and enhance therapeutic effect.

   Approximately 30% of the patients with cognitive disorder are accompanied with depression. Although they lost a lot, even dignity, they are not sober and can realize that their intelligence declines and there are cold receptions. Therefore, all the person who contact with the patients should protect and respect their own value and self-esteem. The patients should be treated with courtesy. Obviously, if the patients are sloppily dressed, it can damage self-image and influence the disease state badly. Maslow's hierarchy of needs are suitable for the patients with cognitive disorder.

Therefore, the therapists should give psychological counseling to the patients with cognitive disorder in patience to eliminate inferiority complex. The therapists should create an environment of respecting the patients, friendly affection and no discrimination to make the patients devote to rehabilitation training joyfully.

6. Music therapy can transform sound energy from regular sound vibration to the power that can promote the functional recovery of disordered brain cells.

   Aristotle is the first person who proposed the relationship between music and body-mind and think that music can go deep into soul, purify spirits, keep the balance between body and mind and promote body health. After World War II, American military hospital use music to help the therapy of insomnia, depression and psychoneurosis in soldiers. In medical field, music is combined with physiological phenomenon to promote therapeutic effect.

   Hebb proposed that music can act on non-specific reflecting system under brain cortex and reticular formation of brain stem through auditory system to influence cortex functions in order to regulate nervous system functions. Sound energy from regular sound vibration can be transformed into the power that can promote functional recovery of disordered brain cells. Therefore, different kinds of music have different therapeutic effects. Song at the Frontier, moonlight of spring river and waltz can be used for the patients with unstable mood.

   Clinical experience demonstrated that music therapy can enhance the feeling of reality in the patients with cognitive disorder. The feeling of reality can provide real information, improve self-perception and increase independence. The patients are asked to listen to or sing the songs associated with current time, season, environment and event to change confusion of the patients. In addition, music can improve long-term memory, short-term memory and other cognitive functions of the patients. During the training, according to disease state and physical truth of the patients, the therapists select proper background music to relax the environment, delight patients' mood and enhance therapeutic effect.

7. There are several considerations in the training process of memory:
   (a) The training difficulty should be mild. According to actual condition of the patients, it is important to select proper difficult training content. The training principle should be from easy to difficulty. If the therapists choose the difficult therapy item, the patients cannot complete it, which can aggravate mental burden of the patients. The patients usually refuse the training, even generate unhealthy psychology.
   (b) The selection of picture type should be proper. According to the memory disorder type of the patients, the therapists choose proper picture to do specific training. For the patients with figure memory disorder, the therapists choose figure picture to do memory training. For the patients with memory disorder of daily supplies, the therapists should choose picture of daily supplies to do the training.
   (c) Picture type and difficulty are proper. According to the memory disorder type of the patients, the therapists choose pictures with proper type and difficulty. For the patients with slight memory impairments, the therapists can select some scenery and animal pictures. For the patients with severe memory impairments, the therapists can select some pictures of daily supplies. For the patients with severe memory damage, the therapists can choose family picture, because this kind of picture can strongly stimulate the patients, which is good for the memory function recovery of the patients.
   (d) Familiar and unfamiliar pictures can be mixed for training. The recovery effect of familiar pictures is poor, but unfamiliar pictures have better stimulation effect. However, the difficulty can make the patients lose confidence. Therefore, the

therapists combine them and utilize them to keep the effect of memory training and the confidence and enthusiasm of the patients.

(e) Focus on error-free learning method: error-free is the method to eliminate error in learning. The learner should start from the item that is easy to discriminate and increase the difficulty gradually to let themselves learn the content without failure. The important characteristics are as follows: Error-free learning is a technique. Error-free learning is not some kind of therapeutic method, but a training technique that run through the learning process. When receiving this kind of learning, the therapists shouldn't give the trainee opportunity to make a mistake. In traditional learning process, the wrong reaction can be avoided. The patients should try not to make mistakes. The therapists can give the right answer to the learner directly or let the patients easy to complete it without make a mistake.

Standardized error-free learning is that the therapists directly tell the patients the right answer and ask them to remember it. Improved error-free learning is that the therapists use abundant semantic words to describe the question and use semantic words to induce the patients to say the right answer. This process avoids the interference of correct information on wrong information and makes the patients are engaged in learning training. The more correct information the patients get in the learning, the better the effect of improving memory capacity.

15.2.3 Cognitive Training Device Development of Neurological Training

Researches show that biofeedback therapy (BF) is a training method to recover neurons and synaptic conduction function, which may improve cholesterol metabolic disorders in hippocampus and injury of synaptic plasticity in order to increase cognitive function of the patients. On the basis of that, the author developed training device for Daoyin technique cognitive training in traditional Chinese medicine.

1. Design principle of cognitive training device: the device can use plasticity of central nervous system to display the results of cognitive training with Daoyin technique real-timely to further enhance the effect of Daoyin technique through biofeedback function.

   At present, in cognitive training method at home and abroad, scenery pictures or pictures of daily supplies are used for memory training. The method is single and not interesting. Existing cognitive training device is mainly used for cognitive function examination and assessment. The therapy is presenting pictures and there is no biofeedback function. The training is at will. Without the process of regulation of mind and breathing in Daoyin technique, the training effect may be affected. If the equipment can enhance the effect of cognitive training on the basis of regulation of mind and breathing in Daoyin technique and make the patients do the training with purpose through biofeedback, it can increase the interests of the training and enhance the training effects.

   Cognitive training system of neurological training is that in an environment with light music, the therapists display the results of cognitive training with Daoyin technique in the previous training on screen in a horizontal line and use this as surpassing goal. The patients are guided to surpass the goal, just like archery training that the archer should shoot at the center of the target. The system provides the patients visual feedback information real-timely to make them do the training with purpose. When the patients meet the requirements, twinkling curve, exploded fireworks and congratulatory sound are given to the patients to encourage them and increase training interests. Clinical applications indicated that although the system requires some improvements, it reaches the goal and obtains satisfying effect.

(a) Design principle of the system: BF is an independent interdisciplinary subject including physical medicine, contrology, physiology, anatomy, psychology and other rehabilitation medicine knowledge. The system is based on biofeedback. During the training process, the system can provide the patients real-time biofeedback signal to enhance cognitive training with a purpose. Positive feedback addition technique can increase cognitive capacity of the patients, develop central neural potential and enhance training effect (Fig. 15.2).

(b) Developing plasticity of nervous system and achieving functional reorganization: After cerebral injury, the adults have the ability to reorganize in structure or function to replace lost function, which can complete functional reorganization. In this process, orient induction proper method can complete the process. Biofeedback cognitive training system is designed according to this goal.

(c) Basic function of system: according to clinical requirements, functional block diagram refers to Fig. 15.3.

2. The content of cognitive training device includes three parts.

The content of operation and design of cognitive training device are compiled in the Chinese interface software that can be operated in Windows through DELPHI 7 programming language. According to the requirements of clinical training, the functions of three parts are achieved. There are two displays so that the control information cannot affect trainee in the system control process. The specific functions of the system are as follows:

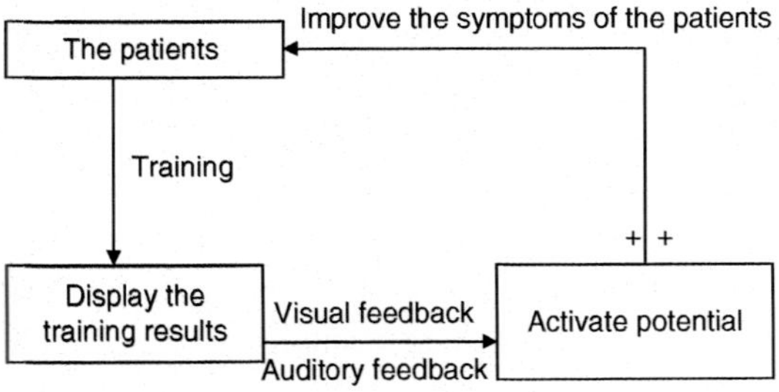

Fig. 15.2 Sketch map of cognitive training device: positive feedback of enhancing effect

(a) Medical record processing: DELPHI is applied to process text and call external program technique and various functions in text of windows to realize the functions of input, modification, save and print of medical record file.

(b) Assessment of cognitive disorder: the system use cognitive dysfunction examination simple scale released by ministry of health. The therapists input the questions into database and then the questions are called randomly by computer program in the functional assessment of the patients. After examination, the computer calculates the score automatically and realizes the function of assessment of cognitive disorder.

(c) Biofeedback cognitive training: memory training is a very important part in the therapy of the patients with cognitive disorder. The key point of memory training of the patients with cognitive disorder is the brain development of the patients. In addition, the training difficulty shouldn't be too high. The therapists should select the difficulty according to the actual condition of the patients. In the process of memory training, this system adopts improved error-free learning method. The therapists use abundant semantic words to describe questions and use semantic tips to induce the patients to say the right answer. The patients can actively involve in the training and get more correct stimulus from the learning and better memory capacity. In order to assure the flexibility of memory training, the system provides automatic memory training and manual memory training. Training content includes pictures, numbers, family image memory training and memory training auxiliary game. The methods include instant memory training, short-term memory training, sequential memory training, attention training, rehearsal, commander

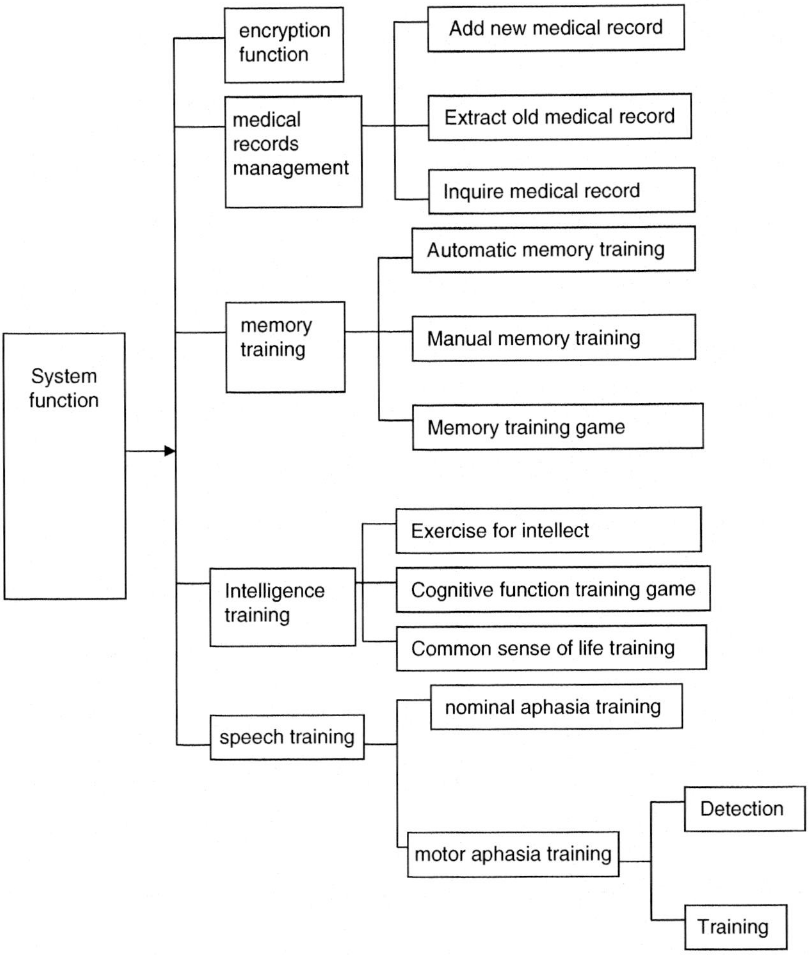

Fig. 15.3 Functional block diagram of cognitive training device

execution. The information is added to the training gradually. Intelligence recovery training can promote improvement of memory capacity and memory capacity improvement can further promote the recovery of the patients with cognitive disorder, which enters into a good circle. Intelligence training in this system is divided into outsight, natural things group ability, figure and mathematical calculation ability, visual spaces identification ability and imagination. In order to increase pertinence and validity of the training and increase the enthusiasm of the patients in the training, the therapists complied a series of Flash animation that are used for the daily life ability of the patients with cognitive disorder. The system provides some games for functional training of right hemisphere such as mahjong, Ninth-Game, Chinese checkers and Chinese chess. The patients can do excitation training of brain to give sensory stimulation to right hemisphere to improve functions.

In addition, the system designs verbal rehabilitation training such as anomic aphasia and motor aphasia. In the training process of verbal rehabilitation of the patients with motor aphasia, there are several procedures: the detection of phonic function, phonic basic training of the patients, phonic training of words and phonic training of single sentence. The training standard is that the accuracy rate of phonic training in every step is 80%.

After that, the patients can do the next training.

3. Background music to enhance training effect.

   The effects of music therapy mainly come from environmental atmosphere to alleviate uneasy and nervous mood of the patients in order to enhance training effect. Music therapy is integrated into rehabilitation training of the patients with cognitive disorder. The patients are asked to listen to or sing the song associated with current time, season, environment and event to ease body-mind and stabilize mood.

   In addition, music can stimulate the patients to recover long-term memory of the patients and improve short-term memory and other cognitive functions. Therefore, the system is equipped with many kinds of background music. According to the condition of the patients, the therapists choose proper music to enhance therapeutic effect.

4. System function, operational approach, indications, contraindications, therapy course and problems to be solved.
   (a) Function: the system includes 340 selected pictures, 30 cognitive function training games and 30 well-designed flash animation for daily life ability training of the patients with cognitive disorder. The patients do the training in an easy, imagery, vivid environment.
   (b) Operational approach: there are two displays in the system. One screen displays control menu and the other displays pictures of therapy training and feedback of the results. In the therapy process of the patients, the patients can see a perfect picture without interference of the control menu. During therapy process, improved error-free learning method is used to help the patients to establish a normal thinking model through effective induction way to avoid the interference of the wrong information on correct information.
   (c) Therapy course: the training way is one-to-one. The training time is 30 min (once a day) and one therapy course takes 3 months. The patients can receive multiple therapy courses.
   (d) Indications: it is suitable for the patients with cognitive disorder, including the patients with senile dementia. It is also suitable for cognitive dysfunction induced by cerebrovascular diseases, cerebral trauma, cerebral palsy, encephalitis, Parkinson's disease, cerebral degenerative disease and carbon monoxide toxic encephalopathy and rehabilitation training of the patients with verbal disorder.
   (e) Contraindication: there is no obvious contradiction.
   (f) Problems to be solved: announcements: the response and disposition of the patients: because the users of the system are the patients with cognitive disorder, the operation is very important. Generally, the patients with cognitive disorder make an oral account and the therapists help them to click the mouse to answer the questions. In order to let the patients answer the questions by themselves, touch screen is a good method. Voice setting: our country is a multiracial country and there are many regional dialects. The ideal way is to use mother tongue to train the patients with aphasia. At present, this system is attached to the system with mandarin pronunciation. With technique development, the therapists can change voice setting to adapt to the training of the patients with different dialects. Tone training: Chines is a kind of tone language. Same pronunciation with different tones means different meanings. Therefore, tone is an important part of rehabilitation training of motor aphasia in the patients with cognitive disorder. Because of technical reason, there is no tone training in the rehabilitation training of aphasia in this system. With the development of computer technology, tone training is certain to be integrated into this system. Teletherapy: with the development of computer and network technology, network resource and clinical resources can be applied and some patients in remote and border areas can

receive some instructions from famous doctors through network resources to increase application rang and cognitive training effect.

In short, according to the degrees and types of cognitive disorder and the process of rehabilitation training, the system is compiled. The interface is clear, the structure is rational and the content is integral. It fully considers the characteristic of the patients with cognitive disorder. Rehabilitation training is classified. According to the requirements of different users, the system is divided into single-screen display and double-screen display. Single-screen display system is suitable for family use and double-screen display is suitable for rehabilitation department.

When the system is applied in clinic, the author will summarize the suggestions and requirements from the patients with cognitive disorder, their family, rehabilitation therapy physicians and doctors. The author rectifies shortcomings, enriches content, and improves functions so that rehabilitation training of cognitive disorder may be more scientific, rational and systematic to enhance the effect of rehabilitation training of cognitive disorder.

Reference

1. Brand M, Labudda K, Markowitsch HJ. Neuropsychological correlates of decision-making in ambiguous and riskv situatioas. Neural Netw. 2006;19(8):1266–76. https://doi.org/10.1016/j.neunet.2006.03.001.
2. Prigatano G. Neuropsychological rehabilitation after brain injury. Baltimore: Johns Hopkins University Press; 1986. p. 29–50.
3. Pennington C, Newson M, Hayre A, et al. Functional cognitive disorder: what is it and what to do about it? Pract Neurol. 2015;15(6):436–44.
4. Brook N, Campsie L, Symington C, et al. The five years outcome of severe blunt head injury: a relatives view. J Neurol Neurosurg Psychiatry. 1986;49:764–70.
5. Wade DT. Measurement in neurological rehabilitation. Oxford: University Press; 1990. p. 135.
6. Jacobs JW. Screccrning for organic mental syndromes CCSE in the medically ill. Ann Intern Med. 1997;86:89.
7. Wilson BA, Cockburn J, Baddeley A. The Rivermead Behavioural Memory Test second edition. London: Thames Valley Test Company; 2003.

16 Rehabilitation Therapy of Neurological Training of Swallowing Dysfunction

16.1 The Mechanism of Swallow and Dysphagia

16.1.1 The Mechanism of Swallow

Swallow is an essential functional movement for eating and drinking. It is a combined movement of voluntary and involuntary movement dominated by central nerves. Finally, manducatory food and liquid in mouth are delivered into stomach for food digestion and nutrition supply through esophagus [1]. Swallow is one of the basic vital movements of human.

Randomness of swallow movement means whether the person want to swallow or not. For example, the people can keep food or liquid in the mouth, don't push them to posterior pharyngeal wall to avoid swallow reflex and put food or liquid into stomach. For the swallow movement, bolus formed by chewing the food is pushed to posterior pharyngeal wall and then into stomach [2]. This is an involuntary reflex that is induced by specific stimulus. During swallowing, bolus stimulate pharyngeal receptor, soft palate rise and posterior pharyngeal wall protrude to seal nasopharynx in order to avoid foot enters into nasal cavity. Meanwhile, vocal cords adduct, throat rises, and move forward to epiglottic cartilage to seal throat and stop breathing in case of astray food and water.

Swallowing dysfunction is one of the common complications in the patients with stroke. Swallowing dysfunction is induced by true bulbar paralysis and pseudo bulbar paralysis. True bulbar paralysis is induced by nuclear lesion or sub nuclear lesion of glossopharyngeal nerve, vagus nerve and hypoglossal nerve and pseudo bulbar paralysis is induced by injuries of bilateral cerebral cortex or corticobulbar tract. Pseudo bulbar paralysis is more common [3, 4] in clinic. The main manifestations of swallowing dysfunction are start time delay of voluntary tongue movement and coordination decrease of swallow movement. There are feed difficulty, bucking and asophia in the patients. Water and electrolyte disturbance and other nutrition insufficiency, even albumin decrease are induced by insufficiency of intake. Astray food and water can induce aspiration pneumonia, even suffocation. Researches show that in the patients with clear consciousness in acute phase, 64–90% of the patients have dysphagia, 22–42% pf the patients have miss inhalation, which are the important factors to increase the case fatality rate of the patients with stroke.

16.1.1.1 Muscles and Nerves Involved in Swallow

1. Muscles involved in swallow include suprahyoid muscles and infrahyoid muscles.
   (a) Suprahyoid muscles is located between hyoid and lower jawbone with basis cranii. There are four muscles in each side including digastric muscles, mylohyoid

W. Zhao, *Rehabilitation Therapeutics of the Neurological Training*,
https://doi.org/10.1007/978-981-13-0812-3_16

muscle, stylohyoid muscle and geniohyoid muscle.

The functions of suprahyoid muscles are to life hyoid to elevate tongue and help bolus enter into pharynx. When hyoid is fixed, mylohyoid muscle, geniohyoid muscle and muscle belly of digastric muscles pull lower jawbone downward to open mouth.

(b) Infrahyoid muscles are located in anterior region of the neck. There are four muscles in each side. It is located in the two sides of the middle line under hyoid, in the front of throat, trachea and thyroid. There are deep layer and superficial layer. They are all named by the starting and ending points. Infrahyoid muscles include sternohyoideus, musculus omohyoideus, sternothyroid 和 thyrohyoid muscle.

The functions of infrahyoid muscles are to lower hyoid and throat. When in swallow, musculus thyrohyoideus lift throat to hyoid.

2. The phase and movement of swallow: The involved muscles and nerves refer to Table 16.1.

Table 16.1 The phase and movements of swallow

The phase and movements of swallow	Muscles	Dominant nerves
Oral cavity phase		
Lip closes	Orbicular muscle of mouth	VII
Control cheek	Buccinator	VII
Chew vertically	Temporalis	V
	Masseter	V
	Interior alary muscle	V
Chew horizontally	Exterior alary muscle	V
Mix food by tongue	Lingual intrinsic muscles	XII
	Genioglossus	XII
	Styloglossus	XII
Pharynx phase		
Tongue and palate close	Styloglossus	XII
Velamen closes	Staphylinus externus	V
Velamen closes	Levator muscle of velum palatinum	IX, X
Pharynx oppress	Styloglossus	XII
	Musculus hyoglossus	XII
	Stylopharyngeus	IX, X
	Upper stegnosis muscles	IX, X
	Middle stegnosis muscles	IX, X
	Lower stegnosis muscles	IX, X
Epiglottis inclines	Aryepiglotticus	IX, X
Throat moves upward	Thyrohyoid muscle	XII
	Musculus hyoglossus	VII
	Stylohyoid muscle	VII
	Posterior digastric muscles	XII
Move forward	Geniohyoid muscle	C_{1-3}
	Genioglossus	XII
Glottis closes	Cricoarytenoid muscles	IX, X
Airflow stops	Intercostal muscles (inhibition)	T_{1-12}
	Diaphragm inhibition	C_{3-4}
Pharynx and esophagus reflex	Cricopharyngeus muscle inhibition	IX, X
Esophagus phase		
Esophagus contracts	Striated muscle fiber	X
	Smooth muscle fiber	X

The list of the involved muscles and nerves

16.1.1.2 The Mechanism of Swallow

Swallow movements are divided into three time phases in mouth, pharynx and esophagus and six stages.

1. Cognition of food is the process to distinguish food and select eating ways.

The information is feedback to brain through visual sense to distinguish the food kinds such as solid, fluid and soft or hard. According to the information, people decide to eat the food or not and adjust consciousness. The person who is in low level of consciousness, cannot concentrate on something, or are indifferent to the food, there is aspiration in eating.

2. Eating is the process to intake food into mouth.

People adjust mouth, lip and foretooth to adapt to the form of food and tableware. After that, people take food into mouth. The patients with lips closure disturbance cannot take food into mouth. The food is easy to leak out even taken into mouth.

3. Food chewing and bolus forming is the process that food in the mouth are grinded through chewing, mixed with saliva and form bolus for swallow.

In the mouth, food mixed with saliva, forming bolus that is easy to swallow. The process is different because of the shape of the food. Liquid diet is easy to swallow. Semiliquid food such as jelly and porridge form bolus through pushing and chewing. The body of tongue fluctuates to make the food are pushed and grinded between tongue and hard palate. Solid food not only requires pushing and chewing, but also requires teeth to chew and grind to form bolus. During chewing, lower jaw fluctuates and rotate. Meanwhile, cuff segment between soft palate and root of tongue is closed to prevent food into pharynx. If masticatory movement, the formation and maintenance of food cannot be completed, the food may be swallowed without thinking and flow into pharynx before inducing swallow reflex.

4. Food enters into pharynx, which is called phase of oral cavity. It is the process that bolus enter into the part that can induce swallow reflex (Fig. 16.1).

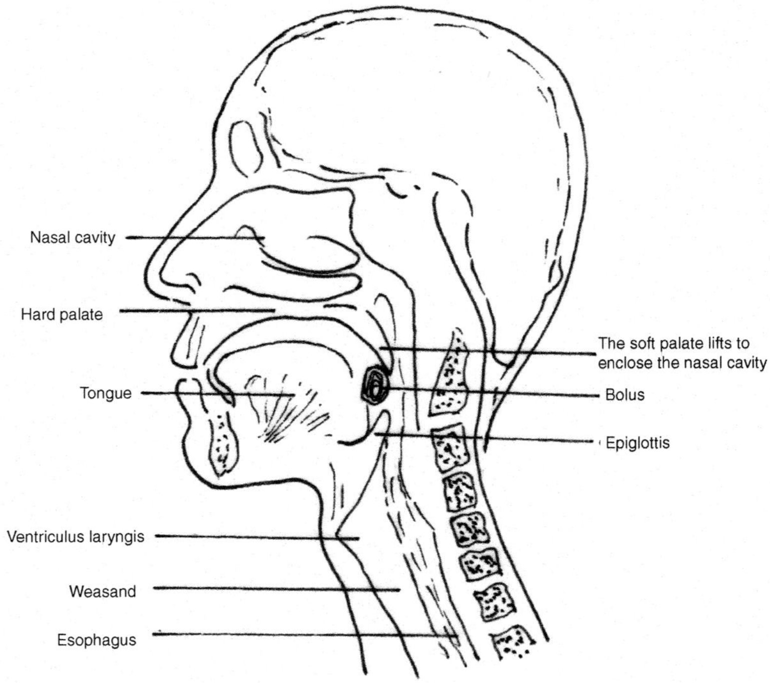

Fig. 16.1 Phase of oral cavity: the process of bolus formation

After formation of bolus, tongue rises to push bolus to root of tongue through hard palate until bolus reaches the part that can induce swallow reflex. Lips close and lower jaw holds still, which generate swallow movement. If bolus cannot reach root of tongue, the patients can throw their head back or be in supine position to make bolus enter into pharynx using action of gravity.

5. Bolus goes through pharynx, which is called pharyngeal phase. It is the process of inducing swallow reflex and bolus enters into esophagus (Fig. 16.2).

Pharyngeal phase is an important stage to induce erroneous deglutition. After bolus reaches pharynx, soft hip seals the channel between pharynx and nasal cavity and epiglottis seals the channel between pharynx and trachea, which immediately induce instant swallow respiratory arrest. Meanwhile, root of tongue oppresses posterior pharyngeal wall and pharyngeal wall generates peristalsis to push bolus into esophagus.

The above process is swallow reflex. The time of completing the reflex in normal people is about 0.5 s. Incapacity of swallow leads to incomplete food swallow and food left on pharynx enters into trachea during inspiration or incoordination of swallow reflex leads to incomplete lockout of trachea, which induce erroneous deglutition.

6. Bolus goes through esophagus which is called esophagus phase. It is the process that bolus enters into stomach through esophagus.

After bolus enters esophagus, smooth muscles of esophagus start peristalsis to make bolus enter into stomach through esophagus. Until now, the swallow process is completed.

Just as the above mentioned, swallow is the same as respiration, urination and defecation. They are all voluntary movements and complicated movements. Before esophagus phase, swallow is voluntary movement. The patients can start, accelerate or stop swallow at will. When bolus induces swallow reflex and enters into esophagus phase, swallow is involuntary reflex movement.

During esophagus phase, esophagus peristalsis is reflex impulse induced by stimulation of receptors in soft palate, pharynx and esophagus by bolus. Afferent nerve of this reflex is sensory fiber of pharynx and esophagus mucosa, including branches of glossopharyngeal nerve, nervi

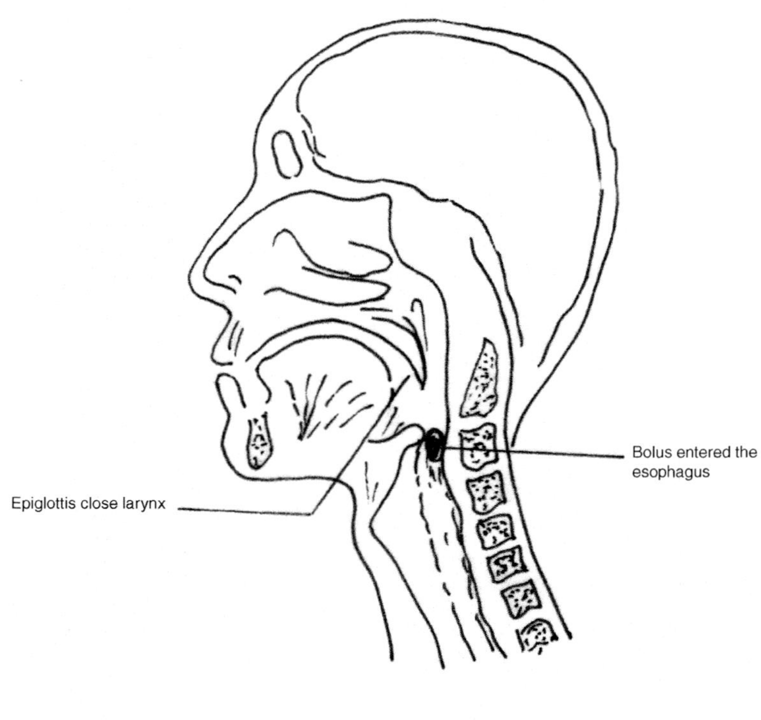

Fig. 16.2 Pharyngeal phase: the process that bolus enter into esophagus

trigeminus, nervi vagus and its upper throat branches. Motor nerve includes hypoglossal nerve, nervi trigeminus, glossopharyngeal nerve, nervi vagus and accessory nerve. They dominate the muscles involved in swallow. Its center locates in medulla oblongata.

16.1.2 Dysphagia

16.1.2.1 The Definition of Dysphagia

Dysphagia is the clinical manifestation after disorder in the process that food enters into stomach through oral cavity. Except for the diseases of mouth, pharynx and esophagus, the inducing factors include cranial nerve lesion, medulla oblongata lesion, pseudobulbar paralysis, extrapyramidal diseases and myopathy.

16.1.2.2 Classification of Swallowing Disorder

1. According to the disorder part, dysphagia is divided into oropharynx dysphagia and esophagus dysphagia.
2. According to handicapped degree, swallow disorder includes lesion, disability and handicap.
   (a) Lesion: central functions disorder of the structure, power, motor, afferent nerve, efferent nerve, involuntary movement or voluntary movement is induced by pathogenic factors. The patients are afraid of swallow, but the swallow function is normal.
   (b) Disability: lesion has certain or irreversible effects on the individual swallow function.
   (c) Handicap: because of lesion and swallow function disorder, the patients cannot have meals with friends and colleagues. They cannot meet the requirements of regular work and society.
3. According to therapeutic requirements, there are three feeding classifications of dysphagia.
   (a) Mild: when the patients eat liquid food or drink water, there is irritating cough, even erroneous deglutition. The patients can eat semiliquid food or solid food. There is no obvious disorders of chewing function and tongue function. There is hypaesthesia of posterior pharyngeal wall, but stimulation of posterior pharyngeal wall can induce vomiting reflex.
   (b) Moderate: the patients cannot eat liquid food or drink water, but can eat solid food. There is usually irritating cough, even erroneous deglutition. Chewing function and tongue function decline. There is hypaesthesia of posterior pharyngeal wall, but only strong stimulation of posterior pharyngeal wall can induce vomiting reflex.
   (c) Severe: The patients are difficult to eat solid food and cannot complete swallow. If there is irritating cough or erroneous deglutition, difficulty of chewing and tongue movement, unconspicuous sensation of posterior pharyngeal wall, strong stimulation cannot induce vomiting reflex.

16.1.2.3 Assessment of Swallowing Disorder

General inspection includes myodynamia, movement and swallow reflex.

1. Inspection of muscles and joint in oral cavity: Movements of lower jaw, lips, tongue, soft palate and buccinators; occlusion and power of teeth.
2. Inspection of swallow: the patients simulate swallow movement or swallow saliva and the therapists inspect chewing movement, lips close, whether there is throat uplift, time limit and neck movement or not during swallow.
3. Swallow ability test: The patients are in sitting position. The patients should relax if they are in bed. The therapists put thumb and index finger on the two sides of neck, Adam's apple and hyoid of the patients and let the patients swallow saliva quickly and repeatedly. The therapists observe the Adam's apple and hyoid cross the fingers and go down with swallow movement and record the times of swallow in 30 s it is normal that there are three times of swallow in 30 s.

4. Swallow provocative test [5]: The therapists put index finger between thyroid cartilage and hyoid and use iced cotton swab with ice water to dampen lips, the tip of the tongue, lingual surface, back of the tongue and mucosa of oral cavity. After that, the therapists slightly stimulate pillars of fauces, root of tongue and posterior pharyngeal wall to induce swallow reflex. If thyroid cartilage crosses the fingers, it is defined that there is swallow movement.
5. Water drinking test is the most commonly used identification method [6]. The patients are in sitting position. The therapists take 30 mL warm water, ask the patients to drink, observe the drinking process and record the time. There are five conditions.
   - The patients drink off and there is no irritating cough.
   - The patients drink it for two times and there is no irritating cough.
   - The patients drink off and there is irritating cough.
   - The patients drink it more than two times and there is irritating cough.
   - There is irritating cough for many times and the patients cannot drink the water.
   - Diagnostic criteria:
   - Normal: the patients drink it in 5 s.
   - Suspicious: the patients drink it more than 5 s or drink it off and there is irritating cough.
   - Abnormal: the patients drink it more than two times and there is irritating cough or there is irritating cough for many times and the patients cannot drink the water.
6. Imaging examination: X-ray photo and X-ray video examinations can be used to know the structure and movement of swallow. They not only can be used for analysis of dysphagia degree, but also can be used for analysis of the reasons of dysphagia and erroneous deglutition such as tongue function decline, swallow reflex attenuation, poor closure of throat, cricopharyngeus muscle hypotonia.
7. Other assessments:
   - Normal reflex: vomiting reflex and cough reflex.
   - Abnormal reflex: occlusion, sucking and swallow reflex.
   - Motor ability and sensation: motor control ability of head, neck and tongue and sensation of tongue, palate and face.
   - Swallow ability of different food: swallow ability of liquid, semiliquid and solid food.
   - Others: whether there is food retention in the mouth or not and there are salivation and choking.
   - Through functional assessment, the therapists can judge the following items:
   - The best position of swallow training: the patients sit erectly and put the head forward slightly.
   - The best location of food in the mouth: the patients push the food to the side with complete sensation and motor function.
   - The kinds of food tolerance: solid, liquid and stickiness of liquid.

16.2 Rehabilitation Therapy of Swallowing Disorder

16.2.1 Principle and Method of Rehabilitation of Neurological Training of Swallowing Disorder

16.2.1.1 Principle of Rehabilitation of Neurological Training of Swallowing Disorder

Through the training of active movement, central nerve system potential can be developed and autonomous contraction ability of swallow muscles is recovered gradually. The training can loose tissue adhesion, recover the range of joint motion, enhance myodynamia, prevent erroneous deglutition, recover or improve swallow function.

In order to prevent aspiration pneumonia, for the severe patients with erroneous deglutition, eating and drinking are forbidden. Liquid food is given through stomach tube. After recovery of swallow function, eating and drinking can be recovered gradually. For the patients with swallowing disorder and cognitive disorder, gastrostomy can be considered and the patients can eat through fistula.

16.2.1.2 Rehabilitation Method of Swallowing Disorder

According to assessment results, dysphagia site and degree, different methods are used for the training.

1. Rehabilitation of neurological training of swallowing muscles: Neurological training device is used for the training. The patients are in sitting position or semireclining position. The therapists paste surface electrode and use normal method or the method of guiding collaterals through meridians to guide the patients to enhance the intensity of motor program signal of suprahyoid muscles and infrahyoid muscles, develop central nerve potential and reestablish motor program of swallow.
   (a) Electrode place of suprahyoid muscles training: these muscles are located between hyoid and lower jawbone and basis cranii. These functions are to life hyoid, elevate tongue and push bolus into pharynx. When hyoid is fixed, these muscles pull down lower jawbone to make the mouth open. The antagonistic muscle of opening mouth is masseter. Therefore, during the training of suprahyoid muscles, surface electrode is placed on the bottom of lower jaw. The other electrode is on the same part of uninjured side (Fig. 16.3). The purpose is that the training goal of injured side is the signal intensity in uninjured side. The electrode can also be placed in masseter on the same side (Fig. 16.4). The purpose is that the antagonistic muscles of opening mouth motor program reestablishment is masseter. The anti-resistance methods of two forms are the same, which are that palm is used to support lower jawbone (Fig. 16.5). During training, the patients should enhance motor program signal of suprahyoid muscles and decrease motor program signal intensity of masseter.
   (b) Electrode place of infrahyoid muscles: These muscles are before neck and there are four muscles in each side. These muscles are in two sides of middle line under hyoid. Its function is to life throat during

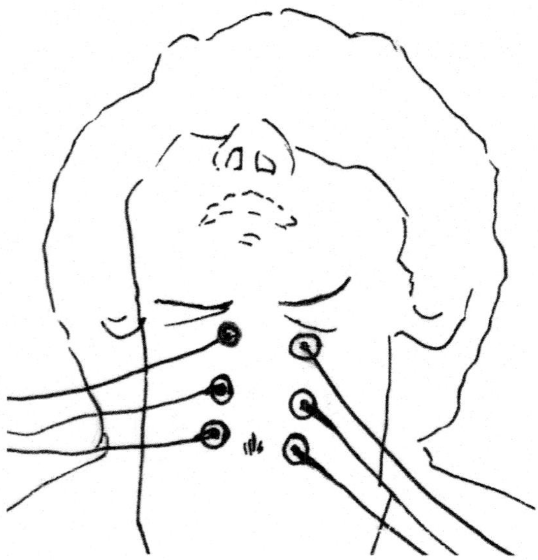

Fig. 16.3 Sketch map of electrode place part of suprahyoid muscles

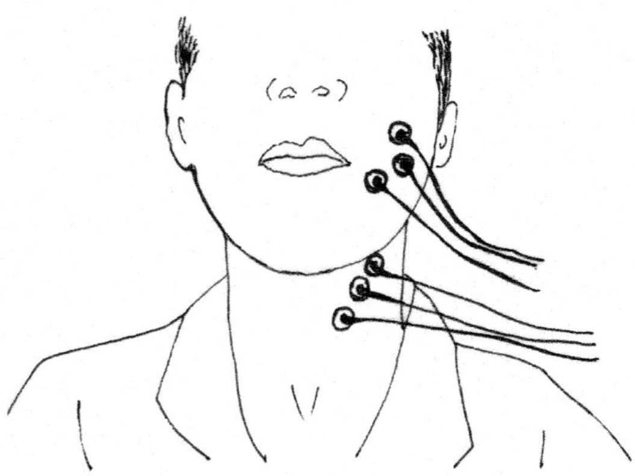

Fig. 16.4 Sketch map of electrode place part of suprahyoid muscles such as masseter

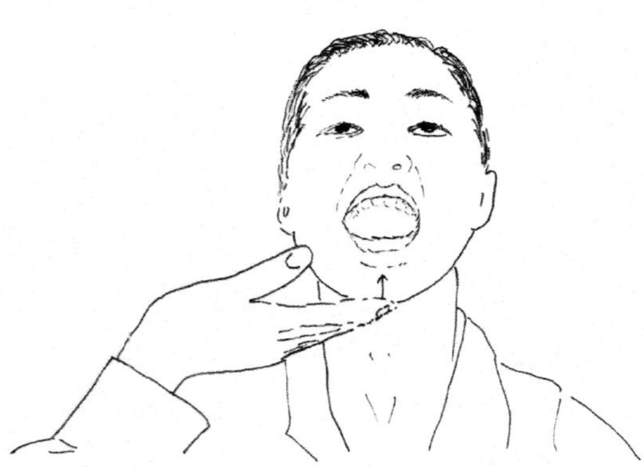

Fig. 16.5 Sketch map of anti-resistance of suprahyoid muscles in swallow

swallow. Reception electrode is below hyoid and beside trachea (Fig. 16.6). The anti-resistance way is to use index finger and finger pulp of thumb to press on Adam's apple. When the Adam's apple moves upward in the beginning of swallow, the patients exert resistance slightly without affect respiration and inducing other discomfort (Fig. 16.7).

When the patients do motor program reestablishment training of infrahyoid muscles, suprahyoid muscles are antagonistic muscles. Electrodes are separately placed on the skin surface of suprahyoid muscles and infrahyoid muscles at the same side (Fig. 16.8). The patients should enhance motor program signal intensity of infrahyoid muscles and attenuate motor program signal intensity of suprahyoid muscles to reestablish motor program of swallow in order to recover swallow function.

The training time is 50 min (once a day) and there are 30 times in one therapy course. The patients can do multiple therapy courses.

(c) Virtual reality training of neurological training: virtual reality training system is used for potential development and motor program reestablishment of suprahyoid muscles and infrahyoid muscles.

The training time is 50 min (once a day) and there are 30 times in one therapy course. The patients can do multiple therapy courses.

2. Actual swallow training the therapists ascertain the optimum eating pattern through assessment and then give the patients actual swallow training.

The specific method: the patients use the optimum eating position such as sitting position or semireclining position. The patients concentrate to open mouth and contain one spoon of powdery apple in the mouth. On the basis of regulation of mind and breathing, the

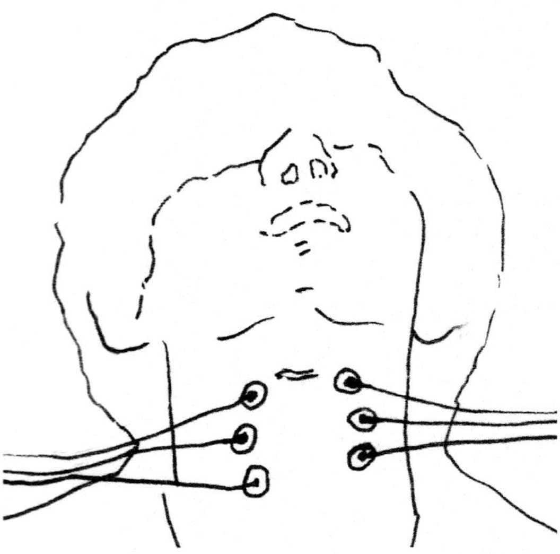

Fig. 16.6 Electrode place part of infrahyoid muscles

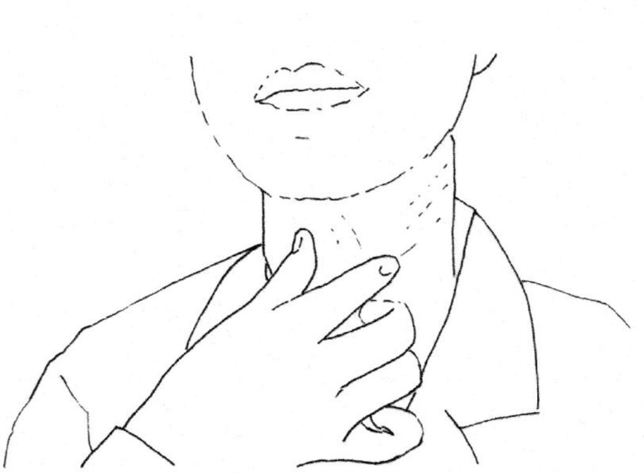

Fig. 16.7 Sketch map of anti-resistance of infrahyoid muscles in swallow

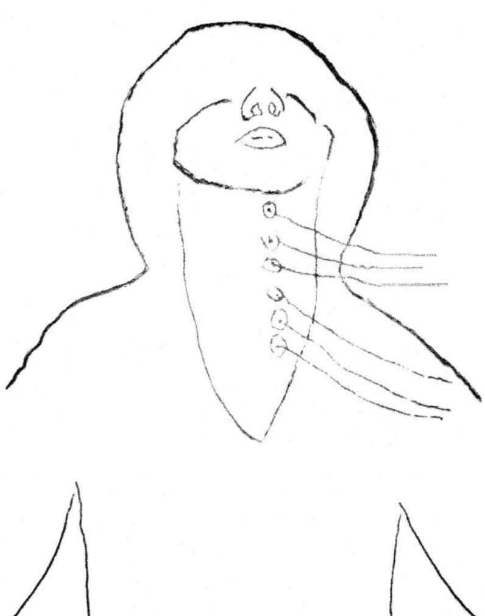

Fig. 16.8 Sketch map of swallow training of suprahyoid muscles and infrahyoid muscles

patients are guided to induce suprahyoid muscles contraction to make bolus reach pharynx, induce infrahyoid muscles contraction to lift head and extend neck in order to induce swallow reflex. Therefore, bolus can enter into esophagus and swallow movement is completed.

When the patients can smoothly complete the swallow movement of powdery apple and there is no irritating cough and erroneous deglutition, the patients used the same method to do the swallow training of eating mushy apple swallow. When the patients can smoothly complete the swallow movement of mushy apple and there is no irritating cough and erroneous deglutition, the patients start the training of eating apple juice until they use liquid for swallow training.

The training time is 20 min (once a day) and there are 30 times in one therapy course. The patients can do multiple therapy courses.

3. Electrical stimulation to increase the excitability of swallow muscles, improve blood circulation of muscle and promote functional recovery [7].

   Conventional wisdom may suggest that electrical stimulation is not suitable for neck because it may lead to throat spasm. In addition, when electrical stimulation act on internal carotid sinus and nerve plexus around branches of carotid artery, it may lead to bradycardia. Therefore, the electrode should be placed vertically in two sides of middle line of neck, but not away from middle line in case of stimulation carotid artery.

(a) Swallow stimulation device therapy: its mechanism is to stimulate suprahyoid muscles with medium-frequency electricity to induce muscle contraction to lift tongue and make saliva enter into throat and pharynx and then induce swallow reflex. Meanwhile, it can stimulate salivary gland and salivary glands to secret saliva that enter into pharynx to induce swallow reflex.

Electrode place part: after ungrease treatment of skin, the positive electrode is placed in the seventh cervical vertebra and negative electrode is placed between lower jaw before neck and cricoid cartilage. Electrode slice is fixed with band and the tightness is proper. Square-wave pulse stimulation is used to get value A and triangular form wave pulse stimulation is used to get value B. The formula is as follows.

Injury degree of swallow muscles $\propto = B/A$.

According to exact value of $\propto$, the therapists select the ration of low-frequency time (T) and rest (R). The stimulation time is usually 1 s and the rest time is 3 s. Current intensity vary with each individual. It is optimum that the patients can tolerant the current and it can induce swallow movement. During stimulation, the therapists ask the patients try to do swallow movement.

Current intensity should not be too strong lest the patients feel uncomfortable or it induces throat spasm.

The training time is 20 min (1–2times per day) and there are 15 times in one therapy course. If there is no excessive muscle excitability, the patients can receive the next therapy course.

(b) Medium-frequency electrical stimulation: Suprahyoid and infrahyoid muscles are separately stimulated. The electrode is placed in suprahyoid infrahyoid muscles on the same side. The electrode can also be placed beside trachea in the level of Adam's apple to enhance excitability of swallow related muscles and improve swallow function.

The training time is 20 min (once a day) and there are 15 times in one therapy course. If there is no excessive muscle excitability, the patients can receive the next therapy course.

4. Infrared therapy infrared lamp is used to irradiate submentum and throat to increase blood circulation of swallow muscles.

   The training time is 20 min (once a day) and there are 15 times in one therapy course. The patients can do multiple therapy courses.

5. Loosen of tissue adhesion manipulation is used to loose tissue of tongue, mouth and neck.
   (a) Adhesion release of tongue muscles and perioral muscles: through traction, malaxation and passive movement, the adhesion

of lingualis and masseter is loosened to increase the movement range and flexibility of tongue, alleviate adhesion of mandibular joint, promote movement of mandibular joint and recovery of chewing function.

(b) Adhesion release of suprahyoid and infrahyoid muscles and their peripheral tissue: manipulation traction, strings, malaxation, active and passive movements can increase range of submandibular joint motion, degree of excursion of Adam's apple and flexibility of movement, loosen adhesion of submandibular tissue and throat tissue to recover movements of submandibular joint and swallow.

The training time is 20 min (once a day) and there are 15 times in one therapy course. The patients can do multiple therapy courses.

6. Acupuncture and massage acupuncture can dredge the channel and regulate of qi and blood and massage can tease muscles and loosen adhesion.
   (a) Acupuncture: The acupuncture points are different. According to the condition of the patients, the therapists select points through different syndromes and treat people individually.

   Major acupuncture points:
   - Double Fengchi: The point of a needle is inclined downward and is inserted into the skin towards Adam's apple about 1.5 Cun (one third decimetre). The needle should not be inserted too deep in case injuring medulla oblongata.
   - Double Gongxue acupoint (extra nerve points): 1.5 Cun below Fengchi in the level of lips, the point of a needle is inserted into skin about 1.5 Cun deep towards offside lips.
   - Double Yiming: the point of a needle is inserted into throat 1.5 Cun deep.

   Adjunct acupuncture points:
   - Double Tunyan: they are located between hyoid and Adam's apple, in the sunken 0.5 Cun beside middle line. The therapists use hand to push arteria carotis communis outward. The needle is inserted inward and is twirled for 5–10 s. The needle cannot be inserted outward in case of injuring superior thyroid artery.
   - Lianquan: the needle is inserted oblique 1.2 Cun deep towards root of tongue andis twirled for 10 s.
   - Zhiqiang (extra nerve points): it is between hyoid and incisura thyreoidea superior. The needle is inserted 0.5 Cun deep towards root of tongue and is twirled for 5–10 s. if there is facial flush and dyspnea, the needle should be withdrawn immediately.

   (b) Massage: soft and slight massage manipulation is used for the massage of facial muscles, tongue muscles, suprahyoid muscles and infrahyoid muscles to loosen adhesion, increase blood circulation and promote functional recovery of muscles involved in swallow movement.

16.2.2 Other Common Rehabilitation Training Methods

16.2.2.1 Therapeutic Purpose

Recovering swallow function: the patients try to eat food with mouth but not through nasal tube, pharynx fistulization, esophagus fistulization, stomach fistulization or jejunal fistulization.

Improving swallow function of food with different consistence.

Avoid aspiration.

16.2.2.2 Methods

1. The training of indirect eating induces swallow movement: It is the training method that swallow movement is induced not through eating.

   Indirect eating training is the training methods that swallow movement are induced not through eating. This method is impossible to induce erroneous deglutition and choke. Therefore, it is safe. Rehabilitation training method of neurological training belongs to this kind of method and can be used for swallowing disorder to varying degrees. The specific methods are as follows:

(a) Movement training of perioral muscles:

The training of oral cavity and facial muscles: the patients can do expression movement training such as frown, closing eyes, blowing cheek and smiling. The patients can also do self-exercise before the mirror.

Movement training of submandibular joint: active movement training of submandibular joint is good for masticatory movement. The patients use cheek tooth to chew gum to enhance the myodynamia of masseter.

Movement training of tongue: movements of tongue protraction, retraction and lateral movement; active movements of cheek massage, cleaning teeth and scrolling with tongue; anti-resistance movement of tongue, the therapists use tongue depressor to oppress and slide on the tongue and do anti-resistance training. Pronunciation training can promote movements of lingual muscles.

Adhesion release of lingual muscles [8]: traction and malaxation: the therapists use wet saline gauze to wrap the tip of the tongue, use one hand to hold the tongue, tract it to all the directions slowly, use the other hand to hold the tongue and malaxate the tongue from the tip of the tongue to root of tongue to loosen adhesion of lingual muscles. The therapists use the convexity surface of the spoon to oppress the center of tongue to loosen tongue tissue and deepen the sunken, which is good for the formation, maintenance and delivery of bolus.

(b) The training of improving the range of cervical joint motion: the patients do myodynamia enhancement and relaxation training of cervical flexor to improve the degree of flexion and extension and flexibility of neck. Flexed position of the neck is easy to induce swallow reflex and relaxation of the neck is good for prevention of erroneous deglutition.

(c) The training of improving swallow reflex: cold-stress stimulation can increase sensitiveness of soft palate and pharynx effectively to induce swallow reflex. The specific methods are as follows: the therapists use small mirror that was soaked in cold water for 10 sec used for ear-nose-throat department to press on soft palate arch or use iced wet cotton swab to stimulate soft palate, pillars of fauces, posterior pharyngeal wall and the back of the tongue for 5–10 times. The therapists can also let the patients swallow small iced cube or swallow stomach tube for 2–3 times a day from oral cavity to accelerate swallow reflex. For the patients who are already eat food from oral cavity, cold stimulation cleaning of oral cavity before meal not only can improve sensitivity of pharynx to bolus, but also can induce swallow reflex.

(d) The training of opening and closing vocal cords is to increase femininity of vocal cords, sensitivity of opening and closing, and strictness of closing to prevent erroneous deglutition. The specific method are as follows: the patients press on the wall or desk and yell out or hold their breath. The patients cross their hands before the chest, use hands to push the chest, yell out or hold their breath.

(e) Swallow training above glottis is the training of simulating swallow. The patients take a deep breath, hold their breath, swallow saliva, expire and cough. It is suitable for the patients who are easy to have erroneous deglutition.

For the patients whose throat is difficult to move upward during swallow, thyroid cartilage can be moved passively. The patients are asked to swallow saliva and lift throat.

(f) The method to promote swallow: for the patients who cannot swallow with food in the mouth, the therapists use fingers to rub the skin from thyroid cartilage to lower jaw, which is good for up-and-down motion of lower jaw and front and back motion of the tongue and then induce swallow reflex.

(g) Respiratory training and cough training: abdominal respiration training can increase myodynamia of diagram, enhance control respiration breath and increase glottis closure. Voluntary cough training can enhance glottis closure, which is good for cough up the food of erroneous deglutition.

2. Swallow movement training during eating is the training that food induce swallow reflex directly.

   If the patients are conscious, stable, with pharyngeal reflex and can cough at will, the training can be done.

   According to the assessment results, the patients choose the position for safe eating and do eating training of various kinds of food gradually. The sequence of food eating is soft food, semisolid, solid and liquid. All kinds of food refer to Table 16.2 and the specific training methods are as follows:

(a) The position of eating: when the patients start eating, the trunk is inclined backward and the neck is ante flexed.

(b) Time-phased eating training: the therapists choose movable food in oral cavity and the food is difficult to induce erroneous deglutition for training. Jelly-like and homogenous pasty food is the best such as soft egg custard, homogenous paste and congee. The patients should use this kind of food for training and then use normal food and water.

   The amount of eating should be started from a little bit about 3–4 mL and the patients can find proper amount for training. if the patients eat too much in one mouth, bolus retention in pharynx can aggravate the danger of erroneous deglutition. However, if the patients eat too little in one mouth, food is difficult to form bolus and cannot induce swallow reflex. For the patients who are easy to have erroneous deglutition, the eating speed should be too fast during training.

(c) The training method to eliminate food retention in pharynx: during training, there is usually food retention in pharynx. The following methods can be used for dealing with this condition: empty swallow repeatedly: empty swallow is that the patients swallow saliva without food. When there is residual food in pharynx, if the patients continue to eat, it is easy to induce erroneous deglutition. Therefore, after swallowing food every time, empty swallow can make the bolus enter into stomach in order to eliminate food in pharynx. Alternative swallow: the patients are asked to swallow solid food and liquid food alternatively. When there is residual food, the patients can drink a little bit water (1–2 mL) after every swallow, which is good for inducing swallow reflex and eliminating residual food. Nodding swallow: there is usually residual food in epiglottic vallecular. When the neck is inclined backward, the epiglottic vallecular becomes narrow, which can squeeze out residual food. After that, the patients ante flex neck, lower their head and swallow saliva to eliminate residual food. Lateral swallow: Piriform recess beside pharynx is the most common place for residual food. The patients are asked to rotate chin to two sides or incline neck to do lateral swallow, which make the offside piriform recess become narrow to squeeze out residuals. Meanwhile, piriform recess on the other side becomes shallow to eliminate residual food in piriform recess.

Table 16.2 Liquid and solid food used for the training of the patients with dysphagia

Classification	Degree
Solid	Single ingredient: bread, steamed bun, muddy flesh, mashed potato, banana, egg salad
	Particle: roast fish, chicken salad, Hamburger
	Multiple ingredients: roast potatoes, carrot, pea, rice and noodle, bottled
Fruits	Liquid sparseness: clear soup, coffee, fruit juice, tea, milk, gelatin
	Viscosity: nectar, hot frumentum, cream soup, milk and egg alcohol, viscous drink
	Viscosity: porridge, sour cream, pudding, milk cake

16.2.2.3 Considerations

1. Reducing the risk of aspiration: When the patients eat food through oral cavity, the therapists should know the actual condition of the patients thoroughly and choose optimum swallow method and safe food. Acid food and lardy food are easy to induce pneumonia after erroneous deglutition. The therapists try not to select this kind of food.

2. Keeping oral cavity clean to reduce aspiration and gastric regurgitation. After eating, the patients raise their head and keep in sitting position for 20–30 min to prevent esophagus backflow and erroneous deglutition.
3. Improving general body state to prevent pneumonia: for the patients who eat too less, they should use nasal feeding or intravenous drip to supply nutrition in order to prevent malnutrition.

16.2.2.4 Disposition of Special Problems

During training, there are some unwieldy problems that can influence training effect directly and are the key point of training.

(a) Poor occlusion of lips and lower jaw: when there is poor occlusion of lips and lower jaw, the patients cannot keep bolus in oral cavity and are difficult to do swallow training. In this case, the therapists use one hand to support lower jaw to make it close and use the other hand to stimulate perioral tissue. If the lips close asymmetrically, the therapists can stimulate the unclosed side. If buccinators spasm influences lips closure, the therapists can put index finger on the inner surface of chin, thumb on the out surface, malaxate the chin inward and tract it towards the orientation of lips closure.
(b) Tongue movement and poor swallow: the patients can lift the last third of the tongue to push bolus into pharynx. If there is poor tongue movement, the therapists use index finger to press and push backward the first third of the tongue to stimulate the elevation of the last third of the tongue and closure of posterior oral cavity. Under normal circumstance, outer edge of the tongue rolls up to make food form bolus. In order to stimulate the outer edge of the tongue roll up, the therapists can use middle finger to support outer edge of the tongue and press and vibrate it towards diagonal orientation, which is good for stimulating the outer edge of the tongue roll up. The therapists use the convexity surface of the spoon to oppress the center of tongue to stimulate lingualis contraction and deepen the sunken, which is good for the formation of bolus.

The above methods can be used repeatedly and alternatively. The therapists oppress on the part of root of tongue in the lower jaw and use the back of the hand to slap lower jaw to stimulate swallow.

(c) Hypaesthesia of oral cavity: Hypaesthesia of oral cavity is bad for chewing and saliva secretion. The patients can malaxate exterior face of gingiva, inner surface of chin or oppress on tongue to improve the sensation of oral cavity.
(d) Irritability of oral cavity: the therapists should oppress on the most insensitive area and decrease unhappy reaction to touch. The patients close lower jaw and malaxate lower jaw towards the orientation of lips closure. After the patients can tolerate it, the therapists put finger into mouth and use force to rub gingiva from outside to inside. Pressure on tongue can increase desensitization.
(e) Abnormal reflex: cough hyperreflexia: for the patients who are with cough hyperreflexia, desensitization should be used for the therapy. Vomiting dysreflexia: for the patients who are easy to inhale food or liquid, malaxation of gingiva and inner surface of chin and oppression of tongue are used for therapy. Hypaesthesia of uvula and soft palate: banister brush or cotton swab is used to stimulate the uvula and soft palate. Cotton swab stimulation should be cooperated with closure training of lips and lower jaw. Positive occlusion reaction: after putting bite block, the therapists use finger to rub the outer surface of gingiva for desensitization. During eating, the therapists cannot press the bottom of lower jaw in case of inducing occlusion reaction. Difficulty in opening mouth: the therapists use thumb to oppress temporomandibular joint continuously or malaxate it from nose to mouth.
(f) Poor facial expression: through facial massage, adhesion tissue release and active movement training of facial muscles, poor facial expression can be alleviated.
(g) The method to help the patients to eat and drink: before meal, the food should be provided from middle line and the patients

can smell it and see it in order to make a preparation. When the spoon enters into mouth, the therapists press on the first third of the tongue and then exert great force downward and backward to stimulate it in order to pour out food. After that, the therapists withdraw the spoon and help the patients to close lips and lower jaw and slightly flex head for swallow. The food should be delicious and fragrant, which is in accordance with the eating habit of the patients. Viscous food is safe and can stimulate the touch and pressure sense of tongue and oral cavity, saliva secretion. It is easy to swallow. The therapists can put gum into cheek tooth to stimulate chewing. Liquid is easier to be inhaled into trachea than solid. The patients should use plastic cup with curved lip for drinking liquid. The patients flex the head slightly, use lower lip to touch the cup lip, drink a little bit liquid, close lips and lower jaw for swallow. If there is incomplete lips closure, cup lip can be used for stimulation. If possible, the patients are asked to eat by themselves for promoting further functional recovery of swallow.

References

1. Hamdy S, Rothwell JC. Cut feeling about recovery after stroke: the organization and reorganization of human swallowing motor cortex. Trends Neurosci. 1998;21(7):278–82.
2. Han TR, Paik NJ, Park JW. Quantifying swaiiowing function after stroke: a functional dysphagia scale based on vide ofluoroscopic studies. Arch Phys Med Rehabil. 2001;82(3):677–82.
3. Work SS, Colamonico JA, Bradley WG, et al. Pseudobulbar affect: an under-recognized and under-treated neurological disorder. Adv Ther. 2011;28(7):586–601.
4. Teasell R, Foley N, Dohetty T, et al. Cinicai characteristics of patients with brainstem strokes admitted to a rehabilitation unit. Arch Phys Med Rehabil. 2002;83(7):1013–6.
5. Martino R, Pron G, Diamant N. Screening for oropharyngeal dysphagia in stroke: insufficient evidence for guidelines. Dysphagia. 2000;15(1):19–30.
6. Smith HA, LeeSH, O' Neill PA, et al.The combination of bedside swallowingassessm ent and oxygen saturation monitoring of swallowing in acute stroke:a safe and humane screening tool.Age Ageing, 2000,29(6):495–499.
7. Burnett TA, Mann EA, Cornell SA, et al. Laryngeal elevation athieved by neuromuscul ar stimulation at rest. J Appl Physiol. 2003;94:128–34.
8. Langmore SE, Miller RM. Behavioral treatment for adults with oro-pharyngeal dysphagia. Arch Phys Med Rehabil. 1994;75:1154–60.

17 Rehabilitation Therapy of Neurological Training of Sphincter Dysfunction

17.1 Micturition Dysfunction

Micturition dysfunction is the common complication of the paraplegic patients. It belongs to neurogenic bladder including dysfunction of sphincter vesicae and urethral sphincter. The early manifestation is retention of urine. The final manifestation is uroclepsia or urinary retention with overflow incontinence. It is difficult to be treated in clinic [1].

17.1.1 Innervation of Micturition

Micturition is the process that urine generated in kidney is stored in bladder to a certain capacity and discharged out under the control of central nervous system through urethra.

17.1.1.1 Functions of Bladder and Urethra

There is net detrusor interweaved by smooth muscle fibers in outer layer of bladder wall. In the joint between bladder and urethra, muscular loop interweaved by smooth muscle fibers is called internal urethral sphincter. It function is sphincter, but it is not circular sphincter. Urethra is wrapped by circular striated muscle fiber to form striated muscle loop when it goes through urogenital diaphragm, which is called external urethral sphincter.

Bladder and urethra belong to the same unit in structure and function. When bladder detrusor relax and urethral sphincter shrink, urine in bladder cannot flow out. During micturition, when bladder detrusor shrink and urethral sphincter relax, urine is expelled from bladder through urethra. When the volume of urine exceeds 400–500 mL in bladder, the tonicity of detrusor is increased with rhythmic contraction and relaxation, which can induce micturition. Physiological characteristics of detrusor make the bladder store a certain volume of urine without innervation and induce automatic micturition. However, out of control of neural center bladder, urine in bladder cannot be drained and there is always 200–300 mL urine in bladder, which is residual urine volume that is the important factor to induce urinary system infection and renal dysfunction.

17.1.1.2 Nerves of Micturition

There are three pairs of composite nerve trunks to innervate bladder and urethra. Every trunk is composed of afferent fiber and efferent fiber.

1. Hypogastric nerve: The efferent fibers are from funiculus lateralis in T_{12}–L_{1-2} of spinal cord and belong to sympathetic nerve. They mainly innervate bladder detrusor and internal urethral sphincter. Their function is to shrink internal urethral sphincter and relax bladder detrusor to store urine in bladder. The afferent

W. Zhao, *Rehabilitation Therapeutics of the Neurological Training*,
https://doi.org/10.1007/978-981-13-0812-3_17

fiber is responsible for the conduction of bladder algesia.

2. Pelvic nerve: The afferent fiber is responsible for the conduction of sensation of bladder and internal urethral sphincter. The efferent fiber is from funiculus lateralis in S_{2-4} of spinal cord and belongs to parasympathetic nerve. They mainly innervate bladder detrusor and urethral sphincter to shrink detrusor and relax urethral sphincter in order to expel urine and empty bladder.
3. Pudendal nerve: The afferent fiber is responsible for the conduction of urethral sensation including algesia. The efferent fiber is from anterior horn motor neuron in S_{2-4} of spinal cord and belongs to somatic nerve to innervate external urethral sphincter and striated muscle of perineum. Its function is to shrink external urethral sphincter and stop bladder micturition. During micturition, catatonic excitement of pudendal nerve is inhibited to weaken tonicity of external urethral sphincter. Urine is driven by detrusor and flow out through relaxed urethra. During micturition, people can excite it consciously at any time and shrink external urethral sphincter to stop micturition. After stopping micturition, this nerve can recover catatonic excitement to maintain tonic contraction of external urethral sphincter.
4. Micturition reflex: Primary irritation of micturition is from dilated bladder. The stretch receptor in bladder wall is stretched to generate distention. With the increase of urine volume, stretch tension is increased and distention becomes stronger. In addition, hyperinflation and contraction of bladder can stimulate bladder algesia ending to induce pain, micturition reflex, bladder evacuation, uncomfortable feelings such as distention and pain.

Basic reflex center of micturition is located in spinal cord is composed of two associated reflex movements.

(a) Afferent and efferent information of sympathetic nerve: Afferent information: sensory impulse information of bladder distention is introduced into micturition center located in lateral column of S_{2-4} of spinal cord through pelvic nerve. Efferent information: micturition center competition and micturition information can induce contraction of detrusor and internal urethral sphincter through pelvic nerve. Posterior urethra is broadened and the resistance is decreased, which press urine in to posterior urethra.
(b) Afferent and efferent information of parasympathetic nerve: Afferent information: urine enters into posterior urethra and stimulates receptor. Impulse information enters into micturition center of spinal cord through pelvic nerve. The information is integrated in spinal micturition center and give out information to inhibit anterior horn cells located in S_{2-4}. Tonic efferent impulse of pudendal nerve decreases and external urethral sphincter relaxes, which expel out urine through urethra.

After transverse injury of inferior spinal cord, detrusor relaxes in the beginning, bladder dilates, micturition reflex disappears and urine is in bladder. However, if there is complete neural connection between micturition center of sacrum and bladder and urethra, micturition reflex can be recovered and there is frequent micturition [2]. One hundred and fifty milliliter urine in bladder can induce micturition, but cannot be expelled out. During micturition, there is no micturition desire and the patients cannot control micturition at will, which is called uroclepsia. Therefore, plenty of urine reservoir and complete evacuation in bladder, micturition desire and voluntary control of micturition are all controlled by higher center in the brain.

5. The regulation of micturition by brain and voluntary movement in micturition.

Detrusor contraction enhances the stimulation of interoceptor in bladder and urine enhances the stimulation of interoceptor in posterior urethra. Impulse is conducted into spinal through pelvic nerve, hypogastric nerve and pudendal nerve, and then is projected to brain through spinothalamic tract and thalamus. It is the conduction pathway of voluntary movement in micturition [3].

Micturition process is inhibited voluntarily by brain cortex. If the situation is improper, people can suppress the urine. Human can suppress urine to 600 mL without pain and can suppress urine to 800 mL painfully. During micturition, human can shrink external urethral sphincter and perineum muscles at will to close posterior urethra, inhibit micturition reflex induced by stimulation of posterior urethra by urine, push urine back to bladder and relax bladder detrusor gradually.

However, inhibitory area of micturition cannot be located in brain exactly. Its downward pathways are corticospinal tract and extrapyramidal pathway. It can inhibit micturition center in spinal cord and excitability of motor neuron to inhibit micturition.

Cerebral function of children is not developed well so that the inhibitory effect on basic micturition center is weak. Therefore, there is micturition frequency. There is usually enuresis at night, even urinary incontinence. For the adult in coma or old people with cerebral hypofunction, they are easy to have urinary incontinence.

6. The factors of micturition: There are many factors to influence micturition such as age, weather and habit.
   (a) Age and gender: Micturition in baby is a reflex movement and cannot be controlled consciously. After 3 years old, they can control it by themselves. For old people, there is usually frequent micturition because of bladder tension decrease. Benign prostatic hyperplasia in old male can oppress urethra and lead to urine drip and micturition difficulty. In the menstrual period and gestation period, micturition morphology is changed.
   (b) Diet and weather: if there are a lot of water in food or people drink a lot of water, urine volume can increase. Diuretic action of coffee, tea and alcohol can increase urine volume. More sodium salt in food can lead to water and sodium retention and decrease urine volume. If the temperature is high, respiration rate increases, people sweat more and urine volume decreases.
   (c) Micturition habit: micturition time is related to work and rest time such as micturition when getting bed and before sleep. If the micturition gesture or micturition environment is not proper, they will influence micturition movement.
   (d) Therapeutic factors: diuretic can increase urine volume. Anesthetic in surgery and pain after surgery can lead to retention of urine.
   (e) Diseases: Disturbance of consciousness of neural conduction and control induced by damage of nervous system can lead to urinary incontinence. Kidney disease can lead to dyspoiesis of urine, oliguria or anuria. Lithiasis in urinary system, tumor, stenosis can lead to tract disturbance of micturition, even retention of urine.
   (f) Psychological factors: emotion changes such as tension, anxiety and fear can lead to frequent micturition, urgent urination or retention of urine because of inhibition of micturition. Implication can also influence micturition. Auditory sense, visual sense and sensory irritation of other parts can induce micturition.

17.1.2 Classification of Micturition Dysfunction

Traditional neurogenic bladder is divided into sensory paralytic bladder, motor paralytic bladder, reflex bladder and uninhibited bladder. At present, the classification can be done according to the combination of urodynamics with the functions of bladder and urethra.

1. Superexcitation type of detrusor and sphincter: Sphincter excitation usually lead to big bladder volume. Meanwhile, detrusor excitation can male urine flow out when there is a certain urine volume in bladder, which is called overflowing urinary incontinence (reflex bladder).
2. The type of detrusor excitation and sphincter relaxation: the urine cannot be stored in

bladder and the ability of storing urine decreases, which lead to small bladder, even contracted bladder.

3. The type of detrusor relaxation and sphincter excitation: Dysuresia lead to big bladder volume or retention of urine. High tension in bladder leads to increase of urethral pressure. Long-term pressure increase can lead to pyelectasis and hydronephrosis. When it is severe, it can damage kidney function. This type is also called motor paralytic bladder.
4. Relaxation type of detrusor and sphincter: This type is called uninhibited bladder. Cerebral cortex lesion makes spinal micturition center break away from inhibition of cerebral cortex center, which can lead to uninhibited bladder. Lesion is located in paracentral lobule of two hemispheres or its descending tractus pyramidalis. The main clinical manifestations are frequent micturition, urgent urination, small urine amounts every time and urinary incontinence. This type is difficult to be treated.

17.1.3 Assessment Method of Micturition Dysfunction

Urodynamics is the important method to assess bladder function. Hydromechanics, electrophysiology and neurophysiology are used to assess bladder function [4].

1. Urine flow rate: The exhaust urine volume in unit time (mL/s). It is the manifestation of the interaction between detrusor and urethral sphincter during micturition, which is the total function condition of lower urinary tract. Major parameters include maximum urine flow rate, urine flow time and urine volume. Urine flow rate is affected by gender, age and micturition.
2. Bladder pressure-volume includes bladder pressure, rectum pressure (abdominal pressure) and detrusor pressure (bladder pressure minus rectum pressure). Normal pressure-volume: There is no residual urine. Internal pressure is maintained at 5–15 cm H_2O in filling period of bladder with good elasticity. There is no uninhibited contraction. During the filling process of bladder, people have the feeling of micturition when the urine volume is 100–200 mL. The total bladder volume is 400–500 mL. People can control micturition at will.
3. Urethral pressure distribution: major parameters include maximum urethral occlusion pressure: The normal is 50–130 cm/H_2O (60–70 cm H_2O in female). Functional urethral length is 5.4 ± 0.8 cm in male and 3.7 ± 0.5 cm in female.

   Sphincter electromyography: Surface electrode can be inserted into anus to test the myoelectric activity signal of sphincter ani. Pin electrode can be directly inserted into external urethral sphincter through perineum to record electromyographic signal of external urethral sphincter. People should know the coordination movement of external urethral sphincter during detrusor contraction.
4. In the filling period of bladder of the normal micturition cycle, external urethral sphincter is activated continuously and the myoelectric activity is stopped during micturition. After micturition, myoelectric activity reappears. Abnormal conditions include: when detrusor shrinks, electromyographic signal of sphincter is enhanced at the same time, which demonstrates that the coordination movement between detrusor and sphincter is lost. During the filling period of bladder, electromyographic signal of sphincter suddenly disappears, which means there is involuntary urine leakage in bladder.
5. Urodynamics, B ultrasonic or X-ray: diluted iodine solution is used to replace saline to fulfill bladder for understanding the morphology of urodynamics, bladder and urethra in the urodynamics test.

17.1.4 Rehabilitation Therapy of Micturition Dysfunction

17.1.4.1 The Main Purpose of Rehabilitation Training of Micturition Dysfunction

The main purpose of rehabilitation training is to recover voluntary skeletal muscles dominated by motor center in brain cortex, including external urethral sphincter, urethrovaginal sphincter muscle and musculus sphincter ani externus. Reflex center of involuntary muscles such as internal urethral sphincter and musculus sphincter ani internus is located in spinal cord just as that of patellar tendon reflex and Achilles tendon reflex. They all belong to lower neural center. In most cases of micturition and defecation dysfunctions, this center is not injured. Therefore, recovering the function of involuntary muscles is the fundamental measure and ultimate rehabilitation goal of recovering functions of defecation and micturition.

Although there are different nerves to dominate micturition and defecation, the two processes can be controlled separately. There is close relationship between the two processes. For example, defecation is easy to induce micturition. Because the reception of signal of external urethral sphincter is difficult through skin surface electrode, for the male with long urethra, internal electrode is hard to be placed exactly and is easy to induce injury of urethral mucosa.

Urethral sphincter, sphincter vaginae and sphincter ani of perineum belong to pelvic floor muscles and are controlled by pudendal nerve. The perineum is generally defined as the surface region in both males and females between the pubic symphysis and the coccyx. The perineum is below the pelvic diaphragm and between the legs. It is a diamond-shaped area that includes the anus and, in females, the vagina. Its definition varies: it can refer to only the superficial structures in this region, or it can be used to include both superficial and deep structures. The perineum corresponds to the outlet of the pelvis. There is urogenital muscles to seal foramen of pelvic diaphragm, enhance pelvic floor and perineal central tendon such as superficial transverse muscle of perineum, ischiocavernosus, bulbocavernosus muscle, deep transverse muscle of perineum, external urethral sphincter around urethral membrane. In female, urethral sphincter is around vagina, which is called urethrovaginal sphincter muscle. Urethral sphincter contractions can crimple urethra and vagina.

In addition, defecation and micturition time overlap. External urethral sphincter and pelvic floor muscle are called spring bed of pelvic floor. They are like a net to support pelvic organs such as bladder, uterus and rectum. The muscles can control micturition, defecation and compressicity of vagina. Therefore, male can use sphincter ani signal and female can use sphincter vaginae signal or sphincter ani signal to replace external urethral sphincter signal for neurological training. During training, the patients are guided to concentrate on the contraction and relaxation of urethral sphincter.

17.1.4.2 Therapeutic Principle

Rehabilitation therapeutic principle of micturition dysfunction is to keep the bladder volume at 300–500 mL through recovering autonomous contraction of external urethral sphincter and recovering coordination movement of bladder detrusor and sphincter in case of urinary incontinence, retention of urine and urinary system infection.

17.1.4.3 Rehabilitation Training Methods

Rehabilitation training method of micturition dysfunction includes rehabilitation training method of neurological training, the common rehabilitation training method and electrical stimulation.

1. Rehabilitation therapy of neurological training of external sphincter dysfunction: Six-step Daoyin technique combined with biofeedback is used for the training of external sphincter, development of neural potential of external sphincter to recover voluntary self-control ability of external urethral sphincter.

   Main and collateral channels of six-step Daoyin technique of guiding collaterals through meridians is Ren channel (Fig. 17.1). Ren channel is on the center of chest and abdomen. The top is chin. It can regulate Qi of Yin channel in the whole body. The pathway of regulation of mind with six-step Daoyin technique is that Qi from Chengqi goes down along anterior middle line of the trunk through

Fig. 17.1 Sketch map of Ren channel

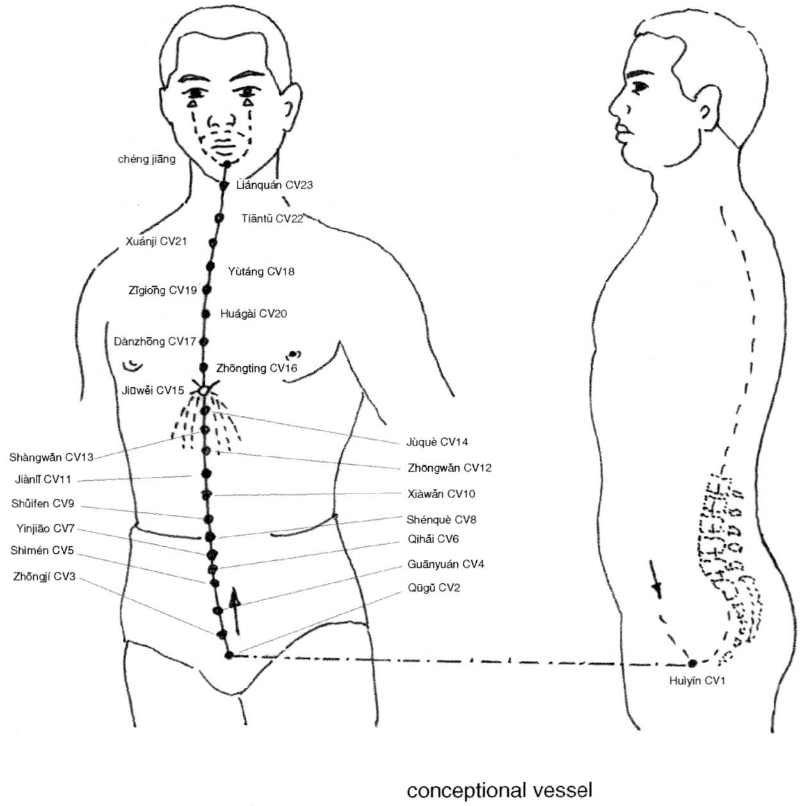

Chengjiang and reach Huiyin through Xuanji, Tanzhong, Jiuwei, Zhongwan, Yinjiao and Qugu to stimulate the contraction and relaxation training of urethral sphincter.

(a) Bare hand training of external sphincter: Before therapy, the patients should defecate. The patients are in knee-chest position, separate two legs to expose anus. The therapists wear sterilized gloves, use thumb and index finger of left hand to separate anus akin, insert index finger of right hand with liquid paraffin into anus and extend around to relax sphincter ani. After that, the therapists insert sterilized anus training probe with liquid paraffin into anus slowly (Fig. 17.2). The patients are help to lie in lateral position for the training.

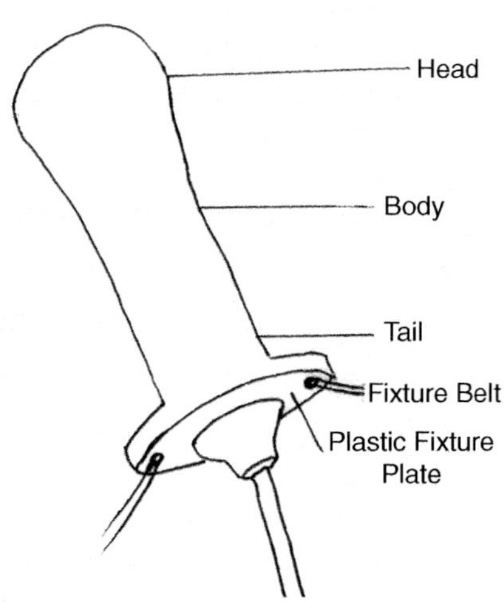

Fig. 17.2 Sketch map of training probe of sphincter ani

The training is divided into two procedures. Contraction training: the therapist should use normal of six-step Daoyin technique of guiding collaterals through meridians to guide the patients after regulation of mind and breathing. The patients are asked to concentrate on external urethral sphincter. The specific method is to shrink urethra. After deep inspiration, the patients are asked to try to shrink urethra and clamp anus training probe for 6 s. After that, the patients take a deep breath and expire slowly. The ratio between inspiration time and expiration time is 1–2. Relaxation training: after regulation of mind and breathing, the therapists guide the patients to concentrate on external urethral sphincter. After taking a deep breath, the patients try to adjust body and mind. During the process of relaxing external urethral sphincter, the patients relax musculus sphincter ani externus for 6 s. After taking a deep breath, the patients expire slowly. The ratio between inspiration time and expiration time is 1–2.

Contraction training and relaxation training is done alternatively and repeatedly.

The training time is 30 min (once a day) and there are 30 times in one therapy course. The patients can do multiple therapy courses.

(b) Rehabilitation training of neurological training of external sphincter: Before therapy, the patients should defecate. Signal reception probe of neurological training is inserted into anus (Fig. 17.3). The operational approach is the same as the mentioned above. The patients are in lateral position or knee-chest position (Fig. 17.4). Reception electrode is connected with the first lead of neurological training device. Motor program signal of sphincter ani from central nervous system is displayed in single screen and the training can be started.

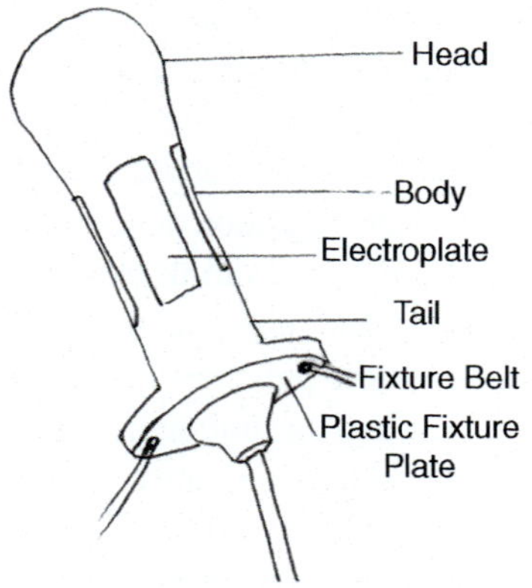

Fig. 17.3 Sketch map of sphincter ani used for neurological training

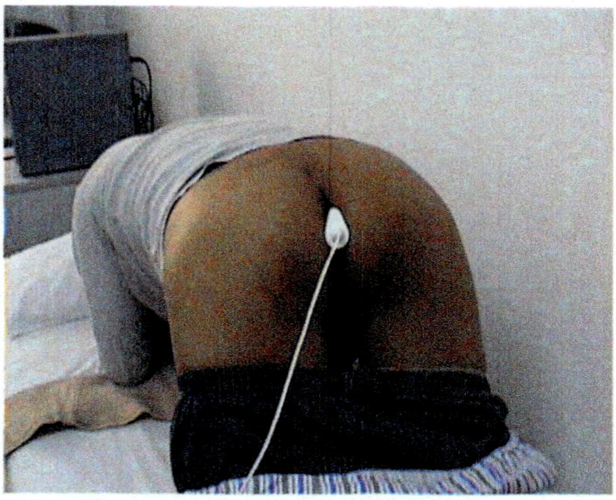

Fig. 17.4 Training position of sphincter ani of neurological training

The training is divided into two procedures. Contraction training: After regulation of mind and breathing, the therapists guide the patients to concentrate on external urethral sphincter. The specific method is to shrink urethra. After taking a deep inspiration, the patients are guided to try to shrink urethra and anus. The patients are asked to stare at the signal curve on the screen to increase signal intensity for 6 s. After that, the patients take a deep inspiration and expire slowly. The ratio between inspiration time and expiration time is 1–2. Signal intensity of the first time is the baseline (Fig. 17.5) and is used as surpassing target. In the next training, the patients are guided to make signal intensity surpass the previous time (Fig. 17.6). The rest can be done in the same manner. Relaxation training: if the patients have external urethral sphincter spasm, the signal intensity is stronger than that of baseline and cannot be reduced to zero. The patients can do this training. After regulation of mind and breathing, the therapists guide the patients to concentrate on signal curve on screen. After taking a deep inspiration, the patients are guided to regulate body and mind to relax external urethral sphincter and musculus sphincter ani externus in order to decrease curve for 6 s. After that, the patients take a deep inspiration and expire slowly. The ratio between inspiration time and

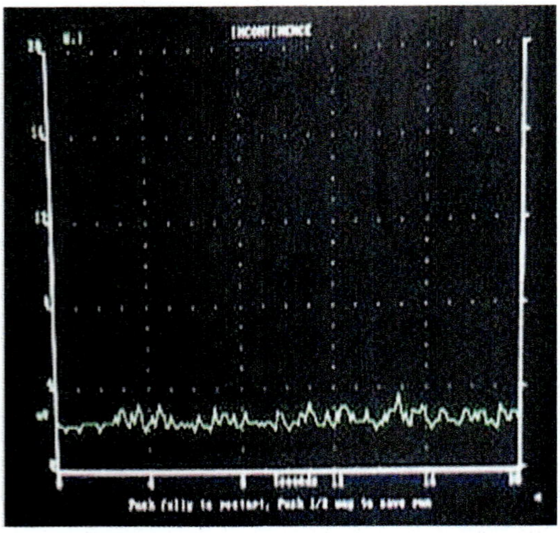

Fig. 17.5 The signal is zero at the beginning of training

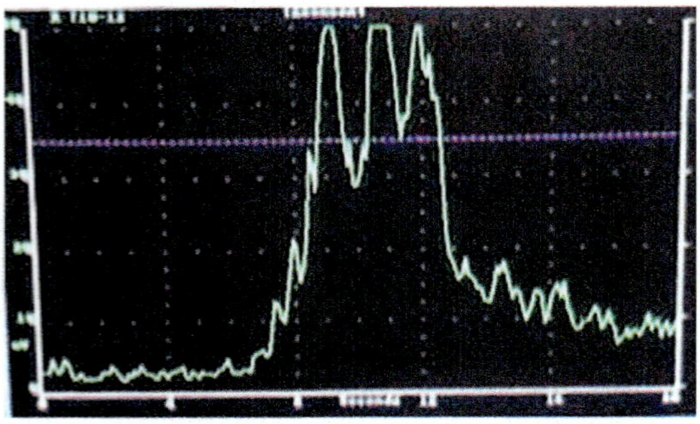

Fig. 17.6 The surpassing goal is the signal intensity of the previous time

expiration time is 1–2. Contraction training and relaxation training is done alternatively. If there is no external urethral sphincter spasm in the patients, the patients can merely do contraction training. Contraction training can enhance the training feeling and is good for the effect. In addition, recovering active contraction function of muscles is the premise and basis of active relaxation of muscles.

The method of guiding collaterals through meridians can be used for the training.

The training time and therapy course: double training of contraction and relaxation: The training time is 50 min (once a day) and there are 30 times in one therapy course. The patients can do multiple therapy courses. Single training of contraction: The training time is 25 min (once a day) and there are 30 times in one therapy course. The patients can do multiple therapy courses.

(c) Virtual reality training of neurological training: Before, the patients should defecate. Training probe of sphincter ani is inserted into anus. The patients lie in lateral position or knee-chest position. The placement of training probe and training method are the same as these of rehabilitation training of neurological training of external sphincter. The only difference is virtual reality training device.

The training time and therapy course: double training of contraction and relaxation: The training time is 50 min (once a day) and there are 30 times in one therapy course. The patients can do multiple therapy courses. Single training of contraction: The training time is 25 min (once a day) and there are 30 times in one therapy course. The patients can do multiple therapy courses.

Every week, neurological training device is used to detect the signal of external urethral sphincter to know the actual therapeutic effect and instruct therapeutic schedule.

(d) Self-exercise method of pelvic floor muscles: the patients who received rehabilitation training of neurological training of external urethral sphincter in rehabilitation department of hospital are already know the method of training active movement of external urethral sphincter with Daoyin technique and are impressed by the relationship between contraction and signal line. After discharge or during the therapy internal, the patients can do self-exercise of external urethral sphincter. On the basis of regulation of mind and breathing, the patients shrink external urethral sphincter and imagine the signal curve change in the previous therapy course for 6 s. During the training, training probe can be placed in anus to consolidate therapeutic effect.

The time of self-exercise is 30 min and there are 2–3 times a day. The patients can do it for a long time.

(e) Acupuncture therapy: Acupuncture can treat difficult urination or urinary incontinence. The therapists can select Huiyin of Ren channel. Huiyin is located at the midpoint between scrotum root and anus in males. In females, it is located at the intersection of the midpoint of labium majus pudenda posterior commissure and anus.

The therapy frequency is once a day and there are 15 time in one therapy course.

2. Other rehabilitation therapeutic methods include biofeedback therapy and clean urethral catheterization technique.

(a) Electromyographic biofeedback therapy: biofeedback therapy is that through gathering electromyographic signal of musculus sphincter ani externus, when signal intensity cannot reach contraction threshold, the major processor of biofeedback therapy device in pelvic floor can change into stimulation mode automatically to stimulate nervous system intermittently through regulation technique of micro-current in order to make motor neurons generate action potential. The action potential is conducted to muscular tissue and the contraction movement is completed [5]. Repeated stimulation can decrease spasm of pelvic floor muscles and recover autonomous contraction function.

However, because the electrical stimulation helps the patients to complete contraction movement, the patients cannot try to develop central nerve potential by themselves and the therapeutic effects may be affected.

The training time is 20–30 min (once a day) and there are 15 times in one therapy course.

(b) Electrical stimulation therapy: in the electrical stimulation therapy of pelvic floor muscles, according to specific condition, the therapists choose proper electrical stimulation schedule and tome. The patients should tolerate the electrical intensity and don't feel painful. If the patients are not sensitive to electrical stimulation, the therapists cannot increase electrical intensity blindly, but should increase pulsative index.

Because there is tolerance in electrical stimulation, the therapists should increase electrical stimulation parameter in the therapeutic process to achieve better effect. The increased range should be 1–5%.

Similarly, electrical stimulation is passive. In the early phase of disease, it can activate undead cells in injured area and promote functional recovery of shock cells, which has a certain therapeutic effect. In the late phase of disease, electrical stimulation can increase excitability of muscles, but it is not active movement so that it cannot develop central neural potential and the therapeutic effect is poor.

The training time is 20–30 min (once a day) and there are 15 times in one therapy course.

(c) Timing and quantitative drinking water and timing micturition: The drinking water volume is 400 mL every time and the patients should urinate 2–4 h after drinking water.

(d) Clean catheterization technique: Clean catheterization is also called intermittent catheterization. Non-medical staffs such as the patients, family or caregiver do catheterization method without indwelling catheter to prevent urinary system infection, decrease the dependence of the patients on medical staffs and increase life independence of the patients. It is widely applied abroad.

Indications: the patients cannot urinate autonomously or the patients can urinate autonomously but the micturition is not sufficient (residual urine exceeds 80–100 mL). The patients with spinal cord injury or other neural paralysis are conscious and can cooperate with therapy actively.

Contraindications: the patients with severe urethral injury, infection or urethral pressure sores; the patients with unconsciousness or who don't cooperate with the therapy; the patients who are receiving a great quantity transfusion; the patients with general infection or extremely low immunity; the patients with notable bleeding tendency; the patients with notable prostatic hyperplasia or tumor.

Specific operation: the minimum catheter or specific catheter with enough length is chosen and the procedures are as follows: 0.9% sodium chloride solution or other medical disinfectant without mucosa irritation such as benzalkonium bromide is used to wash catheter for preparation. Soap or cleaning solution is used to wash the patients' perineum and the operators wash their hands. The patients hold the catheter and insert it into slowly until urine flows out from catheter. For male patients, the therapists should make urethra orifice towards abdomen in case of urethral isthmus injury. Before insertion, the outer surface of catheter should be smeared with lubricating oil such as paroline to reduce resistance. After completing catheterization, the catheter should be removed immediately. The catheter should be washed with clean water and then is put into medical disinfectant without mucosa irritation or 0.9% sodium chloride solution. It can also be disinfected with boiling method. Frequency of utilization: if the patients cannot urinate autonomously, catheterization can be used 3–4 times every day. If the patients can urinate partially, catheterization can be used 1–2 times every day. Urine volume after every catheterization is about 400 mL (physiological bladder volume). If residual urine volume is less than 80–100 mL, the catheterization is stopped.

If the patients can urinate more than 100 mL between two catheterizations and residual urine volume is 300 mL or less, the catheterization can be used once 8 h. If the patients can urinate more than 200 mL between two catheterizations and residual urine volume is less than 200 mL, the catheterization can be used once half a day. If the residual urine volume is less than 80–100 mL, the catheterization should be stopped.

Precautions: the patients should drink water on time and quantitatively, urinate on time can choose proper catheterization time. The patients drink water that is less than 2000 mL every day and the urine volume should be maintained at 800–1000 mL/day. When the catheter is inserted, the movement should be gentle. The catheter cannot be inserted violently in case of urethral injury.

(e) Bladder control training: bladder control training is used for rehabilitation training of the patients with upper motor neuron injury syndrome accompanied with bladder dysfunction.

Indications: it is used for the patients with upper motor neuron injury syndrome accompanied with bladder dysfunction including spinal cord injury, stroke and cerebral trauma. When the patients' hand function is well, the patients can do it by themselves or it can be completed by caregivers with active cooperation of the patients.

Contraindications: the patients with unconsciousness or who don't cooperate with the therapy; the patients with severe bladder or urinary infection; the patients with notable prostatic hyperplasia or tumor.

Specific methods: bladder sphincter control training: the patients usually use exercise method of pelvic floor muscles to shrink sphincter ani actively for ten times (10 s per time). The training can be done 3–5 times a day. Micturition reflex training: the patients can find out or induce trigger point and use reflex mechanism to induce detrusor contraction and promote active micturition. The common trigger points of micturition reflex are tapping suprapubic area, pulling pubes, rubbing inner thigh or squeezing penis and glans penis. The patients can use auxiliary measures such as listening to bicker, hot drinks and lukewarm bath. Tapping should be soft and quick in case of heavy tapping. Heavy tapping can induce bladder and urethra dysfunction or bladder mucosal hemorrhage. The tapping frequency is 50–100 times per min. The total tapping number is 100–500. Reflexive micturition usually can be recovered in higher spinal cord injury. The therapists use hand to stimulate rectum. The electrical stimulation is used. The acupuncture points of the first group include Sanyinjiao, Shenyu, Weiyang and Xiajiaoyu. The second group is Shuidao. The two groups are used alternatively. High-frequency modulated impulse electricity is used for the therapy.

(f) Compensatory micturition training: the patients use manipulation and increasing abdominal pressure to promote micturition.

Valsalva method: the patients are in sitting position, relax abdomen, incline body, hold the breath for 10–12 s, use force to make abdominal pressure reach to bladder, rectum and pelvic floor, flex hip joint and knee joint to make thigh close to abdomen in order to prevent abdominal bulge and increase abdominal pressure to help urine flow out. Credè manipulation: the patients put two thumbs on crista iliaca, put other fingers on the top of bladder (below the navel), press inward and downward gradually. The patients can also use fist to press from umbilical region to pubis, but compression should be slow and gentle in case of compression on the pubis with violence. If bladder pressure is too high, the bladder may be injured or urine may flow back to kidney. The control training of intake and output water volume: the system of timing and quantitative drinking water and timing micturition should be established, which is the basic measures of bladder training. Because the physiological bladder volume is about 400 mL, water intake volume is 400–450 mL to make bladder volume reach about 400 mL. Interval time between drinking water and micturition is usually 1–2 h and is related to body position and temperature. When the patients are in clinostatism and the temperature is low, interval time of micturition is short. Otherwise, the interval time is long. The total urine volume is 800–1000 mL every day.

Considerations: when the patients start training, the therapists should watch bladder residual volume to avoid retention of urine. The therapists should avoid that bladder overfilling or manipulation compression induces urine backflow. The appearance of bladder reflex requires a certain time. The training should be step by step. Especially, the therapists should explain the training to the patients and their family. When the patients are accompanied with spasm, there is close relationship between bladder evacuation and convulsive seizure. The therapists should the relationship between micturition and relieving muscle spasm.

(g) Disposition of lithangiuria: Bladder stone is usually observed in paraplegic patients. The forming reason is related to infection and micturition difficulty.

Therapeutic principle: upper urinary tract calculi: extracortoreal shock wave lithotripsy percutaneous pyeloscope calculus removed. Bladder stone: cystoscope is used for electric hydraulic broken stone. A few patients require calculus removed by surgery. Medicine: Cholinergic preparations such as carbamoyl methylcholine (40–100 mg/day) can increase detrusor tension and promote bladder contraction, which can be used to treat detrusor relaxation. Anticholinergic drug such as atropine can decrease detrusor tension, promote bladder contraction and sphincter tension, which can be used for the patients with bladder spasm. Baclofen can be also used to inhibit bladder spasm. Sphincter relaxant: α adrenergic agents and β receptor stimulant such as ephedrine (25–100 mg/day) can be used to increase sphincter tension.

(h) Bacteriuria and urinary system infection: Bacteriuria and urinary system infection are the common complications of the patients with spinal cord injury. Bacteriuria and urinary system infection can also be observed in the old patients who are older than 65 (10–25%) and the patients who receive home nursing (25–40%). If there is no symptom in the patients with bacteriuria, antibiotic therapy is not required and preventive use is not advocated.

If there are symptoms in the patients with urinary system infection, the therapists should ascertain bacterial species and sensitive medicine in urine culture and use powerful antibiotics intravenously. Four hundred milliliter normal saline is used to wash bladder for 10–15 min. During the therapy, there is slight tremor in bladder area of lower abdomen, which is good for eliminating precipitates and infectious materials.

(i) Surgery: According to bladder dysfunction, sacral posterior rhizotomy, transurethral resection of the bladder neck, Y-V bladder cervicoplasty and artificial sphincter implantation are used in clinic.

17.2 The Mechanism of Defecation Dysfunctions

17.2.1 The Process of Forming Defecation Reflex

17.2.1.1 Faeces Reaction

Before inducing defecation reflex, there is faeces reaction.

After eating, the food are digested and assimilated by stomach and intestinal tract. Unassimilated residue form faeces and enter into colon to stimulate colon peristalsis and contraction so that faeces is pushed to distal colon. This kind of peristalsis is started from hepatic flexure and is pushed to (2–3 time a day and 1–2 cm/min) left semi-colon until the faeces is left in colon sigmoideum.

After eating or getting up in the morning, gastrocolic reflex or body position easily induce colon peristalsis rush. Peristalsis rush can move forward with the speed of 10 cm/h and the propulsive force is strong. It can push faeces stored in colon sigmoideum into rectum. When faeces reaches a certain quantities (about 300 g) in rectum, it can generate great pressure on intestinal wall and induce defecation reflex.

17.2.1.2 Defecation Reflex

When the rectum is full of faeces, it can stimulate receptor in intestinal wall and impulse is conducted into lower defecation center in sacral cord. Meanwhile, impulse is transmitted into cerebral cortex and generate desire to defecate. Cortex gives out impulse to enhance the excitability of defecation center and generate defecation reflex. Colon sigmoideum and rectum contract and sphincter ani relax. The patients can increase thoracic pressure consciously, lower diagram, shrink abdominal muscles to increase abdominal pressure to discharge faeces out of the body through anus.

If the surroundings is not proper, impulse from hypogastric nerve and pudendal nerve induces external sphincter of anal tube contraction to stop excretion. Because compression force of external sphincter is 30–60% stronger than that of internal sphincter, it can antagonize defecation reflex, stop excretion, induce colon anastalsis and make faeces return to colon descendens and colon transversum. After a period of time, faeces in rectum can return to colon sigmoideum and colon descendens under the pressure of colon peristalsis and then induce the next defecation reflex.

Colon anastalsis is a protective mechanism to prevent excretion in improper time. If people frequently inhibit desire to defecate, the stimulation sensitivity of rectum to faeces is decreased. The induction of defecation reflex is difficult. Faeces stays in large intestine for a long time and becomes hard and dry because of water hyperabsorption, which can induce difficult defecation and is one of the causes of constipation. Therefore, people should defecate in definite time. Getting up in the morning easily induces postural reflex and post jentaculum may induce gastrocolic reflex. Both can promote the generation of colon peristalsis rush and induce defecation reflex. Therefore, people should defecate in the morning or after breakfast, which can prevent diseases of anal tube and rectum.

17.2.2 Pathogenesis and Classification of Defecation Dysfunctions

Defecation dysfunctions include constipation and incontinence of feces. Constipation is usually observed in the patients with intestinal motility disorder to varying degrees after spinal cord injury. Incontinence of feces usually is induced by central nervous system diseases, sphincter injury and intestinal system disease. The most common complications are perineum, inflammatory change of sacrococcygeal region and perianal skin. There are retrograde urinary tract infection, kysthitis, skin red and swollen and skin fester in some patients [6]. All these are induced by stimulation of skin by faeces. If they are not handled properly, they can induce retrograde urinary tract infection or kysthitis through urethra.

17.2.2.1 Constipation

1. The definition of constipation: Constipation means that excretion time is decreased but

faeces is hard and dry, which is difficult to defecate. If there are two or more symptoms, it can be diagnosed as symptomatic constipation. If the disease history is more than 6 months, it can be diagnosed as chronic constipation.

Constipation is rectum dysfunction induced by neurogenic rectum (neurogenic bowel). The injury of central nerve that control rectum function or peripheral nerve can induce constipation. The patients with fecal incontinence are rare.

The manifestation of constipation is defecation frequency decrease. The patients usually defecate once in 2–3 days or more time (defecation time is less than three times a week), which is called constipation. The faeces are half molded or sausage-like. Therefore, the doctors can make a correct diagnosis according to the characteristic of faeces, individual defecation habit and defecation difficulty.

2. Cardinal symptoms of constipation include lack of desire to defecate, abdominal distension, abdominal pain, lacking in strength and loss of appetite. All these symptoms are related to the following causes.
   (a) Sphincter ani spasm and lack of desire to defecate: Most patients are lack of desire to defecate who are with abnormal defecation autonomic regulation and sphincter ani spasm, which can lead to intestinal peristalsis evacuation disorder and increase defecation resistance. Faeces stay in large intestine for a long time and become hard and dry because of water hyperabsorption.
   (b) Neural injury and defecation motility disorder: in spinal shock, the early phase of cerebral injury and perineal nerves injury, defecation motility disorder make faeces in intestinal tract for a long time and induce constipation. If the constipation is accompanied with sphincter ani incontinence and intestinal tract irritation such as infection or injury, there may be fecal incontinence.
   (c) Long-term constipation complications: Long-term constipation may lead to abdominal distention, abdominal pain, lacking in strength and loss of appetite. Long-term lying in bed may slow intestinal peristalsis and induce dry stool, which can induce constipation. The early manifestation of constipation is hyperactive bowel sounds to promote defecation. In the late phase, intestinal muscular fatigue leads to hypoactive bowel sounds.
3. The cause for judgement or assessment of constipation: There are many methods to judge or assess the cause and degree of constipation.
   (a) Sphincter ani tension examination: Digital rectal examination is used to determine the function of sphincter ani. The sensation of anus and perineal region can helps to ascertain the level of neural injury and injury degree. Bulboanal reflex is used to judge whether there is spinal shock or not.
   (b) Rectum touch: There is anus relaxation in complete incontinence. When the patients shrink anal tube, the contraction of sphincter ani and anorectal circular muscle is not obvious or completely disappear. In incomplete incontinence, contractility of sphincter ani weakens.
   (c) Splanchnoscopy is used to watch deformity of anal tube, morphology of skin mucosa in anal tube and anal occlusion. Fiber enteroscopy can be used for colonitis, Crohn's disease, polyp and cancer.
   (d) Defecography (DFG): Contrast medium is injected into rectum and is expelled in defecation. Combined with anorectal dynamic and static examination, it can show the functional and pathological disease in anorectal area and provide the basis of diagnosis and therapeutic method of clinical constipation.
   (e) Anal manometry: The pressure of internal, external sphincter and puborectalis muscle should be examined. The therapists should know anorectal inhibition reflex, anorectal basic pressure, contrac-

tion pressure and rectal distention tolerance capacity. Basic pressure and contraction pressure of anal tube in the incontinence patients decrease. Internal sphincter reflex disappears and rectum distention tolerance capacity decreases.

(f) Electromyography measurement can be used to measure envelop of sphincter function and assess voluntary muscles, involuntary muscles, their neural injury and recovery degree.

(g) Ultrasonic inspection of anal tube can show anorectal submucosa, internal and external sphincter, and peripheral tissue clearly, which is good for injury degree of incontinence of feces and sphincter.

17.2.2.2 Incontinence of Feces

If the patients are in clear consciousness, incontinence of feces is that there is involuntary exsufflation and loose stools. Incontinence of feces is one of the symptoms of defecation dysfunction. The patients lose control of exsufflation and defecation. If it is not handled properly, it is easy to induce complication, cause pain in body and spirit and influence life quality [7].

1. Pathogenesis of incontinence of feces: The common causes of incontinence of feces are nervous system diseases, sphincter injuries and intestinal system diseases [8].
   (a) Nervous system diseases such as central nervous system diseases, spinal and sacral nerve injuries, infection, spinal cord tumor, tractive injury of pudendal nerve and anorectal neural dysfunction
   (b) The diseases of anal tube, rectum and colon are usually observed in the patients with rectum tumor and inflammatory diseases. Tumor can infiltrate and destroy sphincter. Inflammatory diseases such as ulcerative colitis and Crohn's disease can induce rectal inflammation and lead to long-term diarrhea. Complete rectal prolapse can lead to anal relaxation and the defecation control ability is lost.
   (c) Anal trauma is mainly sphincter injury, which is usually observed in anorectal surgery and birth injury, especially high anal fistula surgery. In addition, when the surgeries of internal hemorrhoids, anal fissure, rectal prolapse and rectal tumor are not handled properly, or the tissue of anal tube is suffered with external violence, medicine injection, burn and cold injury, all these can lead to sphincter ani injury and then induce incontinence of feces.
   (d) Anorectal congenital malformation is one of the causes for incontinence of feces.
2. The classification of incontinence of feces: The classification is according to incontinence degree, severity and pathological lesion degree.
   (a) Incontinence degree: complete incontinence: the patients cannot control defecation at will and the defecation time is not definite. If there is intestinal peristalsis, faeces flows out of anus, even in cough, squatting, walking or sleeping. Incomplete incontinence: if the faeces is wishy-washy and cannot be controlled, there may be incontinence. Otherwise, there is no continence. Sensory incontinence: if faeces is wishy-washy and the movement is slow before defecation, faeces may flow out unconsciously.
   (b) Severity:
      – First degree: Faeces flow out by accident and involuntarily.
      – Second degree: the patients cannot control faeces. Faeces usually flow out in the incontinence patients accompanied with exsufflation.
      – Third degree: the patients are with complete incontinence. The patients cannot control defecation and exsufflation voluntarily. Faeces flow out involuntarily. During sleeping, faeces are expelled.
   (c) Pathological lesion degree: both internal sphincter and puborectalis muscle are injured, which can induce complete incontinence. Miopragia of external sphincter and puborectalis muscle can

induce stress incontinence. When abdominal pressure is suddenly increased such as cough or sneezing, there are loose stools or liquid.

17.2.3 Rehabilitation Therapy of Defecation Dysfunctions

17.2.3.1 The Main Purpose of Rehabilitation Training

The purpose is to recover voluntary movement and defecation control ability of musculus sphincter ani externus, maintain regular defecation, decrease persistence time of faeces in intestinal tract, and prevent constipation, fecal incontinence and other complications.

17.2.3.2 Therapeutic Principle

The main principle of rehabilitation therapy of defecation dysfunctions is to recover contraction function of musculus sphincter ani externus through rehabilitation training, recover defecation coordination movement and prevent fecal incontinence, constipation and complications.

17.2.3.3 Rehabilitation Training Method of Neurological Training

Rehabilitation training of defecation dysfunctions includes rehabilitation training of constipation and fecal incontinence.

1. Main and collateral channels of rehabilitation training of defecation dysfunctions: Six-step Daoyin technique or Daoyin feedback technique of guiding collaterals through meridians is used for the training of musculus sphincter ani externus to recover voluntary autonomous contraction ability.

   Sphincter ani belongs to Du channel. Du channel is started from uterus in abdomen, go out of perineum, move backward along with the center of lumbar spinal cord to Changqiang in sacrococcygeal region. It goes upward along with spinal cord to Fengfu through the back of neck and then enters into brain. It goes upward along with middle line of head to Baihui point and then go downward to Suliao in apex nasi through forehead and nasal septum. After passing through Renzhong, it reaches Yinjiao point (Fig. 17.7).

   The pathway of regulation of mind in six-step Daoyin technique: the method of guiding collaterals through meridians is used. The idea of regulation of mind is started from the endpoint of collaterals but not the starting point of meridians. The patients are guided to make mind from Yinjiao of Du channel to Changqiang through Suliao, Shenting, Baihui, Dazhui, Zhiyang, Xuanshu, Yangguan and Yaoshu. After regulation of breathing, the patients do contraction and relaxation training of musculus sphincter ani externus.
2. Rehabilitation methods of constipation treated by neurological training include bare hand training, Daoyin feedback method, electrical stimulation and self-exercise method.
   (a) Bare hand training of musculus sphincter ani externus: Before therapy, the patients should defecate. The patients are in knee-chest position, separate two legs to expose perineum. The placement of anus probe is the same as the previous segment. The patients are helped to lie in lateral position and to start the training. Contraction training: the therapist should use normal of six-step Daoyin technique of guiding collaterals through meridians to guide the patients after regulation of mind and breathing along with Du channel. The patients are asked to concentrate on musculus sphincter ani externus. The specific method is to shrink anus. After deep inspiration, the patients are asked to try to shrink musculus sphincter ani externus and clamp anus training probe for 6 s. After that, the patients take a deep breath and expire slowly. The ratio between inspiration time and expiration time is 1–2. Relaxation training: after regulation of mind and breathing along with Du channel, the therapists guide the patients to concentrate on musculus sphincter ani externus. After taking a deep breath, the patients try to adjust body and mind to

relax anus for 6 s. After taking a deep breath, the patients expire slowly. The ratio between inspiration time and expiration time is 1–2. The contraction and relaxation training can be done alternatively.

The training time is 30 min (once a day) and there are 30 time in one therapy course. The patients can receive multiple therapy courses.

(b) Rehabilitation training of neurological training of musculus sphincter ani externus. Before therapy, the patients should defecate. Signal reception probe of neurological training is inserted into anus. The operational approach is the same as the mentioned above. The patients are in lateral position or knee-chest position. Reception electrode is connected with the first lead of neurological training device. Motor program signal of sphincter ani from central nervous system is displayed in single screen and the training can be started.

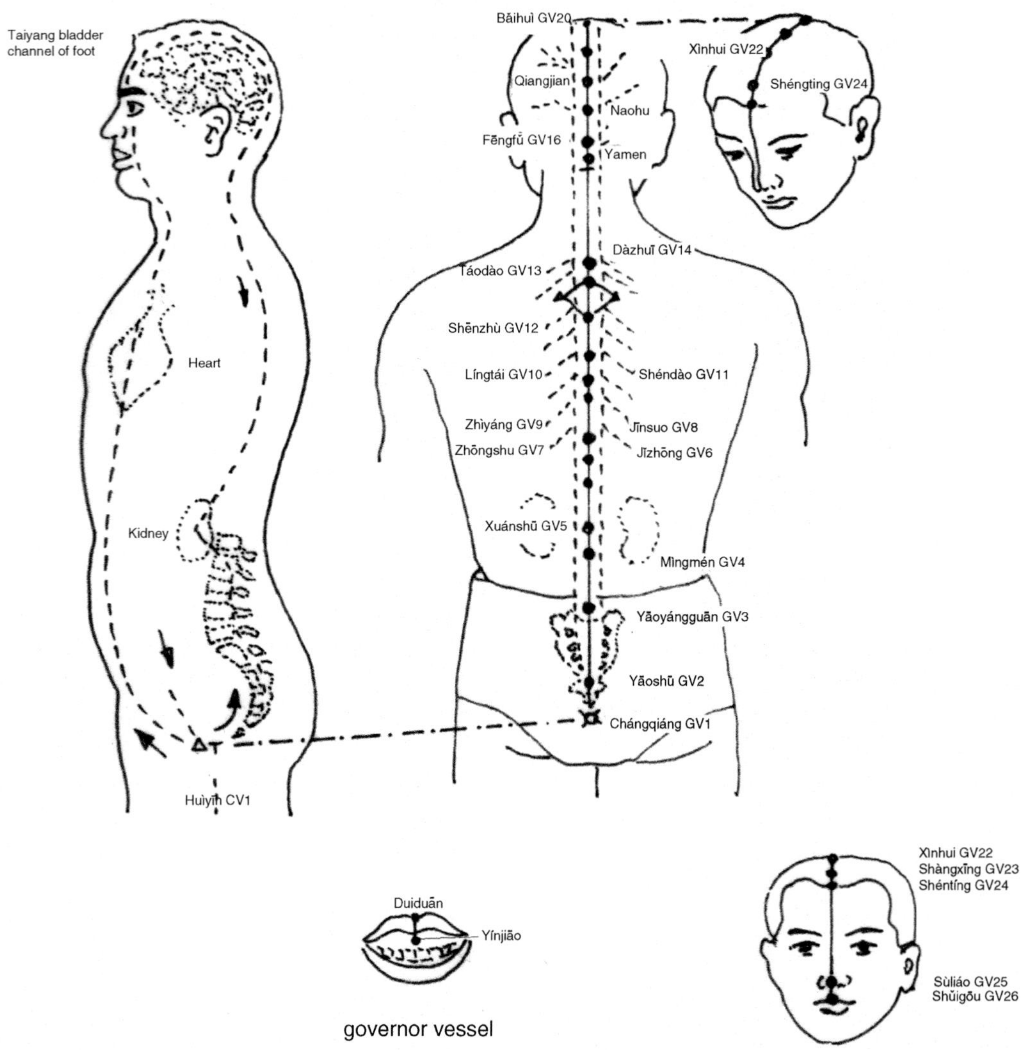

Fig. 17.7 Sketch map of Du channel

The training is divided into two procedures. Contraction training: After regulation of mind and breathing along with Du channel, the therapists guide the patients to concentrate on musculus sphincter ani externus. The specific method is to shrink anus. After taking a deep inspiration, the patients are guided to concentrate on signal curve on the screen but not to shrink urethra and sphincter ani. The patients are asked to increase the altitude of signal curve on the screen to increase signal intensity for 6 s. After that, the patients take a deep inspiration and expire slowly. The ratio between inspiration time and expiration time is 1–2. Signal intensity of the first time is the baseline and is used as surpassing target. In the next training, the patients are guided to make signal intensity surpass the previous time. The rest can be done in the same manner. Relaxation training: if the patients have musculus sphincter ani externus spasm, the signal intensity is stronger than that of baseline and cannot be reduced to zero. The patients can do this training. After regulation of mind and breathing along with Du channel, the therapists guide the patients to concentrate on signal curve on screen but not on the contraction of urethra and sphincter ani. After taking a deep inspiration, the patients are guided to regulate body and mind to relax musculus sphincter ani externus in order to decrease curve for 6 s. After that, the patients take a deep inspiration and expire slowly. The ratio between inspiration time and expiration time is 1–2. Contraction training and relaxation training is done alternatively. If there is no external urethral sphincter spasm in the patients, the patients can merely do contraction training. Contraction training can enhance the training feeling and is good for the effect. In addition, recovering active contraction function of muscles is the premise and basis of active relaxation of muscles.

The training time and therapy course: double training of contraction and relaxation: The training time is 50 min (once a day) and there are 30 times in one therapy course. The patients can do multiple therapy courses. Single training of contraction: The training time is 30 min (once a day) and there are 30 times in one therapy course. The patients can do multiple therapy courses.

(c) Virtual reality training of neurological training: Before therapy, the patients should defecate. Training probe of sphincter ani is inserted into anus. The patients are in lateral position or knee-chest position. The placement of training probe and training method are the same as these of rehabilitation training of neurological training of musculus sphincter ani externus. The only difference is virtual reality training device.

The training time and therapy course: double training of contraction and relaxation: The training time is 50 min (once a day) and there are 30 times in one therapy course. The patients can do multiple therapy courses. Single training of contraction: The training time is 30 min (once a day) and there are 30 times in one therapy course. The patients can do multiple therapy courses.

Every week, neurological training device is used to detect the signal of musculus sphincter ani externus to know the actual therapeutic effect and instruct therapeutic schedule.

(d) Self-exercise method of pelvic floor muscles: the patients who received rehabilitation training of neurological training of musculus sphincter ani externus in rehabilitation department of hospital are already know the method of training active movement of musculus sphincter ani externus with Daoyin technique and are impressed by the relationship between contraction and signal line. After discharge or during the therapy internal, the patients can do self-exercise of musculus sphincter ani externus. On the basis of regulation of mind and breathing, the patients shrink external urethral sphincter and imagine the signal curve change in the previous therapy course for 6 s. During the training, training probe can be placed in anus to consolidate therapeutic effect.

The time of self-exercise is 30 min and there are 1–2 times a day. The patients can do it for a long time.

(e) Acupuncture therapy: Du channel governs the Yang Qi of all the body. If Yang Qi is weak, the therapists can choose proper acupuncture point in Du channel for therapy. For constipation patients, the therapists select Changqiang that is the midpoint between tailbone and anus 0.5 in. below tailbone. Acupuncturing this point can relieve muscular spasm and dizziness, clear heat, promote diuresis, solid doff and cure diarrhea. It is suitable for the patients with diarrhea, hematochezia, constipation, haemorrhoids and rectocele.

The training time is 15 min (once a day) and there are 15 times in one therapy course.

(f) Electrical stimulation therapy: Because of long-term constipation, intestinal peristalsis of the patients weaken, which can further aggravate the symptoms of constipation. Medium-frequency electrical stimulation can increase excitability of intestinal smooth muscle, promote recovery of intestinal peristalsis and defecation.

Electrode placement: the electrodes of medium-frequency electrical stimulation can be placed on left and right abdomen or separately in abdomen and back. The patients should tolerate the electrical intensity and don't feel painful. If the patients are not sensitive to electrical stimulation, the therapists cannot increase electrical intensity blindly, especially for the patients with hypaesthesia.

The training time is 20–30 min (once a day) and there are 15 times in one therapy course.

3. Other rehabilitation therapeutic method means the common therapeutic method in clinic at home and abroad [9, 10].

(a) Electromyographic biofeedback therapeutic method is the same as that of urinary incontinence introduced in the first segment.

The training time is 20–30 min (once a day) and there are 15 times in one therapy course.

(b) Changing dietary structure: The patients should try to eat crude fiber food and avoid irritant and heavy food so that the faeces are soft and easy to be expelled.

(c) Improving defecation way and establishing timing defecation habit: There are several methods as follows: Action of gravity is used for defecation. The patients should use sitting position to defecate. The old or severe patients can use lying and sitting position. Anus stretching is used to relieve sphincter ani spasm. For example, middle finger is put on fingerstall, is smeared with paroline oil and is inserted into anus slowly. The therapists use middle finger to stretch rectal wall to anus slowly. Ring stretching way is used to alleviate sphincter ani internus and externus and expand rectal cavity to induce intestinal tract reflex. Timing defecation habit: postural reflex after getting up and defecation reflex easily induce defecation so that the patients should defecate in the morning. During defecation, the patients should concentrate in case defecation reflex cannot be induced because of attention diversion.

(d) Appropriate exercise: the patients can do appropriate physical activities such as swimming, playing ping-pong and abdominal massage, which can promote efferent and afferent reflex of feedback of intestinal tract sensation and promote intestinal peristalsis motility to prevent constipation.

(e) Defecation tips: Constipation is a common problem, especially in old people. People summarize defecation tip in daily life for personal use. Necessary preliminary motion such as intermittent abdominal curl movement before defecation is good for induction of intestinal peristalsis and moving down of faeces. Abdominal massage: the therapists put hand on the peripheral of abdomen and do massage clockwise, which is good for intestinal peristalsis and moving down of faeces. Acupressure: the therapists use four fingers of right hand (except little finger) to press on four spots in rectangle around navel. The four spots are located two fingers to navel (Up, Down, Left, Right). Acupressure can induce defecation reflex. Tail end of finger pressure: the therapists can press two sides of tail end of fingers alternatively to induce desire to defecate. Intermittent active contraction of sphincter ani: the patients sit on closestool to do active contraction and relaxation of sphincter ani intermittently to induce defecation reflex.

(f) Drug therapy includes purgative prescription and gastrointestinal motility promotion drug. Bulk cathartic includes soluble fiber such as pectin, plantain herb and oat bran and insoluble fiber such as plant fibre and lignin. The effect is slow but they are safe and with less side effect. They are suitable for constipation in gestation or slight constipation, but not suitable for fast free movement of the bowels. The major effect of lubricant cathartic is to lubricate intestinal wall and soften faeces so that faeces are easy to be expelled. This kind of medicine is easy to use such as glycerine enema, mineral oil or liquid paraffin. Salt cathartic such as magnesium sulfate and magma magnesiae can occasionally induce severe adverse reaction and they should be used with precaution. Osmotic cathartic includes lactulose, sorbitol and polyethylene glycol 4000. They are suitable for faecea block or chronic constipation. They can also be used for the patients if the therapeutic effect of bulk cathartic is not good. Irritant cathartic includes plant cathartic (anthraquinone) such a rheum officinale, folium sennae and aloe, phenolphthalein, castor oil and diesters bisoxindole. They are suitable for the condition that other cathartics are useless and cannot be used for a long time. Long-term use of anthraquinone cathartic may lead to colon melena or cathartic colon, atrophy of smooth muscle and intestinal myenteric nerve plexus injury, which can aggravate constipation, but the symptoms disappear after drug withdrawal. Gastrointestinal motility promotion medicine such as mosapride and itopride can promote gastrointestinal motility. Prucalopride mainly act on colon and can be used as the circumstances may require.

4. Rehabilitation therapy of incontinence of feces: Incontinence of feces is the same as constipation and both belong to defecation dysfunctions and may be related to different parts of neural injury. One of the causes of constipation is musculus sphincter ani externus spasm. The injured segment of spinal cord cannot transmit: signal from upper central nerve to the spinal cord segment below the injured segment so that the spinal cord segment below the injured segment are excited because they break away from the inhibition of upper central nerve. Therefore, spasm of musculus sphincter ani externus leads to that faeces in intestinal tract cannot be expelled in time. Water is absorbed too much so that faeces becomes hard. One of the causes of incontinence of feces is musculus sphincter ani externus paralysis. When spinal cord is injured, the nerve root that dominate musculus sphincter ani externus is injured. Therefore, musculus sphincter ani externus is out of control and there is soft paralysis, relaxation of musculus sphincter ani externus, which lead to that intestinal contents in rectum flow out of anus without control.

Therefore, there is no musculus sphincter ani externus spasm in incontinence of feces. Rehabilitation training should enhance muscular excitability and recover autonomic innervation.

(a) Main and collateral channels of rehabilitation of neurological training of incontinence of feces: The method of guiding collaterals through meridians is used. The idea of regulation of mind is started from the endpoint of collaterals but not the starting point of meridians. The patients are guided to make mind from Yinjiao of

Du channel to Changqiang through Suliao, Shenting, Baihui, Dazhui, Zhiyang, Xuanshu, Yangguan and Yaoshu. After regulation of breathing, the patients do contraction training of musculus sphincter ani externus.

(b) Bare hand training of musculus sphincter ani externus: Before therapy, the patients should defecate. The placement of anus probe is the same as the previous segment. The patients are helped to lie in lateral position and to start the training of musculus sphincter ani externus. Contraction training: the therapist should use six-step Daoyin technique of guiding collaterals through meridians to guide the patients after regulation of mind and breathing along with Du channel. The patients are asked to concentrate on musculus sphincter ani externus. The specific method is to shrink anus. After deep inspiration, the patients are asked to try to shrink musculus sphincter ani externus and clamp anus training probe for 6 s. After that, the patients take a deep breath and expire slowly. The ratio between inspiration time and expiration time is 1–2.

The training time is 30 min (once a day) and there are 30 times in one therapy course. The patients can do multiple therapy courses.

(c) Rehabilitation training method of neurological training of musculus sphincter ani externus: Before therapy, the patients should defecate. Signal reception probe of neurological training is inserted into anus. The operational approach is the same as the mentioned above. The patients are in lateral position or knee-chest position. Reception electrode is connected with the first lead of neurological training device. Motor program signal of sphincter ani from central nervous system is displayed in single screen and the training can be started.

Contraction training: After regulation of mind and breathing along with Du channel, the patients are asked to concentrate on musculus sphincter ani externus. The specific method is that after deep inspiration, the patients are asked to stare at the screen and concentrate on signal curve to increase signal line altitude but not concentrate on anus contraction for 6 s. After that, the patients take a deep breath and expire slowly. The ratio between inspiration time and expiration time is 1–2. Signal intensity of the first time is the baseline and is used as surpassing target. In the next training, the patients are guided to make signal intensity surpass the previous time. The rest can be done in the same manner.

The training time is 50 min (once a day) and there are 30 times in one therapy course. The patients can do multiple therapy courses.

(d) Virtual reality training of neurological training: Before therapy, the patients should defecate. Training probe of sphincter ani is inserted into anus. The patients lie in lateral position or knee-chest position. The placement of training probe and training method are the same as these of rehabilitation training of neurological training of musculus sphincter ani externus. The only difference is virtual reality training device.

The training time is 50 min (once a day) and there are 30 times in one therapy course. The patients can do multiple therapy courses.

Every week, neurological training device is used to detect the actual signal of musculus sphincter ani externus to know the actual therapeutic effect and adjust the therapeutic schedule.

(e) Pelvic floor muscle exercise of neurological training: it is a modified form of Kegel method. The specific method is as follows: The patients are in sitting position or standing-sitting position. In standing position, the space between two feet is the same wide as two shoulders. The whole body is relaxed. The patients are guided to make mind from Yinjiao of Du channel to Changqiang through Suliao, Shenting, Baihui, Dazhui, Zhiyang, Xuanshu, Yangguan and Yaoshu. After taking a deep inspiration, the patients shrink anus, count for 6 s and relax anus.

The frequency of self-exercise is 15–30 min per time and there are 2–3 times a day. One therapy course takes 2 months and the patients can do multiple therapy courses, even do exercise for a long time as health protection measures.

Considerations: during self-exercise of pelvic floor muscles, there are several key points. Strength: the patients should try to increase maximum tension of muscle contraction. Velocity: the patients should try to shorten the time to get to maximum tension of muscle contraction. Duration time: the patients should maintain the time of maximum tension of muscle contraction as long as possible. Repeatability: the patients try to reduce the number of times to get to maximum tension. Fatigue: the patients should try to reduce fatigue degree after muscle contraction.

(f) Acupuncture therapy: Changqiang point is selected and the method is the same as acupuncture therapy of constipation.

The frequency is once a day and there are 15 times in one therapy course.

(g) Other rehabilitation methods: Electromyographic biofeedback therapy is the same as that of urinary incontinence in the first segment. The training time is 20–30 min (once a day) and there are 15 times in one therapy course. Electrical stimulation is usually set in neurogenic incontinence of feces. Caldwell in 1963 placed stimulation electrode in musculus sphincter ani externus and induce regular contraction and sensory feedback of sphincter ani to improve function. The training time is 20–30 min (once a day) and there are 15 times in one therapy course. Defecation promotion: the patients should treat inflammation of colon and rectum actively in case of diarrhea. They should try not to eat irritant food and try to eat food with fruitful fiber. Surgery is suitable for the patients with local defect of sphincter induced by surgery injury, birth injury or violent injury. In addition, congenital disease and anal sphincterectomy require surgery. Operation mode includes sphincter neoplasty, rectovaginal internal sphincter neoplasty, plication operation of sphincter, skin transplantation tuboplasty and sphincteroplasty.

(h) Precautions of incontinence of feces: establishing normal dietary habit: the patients should eat less greasy food and eat more light food with vitamin such as fresh vegetable and fruit including mung bean, radish and wax gourd. If the patients cannot be cured for a long time, they should eat more food with high protein such as lean meat, beef and mushroom. The patients should keep anus clean. After defecation, the patients should wash anus or they can wash anus morning and evening to keep anus clean. Timing defecation: the patients should develop a habit of timing defecation to prevent injuring anal tube skin and infection.

(i) Nursing materials of incontinence of feces: disposable urinal pad is nursing material suitable for the patients with incontinence of feces. It can shorten damp and pollution scope and decrease injury degree of skin. Control valve plug of anus is made of polyurethane sponge and is placed between anus and rectum. This kind of sponge can swell after encountering water so that it can prevent flowout of faeces. Anal tube: thick anal tube with gauge 22 is inserted into anus 18–22 cm in depth until it reaches the middle of colon sigmoideum. It is not fixed around anus and the exposed terminal of anal tube is connected with plastic bag. After defecation, the patients should change plastic bag to keep anus clean. Disposable gasbag catheter is inserted into rectum 16–20 cm in depth. The gasbag is located in the interface of rectum and colon sigmoideum. Gasbag is inflated to prevent flow of faeces in to rectum. In addition, in the interface of rectum and colon sigmoideum, there is no receptor of defecation reflex ao that it is difficult to induce defecation reflex, which is good for the fixation of catheter.

References

1. Schmidt RA, Jonas U, Oleson KA, et al. Sacral nerve stimulation for treatment of refractory urinary urge incontinence. J Urol. 1999;162:352–7.
2. Goodwin RJ, Swinn MJ, Fowler CJ. The neurophysiology of urinary retention in young women and its treatment by neuromodulation. World J Urol. 1988;16:305–7.
3. Finazzi Agro E, Peppe A, Damico A, et al. Effects of subthalamic nucleus stimulation on urodynamic finding in patients with Parkinson' disease. J Urol. 2003;169(4):1391.
4. Fall M, Lindstrom S. Electrieal stimulation. A physiologic approach to the treatment of urinary incontinense. Urol Clin North Am. 1991;18(2):393–407.
5. Bazanova M, M Mernaia EM, Shtark MB. Biofeedback in psychomotor training. Electro physiological bases. Ross Fiziol Zh Im I M Sechenova. 2008;94(5):539–56.
6. Lynch AC, Antony A, Dobbs BR. Bowel dysfunction following spinal cord injury. Spinal Cord. 2001;39(4):193–203.
7. Christiansen J. Modern surgical treatment of anal incontinence. Ann Med. 1998;30:273–7.
8. Vaizey CJ, Kamm MA, Nicholls RJ. Recent advances in the surgical treatment of faecal incontinence. Br J Surg. 1998;85:596–603.
9. Rezvan A, Jakus-Waldman S, Abbas MA, et al. Review of the diagnosis, management andt reatment of fecal incontinence. Female Pelvic Med Reconstr Surg. 2015;21:8–17.
10. Halland M, Talley NJ. Fecal incontinence: mechanisms and management. Curr Opin Gastroenterol. 2012;28:57–62.

18 Rehabilitation Therapy of Neurological Training of Visual Impairment

18.1 Visual Structure and the Mechanism of Visual Formation

18.1.1 Visual Structure

Eye is an ocular organ of human and animals.

Eye can be used for reading, learning, watching pictures and enjoying the view. Human can use eye to distinguish different colors and lights and change these visual image into neural signal that are transmitted to the brain to form vision.

Eye is composed of eyeball and appendant organ of eye. It includes the following important parts [1, 2].

1. Eyeball includes eyeball wall, intraocular cavity and contents, nerves and blood vessels (Fig. 18.1). Intraocular cavity includes anterior chamber, posterior chamber and vitreous cavity. Eye contents include aqueous fluid, crystalline lens and vitreous body. They are all transparent materials. They three and cornea are called refracting media. Aqueous fluid is generated by ciliary processes. It can provide nutrition for cornea, crystalline lens and vitreous body, and maintain intraocular pressure. Crystalline lens is elastic transparent body behind iris and pupil, and before vitreous body, which is like biconvex lens. Vitreous body is transparent colloid body that occupies posterior four fifth of the whole eyeball. The major ingredient is water, which can refract light and support retina. Optic nerve can transmit visual information from retina to neural pathway of brain. Visual pathway is the neural impulse conduction pathway from retina to brain cortex.
2. Accessory organs of eye include seven extraocular muscles of eyeball movements (Fig. 18.2). They are all skeletal muscles. There are four rectus such as superior rectus, inferior rectus, medial rectus and lateral rectus. They all originate from common tendinous ring around canalis opticus and end forward in four surfaces (Upward, downward, inward and outward) of the front of equator of sclera. There are two oblique muscles including superior oblique and inferior oblique. Superior oblique originates from common tendinous ring and ends in lateral surface behind the eyeball through tendon trochlea in anterior and superior medial wall of orbit. Inferior oblique originates from medial part of inferior orbit and ends in posterior lateral surface of eyeball. Levator palpabrae muscle originates from common tendinous ring of aobital apex and the middle part of it ends in the bottom of tarsus and corresponding skin tissue. Bilateral fibers attach to medial canthus ligament zygomatic tubercle through tendon to elevate upper eyelid.

The effects of all the muscles: Superior rectus can turn pupil inward and upward.

W. Zhao, *Rehabilitation Therapeutics of the Neurological Training*,
https://doi.org/10.1007/978-981-13-0812-3_18

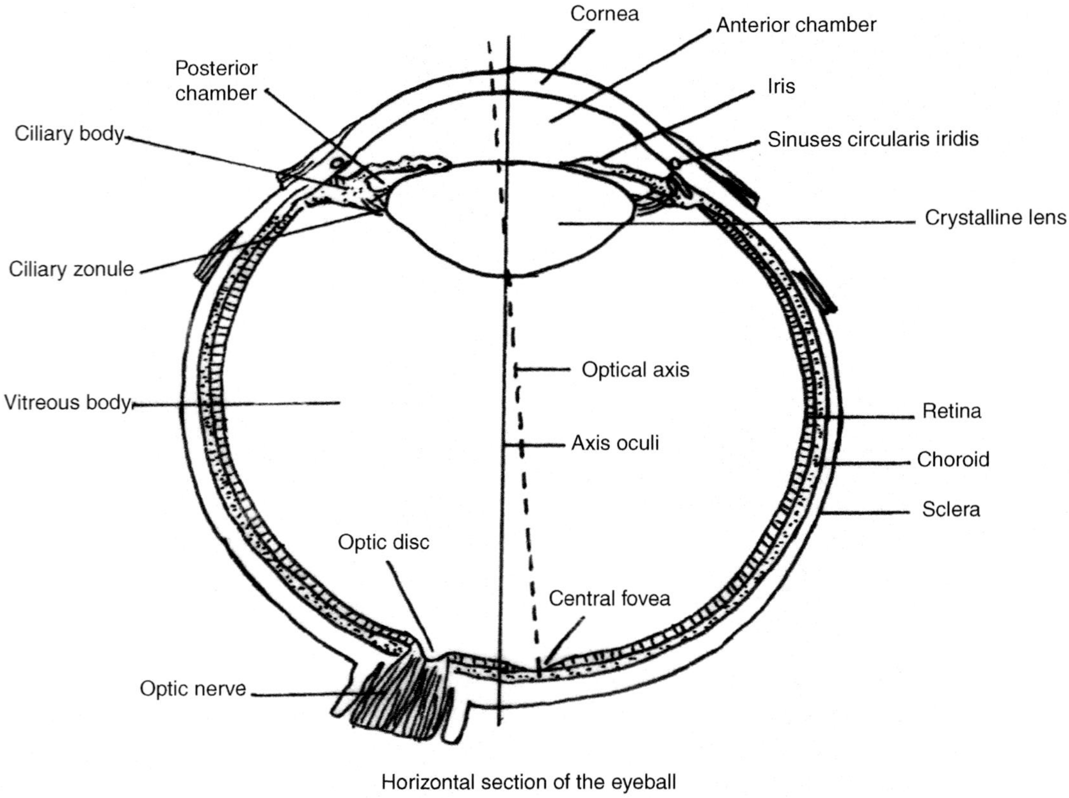

Fig. 18.1 Sketch map of eyeball structure

Fig. 18.2 Peripheral muscles of eyeball

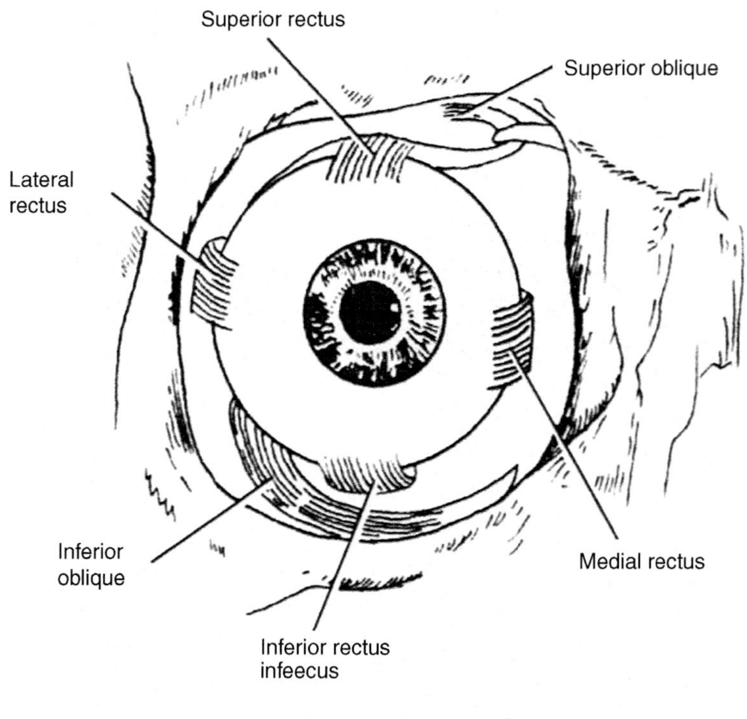

Inferior rectus turns pupil downward and inward. Medial rectus turns pupil inward. Lateral rectus turns pupil outward. Superior oblique turns pupil downward and outward. Inferior oblique turns pupil upward and outward.

The normal movement of eyeball must be completed by the collaboration of many muscles. During side view, lateral rectus of one eye and medial rectus of the other eye should contract simultaneously to complete it.

3. Distance of distinct vision is that people can read the book in this distance for a long time but cannot get tired. Distance of distinct vision of emmetropia is 25 cm and distance of distinct vision of myopic eye is 10 cm.

18.1.2 The Mechanism of Visual Formation

18.1.2.1 Image-Forming Principle

The light form outer objects (the objects we see) are refracted through ocular refraction system and form clear image in retina. Photoreceptor cell in retina can receive the visual information and transmit it into optic center through action potential of neural fiber. Finally, vision is formed in optic center of cortex.

In the process of vision formation, because of the different distance between objects and eye, refraction adjustment is required through crystalline lens, pupil and binoculus convergence to make objects form clear image in retina. Therefore, people can see these objects clearly. Therefore, crystalline lens, pupil and binoculus convergence are important factor to affect visual quality, especially crystalline lens.

1. Crystalline lens: eye can adjust degree of crook of crystalline lens (refraction) to change focal length of crystalline lens in order to obtain upside-down and contractible real image. The farthest point people can see is called far point of accommodation. The far point of emmetropia is extremely far. The nearest point people can see is called near point of accommodation. The distance between the two points is called accommodation range. The normal near point is about 10 cm away from eye. People see something in this distance for a long time, which can generate eyestrain. The manifestations of eyestrain are eye sour, dry and swell, headache, and blurred vision.

Crystalline lens is between iris and vitreous body (Fig. 18.3), which is like biconvex lens, elastic and is main portion of refraction system of eyeball. Its periphery is connected to ciliary processes through ciliary zonular fibers. The better the elasticity of crystalline lens is, the stronger the regulation ability is, the closer people can see the objects clearly. The maximum adjustment ability of crystalline lens is expressed by the near point.

The near point is the nearest distance that people can see the objects clearly when eyes exert maximum adjustment ability. The shorter the distance is, the better the elasticity of crystalline lens is. The near point of the 8 years old children is about 8.6 cm. The near point of 20 years old young man is 10.4 cm. The near point of old people is 83.3 cm.

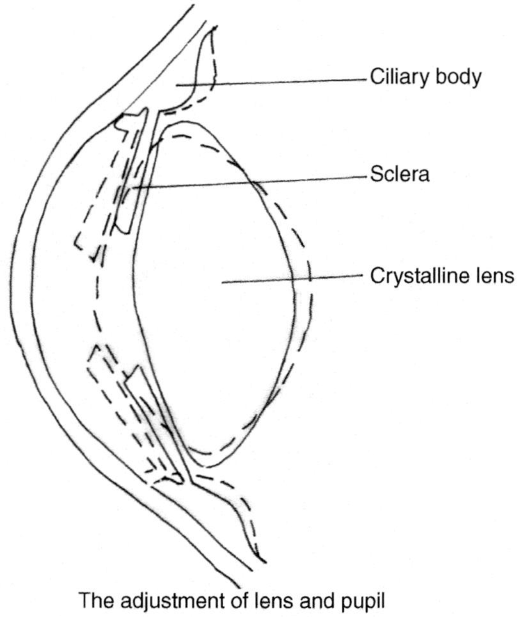

Fig. 18.3 Sketch map of crystalline lens structure

The adjustment of crystalline lens is achieved through contraction and relaxation of smooth muscles in ciliary body. Ciliary body is the fleshiest part of middle membrane and is on the inner surface of sclera and cornea migration. There are many protruded plica in the front, which is called ciliary processes that give out ciliary zonular fibers to connect crystalline lens (Fig. 18.4). The smooth muscles in ciliary body are called ciliaris that are dominated by parasympathetic nerve of oculomotor nerve. The contraction and relaxation of ciliaris can lead to relaxation and tension of ciliary zonular fibers separately. The contraction of ciliaris leads to relaxation of zonular fibers. Crystalline lens can lengthen anteroposterior axis through self-elasticity, increase degree of convexity and enhance refractive index. When ciliaris relaxes, zonular fibers are strained, which make crystalline lens become flatten and decrease refractive index. Refractive index is regulated through adjusting curvature of crystalline lens.

2. Adjustment of pupil: The diameter of pupil is 1.5–8.0 mm. there are two kinds of adjustment of pupil. Near reflex of pupil: when people see the near objects, it can reflexively induce contraction of pupil sphincter to shrink pupil in order to decrease spherical aberration and chromatic aberration of refraction system so that the image in retina is clearer. Light reflex of pupil: under strong light exposure, pupil shrinks and dim light can reflexively induce contraction of dilator pupillae to enlarge pupil and increase amount of light. This reflex can adjust the amount of light in case retina is injured in strong light and dim light affect the quality of vision imaging. The center of light reflex of pupil is in midbrain.
3. Binoculus convergence: when two eyes stare at an object from far to near, optical axis of two eyes close to nasal side under the action of ocular medial rectus, which is called binoculus convergence or convergence reflex. When people see near objects with two eyes, convergence reflex makes image on symmetry point of retinas of two eyes and form clear single visual objective image but not double image.

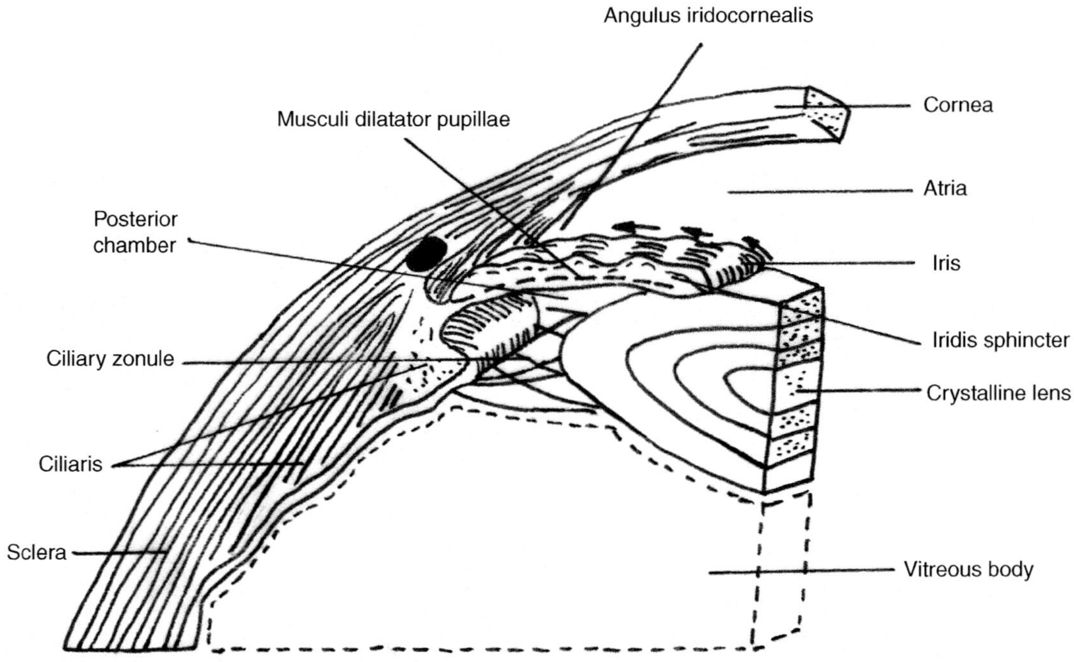

Fig. 18.4 Sketch map of relationship between ciliaris and crystalline lens

18.1.2.2 Eyesight

Eyesight is visual acuity. It is the resolving power of eye for miniature structure of objects. The measurement criterion is minimum visual angle of eye. Visual angle is that the lights from two point of the object enter into eye and form the angle through node. The size of visual angle is in direct proportion to the size of objective image in retina.

For example, 5 cm before the eye, the lights from two spots whose space is 1.5 mm (the space between two "E" in 1.0 row of international standard visual acuity chart) can form 1 min of angle and the objective image in retina is about 4.5 μm (the diameter of one cone cell). If there are three cone cells in one line of retina, the cone cells in two end of the line receive light exposure and the cone cell in the middle doesn't receive light exposure. The eye can distinguish two spots. International standard visual acuity chart is designed according to this principle. In fact, the eye of normal people can distinguish smaller visual angle, which means eyesight can be 1.0, 1.5 or bigger. This may be related to the fact that the diameter of cone cell is merely 1.5–2.0 in central fovea of retina.

18.1.2.3 Binocular Vision and Stereoscopic Vision

The vision is formed when two eyes stare at the objects at the same time, which is called binocular vision. When two eyes stare at the objects at the same time, there is a complete objective image separately in retinas of two eyes. Because exquisite coordination effect of extraocular muscles, the light from the same part of the object form image in symmetry point of retinas of two eyes and people can see one object subjectively, which is called haplopia. If there is extraocular muscles paralysis, oppression of tumor or foreign matter in eye, or displacement of eyeball pushed by fingers, objective image is on the asymmetric point of retinas of two eyes so that the patients can see two overlapping objects to a certain extent subjectively, which is called diplopia.

18.2 Visual Impairment

Visual impairment is complete or partial structure or function disorder of visual organ and visual sense due to congenital or acquired factors and the eyes cannot distinguish outer objects [3].

From diminution of vision to blindness, the range of visual impairment is wide. The symptoms include blurred vision, high hyperopia or myopia, colour blindness and tunnel vision. Because there are different nosogenesis, the severity of symptoms and disease progression are different. For example, rapid diminution of eyesight with normal ocular appearance is usually observed in the patients with vascular and neural diseases such as central retinal artery and vein occlusion, optic neuritis, disseminated sclerosis, leukemia, retinal detachment, acute methyl alcohol and quinine poisoning. Rapid diminution of eyesight with ocular congestion or infection is usually observed in acute glaucoma, iridocyclitis, severe eye traumas, keratitis, keratohelcosis and purulent inflammation of entire eyeball. Rapid diminution of eyesight without ocular congestion is due to cataract, cornea degeneration, vitreous opacity and simple glaucoma, optic nerve atrophy, retinoblastoma and melanoma in the early phase. In addition, myopic eye, presbyopia and amblyopia can lead to diminution of eyesight. Slow diminution of eyesight with ocular congestion is usually observed in the patients with keratitis, keratohelcosis, chronic glaucoma, chronic iridocyclitis, alkali burn of conjunctiva and cornea in late phase.

In this chapter, we discuss the cause, mechanism and rehabilitation therapy method of myopia, hyperopia and retrogressive hyperopia.

18.2.1 Ocular Abnormal Refraction

18.2.1.1 Formation Mechanism of Abnormal Refraction

The light of object is refracted to retina through refraction system and form objective image so that the eyes can see the object clearly. If there is abnormity in refraction process, there will be blurred vision.

1. Emmetropia: Without any adjustment, the parallel lights can focus on retina and the eye can see the far object clearly. Through adjustment, the eye can see the near object outside near-point, which is called emmetropia.
2. Non-emmetropia: If there is abnormal refraction or eyeball paramorphia, without adjustment of eye, parallel lights cannot focus on retina, which is called non-emmetropia or ametropia.

18.2.1.2 Classification of Abnormal Refraction

Abnormal refraction includes myopia, hyperopia and astigmatism.

Myopic eye: if the anteroposterior diameter of eyeball is too long or refractive index of refraction system is too big, parallel lights focus on the front of retina and there is unclear objective image on retina. The near-point is shorter than that of emmetropia.

1. Presbyopia: if the anteroposterior diameter of eyeball is too short or refractive index of refraction system is too small, parallel lights focus on the back of retina and there is unclear objective image on retina. The near-point is longer than that of emmetropia. People with presbyopia can see the far object clearly after adjustment and see near object clearly after adjustment to a great degree. Therefore, there is easily eyestrain in presbyopia.
2. Astigmatism: if the curvatures on the surface of cornea are different in different part, parallel lights are refracted by this surface and cannot focus on retina. The lights focus on retina and the planes before or after retina, which generate unclear objective image or metabolic objective image.
3. Diopter.

   Diopter is a unit to measuring refraction phenomenon. Diopter is abbreviated as D. When light is from one object to another object with different optical density, the transmission orientation will deflect, which is called refraction phenomenon. It is measured by diopter. 1D refractive power means that parallel lights can focus on 1 m focal length behind the object after penetrating it.

18.2.2 Myopic Eye

Myopia is a kind of eye disease with blurred vision of far object and clear vision of near object. The pathogenesis is not clear. Tao Yongjian deemed that genetic factor, adjustment theory, blurred theory and biochemical criterion are the major causes of myopia formation. At present, it is widely accepted at home that adjustment is the important factor of genesis and development of myopia. The major basis of adjustment theory is to adjust the effect of intraocular muscles, effect of extraocular muscles induced by three simultaneous controllable axes such as pupil shrink, convergence and adjustment, convergence reflex and intra-ocular pressure change [4].

18.2.2.1 Regulation Theory of Forming Myopia

Regulation theory shows that the formation of myopic eye is the results that contraction of intraocular muscles and extraocular muscles acts on sclera to regulate the curvature of crystalline lens in order to make two eyes focus and imaging when people see the near object. During this process, intra-ocular pressure is increase. If people stare at the near object for a long time, persistent high pressure may lengthen axis oculi and increasing axis oculi may affect refractive index of crystalline lens to make objective image before the retina, which is called axis myopia.

1. The effect of intraocular muscles: if people stare at the near object for a long time, in order to see the object clearly, people should enhance the adjustment of eye. Long-term contraction of ciliaris leads to tension and spasm and may relax zonular fibers further. Crystalline lens can protrude further with its own elasticity to

induce myopic eye. On the other hand, in order to resist the pressure of ciliaris, choroid is stretched excessively and cannot recover the normal state after a long time stretch. The blood vessel in it is oppressed and blood volume is decreased, which can induce malnutrition and atrophy. Choroid gradually lose elasticity and buffer ability. Sclera lack of elasticity starts to deform and finally lead to elongation of posterior pole of axis oculi, which can change refractive index and make objective image focus on retina to form myopia.

2. The effect of extraocular muscles: The contraction and relaxation of four rectus attached to eyeball surface can complete various kinds of eyeball movements to generate mechanical traction and oppression to eyeball. Especially when two eyes do convergence movement, the contraction of medial rectus can lengthen anteroposterior diameter of eyeball to induce myopia.

18.2.2.2 Blurred Theory

In blurred theory, bad imaging quality of retina is the important cause of genesis of development of myopia. Ametropia is the major cause of blurred vision and severe blurred vision induces binocular form deprivation. When there is binocular form deprivation in all distances, it can lead to myopia [5].

18.2.2.3 Biochemical Criterion Change Theory

In recent years, biochemical studies related to myopic eye showed that genesis of myopic eye is related to the change of biochemical substances of retina such as retinal neurotransmitter and retinal growth factor. The former includes retinene, dopamine and acetyl choline. The latter includes transforming growth factor and alkaline fibroblast growth factors β. Retinene is active metabolite of vitamin A and can combine with nuclear receptor of transcription factor to regulate the differentiation and growth of cells. The experiments showed that the change of retinene metabolism plays an important role in the genesis and development of experimental myopia. It is inferred that retinene of retina decreased the synthesis and release of choroid retinene in order to increase the synthesis of protein polysaccharide of sclera. Finally, the length of axis oculi is changed.

Researches show that through changing biochemical criterion, people can control the growth and development of eyeball to provide basis for the medicine therapy of myopia. It is possible that adjustment induces the change of biochemical criterion through blurred vision to affect the growth and development of eyeball. In addition, individual difference, genetic factor, different age, dietary structure and using habit of eye all can affect biochemical criterion of genesis and development of eyeball.

18.2.2.4 Symptoms and Assessment of Myopia

1. Clinical symptoms of myopia: Clinical manifestations of myopic eye are important evidence of diagnosis. After forming myopic eye, there are following manifestations:
   (a) Distant vision decrease: blurred distant vision with normal near vision.
   (b) Asthenopia: if the patients stare at the object for a long time, there are ophthalmic sore, swell and uncomfortable.
   (c) Exophoria or concomitant exotropia: slanting eye is usually one eye of myopia that is more severe. It is induced by imbalance of accommodation force due to excessive adjustment of eyeball by extraocular muscles.
   (d) Vitreous synchesis and opacity: they are usually observed in the patients with high myopia accompanied with cataract, waved black shadow before eye or eyesight decrease.
   (e) Ocular fundus change is usually observed in the patients with high myopia. There are temporal or peripheral ring choroid atrophy of optic nerve papilla in ocular fundus, macular degeneration, haemorrhage, posterior scleral staphyloma, retinal tear and retinal detachment.
   (f) Blunt light reflex is observed in the patients with high myopia. It is induced by long axis oculi accompanied with deep anterior chamber and big pupil.

2. Assessment of myopia includes the degree of eyesight and assessment of diopter.
   (a) Grading of eyesight: The minimum eyesight of naked eye in two eyes is the criterion.
      - Normal eyesight: eyesight is more than 5.0.
      - Mild myopia: eyesight is 4.7–4.9.
      - Middle myopia: eyesight is 4.4–4.6.
      - Severe myopia: eyesight is less than 4.3.
   (b) Pattern visual evoked potential examination: this examination is not affected by subjective response and cognitive competence of the patients and can provide objective condition of visual function. The wave form of this examination is stable. It is easy to be repeated and is highly correlated to graphic eyesight. It is suitable for the eyesight assessment of children.
   (c) According to diopter, there are three grades
      - Emmetropia: refraction range is +0.50 to −0.25D.
      - Low and middle myopia: refraction range is −0.50 to −6.0D.
      - High myopia: refraction range is more than −6.00D.
3. Classification of therapeutic effect: It is classified according to the eyesight of standard logarithmic visual acuity chart or score of diopter.
   (a) There are four grades according to eyesight.
      - Cure: eyesight is recovered to more than 5.0.
      - Excellent: eyesight is recovered to more than 3.0 on the original basis.
      - Effective: eyesight is recovered to more than 3.0 on the original basis.
      - Invalid: eyesight is recovered to less than 0.1 on the original basis.
   (b) There are three grades according to diopter.
      - Cure: refraction range is recovered to +0.50 to −0.25D.
      - Effective: refraction range is recovered to −0.50 to −6.0D.
      - Invalid: refraction range is not recovered.
4. Rehabilitation training and prevention of myopia.

If there are syndromes and symptoms of myopia, the patients should seek therapy in hospital. According to the suggestions of ophthalmologists, the patients should wear appropriate glass to rectify eyesight or use other methods for therapy. In this segment, we only discuss rehabilitation training and prevention of myopia.

1. The mechanism of rehabilitation of neurological training of myopia Six-step Daoyin technique is used for active movement training of ocular muscles to promote synaptic plasticity and functional reorganization of optic center in order to develop potential ability, recover coordinated movement ability among ocular muscles, relieve ciliaris spasm and increase blood circulation of ocular tissue. Virtuous circle of ocular tissue metabolism and adjustment ability are recovered to alleviate myopia.

   Whether adjustment theory and biochemical change theory of myopia or blurred theory and genetic factor, in the early phase of myopia, blurred objective image on retina leads to persistent powerful contraction of ciliaris to increase convexity of crystalline lens and increase refractive index in order to make objective image on retina. The difference is that there are different causes of blurred objective vision. For example, adjustment theory demonstrated that oppression and traction of intraocular and extraocular muscle can lengthen axis oculi. Biochemical criterion change theory thinks there is material deficiency. Genetic factor thinks that there is developmental defect. Blurred theory thinks that there are many factors. Some kind of factor make the object not focus on retina clearly and blurred objective image is transmitted to optic center through optic nerve. Through feedback mechanism, optic center gives out information to activate deep adjustment to make the objective image clear through trigemini movements such as pupil shrink, convergence and adjustment.

In trigemini movements, there are two kinds of involved muscles. Skeletal muscles of voluntary movement include seven muscles around eyeball. Smooth muscles of involuntary movement include ciliaris, sphincter pupillae and dilator pupillae, which are all dominated by parasympathetic nerve of oculomotor nerve.

Extraocular muscles are skeletal muscles of voluntary movements such as medial rectus, superior rectus, inferior rectus, inferior oblique and levator palpabrae muscle dominated by oculomotor nerve, superior oblique dominated by trochlear nerve and lateral rectus dominated by abducens. These cerebral nuclei are correlated with each other and are related to cerebral cortex so that they can complete a series of higher eyeball movements such as voluntary movements of eyeball and stare function of eyeball. Through training, people can complete special voluntary movements of eyeball of cross eye, showing the whites of one's eyes and strabismus.

Voluntary movement function of extraocular muscles can make eyeball do active movement training to develop neural potential that dominates extraocular muscles in order to increase contraction power and suppleness of muscles. Contraction of muscles can increase blood circulation of local ocular tissue, promote metabolism and decrease oppression of eyeball to lengthen axis oculi. Special eyeball movement can rectify esotropia and increase flexibility and correctness of eyeball rotation.

Sphincter pupillae and ciliaris are involuntary muscles dominated by parasympathetic nerve. Through reflex adjustment, these muscles can complete contraction and relaxation movements. However, movement training of conditioned reflex can increase flexibility of reflex adjustment movement, increase blood circulation and nutrition of muscles, and alleviate muscle spasm. Meanwhile, during the process of active movement training of extraocular muscles, oppression of eyeball can be decreased to improve blood circulation of ocular tissue, promote metabolism, promote functional improvement of optic center and promote functional recovery of intraocular muscles.

2. Specific methods of rehabilitation training of neurological training include neurological training, reflexive active movement training and manipulation massage.
   (a) Training methods of neurological training of extraocular muscles: Neurological training device is used. The placement of button surface electrode is outward and upward of paropia (Figs. 18.5 and 18.6). In a warm, quiet and lucifugal room, the patients are in sitting position. The electrode is connected to the first lead of neurological training device. Normal six-step Daoyin technique training: on the basis of

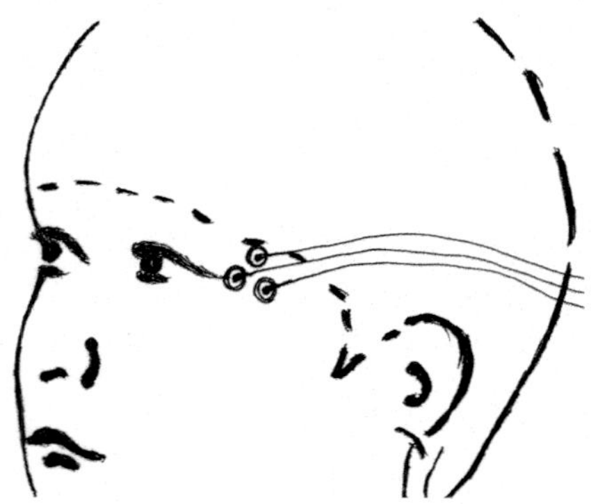

Fig. 18.5 The sketch map of the placement is outward and upward of outer canthus (triangular arrangement)

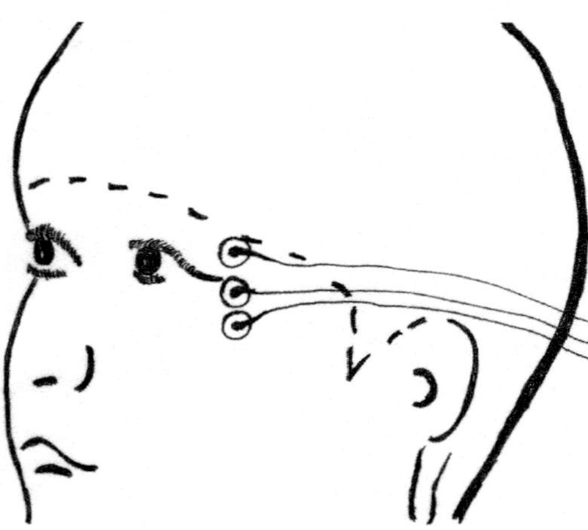

Fig. 18.6 The placement is outward and upward of outer canthus (vertical arrangement)

regulation of mind and breathing, the patients are guided to shrink ocular lateral rectus to make eyeball turn outward (offside eyeball turns inward) until the eyeball reaches the zenith of ocular abduction for 6 s. After that, the patients take a deep breath and expire slowly to relax eyeball. On the basis of the signal intensity in the pervious, the therapists make a transverse line as the surpassing goal of the next training. The therapists can use finger pulp to exert resistance on the negative direction of eyeball movement (Fig. 18.7) to increase signal intensity. The method of guiding collaterals through meridians: the therapists choose Shaoyang in gallbladder meridian and guide the patients to generate mind from Wuhui point on the same side of the trained eye and make Qi upward through Shaoyang in gallbladder meridian, Yangguan, Huantiao, Yuanye, Dazhui and Tianchong to Tongziliao of outer canthus. After taking a deep breathing, the patients activate contraction of extraocular muscles until the eyeball reaches the zenith of ocular abduction for 6 s. After that, the patients take a deep breath and expire slowly to relax extraocular muscles fully. On the basis of the signal intensity in the pervious, the therapists make a transverse line as the surpassing goal of the next training. The therapists can use finger pulp to exert resistance on the negative direction of eyeball movement (outward and upward of outer canthus) to increase signal intensity.

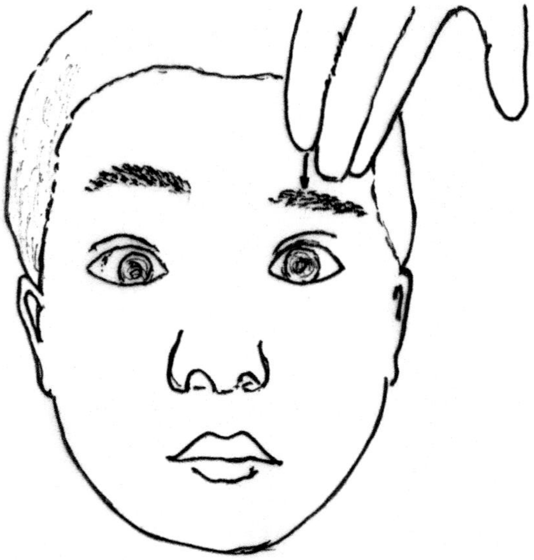

Fig. 18.7 Sketch map of the therapists exert resistance on negative direction of eyeball movement

Through electrode of ocular abduction, the patients can do the training of ocular adduction, up and down movement and convergence movement. The training time is 20 min (once a day) and one therapy course takes 3 months.

(b) Virtual reality of neurological training: Virtual reality of neurological training device is used for training. The method and therapy course are the same as these of neurological training.
(c) Reflexive movement training method is used for ciliaris, sphincter pupillae and dilator of involuntary movement. Through essential condition, conditioned reflex movement can be induced.

The conditions to induce reflexive contraction of ciliaris, sphincter pupillae and dilator include the size of objects, the distance to eye and color. Beijing Xing Cheng Wan You Technology Ltd. designed training system of ciliaris (eye protection device) according to the principle of reversible myopia and hyperopia. This system is composed of optical imaging and massage bar of magnet therapy. Optical imaging is used to exercise adjustment ability and flexibility of ciliaris, sphincter pupillae and dilator pupillae through changing distance and size of dynamic image. Mechanical eye protection device is equipped with image turntable and image movement orbit with six kinds of images that are driven by micromotor automatic control. When one kind of image is on the movement orbit, it can do uniform motion back and forth from far to near or from near to far. Every back and forth movement takes 20 s. After completion of one back and forth movement, this image gets away from image movement orbit automatically and then another image is on the movement orbit. It is in cycle. Image creates the view from 10 cm to infinity through optical effect. The patients watch image and do the training through complex optical lens barrel with the function of eliminating chromatic aberration. Digital eye protection device is equipped with image selection, image quantity and light intensity.

Training method of rehabilitation of myopia: on the basis of regulation of mind and breathing, the trainees are guided to concentrate on one spot of image. When the image is on the blurred critical point from near to far, the patients should see the image clearly until the object is blurred as far as possible. During this process, the patients can train adjustment potential of ciliaris controlled by brain. Meanwhile, object movement from near to far can be used for the training of pupil shrink, relax and convergence adjustment. When the image moves from far to near, the patients can relax and watch panorama of the image to do relaxation training of ciliaris in order to increase entire adjustment ability of ciliaris. When the patients watch the image that is from far to near, it can train pupil dilation and convergence adjustment.

Through a certain condition, the contraction and relaxation of ciliaris, sphincter pupillae and dilator are induced to complete actual muscle contraction, which is called reflex movement and is different from passive movement without muscle contraction. During this process, the muscles controlled by central nervous system can be recovered to different degrees and the myodynamia can be enhanced to promote blood circulation and metabolism of muscles and local tissue, alleviate muscle spasm, promote good circulation and improve functions.

(d) Manipulation massage: The ultimate result of myopia is the elongation of axis oculi. Long-term elongation of axis oculi leads to adhesion and stiffness of eyeball wall and tissue around eyeball. This kind of adhesion and stiffness are like the adhesion of bone and joint, which cannot be relieved by muscle contraction. Manipulation massage is good for the alleviation of adhesion and stiffness of ocular tissue.

Manipulation massage: the therapists use hot cotton cushion that the patients can tolerate (the temperature is 40–45 °C) to soak two eyes. The therapists do massage on one eye at first and it is forbidden to do massage on two eyes. The patients close two eyes. The therapists put pulp of index finger and middle finger on the other palm and rub them warm. After that, the therapists put fingers on the eye and press it for 1 s. The therapists relax and press the eye with stronger intensity. The maximum power is that the patients can tolerate it and don't feel uncomfortable. The therapists massage the eye clockwise or anticlockwise and the patients don't feel uncomfortable. The massage time of every eye is 5 min and the time of two eyes is 10 min (once a day). One therapy course includes 15 times.

During massage, the therapists should pay attention to the force and the feeling of the patients. If there is nausea or other discomfortableness, the therapists should stop massage. Massage cannot be used for the patients with glaucoma, retinal detachment, ophthalmia, hypertension, diabetes mellitus and severe trachoma.

3. Other methods to treat myopia include self-exercise and surgery [6].
   (a) Overlook method: The patients can see grassland or green tree 10 m away. Because wave length of green light is short, it can focus before retina, which can relax ciliaris and alleviate eyestrain. Eyestrain can induce false myopia. Therefore, avoiding eyestrain is the important link to prevention and alleviation of eyestrain.
   (b) Crystalline lens exercise is the exercise of self-rotation of eyeball. The method is that the patients support cheek with two hands and rotate eyeball up, down, left and right for ten times. After that, the patients can rotate eyeball clockwise or anticlockwise for ten times (once a day) and the patients can usually do it.

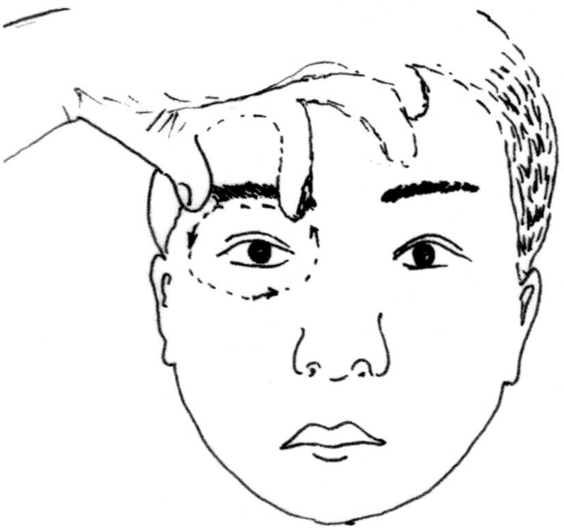

Fig. 18.8 The sketch map of the patients use thumb to press on temple and use index finger to massage acupuncture point around eye

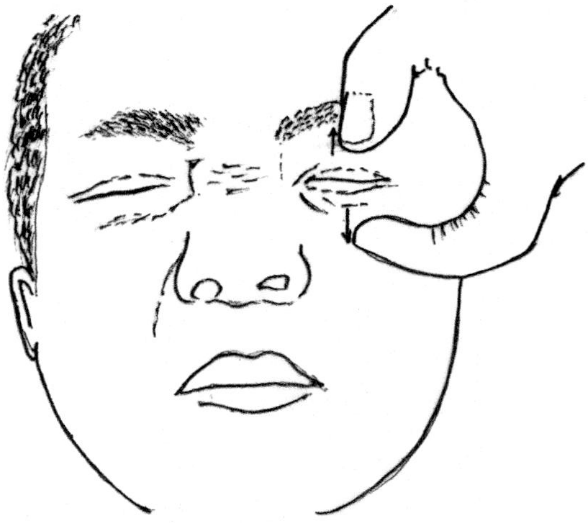

Fig. 18.9 The sketch map of the patients use thumb and index finger to massage acupuncture points around eye

(c) Massage exercise: The patients press on temple and scrape orbit. The patients use thumb to press on temple and scrape orbit up, outside and up, outside and down, inside and down along with the inside surface of the second knuckle of curled index finger (Fig. 18.8). The patients can massage Zanzhu, Yuyao, Sizhukong, Tongziliao, Qiuhou and Chengqi around orbit. This method can be used for treating false myopia and preventing aggravation of myopic eye. The therapy time is 10 min (once a day) and the patients can usually do it.

(d) Acupressure: the patients close two eyes and massage Zanzhu, Yuyao, Sizhukong, Tongziliao, Qiuhou and Chengqi around orbit. Acupoint selection should be precise and the manipulation should be slow. The oppression force makes the patients feel sore (Fig. 18.9). The therapy time is 10 min (once a day) and the patients can usually do it.

(e) The patients can wear Ortho-K lenses at night to increase high and far vision and not change physiological structure of eye. It is safe and easy to be applied.

(f) Excimer laser surgery is used to change the molecular connection of eye to recover normal eyesight.

4. Prevention of myopia [7].

(a) Eye using time in close range should be controlled, which is a good method to prevent myopia in children and adolescent in development phase.

(b) Invigorating health effectively: the patients should do exercise persistently to keep good body condition, which is an important condition to prevent myopia.

(c) Paying attention to nutrition and dietary structure: Nutrition has important effect on occurrence and development of myopia. Proper dietary structure is an effective measure to prevent myopia.

(d) Noticing the distance between eye and book and developing good habit: the distance between eye and book is too short, which is the important cause to generate myopia. The best reading sight distance is 33–50 cm. It is easy to generate myopia if the sight distance is shorter than 20 cm. Intermittent look in the distance should be developed. The patients should improve visual environment and don't read books in movement or with dim light to prevent fatigue and adjustment function decrease of ciliaris because of frequent adjustment.

(e) The patients should use eye scientifically and don't use it excessively: Excessive eye using can induce tension and fatigue of ciliaris. The patients should use eye scientifically and don't use it excessively such as long-term internet game and watching TV. Eyestrain should be alleviated timely and ciliaris spasm can be relaxed gradually to recover normal state.

18.2.3 Presbyopia

Hyperopia is that some reasons make axis oculi become short. Without adjustment, parallel lights focus behind retina through refraction and there is no clear objective image on retina. Therefore, hyperopia requires adjustment to enhance ocular refractive index so that the light into eyeball can converge and form clear objective image on retina, which is easy to generate eyestrain [8].

However, there are many mistakes in the prevention of presbyopia. People think that myopia is better than hyperopia, because people with hyperopia can see far. Wearing glasses is the business of myopic eye. These statements are incorrect. Because the patients with presbyopia cannot see objects clearly whether far or near, it requires frequent adjustment. During the process of convergence adjustment, medial rectus is involved in it. Super contraction of bilateral medial rectus may stretch eyeball inward and induce esotropia of two eyes. When hyperopia of one eye is severe, super contraction of medial rectus in this side can induce unilateral esotropia. There are poor vision, strabismus and amblyopia in the patients with medium and high presbyopia. Therefore, the mechanism of hyperopia is complicated than that of myopia and there are more complications. Hyperopia requires treatment more than myopic eye.

18.2.3.1 The Classification and Pathogenesis of Hyperopia

Hyperopia includes axile hyperopia, curvature hyperopia and refraction hyperopia. Axile hyperopia is usually observed [9].

1. Axile hyperopia is the most common type in abnormal refraction.

   After birth, the average length of axis oculi is about 17.3 mm. It is physiological hyperopia. With the development of infant body, the anteroposterior axis of eye is lengthened until the length reaches the normal length or is close to the physiological length in adult. Genetic and environmental factor can affect eyeball development and the axis oculi cannot reach the normal physiological length, which is called axile hyperopia.

   In addition, axis oculi becomes short because of pathological condition: oppression of tumor or inflammatory mass can induce invagination of posterior pole of eyeball and make it flat. Edema of neoplasm behind eyeball or eyeball wall can put forward macular region of retina and oppress posterior pole of eyeball. Retinal detachment induces displacement to oppress the back of eyeball, even the back of crystalline lens, which can induce obvious change of diopter.
2. Curvature hyperopia: Because the curvature of any refraction object in refraction system of eyeball is small and refractive index becomes big so that objective image focus behind retina, which is called curvature hyperopia. Cornea is the part where the curvature becomes small such as congenital flat cornea, cornea trauma or cornea diseases.
3. Refraction hyperopia is induced by poor refraction of crystalline lens.

   The common cause is physiological degenerative alterations due to age and pathological changes of cornea in the patients with diabetes mellitus [10]. In addition, backward dislocation of crystalline lens is induced by congenital factor or ocular trauma, which can form hyperopia.

18.2.3.2 The Adjustment of Presbyopia

Adjustment is the result that people want to see near or miniature object with eye. Emmetropia is at resting state. People see far object and the objective image focuses on retina clearly without adjustment. When people see near object, the objective image focuses on retina clearly with near reflex mechanism, which is physiological adjustment.

The eye is at resting state because of short axis oculi or poor refractive index due to hyperopia. The far and near objects cannot focus on retina clearly. Unclear objective image is the visual movement stimulation factor of optic center. Ciliaris, pupil sphincter and medial rectus dominated by the third cranial nerve are activated, which forms associated movement of adjustment, convergence and miosis. The adjustment is principal and is non-physiological.

18.2.3.3 Clinical Manifestations

1. Hypopsia: The degree of hypopsia depends on hyperopia degree and the intensity of adjustment ability.
2. Eyestrain: There are blurred vision, swell of geisoma, headache, drowsy, insomnia and hypomnesis.
3. Esotropia: excessive adjustment and convergence movement induce near reflex disorder and then induce esotropia.

18.2.3.4 Assessment of Presbyopia

Except the examination method to assess myopia, there are many examinations such as ocular appearance and adjustment ability of presbyopia.

1. Ocular appearance examination: in diffused light, the therapists examine the size of eyeball, symmetry of face or not, esophoria or not, esotropia or exotropia.
2. Eyesight examination: Correct examination and flexible analysis of far and near eyesight are good for the rapid diagnosis of hyperopia. The teen-age eyes are capable to adjust. In mild hyperopia, the far and near eyesight are normal. There are hypopsia of far and near eyesight in the adolescent with high hyperopia and middle age patients with moderate hyperopia.
3. Ophthalmoscopy examination: The symptoms include small, red and dim optic nerve head. There is faint yellow transparent choroid wart in the patients with high hyperopia. There is defect of field vision if the wart is big. There is crescent-shaped change below the optic nerve head. In addition, gonioscope can also be used for examination.
4. The grade of hyperopia degree: The grade of the severity is according to refractive index of hyperopia.
   (a) Mild hyperopia: The refractive index is less than 3D. The patients with mild hyperopia are adolescent with compensatory adjustment function. The far and near eyesight are normal and people can see objects in any distance clearly. This kind of presbyopia is called false presbyopia.
   (b) Moderate hyperopia: The refractive index is no less than 3D but less than 6D. The adjustment ability of moderate hyperopia or elder patients is poor and cannot be compensated. The residual part after compensation is called dominant hyperopia.
   (c) High hyperopia: The refractive index is more than 6D. The adjustment ability of the patients with high hyperopia is bad, which is called dominant hyperopia.

Both recessive and dominant hyperopia are called entire hyperopia.

18.2.3.5 Rehabilitation Therapy and Prevention of Presbyopia

If there are signs or symptoms of hyperopia in eye, the patients should go to hospital for diagnosis and therapy in time and wear proper glasses to rectify eyesight according to the instructions of ophthalmologists or use other methods for therapy. We only discuss rehabilitation training and prevention of presbyopia.

1. The mechanism of the rehabilitation of neurological training of hyperopia: The mechanism is the same as that of rehabilitation of myopia. Six-step Daoyin technique is used for active movement of ocular muscles to

promote plasticity and functional reorganization of optic center in order to develop potential ability, recover coordinated movement ability between ocular muscles, alleviate ciliaris spasm, increase blood circulation of ocular tissue and recover virtuous circle of ocular metabolism and adjustment ability of eye. Therefore, the aggravation of hyperopia can be alleviated or stopped.

2. Specific methods of rehabilitation of neurological training include neurological training, reflexive movement training and manipulation massage.
   (a) The training method of neurological training of extraocular muscles are the same as these of myopic eye.

      The training time is 20 min (once a day) and one therapy course takes 3 months.
   (b) Virtual reality training of neurological training: Virtual reality training device of neurological training is used for the training. The methods and therapy course are the same as neurological training methods.
   (c) Reflexive movement training method is used for ciliaris, sphincter pupillae and dilator of involuntary dominance. Through essential condition, adjustment reflex movement is induced.

      The conditions to induce reflexive contraction of ciliaris, sphincter pupillae and dilator include the size of objects, the distance to eye and color. The specific method of training with eye protection device is the same as that of myopia. On the basis of regulation of mind and breathing, the trainees are guided to concentrate on one spot of image. When the image is on the blurred critical point from far to near, the patients should see the image clearly until the object is blurred as near as possible. During this process, the patients can train adjustment potential of ciliaris controlled by brain. Meanwhile, object movement from far to near can be used for the training of pupil shrink, relax and convergence adjustment. When the image moves from far to near, the patients can relax and watch panorama of the image to do relaxation training of ciliaris in order to increase entire adjustment ability of ciliaris. When the patients watch the image that is from near to far, it can train pupil dilation and convergence adjustment.

      The differences between this method and training method of myopia are as follows: myopic eye: When the image is on the blurred critical point from near to far, the patients should see the image clearly until the object is blurred as far as possible. Presbyopia: When the image is on the blurred critical point from far to near, the patients should see the image clearly until the object is blurred as near as possible.

      The training time is 15 min (once a day) and the patients can usually do it.
   (2) Manipulation massage of eyeball: Short axis oculi and abnormal refraction are the ultimate result of hyperopia. Long-term short of axis oculi leads to adhesion and stiffness of tissue of eyeball, ocular wall and eye area. The adhesion and stiffness are difficult to be loosened through muscle contraction. Manipulation massage is good for adhesion of ocular tissue and alleviation of stiffness.

Manipulation massage: the therapists use hot cotton cushion that the patients can tolerate (the temperature is 40–45 °C) to soak two eyes. The therapists do massage on one eye at first and it is forbidden to do massage on two eyes. The patients close two eyes. The therapists put pulp of thumb, index finger and middle finger on the other palm and rub them warm. After that, the therapists put fingers on the eye and press inner wall of orbit into eye socket from inward and upward, outward and upward, downward. The therapists put eyeball among the pulps of three fingers (Fig. 18.10) and press it slightly. The maximum power is that the patients can tolerate it and don't feel uncomfortable.

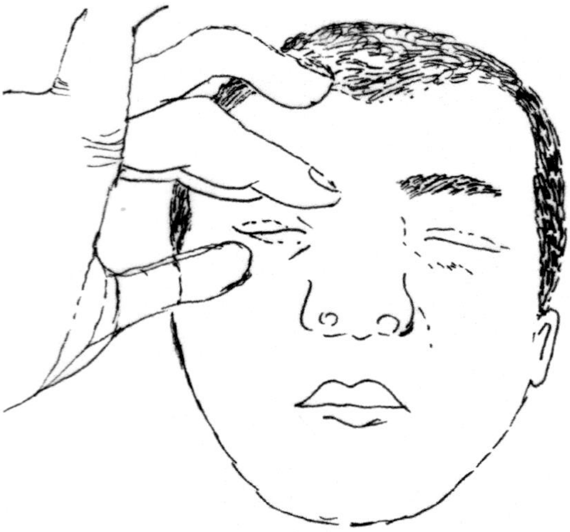

Fig. 18.10 Sketch map of the therapists put eyeball among the pulps of three fingers and press it slightly

The massage time for one eye is 5 and 10 min for two eyes (once a day). There are 15 times in one therapy course.

During massage, the therapists should pay attention to the force and the feeling of the patients. If there is nausea or other discomfortableness, the therapists should stop massage. Massage cannot be used for the patients with glaucoma, retinal detachment, ophthalmia, hypertension, diabetes mellitus and severe trachoma.

3. Other methods to treat myopia include self-exercise and surgery.
   (a) Overlook method: The patients can see grassland or green tree 10 m away. Because wave length of green light is short, it can focus before retina, which can relax ciliaris and alleviate eyestrain for prevention and alleviation of hyperopia.
   (b) Ocular muscles exercise is the exercise of self-rotation of eyeball. The method is that the patients support cheek with two hands and rotate eyeball up, down, left and right for ten times. After that, the patients can rotate eyeball clockwise or anticlockwise for ten times (once a day) and the patients can usually do it.
   (c) Massage exercise: The exercise method is the same as that of myopic eye. The therapy time is 10 min (once a day) and the patients can usually do it.
   (d) Acupressure: The exercise method is the same as that of myopic eye. The therapy time is 10 min (once a day) and the patients can usually do it.
4. Prevention of presbyopia: Self-exercise of ocular muscles is an effective measure to prevent visual impairment. On the basis of meeting the daily functional requirements or existing athletic ability, special additional movement increase functional ability of tissue and organ to supplement the deficiency of functional ability or prepare for the rainy day.
   (a) The patients should use eye scientifically and don't use it excessively: Excessive eye using can induce tension and fatigue of ciliaris and medial rectus. Excessive adjustment oppresses eyeball and elongates axis oculi. The patients should use eye scientifically and don't use it excessively such as long-term internet game and watching TV. Eyestrain should be alleviated timely and ocular muscle spasm can be relaxed gradually to recover normal state.
   (b) Paying attention to eye using environment: people watch books or use eyes in a bad environment or condition such as moving position, clinostatism, dim light, near vision and too small object, which all lead to excessive adjustment of eye. Long-term excessive adjustment easily leads to change of ocular structure, and then induces refractive index and eyesight change. People should watch books in an adequate and mild light with stable sitting position and proper distance between book and eye. People should see far intermittently and do eye exercises.
   (c) Invigorating health effectively: the patients should do exercise persistently to keep good body condition, which is an important condition to prevent myopia visual impairment.

(d) Paying attention to nutrition and dietary structure: Nutrition has important effect on occurrence and development of myopia. Proper dietary structure is an effective measure to prevent hyperopia.

(e) Acupressure: The patients are in sitting position or horizontal position, close two eyes naturally and massage acupuncture points around eye. The acupuncture point selection should be precise and soft until there is sour and swell in this point. People use two thumbs to massage Tianying that is on the interface between the bottom of brows and lateral-superior orbit. People use thumb of one hand to squeeze and press Jingming acupuncture point that is in nasal root and beside inner canthus of two eyes. People should press downward at first and squeeze upward. People use index finger to massage Sibai that is in the center of cheek one transverse finger below inferior margin of orbit.

18.2.4 Presbyopia

Presbyopia is the condition that elder people are difficult to read or work gradually with age in near vision, which is one of the phenomenon of human function aging.

18.2.4.1 Pathogenetic Mechanism of Presbyopia

Presbyopia is induced by many causes such as crystalline lens sclerosis due to increase of age that can make the flexibility and elasticity weaken. Meanwhile, the contraction ability of ciliaris decreases, which can slow down adjustment ability of eye and move far the near-point. People cannot or are difficult to see near object clearly, which is the result of comprehensive factors such as recession of intraocular and extraocular muscles and deformability decrease of crystalline lens.

Presbyopia is also called functional decline syndrome of visual acuity or presbytia, which is usually observed in the people who age is more than 40 years old. People whose age is 40–50 are not called old people so that many people are reluctant to wear presbyopic glasses even if they are presbyopic. Mentally, people in this group don't recognize and feel they are old. Therefore, the author called presbyopia as retrogressive hyperopia, which demonstrate that presbyopia is induced by physiological degeneration of ocular tissue and show respect to the patients and their family. For example, dementia is called cognitive disorder, which can protect the pride of the patients and their family effectively. It is widely accepted by academic world and all sectors of society.

In addition, researches show that retrogressive hyperopia is related to the job of people and reading habit. Therefore, it is very important to cultivate and maintain good reading habit.

18.2.4.2 Clinical Symptoms of Retrogressive Hyperopia

1. Early symptoms: if people cannot see the small handwriting clearly, they can move reading target far to alleviate blurred vision and eyestrain. Even if the patients can see the object clearly without moving the object far, this can also generate eyestrain.
2. Symptoms of formation period: after formation of degenerative presbyopia, the direct manifestations are eyestrain, sour and swell, hyperdacryosis, photophoby, aningeresting and headache that can be relieved after rest when they cannot see object clearly in near vision or reading.
3. Late symptoms: Frequent eyestrain and headache usually decrease work efficiency, even people cannot do the work with small sight distance. Just as many chronic diseases, retrogressive presbyopia in early phase is not taken into account. When it is developed to cataract and severe decrease of eyesight, they receive therapy. This may induce other complications and increase difficulty of healing.

18.2.4.3 The Difference Between Retrogressive Hyperopia and Hyperopia

Although the common symptoms of presbyopia and retrogressive hyperopia include blurred vision of near object and people regard retrogressive presbyopia as presbyopia, there is qualitative difference between two diseases. Retrogressive hyperopia is normal physiological phenomenon with age and is the manifestation of human function aging. Whereas, hyperopia is induced by ametropia and its mechanism is totally different.

Actually, it is easy to distinguish the two diseases. People with hyperopia cannot see far and near objects clearly. People with retrogressive presbyopia only cannot see near object. The differences between the two are as follows:

1. Age: Retrogressive hyperopia is usually observed in the middle and old aged whose age is more than 40. Presbyopia is usually observed in children and adolescent. The degree of retrogressive presbyopia is increased with age (50° per 5 years) until 60 years old when the degree is increased to 250–300°. After that, the degree isn't increased.
2. Pathomechanism: Retrogressive hyperopia is normal physiological phenomenon with age and is the manifestation of human function aging. Presbyopia is that some causes shorten axis oculi and it is an abnormal state.
3. The ability to see far: when people with retrogressive presbyopia see far, with no need for excessive adjustment of ocular muscles, objective image can focus on retina clearly. In presbyopia, anteroposterior diameter of eyeball becomes short, curvature of crystalline lens becomes short, and refractive index decreases. Therefore, objective image can focus behind retina. People with presbyopia cannot see far object clearly.

18.2.4.4 Rehabilitation Therapy and Prevention of Retrogressive Hyperopia

The key points of rehabilitation therapy and prevention of retrogressive hyperopia are as follows: through training, the potential ability of ocular muscles, tissue and nerves is developed to counteract or compensate functional defect induced by ocular tissue regression. Protecting eye and enhancing self-exercise of eye can alleviate aging and regression of ocular tissue.

In daily life, there are many examples that exercise delays senescence. For example, the face of the actors who use mimetic muscles frequently is younger than the peer. The body flexibility of the old person whose age is 70 years old is similar to that of the adolescent because of unremitting exercise. Just as mentioned above, exercise is additional movement on the basis of movements required for daily life. Therefore, exercise can enhance neural functions and myodynamia, maintain tissue vitality and elasticity, and increase functions of organ and tissue.

1. The mechanism of the rehabilitation of neurological training of retrogressive hyperopia: The entire training can recover contraction ability and coordination ability of muscles comprehensively, release adhesion of ocular tissue, maintain and recover flexibility of ocular tissue. Six-step Daoyin technique is used for active movement training of ocular muscles to develop their potential ability, promote synaptic plasticity and functional reorganization of optic center, recover coordinated movement ability between ocular muscles, alleviate ciliaris spasm, increase blood circulation of ocular tissue, recover virtuous circle of ocular tissue metabolism and ocular adjustment ability, rectify the difficulty of seeing near object in retrogressive presbyopia, alleviate or delay the disease.
2. The specific methods of rehabilitation training of neurological training include neurological training, ciliaris reflexive movement training and manipulation massage.
   (a) The training method of neurological training of extraocular muscles is the same as rehabilitation training of neurological training of presbyopia. The training time is 20 min (once a day) and the therapy course takes 3 months.

(b) Virtual reality training of neurological training: Virtual reality training device of neurological training is used for the training. The method and therapy course are the same as the training method of neurological training. Combined with rehabilitation training of neurological training of extraocular muscles, this method has good training effect. The training time is 20 min (once a day) and the therapy course takes 3 months.
(c) Ciliaris reflexive movement training method: through essential condition, reflexive movement training of ciliaris, sphincter pupillae and dilator pupillae of involuntary dominance is induced.
(d) Eye protection device is used for the training. The basic method is the same as training method of presbyopia. The training time is 15 min (once a day) and the patients can insist on it for a long time.
(e) Manipulation massage of eyeball: the method is the same as the training method of myopic eye. The training time is 5 min for one eye and 10 min for two eyes (once a day). There are 15 times in one therapy course.

During massage, the therapists should pay attention to the force and the feeling of the patients. If there is nausea or other discomfortableness, the therapists should stop massage. Massage cannot be used for the patients with glaucoma, retinal detachment, ophthalmia, hypertension, diabetes mellitus and severe trachoma.

3. Other Therapy Methods of Retrogressive Hyperopia Include Self-Exercise and Wearing Glasses
(a) Near vision method: in an environment with sufficient light, the patients use two hands to hold paper or newspaper with colorful character and move it from far to near slowly. When the object reaches the critical point of blurred vision, the patients stop the movement and concentrate to see the object clearly for 6 s after regulation of mind and breathing. The training time is 15 min (once a day) and the patients can insist on it for a long time.
(b) Ocular muscles exercise: active rotation of eyeball can exercise muscles around eye. The patients are in sitting position, support cheek with two hands and rotate eyeball up, down, left and right for ten times. After that, the patients can rotate eyeball clockwise or anticlockwise for ten times (once a day) and the patients can usually do it.
(c) Massage exercise is the same as that of presbyopia. The frequency is once a day and the patients can usually do it.
(d) Acupressure is the same as the exercise method of presbyopia. The frequency is once a day and the patients can usually do it.
(e) Wearing correct glasses: if people wear improper glasses, it may deepen the symptoms. Therefore, optometry should be precise before wearing glasses. The patients should receive optometry every 5 years. Progressive glasses are scientific. The upper part of progressive glasses is used to see far object, middle part of it is used to see object in middle distance and near part of it is used to see near object. The degree is from high to low in these three areas gradually so that the patients can see far and near objects.

The patients cannot buy glasses randomly. Traditional retrogressive hyperopia eye only helps the patients to see near object.

4. Prevention of retrogressive presbyopia: Frequent self-exercise of ocular muscles is effective measure to prevent ocular muscles and ocular structure degradation. The patients should insist on it so that they can obtain desired effect.
(a) The patients should use eye scientifically and don't use it excessively: Excessive eye using can induce tension and fatigue of ocular tissue. The patients should use eye scientifically and don't use it excessively to alleviate eyestrain and maintain blood circulation and elasticity of ocular tissue in order to delay aging of ocular tissue.
(b) Paying attention to eye using environment: people watch books or use eyes in a bad

environment or condition such as moving position, clinostatism, dim light, near vision and too small object, which all lead to excessive adjustment of eye. Long-term excessive adjustment easily leads to change of ocular structure, and then induces refractive index and eyesight change. People should watch books in an adequate and mild light with stable sitting position and proper distance between book and eye. People should see far intermittently and do eye exercises.

(c) Invigorating health effectively: The patients should do exercise persistently to keep good body condition, which is an important condition to prevent retrogressive hyperopia.

(d) Paying attention to nutrition and dietary structure: Nutrition has important effect on occurrence and development of myopia. Proper dietary structure is an effective measure to prevent visual impairment including retrogressive hyperopia.

(e) Acupressure is the same as the method of presbyopia.

(f) Self-exercise: the patients should frequently be in green environment such as grassland and forest and concentrate to see the objects from far to near until they can see the object clearly in the nearest distance. The distance should be recorded. After repeated exercise, they should compare the distance to see the object clearly. This method can develop ciliaris potential and improve retrogressive hyperopia.

18.3 Clinical Application of Rehabilitation Training of Ciliaris in Pupil with Early Myopia

Myopia is a somatopsychic illness to harm the teen-age. The morbidity of myopia in the students of our country is increased consistently, which is the second in the world. The cause of formation is related to such as long-term near vision and bad habits in visual environment. In our country, the patients with myopia usually wear glasses and receive medicine and surgery therapy, but there is no effective rehabilitation training measures. In our study, we used ciliaris training method. In Huajiadi Experimental Primary School Chaoyang District Beijing, from May 22th 2006 to September 27th 2006, we did a 4-month's experiment to observe the rehabilitation effect of early myopia. The results are as follows:

18.3.1 Materials and Methods

18.3.1.1 Clinical Materials

In Huajiadi experimental primary school Chaoyang district Beijing, we choose class five in fourth grade and class four in fifth grade. They are randomly divided into two groups. The training group is class five. There are 39 people (22 males and 17 females) and the average age is 10.4. The control group is class four. There are 37 people (21 males and 16 females) and the average age is 10.3.

18.3.1.2 Training Method

1. Training group: OO brand SU-001 eye protection device produced by Beijing Xingchenwanyou Science and Technology Ltd. is used for ciliaris training. Every student have an eye protection device and do ciliaris training (15 min per time, twice a day in moon break and before sleep. The total training time is 4 months.

   In order to guarantee training quality, the teachers and parents should examine and instruct the training and give the students training notebook. Under the supervision of the parents, the students should fill in the training notebook.
2. Control group: The students only receive propaganda and education of prevention of myopia.

18.3.2 Observational Index

International universal index is used for assessment.

18.3.2.1 Eyesight Detection

Standard logarithmic visual acuity chart of light box is used to test eyesight of naked eye of one eye in 5 m away.

18.3.2.2 Refraction Test

NIDEK-AR600 auto refract keratometer produced by Beijing Xueliang Glasses Company is used to test diopter and astigmatism of every eye.

18.3.2.3 Data Collection and Statistical Analysis

Eyesight and diopter are tested before and after training. The data is recorded and stored. SPSS12.0 statistical software is used for T-test.

Before training, there is no difference of age and myopia between the two groups ($P > 0.05$).

18.3.2.4 Classification of Eyesight and Evaluation Criterion of Therapeutic Effect

International universal classification and evaluation criterion.

1. Classification of eyesight is according to the lower eyesight of naked eye.
   (a) Normal eyesight: Eyesight is more than 5.0.
   (b) Mild myopia: Eyesight is 4.7–4.9.
   (c) Moderate myopia: Eyesight is 4.4–4.6.
   (d) Severe myopia: Eyesight is less than 4.3.
2. Classification of therapeutic effect is according to eyesight from standard logarithmic visual acuity chart.
   (a) Cure: eyesight is recovered to more than 5.0.
   (b) Excellent: eyesight is recovered to more than 3.0 on the original basis.
   (c) Effective: eyesight is recovered to more than 0.1 on the original basis.
   (d) Invalid: eyesight is recovered to less than 0.1 on the original basis.
3. There are three grades of according to diopter.
   (a) Cure: refraction range is recovered to +0.50 to −0.25D.
   (b) Effective: refraction range is recovered to −0.50 to −6.0D.
   (c) Invalid: refraction range is not recovered.

18.3.3 Results

18.3.3.1 Data Analysis

There are 78 eyes of 39 students in training group. After training, the average eyesight is 1.20 ± 0.56 from the eyesight before training (0.71 ± 0.36的). There is significant difference of eyesight before and after training ($P < 0.01$, Table 18.1). There are 74 eyes of 37 students in control group. The average eyesight is 0.71 ± 0.37. Four months later, the average eyesight is 0.71 ± 0.63. There is no significant difference of eyesight before and after the training ($P > 0.05$, Table 18.2. There is significant difference of eyesight between two groups ($P < 0.01$). Two eyes have myopia in control group.

After training, the number of the eyes with normal eyesight is 52 from 27 before training. The increase rate is 92.6%. The number of the eyes with mild myopia is decreased to 17 from 31 before training. The decrease rate is 45.2%. The number of the eyes with moderate myopia is decreased to 8 from 10 before training. The decrease rate is 20%. The number of the eyes with severe myopia is decreased to 1 from 10 before training. The decrease rate is 90%.

In control group, the number of normal eyes is 31 from 33 before intervention. The number of myopic eye is increased to 43 from 41. The increase rate is 12.5%. The number of moderate myopia is increased to 20 from 17. The increase rate is 17.6%. The number of severe myopia is decreased to 5 from 8 before training. The decrease rate is 37.5%.

18.3.3.2 Classification of Therapeutic Effect

Therapeutic effect is measured by the eyesight that is lower than 5.0 before training. There are 51 eyes.

Healing: eyesight of 25 eyes is recovered more than 5.0. The cure rate is 49%.

Excellent: eyesight of 24 eyes is recovered more than 0.3. The excellent rate is 47.1%.

Effective: eyesight of 50 is recovered more than 0.1. The effective rate is 98%.

Invalid: eyesight of one eye is recovered less than 0.1. The invalid rate is 2%.

Table 18.1 Comparison table before and after training of rehabilitation training of eyesight in training group

Side	Degree			
	Normal	Mild	Moderate	Severe
Left eye pre-test	14	16	4	5
Left eye post-test	28	7	4	0
Right eye pre-test	13	15	6	5
Right eye post-test	24	10	4	1
Total pre-test 27 (34.6%)	31 (39.7%)	10 (12.8%)	10 (12.8%)	
Total post-test 52 (66.7%)	17 (27.8%)	8 (10.3%)	1 (1.3%)	

Table 18.2 Comparison table before and after training of eyesight in control group

Side	Degree			
	Normal	Mild	Moderate	Severe
Left eye pre-test	19	6	8	4
Left eye post-test	16	8	11	2
Right eye pre-test	14	10	9	4
Right eye post-test	15	10	9	3
Total pre-test	33 (89.2%)	16 (43.2%)	17 (45.9%)	8 (21.6%)
Total post-test	31 (83.8%)	18 (48.6%)	20 (54.1%)	5 (13.5%)

Table 18.3 Refraction change in training group before and after training

	Emmetropia	Low and moderate myopia	High myopia
	(+0.50 to −0.25D)	(−0.50 to −6.0D)	(> −6.00D)
Before training	61	11	0
After training	63	7	1

After training, the number of the eyes with normal diopter in training group is increased to 63 from 61 before training. The increase rate is 3.3%. The number of low diopter of myopia is decreased to 7 from 11 before training. The decrease rate is 36.4%. One eye is developed to high diopter of myopia before training (Table 18.3).

18.3.4 Discussion

18.3.4.1 Myopia Can Be Recovered Through Increasing Adjustment Ability After Ciliaris Training

There is no method to cure myopia in modern medicine and there is no effective measure to inhibit the progress of myopia effectively. It is widely accepted that long-term near vision is the major factor to form myopia. Excessive near vision induces excessive adjustment of ciliaris and finally leads to spasm, which elongates long ocular axis, increase refractive index of crystalline lens. Therefore, objective image focus before retina and the manifestation is myopic optical defocus. However, with further research, the scientists found that there is no excessive adjustment but adjustment lag in human eyes. When people see the object in a certain distance, if adjustment of ciliaris is insufficient, objective images focus behind retina and the manifestation is hyperopic optical defocus. Atropine eyewash, muscarinic cholinergic receptor blocker, can control myopia, which demonstrated that myopia is related to ciliaris spasm. Atropine eyewash has an effect through alleviating ciliaris spasm. Some researches show that there is adjustment lag of ciliaris in near vision. Marco found that in near vision ciliaris seldom adjust even don't adjust. Long-term no-adjustment of ciliaris leads to retrogressive change and disuse myasthenia, which can decrease adjustment function, aggravate myopia and form vicious circle.

The author deemed that two paradoxical conclusions are the results of ciliaris damage to varying degrees in different phase of myopia development. In the early phase of myopia, because of long-term near vision, persistent excessive contraction of ciliaris can make the objective image on retina, which may induce insufficient blood supply of ciliaris, metabolite accumulation and muscle fiber injury. These can induce ciliaris spasm. In the early phase of myopic eye, there are eyestrain, discomfort, sour and headache in the patients, which are related to spasm after ciliaris injury. For example, people feel muscular soreness after long-distance running and there are sternocleidomastoid spasm and soreness after stiff neck. Because ciliaris is small and in the deep of eye socket and the sensory location is not accurate, the symptoms are slight. This is why Atropine, spasmolytic, is effective in the early phase of myopia. With the development of myopia, people should wear glasses. Although glasses can alleviate myopia, it decreases adjustment change of crystalline lens. After a long time, it may induce disuse myasthenia of ciliaris and worsen adjustment function. Therefore, in the late phase of myopia, there are tension decrease and lacking in strength of ciliaris.

The author deemed that the common characteristic of ciliaris whether with spasm in early phase or tension decrease in late phase is adjustment ability decrease of crystalline lens. Major performance of adjustment ability includes two aspects such as adjustment range and adjustment flexibility. Adjustment range is the change of crystalline lens due to contraction and relaxation of ciliaris. Adjustment flexibility is the times of changed curvature of crystalline lens regulated by ciliaris in unit time. The researches show that ocular refractive error is significantly related to adjustment range of ciliaris, and has no relationship with adjustment flexibility. By this token, the training of adjustment function of ciliaris, especially adjustment range has good effect on the prevention and rehabilitation of myopia. Magnet therapies, medicine such as atropine and hot compress have some effect on myopia in the early phase. These methods can alleviate ciliaris spasm and ocular sourness and promote excretion of metabolite. In the late phase of myopia, these methods have no obvious therapeutic effect. Only training can develop neural potential of nerve that dominates ciliaris and increase its adjustment ability. For example, if a person wants to lift up 100 kg, he must do special exercise.

Skeletal muscles are voluntary muscles. The joint motion generated by contraction and relaxation is obvious, but people are difficult to feel the movement of crystalline lens generated by contraction and relaxation of ciliaris. Therefore, they think that there is no way to train ciliaris. This is a misunderstanding. Although ciliaris is dominated by parasympathetic nerve of oculomotor nerve and belongs to involuntary muscle, reflexive movement can increase its function. The cure rate is 49% and effective rate is 97.4% in training group, which demonstrates the effectiveness of this training method.

18.3.4.2 Adjustment Ability of Ciliaris Is the Important Factor of Negative Refraction Induced by Elongation of Axis Oculi

In all the 78 eyes in training group, there are only 27 eyes with emmetropia measured by logarithmic visual acuity chart and there are 61 eyes with emmetropia measured by refraction test. The number of difference is 34. After training, the cure rate measured by logarithmic visual acuity chart is 49% and the cure rate measured by refraction test is only 7.4%. There is significant difference between the two methods. This phenomenon is related to adjustment ability of ciliaris and the change of axis oculi.

Near vision leads to elongation of axis oculi and the mechanism remains unclear. Someone think that it is a process of active remodeling of eyeball regulated by neural and bioactive substance. Some researchers think that it is trigeminy reflex mechanism of near vision such as adjustment, pupil shrink and convergence. Intraocular and extraocular rectus of eyeball oppress eyeball. Linzhi proposed that elongation of axis oculi is because ciliaris contraction regulated by brain decreases ocular pressure and ocular pressure is too high because this regulation fails. Only elongation of axis oculi can change diopter. In the early phase of myopic eye, adjustment ability of ciliaris decreases, but the axis oculi are not elongated. Although the refraction is normal, because adjustment ability of ciliaris decreases, eyesight measured by visual testing chart is lower than the normal. In the late phase of myopic eye, the adjustment ability of ciliaris decreases with elongation of axis oculi, the eyesight is lower than the normal measured by refraction test and visual testing chart. The former myopia is called adjustment myopia and the latter is called refractive myopia, which is one of the criterions to distinguish false and true myopia. Ciliaris training can recover and increase adjustment ability of ciliaris, but cannot shorten elongated axis oculi. Therefore, eyesight is increased significantly measured by visual testing chart and eyesight is not increased obviously measured by diopter test. The author think that static refraction is not the only golden standard to assess the therapeutic effect of myopia. When one condition is stable, changing another condition can achieve the goal. For example, a person in severe environment can increase his own viability to survive without changing the environment. In addition, potential ability training of ciliaris recovers adjustment myopia and prevent refractive myopia.

18.3.4.3 Correcting Bad Reading Habit Is the Fundamental Guarantee for the Prevention and Rehabilitation of Myopia

The distance between eye and book is too short, which is the important cause to generate myopia. The best reading sight distance is 33–50 cm. It is easy to generate myopia if the sight distance is shorter than 20 cm. If people cannot overcome near vision habit, it cannot maintain the therapeutic effect of myopia rehabilitation. After wearing glasses, myopia is worsened in the eye whose eyesight is rectified. Therefore, the understanding and memory learning method is advocated. Intermittent look in the distance should be developed. The patients should improve visual environment and don't read books in movement or with dim light to prevent fatigue and adjustment function decrease of ciliaris because of frequent adjustment. It is also the fundamental measure to prevent myopia, recover myopia and keep the therapeutic effect.

Rehabilitation training has short-term effects on the pupils with myopia in the early phase. Long-term therapeutic effects are related to whether the pupils can keep the exercise or the near vision habit can be overcome. For the pupils with moderate and high myopia and elongation of axis oculi, the effectiveness of ciliaris training, visual environment changes and unsynchronized longitudinal massage of two eyes requires further verification. In addition, criterion of cure is that the eyesight reaches 5.0 in the assessment of therapeutic effect, but excellent criterion is that the eyesight is increased by 0.3 on the original basis. If the eyesight is from 4.9 to 5.0, it belongs to curative case but not excellent case. The reasonableness that cure rate is higher than excellent rate requires further investigation.

References

1. Bill A. Blood circulation and fluid dynamics in the eye. Physiol Rev. 1975;55(3):383–417.
2. Becker B, Neufeld AH. Pressure dependence of uveoscleral outflow. Glaucoma. 2002;11(6):545–9.
3. Troster H, Brambring M. The play behavior and play materials of blind and sighted infants and preschoolers. J Vis Impair Blind. 1994;88(5):421–33.
4. Jiang BC. Accommodative vergence is driven by the phasic component of the acconmodative controller. Vision Res. 1996;36(1):97–102.
5. Grosvenor T, Goss DA. Role of the cornea in emmetropia and myopia. Optom Vis Sci. 1998;75(2):132–45.
6. Hamelin N, Glacet-Bernerd A, Brindeau C, et al. Surgical treatment of subfoveal neovasculariztion in myopia: macular translocation vs surgical removal. Am J Ophthalmol. 2002;133(4):530–6.
7. Tano Y. Pathologic myopia: where are we now? Am J Ophthalmol. 2002;134(5):645–60.
8. Sawada A, Tomidokoro A, Araie M, et al. Refractive errors in an elderly Japanese population: the Tajimi study. Ophthalmology. 2008;115(2):363–70.
9. Xu L, Lin T. Refractive error in urban and rural adult Chinese in Beijing. Ophthalmology. 2005;112(10):1676–83.
10. Attebo K, Lvers RO, Mitchell P. Refractive errors in an older population: the Blue Mountains Eye Study. Ophthalmology. 1999;106(6):1066–72.

Corollary Equipment of Rehabilitation Training of Neurological Training

19

19.1 The Guiding Ideology of Developing Corollary Equipment of Rehabilitation Training

19.1.1 The Implication of Rehabilitation Training Equipment

Broadly speaking, at present, the definition of equipment is that machine and device can be used for a long time in industry or enterprise and the matter form and material goods are maintained in use. Equipment is the physical means to create wealth, is material and technological foundation of social production and is one of the marks of progress of modern productivity.

Except for the performances mentioned above, the author thinks that equipment is the instrument of implementation method. It can implement the method better and make the best use of the method. In a way, it can broaden the application range of the method to varying degree, even complete the job or mission that human cannot finish. For example, if people want to hit a target far away from their body, the fist can only be used to hit the target in the distance of arm length and the power is limited. Slingshot can be used to hit the target 30 m away and the power is big to harm the target to a certain extent. If bow and arrow are used, people can hit the target 100 m away. The arrow is more powerful than mud ball. If rifle is used, the bullet can damage or kill the target about 200 m away. If guided missile is used, it can hit any target on the earth and damage the target greatly. In this example, the method is hit. Because the instrument is different in the hit, the hit distance and the damaged degree are double. Instrument amplifies the application of method.

In daily productive labor, there are many instruments such as pliers and wrench to cut off steel wire or screw nut that human cannot complete.

These show that instrument can extend the effect of the method to varying degrees to complete the mission that human cannot complete. All the instruments or equipment are good for the better implement of the method, making use of the method, extending the effect of the method to varying degrees and achieving the goal of the method. Therefore, advanced extent of instrument and equipment stands for technological development of modern society and is the important factor to promote production and development and progress of all walks of life.

There are many kinds of equipment with various uses. Medical apparatus and instruments can be uniquely or combined used for human body to obtain certain therapeutic effect or support therapeutic efficacy, including instruments, equipment, apparatus, materials or other goods. At present, medical equipment [1] is divided into diagnostic equipment, therapeutic equipment and auxiliary equipment in medical industry. There

W. Zhao, *Rehabilitation Therapeutics of the Neurological Training*,
https://doi.org/10.1007/978-981-13-0812-3_19

are many subtypes in each class. According to the effect of the equipment, rehabilitation training equipment belongs to therapeutic equipment.

Except for the similarity, rehabilitation training equipment can make full use of training method and show the therapeutic effect. It can make the people who receive the training know the training mechanism, relieve labour intensity of the therapists and decrease treatment cost to enhance training effect.

Therefore, the definition of rehabilitation training equipment is summarized as follows: rehabilitation training equipment can make full use of training method, show the therapeutic effect and extend the effect of the method to varying degrees. It is special instrument that can complete the job or mission that human cannot finish including machine, device and instrument for long-term use. It can relieve labour intensity of the therapists and decrease treatment cost to enhance training effect. It can be used repeatedly and the original form and material can be maintained in use.

19.1.2 Development Mechanism of Corollary Equipment of Rehabilitation Training of Neurological Training

Just as mentioned above, rehabilitation training equipment is to implement rehabilitation method better, make full use of method and increase the effect of rehabilitation training. On the basis of rehabilitation training method, the developed training equipment has actual clinical application value and can enhance effect of rehabilitation training. The equipment must originate from method.

In that way, what is the root of method? Method must originate from theory.

For example, we use rehabilitation training method to recover lost motor function after injury of central nervous system [2]. The major purpose is to recover lost motor function and then we should consider the rehabilitation method to achieve goal. In the method selection, we should analyze the process and mechanism of recovering motor function at first. CNS injury may lead to motor function loss of corresponding part of the body such as limbs and trunk, which demonstrates that CND dominates the body movement. The root of the problem is in CNS but not the limbs or the trunk. Because there is no problem in limbs or trunk, lost motor function is the external manifestation of CNS dysfunction. Therefore, the premise of recovering lost motor function is to recover injured CNS function at first. CNS is lack of regeneration ability, but with plasticity, functional reorganization and skillful use and dependence. Only active movement of the body dominated by brain can promote plasticity and functional reorganization of brain so that the effective rehabilitation method must be active movement. Developed corollary equipment according to the method must meet the application requirements of active movement rehabilitation training method. Therefore, active movement is the method to recover lost motor function. The mechanism and theoretic basis are plasticity and functional reorganization of CNS. The normal method and six-step Daoyin technique of guiding collaterals through meridians used in neurological training are the training methods of active movement that the therapists encourage the patients to do according to these mechanisms.

The author found that methodology promotes CNS plasticity, which is not equal to functional reorganization of CNS. On one hand, it is unclear that how active movement training is used for the disabled without motor function, how to make full use of and enhance the effect of active movement and what is the major effect of active movement. On the other hand, is the motor function recovered by potential development, replacement of injured cells by normal cells around injured area, or reserved conduction pathway is activated? Practice demonstrates that the answer is no. one joint motion should require several muscles and associated movement of many joints requires more muscles. These muscles are dominated by many CNS cells and conduction pathways. Through coordinated and orderly work, these cells can promote or achieve functional reorganization. The process of coordinated and orderly work includes motor program proved in animal experiment and its external manifestation, motor pattern. The method of promoting cerebral functional reorganization must reestablish motor program and remodel motor pattern to recover motor function.

Rehabilitation method of neurological training is that on the basis of regulation of mind and breathing, the patients are guided to complete active joint motion and neurological training device is used to receive the motor program signal real-timely and display is in a curve form. Through the biofeedback mechanism [3] of practicing archery towards target, on the basis of rectifying disordered motor program, normal motor program is reestablished. On the basis of reestablishing motor program, the therapists can adopt the training method that can restrain unnecessary joint motion in body movement effectively and gradually remodel normal motor pattern to realize cerebral functional reorganization and recover lost motor function.

Therefore, neurological training is the method to realize the theory of CNS functional reorganization, display the effect of Daoyin technique real-timely and do reestablishment training of motor program. Neurological training device is the corollary equipment to fully implement this method and make full use of it.

In short, effective rehabilitation training equipment must originate from method so that the rehabilitation method can be implemented well to give full play to the effect of method. Rehabilitation method must originate from theory and the method is the practice of theory. All the methods must meet the requirements of theory so that they become effective methods.

At present, in the research of rehabilitation method and equipment at home and abroad, there is no mechanism of developing method according to theory and developing equipment according to method. Especially in the equipment research, there is no some kind of rehabilitation method and it is not based on some rehabilitation theory or the theory has some defects so that there is blindness in the beginning of the research. The defect is obvious in the automation, complication and expensiveness of the equipment.

Rehabilitation equipment of neurological training is made according to the mechanism that equipment must originate from method. All the equipment are developed according to the actual requirements of rehabilitation method. After clinical application for more than 10 years. We obtained satisfying effects and develop the idea of realizing rehabilitation training equipment. In order to highlight the characteristics of corollary equipment of rehabilitation training of neurological training according to the above law and maintain the original innovation of the inventor, we registered the brand Wenru (Fig. 19.1). The purpose is that we hope the brand can stand for the sign of rehabilitation technique of neurological training, symbol of rehabilitation technique innovation, promise of social honesty, guarantee of technique and product quality and the brand recognized by public. Meanwhile, it stands for the

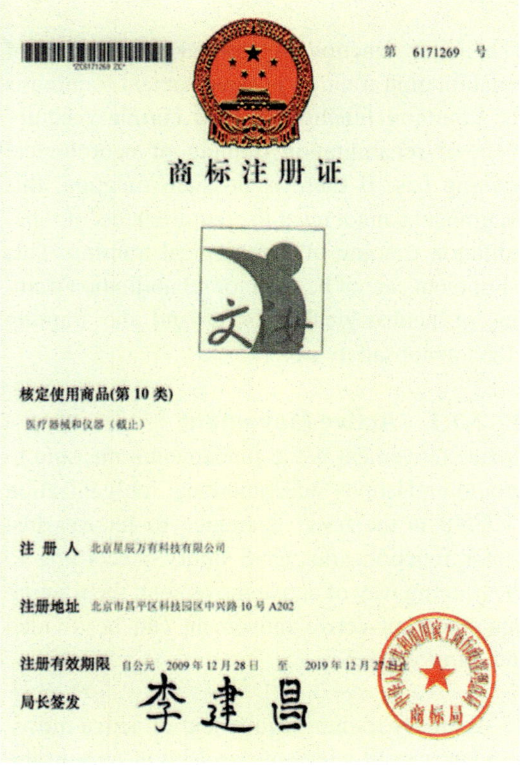
第 6171269 号

商标注册证

核定使用商品(第 10 类)

医疗器械和仪器(截止)

注 册 人 北京星辰万有科技有限公司

注册地址 北京市昌平区科技园区中兴路 10 号 A202

注册有效期限 自公元 2009 年 12 月 28 日 至 2019 年 12 月 27 日止

局长签发 李建昌

中华人民共和国国家工商行政管理总局 商标局

Fig. 19.1 Registered Wenru brand

expectation of renaissance of rehabilitation technique in traditional Chinese medicine and footstone of serving as a modest spur to induce someone to come forward with his valuable contributions.

19.2 The Major Function and Classification of Corollary Equipment of Neurological Training

The basic method of rehabilitation of neurological training is six-step Daoyin technique. The basic method of Daoyin technique is the entire active movement of regulation of movement on the basis of regulation of mind and breathing. Therefore, rehabilitation equipment of neurological training developed according to the method must meet the requirements of all active movement training.

19.2.1 Major Function

The major function of corollary equipment of rehabilitation training of neurological training is the common function that all corollary equipment of rehabilitation training of neurological training has. If there is no such function, this equipment cannot meet the requirements of rehabilitation training of neurological training. This equipment cannot be used for rehabilitation training of neurological training and the training effect is not satisfying.

19.2.1.1 Active Movement

Active movement is the fundamental measure to promote plasticity and functional reorganization of CNS is the basic guarantee to recover lost motor function after CNS injury. According to the training way of active movement, the training equipment of active movement can be divided into three classes.

1. Auxiliary training equipment of active movement can provide safe protection to help the patients to keep some kind of gesture and lose weight so that the patients can complete the training that they cannot finish or are difficult to finish.

This kind of equipment provides essential condition to help the therapists to use normal or six-step Daoyin technique of guiding collaterals through meridians to develop CNS potential through active movement training in the safe imminent danger state created by posture change and speech.

2. Goal training equipment of active movement: the surpassing goal of the patients in the process of neurological training is set in the system of the equipment and the rehabilitation training can be used to develop neural potential [4], reestablish motor program, remodel motor pattern and recover lost motor function with the goal and motive mechanism and Daoyin technique. However, this goal requires the therapists to set through the computer system of the equipment or select virtual goal stored in the equipment. Anti-resistance requires the therapists to exert in the orientation of joint motion.

This kind of equipment usually is equipped with neurological training device (receiving equipment of bio-electricity signal) to receive motor program signal real-timely and display it on the fluorescent screen. The setting digital surpassing goal is showed in a transverse line. The transverse line of agonistic muscle is green and that of antagonistic muscle is pink. During the training process, the therapists use six-step Daoyin technique repeatedly to guide the patients to do anti-resistance training to varying degrees to make signal intensity of agonistic muscle surpass the green transverse line and signal intensity of antagonistic muscle lower than pink transverse line in order to make motor program gradually return to the normal. On the basis of that, motor program of associated movement that multiple joints are involved in are reestablished and lost motor functions are recovered to varying degrees.

3. Automatic equipment of active movement can provide surpassing goal, anti-resistance,

speech guideline of Daoyin technique and instruction of main and collateral channels according to training program automatically after the training is activated so that the patients can be guided to do rehabilitation training to develop neural potential, reestablish motor program, remodel motor pattern and recover lost motor function through goal and motive mechanism.

Automatic equipment of rehabilitation training of neurological training of active movement realizes the function of man-machine conversation so that people can do one-to-one training with the machine. The method of rehabilitation training of neurological training is basically implemented. Therefore, it is possessed with the basic elements of the robot of rehabilitation training, which is called robot equipment of rehabilitation training of neurological training.

19.2.1.2 Weight Support and Protection

Weight support and protection is the premise and basic condition of implementation of rehabilitation method of neurological training, is the guarantee of safe training, is the important channel to alleviate or eliminate the fear or anxiety of the patients, and is the effective method for successful implement of the training that cannot be completed in normal condition.

The purpose of weight support is to lose the weight of the patients according to their actual condition through the weight support system of the equipment in order to reduce the bear load of the lower limbs or the trunk so that the patients can stand, support or walk from the condition that they cannot stand, support or walk. Therefore, the training can be implemented successfully. For example, the patients with paralysis of two lower limbs who cannot stand, cannot do potential development training of lower limbs under normal circumstances. However, through weight support system of potential development training of lower limbs, the patients use hanging belt of thorax and hip to bear the partial body weight of the patients so that the patients are kept in standing position. The therapists are guided and helped to do potential development training of lower limbs to promote plasticity and functional reorganization of cortex motor center [5] that dominates lower limbs.

Through weight support system of the equipment, the therapists use hanging belt of thorax and hip to exert upward traction force to the body of the patients. In the process of weight support, the equipment can prevent falling off or bumping of the patients effectively and avoid training accident so that the training can be safe and reliable. It can alleviate or eliminate the fear or anxiety of the patients, which is good for training effect.

19.2.1.3 Avoiding Unnecessary Joint Motion in Limbs Movements Effectively

Single joint movement is the basis of limbs movements. There is no functional movement with actual significance. Limbs movements with multiple joints and actual significance are the basis of motor pattern of limbs. Abnormal single joint movement is the important cause of abnormal motor pattern of limbs. Therefore, avoiding unnecessary joint motion in limbs movements effectively is the important link of remodeling motor pattern.

In all the equipment of rehabilitation training of neurological training, abnormal joint motion should be prevented in the potential development training, motor program reestablishment and motor pattern remodeling. In the training of abnormal gait rectification weight support device, weight support stride and gait shifting of weight device, weight support walking balance device or motor pattern remodeling [6] device, abnormal joint motion should be rectified and prevented.

19.2.1.4 Daoyin Technique Speech Guide and Setting Surpassing Goal

Six-step Daoyin technique in traditional Chinese medicine is used. In order to realizing standard application of Daoyin technique, give full play to therapeutic effect and alleviate labour intensity of the therapists, we recorded tape of Daoyin technique, put it into the training items of equipment software and play it automatically according to training program. Through operational system of equipment, according to the specific condition of the patients, we can set different therapeutic items, and establish surpassing goal such as archery to the target and high jump with cross bar to guide the patients to do the training with purpose and increase training effect.

19.2.1.5 Automatic Tracking of Main and Collateral Channels and Animation Spot Display

The basic method of rehabilitation training of neurological training is six-step Daoyin technique, especially guiding collaterals through meridians in six-step Daoyin technique according to main and collateral channels. Therefore, whether rehabilitation training device of neurological training is set up independently or is the part of the equipment, automatic tracking of main and collateral channels and animation spot display are used to keep Qi in the correct main and collateral channels.

One of the key techniques of guiding collaterals through meridians and guiding meridians through collaterals is to keep Qi guided in six-step Daoyin technique in correct main and collateral channels. Whether the therapists or the patients, doctors or the patients' family, they know little about correct main and collateral channels. Correct main and collateral channels are the basis of implementing the methods of guiding collaterals through meridians. Animation spot blink technique is used in virtual body. The speed of spot follows the speed of automatic guide speech of Daoyin technique. Animation blink technique is used to mark the Qi in main and collateral channels and its pathway. The patients guide Qi around their body according to the instruction of the spot to clear and activate the channels and collaterals.

19.2.2 The Classification of Rehabilitation Corollary Equipment of Neurological Training

Neurological training is composed of training methods that aim at different diseases or symptoms. Therefore, there are many kinds of corollary equipment. They can be divided according to the way of active movement, the source of feedback signal, major function and mechanical degree.

19.2.2.1 The Way of Active Movement

It can be divided into three classes such as auxiliary active movement, goal active movement and autonomous active movement. There are several subtypes in each class.

1. Auxiliary active movement training equipment are training device of neurological training. The main equipment are as follows:
   (a) Training equipment of potential development include potential development training device of upper limbs, lower limbs, trunk, tibialis anterior muscle and hamstring muscles.
   (b) Training equipment of gait and shifting of body weight include stride and gait shifting of body weight training device, abnormal gait rectification weight support training device, motor pattern remodeling training device, weight support walking training device and gait training footpath.
   (c) Training equipment of balance include weight support balance training device, air or water bag standing balance training device and walking balance training device.
   (d) Induction equipment of active movement include induction training device of rolling active movement, induction training device of weight support crawling autonomic movement, active standing training bed, induction training device of autonomic movement of lower limbs and upper limbs.
2. Goal active movement training equipment are neurological training device that can provide motor program signal, pressure signal or analogue signal to do surpassing goal training through biofeedback mechanism.
   (a) Potential development equipment include potential development training device of upper limbs, potential development training device of lower limbs, potential development training device, potential

development training device of tibialis anterior muscle, potential development training device of hamstring muscles, Daoyin device of myodynamia, Daoyin device of balance potential and Daoyin device of sphincter.

(b) Motor program reestablishment equipment include neurological training device and Daoyin device of muscle tension.

(c) Motor pattern remodeling equipment include neurological training device of motor pattern remodeling, neurological training device of stride gait shifting of body weight and neurological training device of weight support walking, neurological training device of animation gait training footpath, neurological training device of abnormal gait rectification weight support walking and neurological training device of weight support walking.

(d) Comprehensive type includes virtual reality training device of neurological training indicating instrument of guiding collaterals through meridians.

3. Autonomous active movement training equipment are robot equipment of rehabilitation training of neurological training. The equipment can provide feedback signal and surpassing goal. It is equipped with automatic speech guide of six-step Daoyin technique, speech guide of main and collateral channels, and automatic tracking indication system of animation spot. It can do anti-resistance training.

It is divided into several types according to the training part. Rehabilitation training robot of neurological training of shoulder and elbow is suitable for the neural potential development and motor program reestablishment of central nervous system that dominate shoulder and elbow movement to recover autonomic movement, enhance myodynamia and prevent adhesion of soft tissue and joint [7], muscle atrophy and tendon contracture. Rehabilitation training robot of neurological training of wrist and hand is suitable for the neural potential development and motor program reestablishment of central nervous system that dominate wrist and hand joint to recover autonomic movement, enhance myodynamia and prevent adhesion of soft tissue and joint, muscle atrophy and tendon contracture. Rehabilitation training robot of neurological training of head and neck is suitable for the neural potential development and motor program reestablishment of central nervous system that dominates head and neck movement to recover autonomic movement, enhance myodynamia and prevent adhesion of cervical tissue. Rehabilitation training robot of neurological training of lumbosacral spinal cord is suitable for the neural potential training of central nervous system that dominates lumbosacral movement to recover autonomic movement, enhance myodynamia, alleviate and prevent adhesion and pain of lumbosacral tissue Rehabilitation training robot of neurological training of hip and knee is suitable for the neural potential development, motor program reestablishment and motor pattern remodeling of central nervous system that dominate hip and knee joint to recover autonomic movement [8], enhance myodynamia and prevent adhesion of hip joint, knee joint and peripheral tissue. Rehabilitation training robot of neurological training of foot and ankle is suitable for the neural potential training of central nervous system that dominates ankle joint to recover autonomic movement, enhance myodynamia, alleviate and prevent adhesion of ankle joint and peripheral tissue and tendon contracture.

19.2.2.2 The Source of Feedback Signal

It is the source of feedback signal provided by the equipment and can reflect the effect of Daoyin technique. It includes motor program signal, anti-resistance signal and analogue signal guided in real-time.

1. Motor program signal equipment: When Daoyin technique is used to induce autonomous joint motion, the reception equipment of bio-electricity signal can receive the signal intensity and proportion of agonistic muscle or antagonistic muscle involved in joint

motion form CNS and display it in a curve form. The surpassing goal is set on the basis of the intensity of motor program signal. Through biofeedback and goal-motive mechanism, the patients are guided to surpass the goal, develop neural potential and reestablish motor program.
2. Resistance signal equipment: The objective indicator is the strength of resistance. When Daoyin technique is used to induce autonomous joint motion and exert anti-resistance to develop neural potential, the signal source is the strength of resistance and the signal is displayed in a curve form real-timely. The resistance in the previous training is the surpassing goal of the next training. Through biofeedback and goal-motive mechanism, the patients are guided to surpass the goal.
3. Analogue signal equipment: virtual reality training system of the equipment provides analogue motor program signal, surpassing goal and the patients are immersed into virtual environment through immersed technique. Six-step Daoyin technique is used to guide the patients to surpass goal.

19.2.2.3 Major Function

According to training goal and major function of the equipment, the equipment includes the equipment of neural potential development, motor program reestablishment and motor pattern remodeling.

1. Potential development equipment this kind of equipment is named with the body part such as potential development training device or neurological training device of upper limbs, lower limbs, the trunk, tibialis anterior muscle and hamstring muscles.
2. Motor program reestablishment equipment this kind of equipment can receive guided motor program signal, enhance signal intensity of agonistic muscle and decrease signal intensity of antagonistic muscle in order to reestablish motor program.
3. Motor pattern remodeling equipment: on the basis of reestablishing motor program of single joint movement, motor program of associated movement that multiple joints are involved is reestablished such as motor program reestablishment of balance, gait and motor pattern, and training device and neurological device of function transformation.

19.2.2.4 Mechanical Degree

This classification method is simple, intuitional, clear easy to memorize and understand. There are four classes.

1. Training appliance: In order to keep the therapeutic effect of the patients in hospital and at home and improve functions, the training appliance is designed for self-exercise. It is portable, inexpensive, and simple. It is in accordance with the theory and physiological mechanism of active movement and the therapeutic effect is good.
2. Training device belongs to mechanical device without electric appliance and software. The functions include weight support and safe protection. This kind of equipment can be used to do active movement, auxiliary active movement and compulsory active movement.
3. Training instrument is equipped with reception system of bio-electricity signal or muscle tension signal. It can use digital subjective indicator to display the effect of Daoyin technique and provide surpassing goal for the patients. Through biofeedback and goal-motive mechanism, the patients are guided to do the training of neural potential development, motor program reestablishment, stride gait shifting of body weight, gait balance and motor pattern remodeling.
4. Training robot is equipped with the function of man-machine conversation. In this robot, there are many training items for selection, automatic speech guide of Daoyin technique, automatic tracking and display of animation spot of main and collateral channels and anti-resistance function with different strength. The results of comprehensive effects are that this robot can realize or approach the actual operation level of the therapists.

Particularly, all corollary equipment rehabilitation training of neurological training is developed to cooperate with six-step Daoyin technique including normal method and the method of guiding collaterals through meridians. It is a method to implement Daoyin technique and give play to Daoyin technique in order to increase the effect of corollary equipment. Equipment play a supporting role and Daoyin technique is the major therapeutic method. Formulation of rehabilitation goal and establishment of rehabilitation principle are strategic measures to implement rehabilitation of neurological training. Specific rehabilitation method is that various kinds of methods are used properly to obtain the best therapeutic effect. Daoyin technique can clear and activate the channels and collaterals, and develop cerebral potential. Equipment can guarantee the implementation of the method to increase the effect of Daoyin technique, develop cerebral potential and recover lost motor function. However, if we use equipment alone or emphasize on the equipment excessively and don't formulate strategies and tactics of neurological training, the method cannot be used correctly and the anticipated training effect cannot be achieved.

Rehabilitation training of the disabled is like a battle. Advanced weapons are not the key of victory. The prerequisite of victory is correct application of strategies and tactics. Advanced weapons are the instruments to keep the implementation of strategies and tactics.

19.3 Introduction of Partial Corollary Equipment of Rehabilitation of Neurological Training

19.3.1 Training Appliance

Pulmonary function exercise device.
The detailed content refers to Chap. 14.2.
Multifunctional training box of limbs.

19.3.1.1 Design Principle and Essential Structure

1. Design principle: Neurological training is composed of Daoyin technique, active movement and anti-resistance. A series of self-training band is developed. Under the instruction of speech guidance of Daoyin technique, in active joint motion, elastic recoil of elastic band is used unlimitedly. One end of elastic band is fixed on the limbs or some objects such as table leg and trunk and the other end is fixed on the limbs of movable joint so that the therapists can exert resistance in joint motion. Moreover, the strength of resistance is increased with the increase of joint motion angle. Therefore, Daoyin technique can be used to induce anti-resistance training of active movement, which is good for the development and utilization of central neural potential. The results of comprehensive effects are that it can clear and activate the channels and collaterals, develop cerebral potential and recover lost motor function.
2. Essential structure: Multifunctional training box of limbs is composed of elastic training bands that are suitable for active movement of all joints. Training band is black or brown elastic band with 6 or 11 cm in width. Elastic tensile elongation is 2.4 times. The elastic is monolayer except for double layer elastic band of hip abduction. The band is cut into elastic strips with 15 cm in length. The two ends are sewed with black canvas with the same width. The two ends of canvas are fixed with son thread of nylon and mother gluing thread.

   Manufacture of training appliance for special part: for the proximal and distal ends of the training joint that cannot be fixed or is difficult to be fixed, the part of fixing training band such as hip adduction, foot dorsiflexion, strephexopodia and wrist extension, should be fixed on the contralateral limbs for fixing point of training band. Elastic training cushion is made or elastic band is fixed on the training board for anti-resistance of active movement.

   (a) Training cushion of hip adduction: the therapists select cardboard sponge with 11 cm in depth and cut it into trapezoid (the top edge is 10 cm, the bottom edge is 22 cm and the height is 18 cm) with two arch sides. The shape is suitable for the thigh. The outside is wrapped with corduroy soft cloth.

(b) Training board of wrist and hand: The therapists choose wood board (30 cm × 15 cm × 1 cm). The front is like palm. After polishing, five rubber bands are fixed on the front edge. Training elastic band of wrist flexion and extension is fixed on the metacarpophalangeal joints part of training board. Fixing band of forearm is fixed on the wrist joint of training board. It can be used for the training of wrist extension, wrist flexion, finger flexion and finger extension.

(c) Training board of foot dorsiflexion and strephexopodia: the therapists choose wood board (30 cm × 25 cm × 1 cm) and dig a herringbone groove in the middle of the front. The therapists cut two sides and make it like shoe sole. Elastic bands are fixed on the groove and two sides 8 cm away from the front after polishing. It is suitable for the anti-resistance training of active movement of foot dorsiflexion and strephexopodia. During the training of left foot, the patients use right foot to step on the training board for foot dorsiflexion and strephexopodia, vice versa.

The training bands of shoulder abduction, elbow extension and flexion, hip adduction, knee extension and flexion, and foot plantar flexion and training board of special part are sealed in box (Figs. 19.2, 19.3, 19.4, 19.5, 19.6, 19.7, 19.8, 19.9, 19.10, 19.11, 19.12, 19.13, 19.14, and 19.15). There are video of application method and dub disk of Daoyin technique.

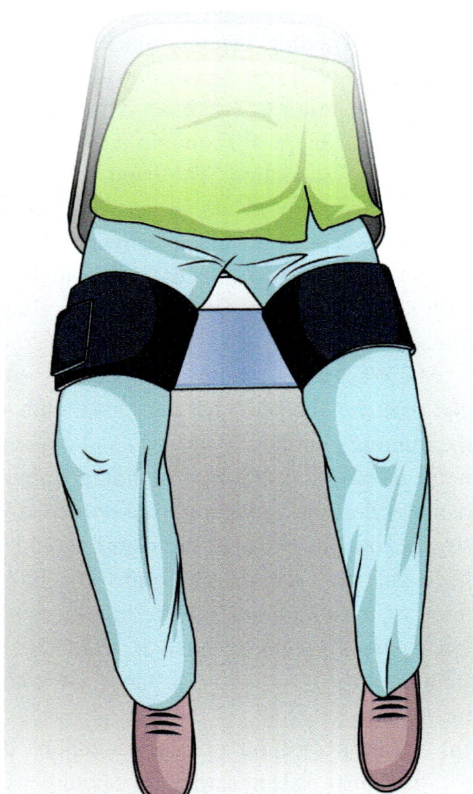

Fig. 19.2 Training band of hip abduction

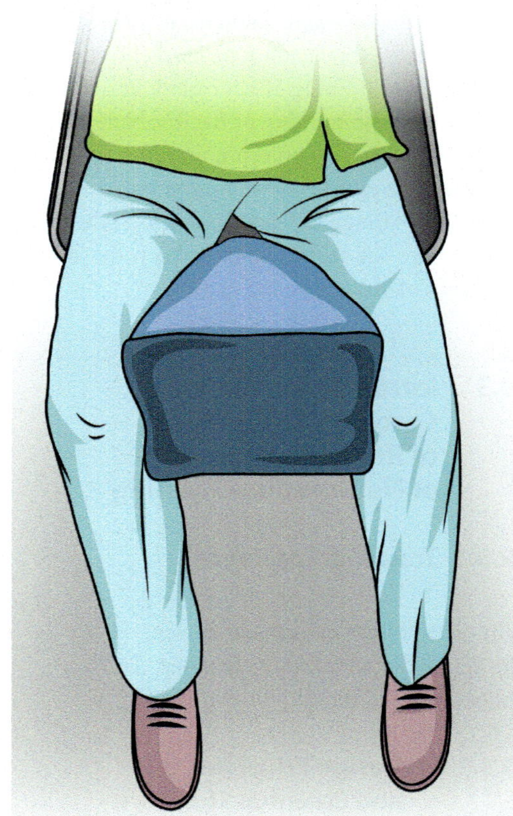

Fig. 19.3 Training cushion of hi adduction

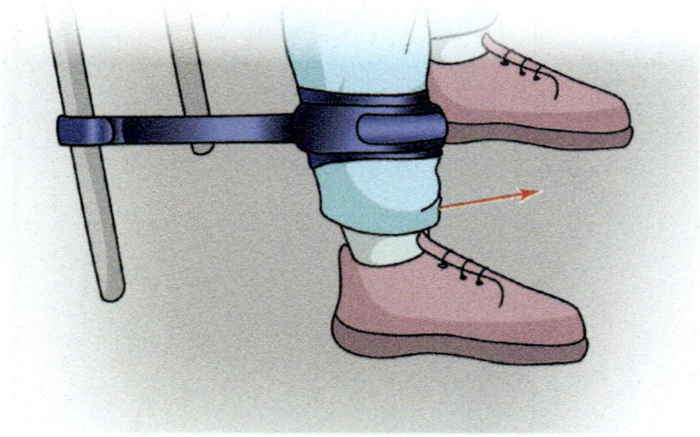

Fig. 19.4 Training band of knee extension

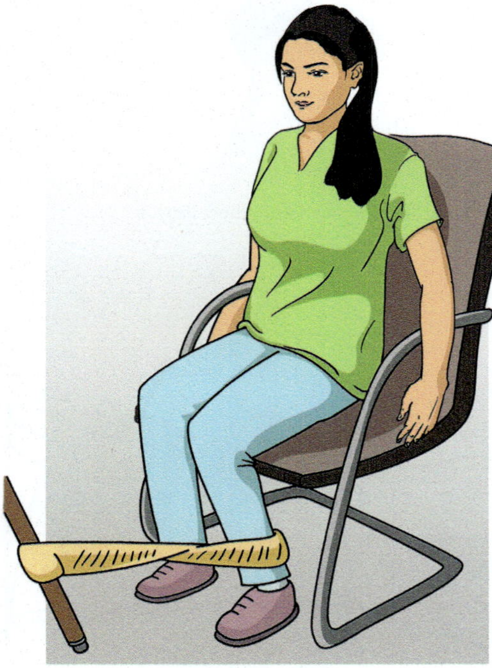

Fig. 19.5 Training band of knee flexion

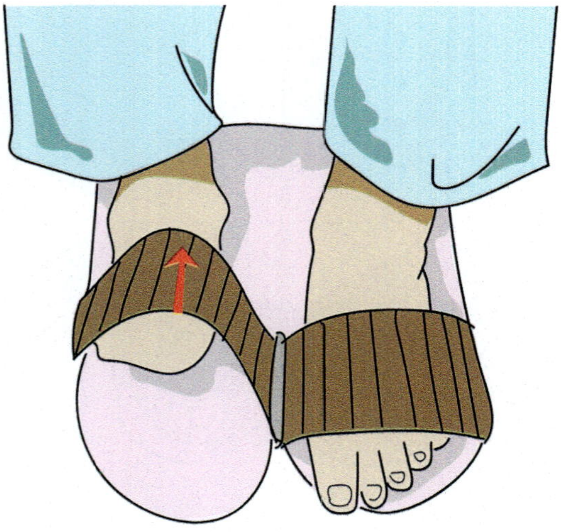

Fig. 19.6 Training band of foot dorsiflexion

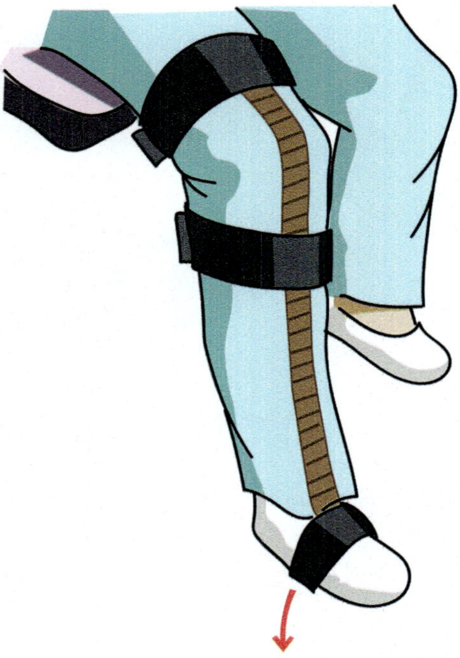

Fig. 19.7 Training band of foot plantar flexion

19.3.1.2 Application Method

The patients can do self-training according to the video of application method.

According to the training part, the patients choose corresponding training band, wear it and fix it. The training procedures are as follows:

1. Regulation of mind: The patients relax body and mind, meditate and concentrate on the contralateral brain. During the training of right limbs, the patients concentrate on left hemisphere, vice versa.
2. Regulation of breathing: The patients sit up, lift the chest, regulate breathing and make the body and mind in ready state.
3. Regulation of movement: The patients should confirm the goal point at first. For example, during the neurological training of foot dorsiflexion, the patients' goal point is tibialis anterior muscle. On the basis of regulation of

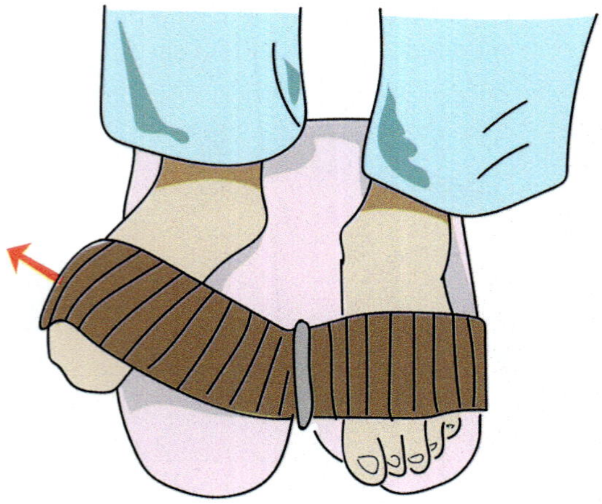

Fig. 19.8 Training band of strephexopodia

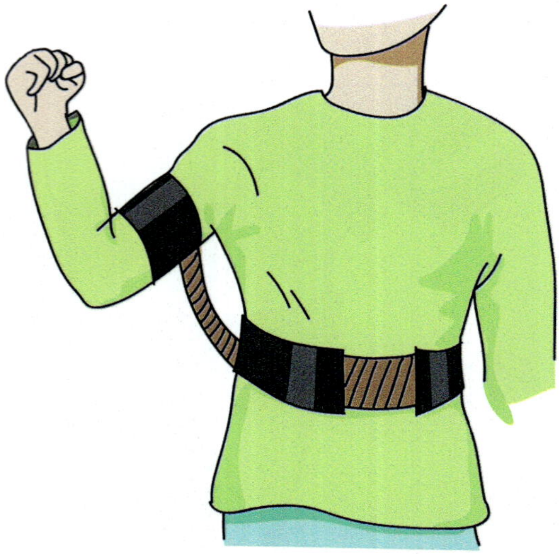

Fig. 19.9 Training band of shoulder abduction

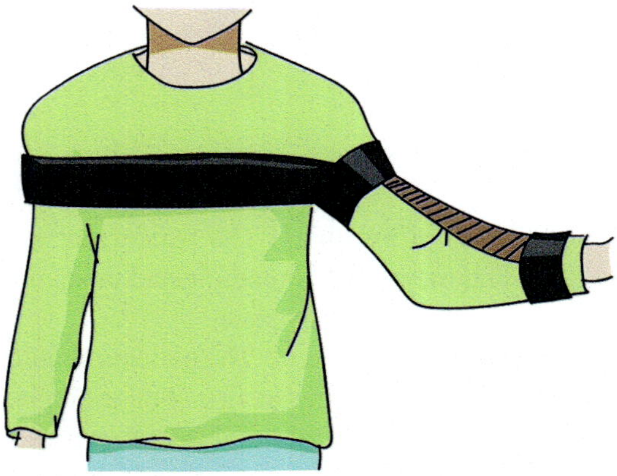

Fig. 19.10 Training band of elbow extension

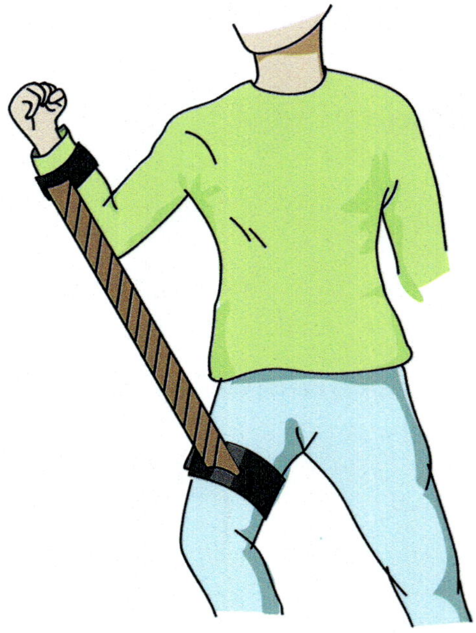

Fig. 19.11 Training band of elbow flexion

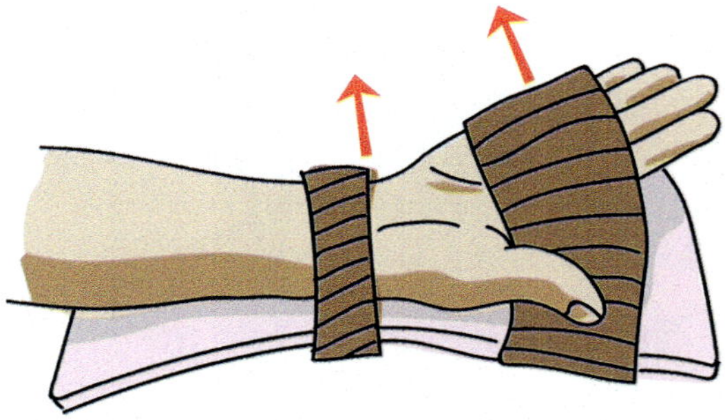

Fig. 19.12 Training band of wrist extension

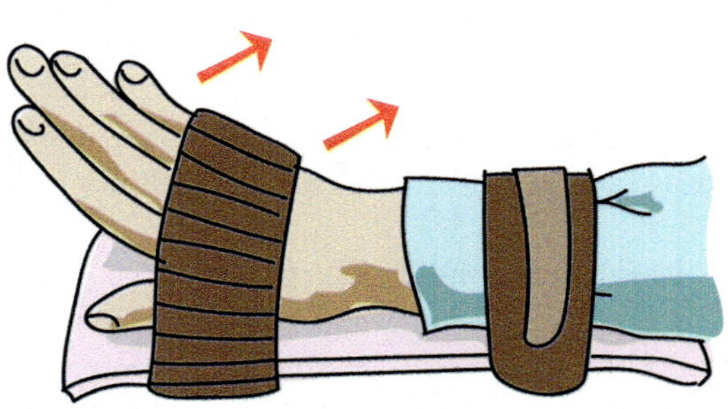

Fig. 19.13 Training band of wrist flexion

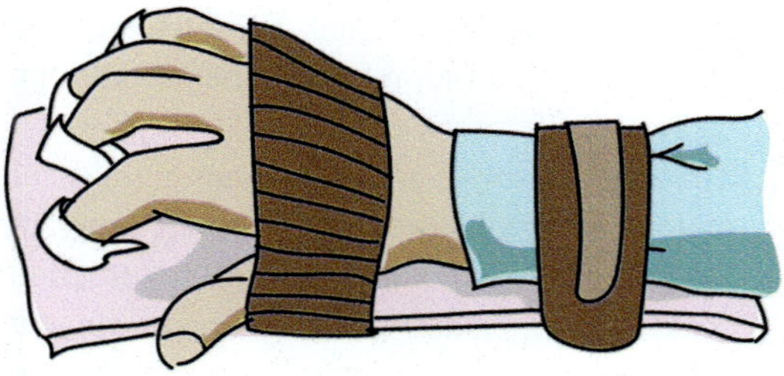

Fig. 19.14 Training band of finger extension

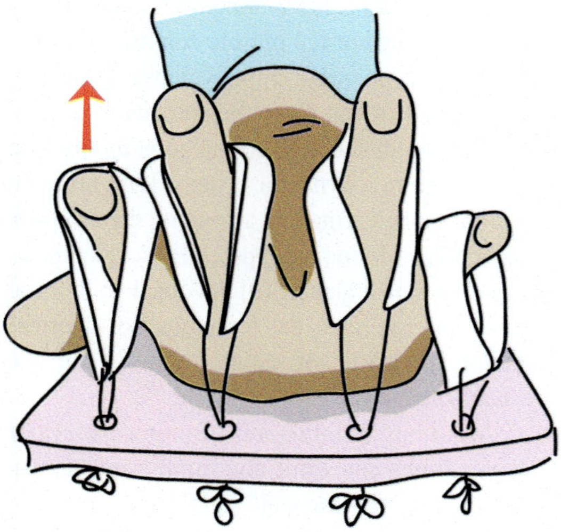

Fig. 19.15 Training band of finger flexion

mind and breathing, the patients use trigger way to shrink tibialis anterior muscle suddenly and increase the angle of foot dorsiflexion to the summit for 6 s. After that, the patients take a deep breathing and expire slowly. They try to relax body and mind to alleviate fatigue. After a break, they start the next training. The training of the same part can be done for 6–8 times. If there is difficulty with the training, the patients can do the training with the help of physical therapists, family or caregiver. The training time is 30 min (1–2 times a day) and they should persist in it.

19.3.1.3 Clinical Indications, Contraindications and Announcements

1. Indications include CNS injury, peripheral nerve injury, bone and joint inflammatory disease.
   (a) Limbs motor dysfunction induced by CNS injuries such as hemiplegia due to cerebral hemorrhage, cerebral infarction, cerebral embolism and subarachnoid hemorrhage, cerebral trauma, acroparalysis after brain surgery, incomplete hemiplegia after spinal cord injury and child cerebral palsy
   (b) Muscle paralysis induced by peripheral nerve injury such as brachial plexus injury and cauda equine injury
   (c) Bone and joint inflammatory diseases such as scapulohumeral periarthritis and pain in waist and lower extremities
2. Contraindications: There is no obvious contraindications. For the people with bone fracture, articular ligament injury, tendon injury and muscle injury, they can do the training with the permission of the doctors.
3. Announcements
   (a) Training environment: The training should be done in a warm and quiet room and the patients should concentrate on the training.
   (b) Training amount: There should be internals in the training and the training frequency shouldn't be too high. The limit is that the patients sweat slightly and breathe smoothly or the training can be done according to the video and tape.
   (c) Set goal point: During training, the patients should concentrate on the agonistic muscle of movable joint, feel slight hotness of muscle contraction and relax antagonistic muscle.
   (d) The patients should persist in the training.

19.3.1.4 Moulding Training Aids of Limbs Motor Pattern

Abnormal motor pattern is the common motor dysfunction after CNS injury and is difficult to be treated in clinic. At present, rehabilitation method widely used at home and abroad cannot effectively restrict unnecessary joint motion in limbs movements, which affect the training effect of rectifying abnormal motor pattern.

The author developed motor pattern moulding training aids of upper and lower limbs to transform previous training results such as neural potential development and motor program reestablishment into motor ability required for daily life through restricting unnecessary joint motion in limbs movements effectively and Daoyin technique that can clear and activate the channels and collaterals, and develop brain potential. Therefore, it can improve motor function of limbs, decrease energy consumption and prevent joint deformity.

Moulding training aids of motor pattern are divided into upper limbs and lower limbs.

Moulding Training Aids of Motor Pattern of Lower Limbs

It is suitable for the motor pattern remodeling training on the basis of normal motor program reestablishment of lower limbs.

1. The composition of moulding training aids of motor pattern of lower limbs: Motor pattern moulding training aids of motor pattern of lower limbs are composed of waistline, joint motion limitor of hip-knee-ankle, aluminium alloy lattice framing, foot orthosis and fixing band. Joint motion limitor can limit the motion range and original angle (15° flexed position) of hip, knee and ankle joints. This limitor only allow the joint motion in the sagittal plane. The hip, knee and ankle joints are connected with double-layer aluminium alloy lattice framing. There is a groove in the center that can be slidable upward and downward. Therefore, the length can be adjustable and can be fixed with adjustable bolt for the patients with different statures. The bottom of artificial ankle joint are connected to aluminium alloy foot orthosis (the domestic type is high temperature thermoplastic board). Bilateral hip joints are fixed on the two sides of waistline made of high temperature thermoplastic board through lattice framing to support and limit adduction and abduction of lower limbs. Foot orthosis can rectify foot drop, strephenopodia and strephexopodia, and don't affect the ankle joint motion in sigittal surface.

   According to the specific condition of the patients, the therapists select corresponding type (Figs. 19.16a, b and 19.17) to restrict abnormal joint motion for that the patients can wear it comfortably.
2. The mechanism of moulding training aids of motor pattern of lower limbs: Motor program can interact with motor pattern. Motor program decides motor pattern and long-term movement with abnormal motor pattern can modify formative motor program in motor center of cortex. On the contrary, normal motor pattern under limitation can restrict abnormal joint motion induced by abnormal muscle contraction effectively and decrease myodynamia gradually. Meanwhile, it can force the patients to use the muscle associated with normal joint motion and strengthen myodynamia. After a long time, on the basis of clearing and activating the channels and collaterals and brain potential development, myodynamia balance [9] involved in normal joint motion can be reestablished. Normal motor program of joint motion can be established in cortex.

   Moulding training aids of motor pattern of lower limbs can limit abnormal joint motion of lower limbs through rigid lattice framing and one-way motion of assistive joint to keep normal motor pattern. In order to use the muscles of correct movement frequently and not to use the muscles of abnormal joint motion, normal motor pattern can be reestablished and solidified and then the patients can walk without assistance.

   The development of moulding training aids of motor pattern of lower limbs allows the patients to walk with the help of weight support and assistance. During the training of potential development [10] and motor program reestablishment in the early stage, the patients should do the training of motor pattern remodeling as soon as possible. It not only can transform developed potential and established motor program into motor function, but also can meet the requirement and desire of the patients to walk to activate the enthusiasm of the patients, increase the effect of rehabilitation training and shorten therapeutic course. In addition, moulding training aids of motor pattern of lower limbs in domes-

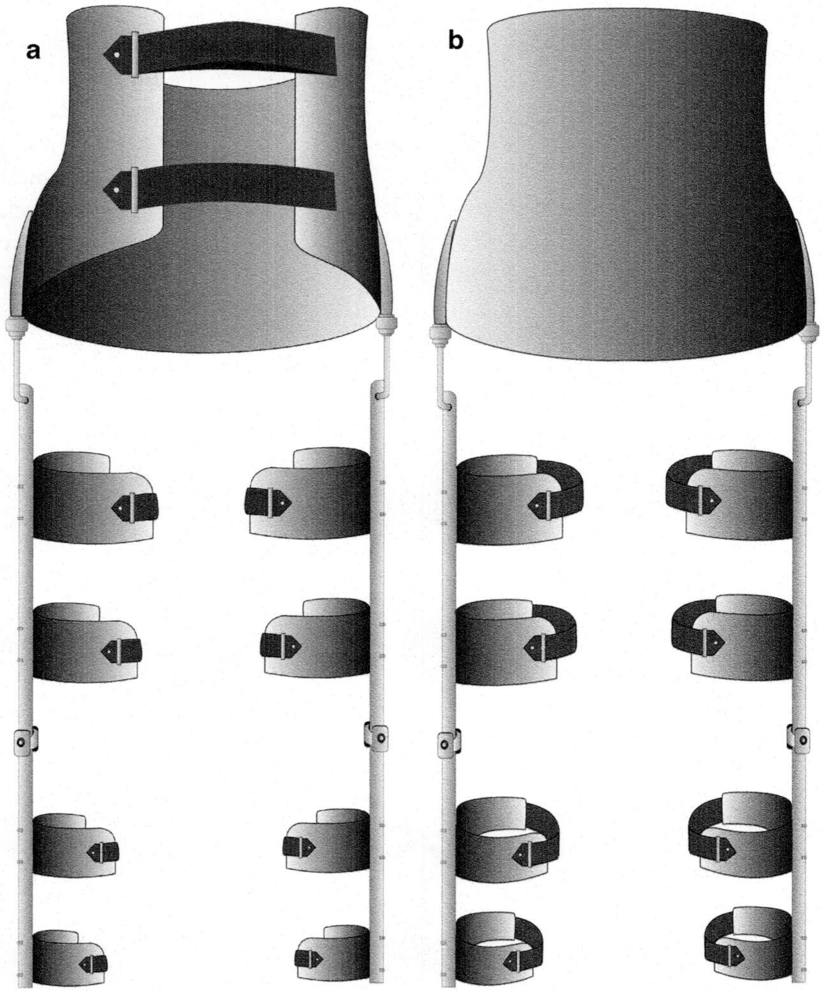

Fig. 19.16 (**a**) Moulding training aids of motor pattern of hip and knee joints (the front). (**b**) Moulding training aids of motor pattern of hip and knee joints (the back)

tic use can guarantee the correctness of self-exercise of the patients, which is good for the solidification of normal motor pattern and prevention of relapse of abnormal motor pattern.

3. The classification of moulding training aids of motor pattern of lower limbs is accordance with usage, limbs part and size.
   (a) According to usage, it includes training type and domestic type. The training type is composed of double-layer assistive aluminium alloy lattice framing with strong anti-bending capacity. There is a groove in the center that can be slidable upward and downward to adjust the length. The length can be adjusted with adjustable bolt for the patients with different statures. This type is firm and durable with heavy weight. It is difficult to wear and it is suitable for the neurological training of rehabilitation hall in the hospital. Domestic moulding training aids of motor pattern of lower limbs is a portable limited device to maintain formative motor pattern during the process of self-exercise of the patients at home who are with abnormal motor pattern due to incorrect method. It is composed of single-layer magnesium alloy. Waistline and foot orthosis are made of thin high temperature thermoplastic board. The characteristics of this type are as follows: it can restrict unnecessary movements in lower limbs movements effectively, but don't affect the joint motion in correct orienta-

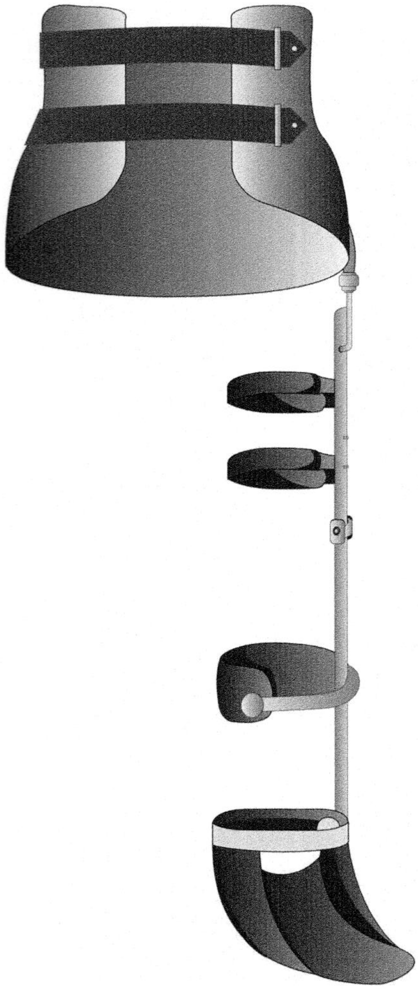

Fig. 19.17 Moulding training aids of motor pattern of hip, knee and ankle joints (the unilateral)

tion. It can rectify abnormal joint position such as foot drop, talipes varus and valgus. The weight of magnesium alloy lattice framing is small, which is one third of that of aluminium alloy lattice framing. It can be assembled or taken apart as requirements. It can be weared in trousers and is easy to wear. It can be weared for a long time, even 6–12 months. The anti-bending ability of this type of training device is poor, which is suitable for self-exercise of the patients whose normal motor pattern is established through the training of motor pattern remodeling.

(b) According to parts, it is divided into double limbs type, single limb type, double limbs of trunk type, single limb of trunk type and local type (Figs. 19.18, 19.19, 19.20, 19.21, 19.22, and 19.23).

(c) According to the size, it is divided into children type and adult type. Children type is made of magnesium alloy lattice framing and thin high temperature thermoplastic board to reduce weight and wear.

The principle and structure of various types are the same. They restrict abnormal position and movement of joint motion through joint motion limitor and lattice framing.

The difference between training type and domestic type moulding training aids of motor pattern are as follows: the training type is used in the early phase of the training for the patients who just start moulding training aids of motor pattern with severe abnormal motor pattern. Moulding training aids of motor pattern is made of double-layer aluminium alloy

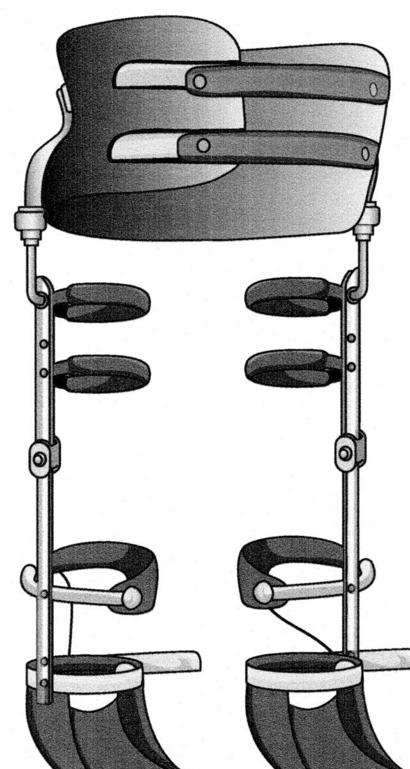

Fig. 19.18 Moulding training aids of motor pattern of bilateral waistline type

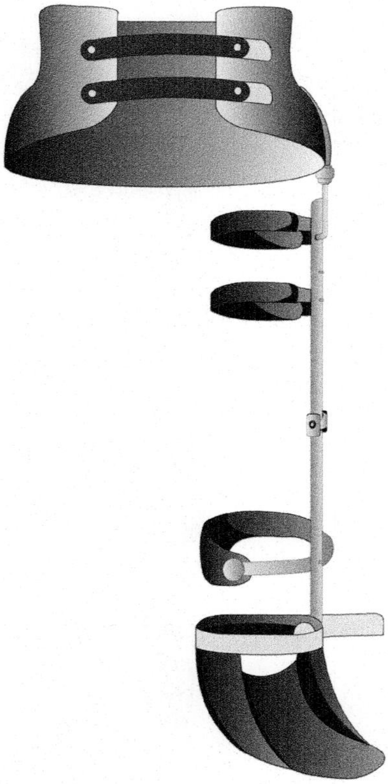

Fig. 19.19 Moulding training aids of motor pattern single limb of waistline

lattice framing that is firm and can support and limit joint motion. It can totally limit abnormal joint motion and is suitable for the training in rehabilitation hall of hospital. It can be weared outside of the clothing. Domestic type is a portable and formative limitation device of normal motor pattern suitable for the patients whose normal motor pattern is established through the training of motor pattern remodeling in order to prevent the relapse in the process of self-exercise. The anti-bending ability of magnesium alloy lattice framing is poor whose weight is one third of that of single layer aluminium alloy lattice framing. Other accessories can meet the requirements that they can restrict abnormal motion. It can be weared in trousers and is easy to wear. It can be weared for a long time, even 6–12 months.

Training method: According to the following procedures, the patients do the motor pattern remodeling training.

(a) Preparation before training: the patients wear moulding training aids of motor pattern of lower limbs and do the training in the abnormal gait rectification weight support training device and gait mark foot path. According to movement prescription, the amount of weight support is adjusted. According to the specific condition of the patients, the therapists can stand one side, the front or the back of the patients. The patients can use two hands to grasp the handrail of weight support device or can walk without grasping the handrail.
(b) The training includes assistive motor and autonomous motor walking training (Figs. 19.24 and 19.25). Assistive motor walking training: exercise therapists push weight support device forward and the patients can step forward according to the footprint on the footpath. Autonomous motor training: during the process of pushing weight support device forward by themselves, the patients practice stepping forward. Daoyin technique gait disassembly slow motion training: exercise therapists use Daoyin technique of six-step method in traditional Chinese medicine (normal method or guiding collaterals through meridians) to guide the patients to do gait disassembly training on the basis of regulation of mind and breathing. The specific procedures are as follows: the patients are guided to regulate breathing, concentrate, put the center of the body on one side, try to flex hip joint of stepping forward, bend the body forward to move foot forward, make the heel touch the ground on the footprint of the foot path and the foot on the footprint. The center of the body moves to this side and the same method is used to do the contralateral stepping disassembly training. The training of control ability of limbs: under the condition of weight support, the patients are guided to do the training of hip flexion, knee flexion and foot dorsiflexion on the spot. The

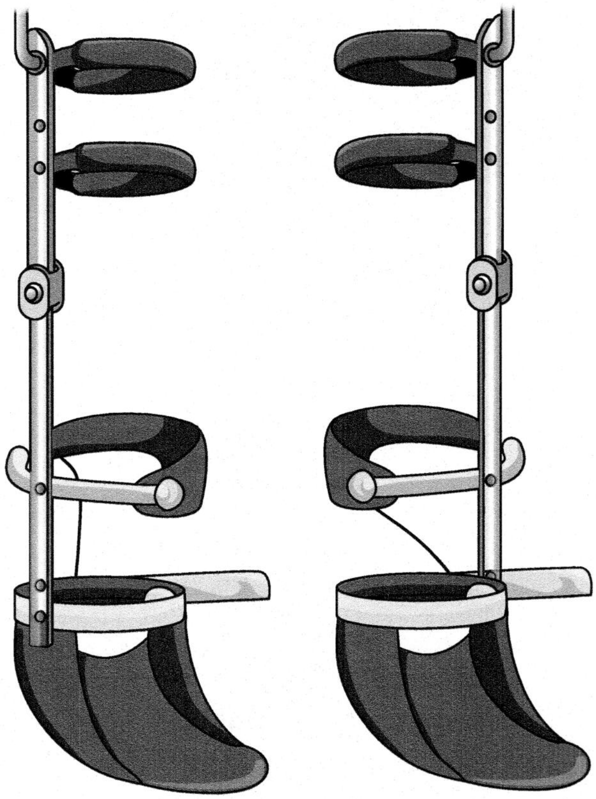

Fig. 19.20 Moulding training aids of motor pattern of double limbs

specific procedures are as follows: the patients are in standing position, move the center of the body to one side. On the basis of regulation of mind and breathing, the patients are guided to flex hip joint, dorsiflex ankle joint and put the foot in the footprint of the footpath after the heel touches the ground. The purpose of this training is to increase the flexibility, starting speed and accuracy of limbs movements. During training, the patients are asked to relax and don't exert the force excessively in case of associated reaction. They are asked to shorten the time of completing the movements. The training time is 30 min (once a day) and there are 90 times in one therapy courses.

With the increase of walking ability, limbs control ability, autonomous control ability and myodynamia of hip flexor, hip abductor tibialis anterior muscle and peroneus longus and brevis of the patients, the patients can decrease the amount of weight support and start walking independently.

Self-exercise at home: after abnormal motor pattern is rectified and normal motor pattern is established, in order to shorten the hospital stays, the patients wear domestic moulding training aids of motor pattern to do exercise after hospital for 6–12 months to maintain the therapeutic effect and normal motor pattern. After the normal motor pattern is consolidated, the exercise can be stopped.

4. Clinical indications, contraindications and announcements
   (a) Indications: It is suitable for motor pattern remodeling training of lower limbs of the patients in recovery phase of hemiplegia, cerebral palsy and paraplegia. It is also used for the abnormal motor pattern train-

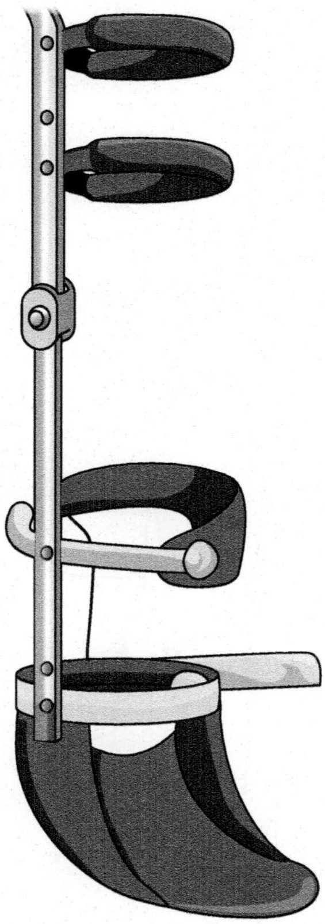

Fig. 19.21 Moulding training aids of motor pattern of single limb

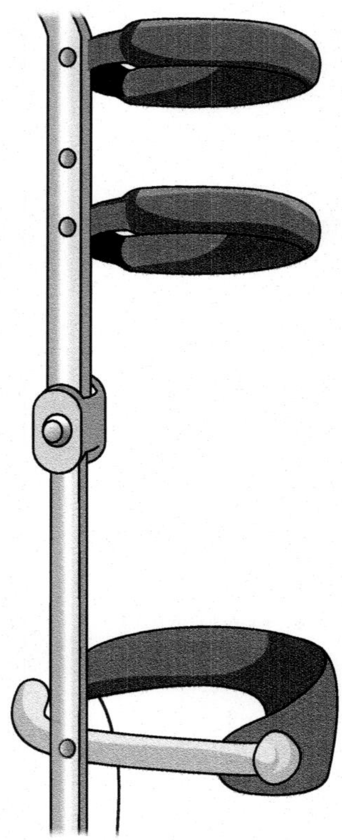

Fig. 19.22 Moulding training aids of motor pattern of simple knee joint

ing of lower limbs of the patients whose rehabilitation method training is invalid.

(b) Contraindications: If there is any one of the following contradictions, the patients should stop or use moulding training aids of motor pattern with caution. The patients with uncontrolled high blood pressure and diabetes mellitus; the patients with unstable state after stroke and cerebral trauma; the patients with unhealed bone fracture of lower limbs, joint cartilage and ligament injuries; the patients with unhealed pelvic fracture or pelvic soft tissue injury

(c) Training considerations: The training should be step by step and it is forbidden to increase training intensity without purpose. The training time should be 30 min. If there is any discomfort in the training, the training should be stopped. The therapists should find out the cause and deal with it. The therapists can control the training intensity through reducing the amount of weight support or shortening the training time. During the training, the therapists should use six-step Daoyin technique in traditional Chinese medicine correctly, activate the enthusiasm of the patients fully, activate training atmosphere, use encouraging words and avoid using scolding words.

Moulding Training Aids of Motor Pattern of Upper Limbs

Moulding training aids of motor pattern of upper limbs is used rehabilitation training device in the process of rectifying the walking to rectify the incoordination of swing movement of double

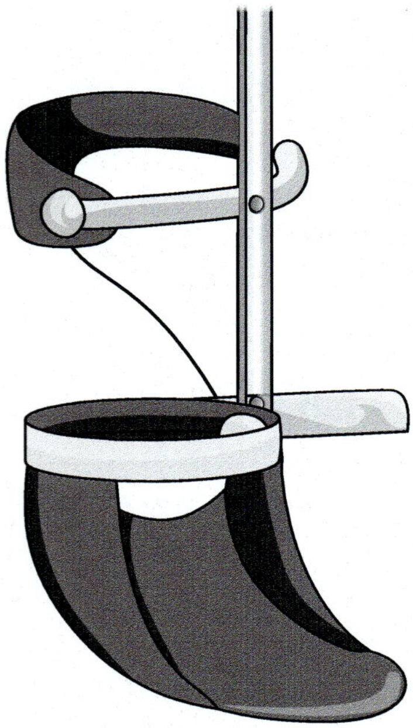

Fig. 19.23 Moulding training aids of motor pattern of simple ankle foot type

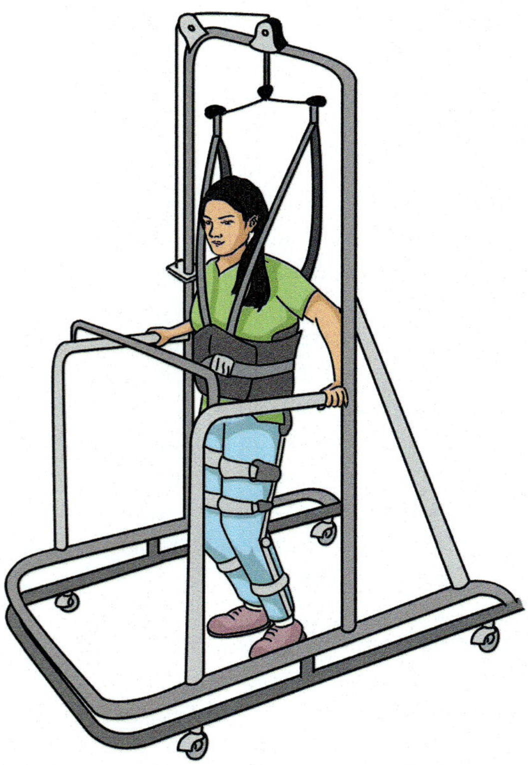

Fig. 19.24 Wear pattern shaping device under the lose weight walking training equipment for training

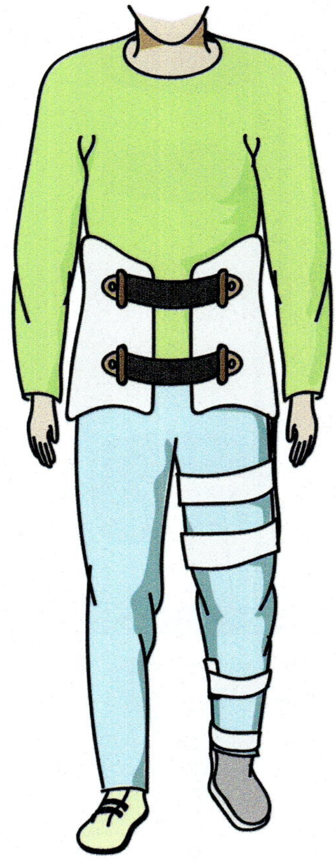

Fig. 19.25 Wear the lower limb motion mode shaping device for training

upper limbs, prevent flexion and spasm of upper limbs and remodel normal motor pattern of upper limbs.

1. Essential structure. It is composed of hand tray, should-elbow joint limiter, lattice framing, movement orientation switch gear, transmission shaft and fixing vest (Fig. 19.26).

   The role of hand tray is to rectify the deformity of hand in flexion position. Should-elbow joint limiter can keep the joint in a normal position and range. The role of lattice framing is to connect hand tray with should-elbow joint. Movement orientation switch gear can transform the movement of upper limb in healthy side into the opposite orientation movement of upper limb in injured side. Transmission shaft can conduct the power of

Fig. 19.26 Moulding training aids of motor pattern of upper limbs

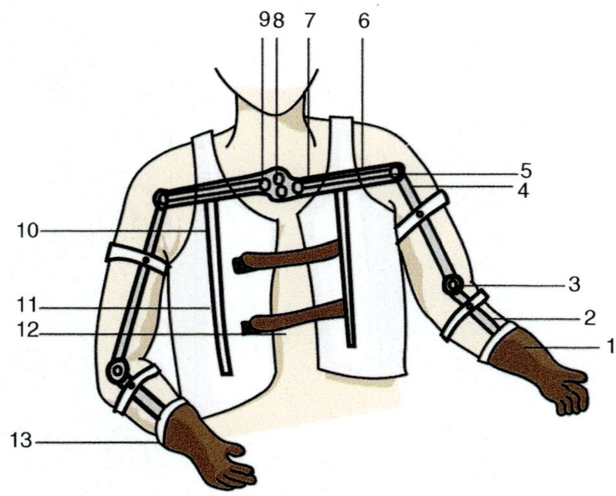

1. Wrist pad
2. Forearm support strip
3. Elbow restrictor
4. The upper arm support strip
5. Shoulder restrictor
6. Drivepipe
7. Transmission shaft
8. Shift gears
9. Drive bearing
10. Drive shaft support strip
11. Fixed vest
12. Linkbelt
13. Upper limb fixed plate

limb swing in healthy side to movement orientation switch gear. Fixing vest can fix movement orientation switch gear and transmission shaft on chest and back.

In short, the characteristics of moulding training aids of motor pattern of upper limbs are summarized as follows: the power from upper limb swing in healthy side can drive the limb in injured side to the opposite orientation. Therefore, the patients can swing double upper limbs coordinately during walking. It can restrict unnecessary movements in the joint motion effectively such as upper limbs flexion, wrist joint flexion and finger flexion in walking. It can rectify adduction of injured limbs, elbow flexion and wrist flexion. It is easy to put on and off according to the requirements. It doesn't affect the normal autonomic movement of upper limbs.

2. The mechanism of moulding training aids of motor pattern of upper limbs. When there is flexion and spasm of upper limbs [11] and walking, no-swing of injured upper limbs or uncoordinated swing of double upper limbs is the common abnormal motor pattern of upper limbs, which is usually observed in the patients with hemiplegia, cerebral palsy and spinal cord injury. The cause is that CNS injury leads to paralysis of some muscles of upper limbs and the patients' upper limbs are in flexion contracture because of muscle paralysis, muscle spasm or tendon contracture, which can lead to motor function loss, hypofunction or uncoordinated movement of upper limbs.

   Moulding training aids of motor pattern of upper limbs can restrict joint deformity position through rigidity of lattice framing. The connection of lattice framing only allows the single orientation of joint motion and restrict unnecessary joint motion of upper limbs movements effectively. Movement orientation switch gear can transform the movement of upper limb in healthy side into the opposite orientation movement of upper limb in injured side. Therefore, during walking, the patients can keep the swing coordination of double upper limbs and normal posture of injured upper limbs. Through repeated training, abnormal motor pattern can be rectified and coordinated motor pattern of upper limbs can be recovered gradually.

   The training time and therapy course: the training time is 20–30 min (twice a day) and there are 60 times in one therapy course.

3. Indications, contraindications and announcements.
   (a) Indications: It is suitable for the patients with hemiplegia, cerebral palsy and spinal cord injury accompanied with abnormal motor pattern of upper limbs.
   (b) Contraindications: the patients with unhealed pelvic fracture or pelvic soft tissue injury; the patients with unhealed

bone fracture of upper limbs, joint cartilage and ligament injuries; the patients with unhealed rib fracture or injuries of chest, spinal cord and pelvis; the patients with unstable state after stroke; the patients with uncontrolled high blood pressure and diabetes mellitus

(c) Considerations: the training should be step by step. It is forbidden to increase the training intensity without purpose. The therapists should activate the enthusiasm of the patients fully, activate training atmosphere, use encouraging words and avoid using scolding words.

Gait footprint training footpath.

Gait footprint training footpath is developed according to biofeedback mechanism. Biofeedback mechanism includes goal and motive mechanism and the mechanism that archery accuracy can be increased through practicing the archery towards the center of the target. It is the assistive device developed for the gait rectification training. The footpath is made of transparent and soft plastic board with the width of 2 mm. The width is 30–50 mm. The length is decided by the size of the rehabilitation hall. Different strides and footprints of adult and children are printed in the footpath (Fig. 19.27). The footprint can be drawn on the floor directly so that the footpath of gait training for different age and stature.

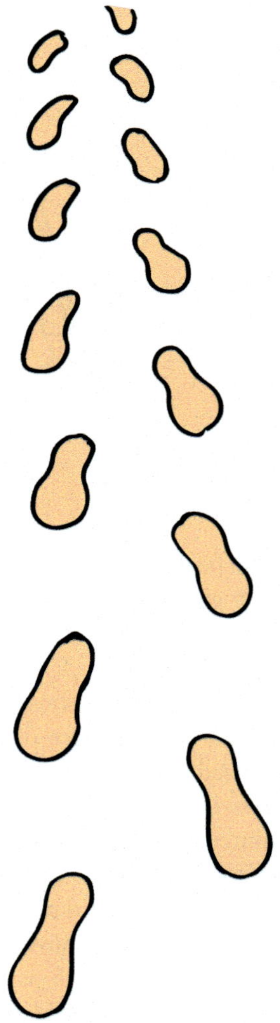

Fig. 19.27 Sketch map of footpath of gait footprint training

During the gait training, the therapists use Daoyin technique to guide the patients to do hip flexion. When the feet step forward, the patients are guided to put feet on the footprint of footpath so that the patients can do gait remodeling training with a purpose to develop CNS potential and promote recovery of normal gait.

19.3.2 Training Device

There are many kinds of rehabilitation training devices of neurological training including CNS potential development, motor programs of all joint motions, the balance of sitting, standing and walking and motor pattern remodeling training devices. These devices not only can be used for the walking training of sober patients, but also can be used for the walking training of the patients in coma or low conscious state. These devices not only can be used for the patients with mild symptoms, but also can be used for the severe patients who even cannot sit. These devices broaden the range of rehabilitation training, alleviate the labor intensity of the therapists and play an important role in the clinical rehabilitation therapy of neurological training.

It is noticeable that all rehabilitation corollary equipment of neurological training is the assistive device for the application of six-step Daoyin technique of guiding collaterals through meridians. It is the method to carry out Daoyin technique better and increase the effect of Daoyin technique. Because there are many kinds of devices, we only introduce the representative training device.

Potential development training device of upper limbs.

They are specially used for the application of Daoyin technique to develop the CNS potential of autonomic movement of upper limbs, promote CNS plasticity and functional reorganization and recover more and more lost motor function.

19.3.2.1 Essential Structure and Design Principle

1. Essential structure: Potential development training device of upper limbs is composed of (Fig. 19.28) expansion board of hand, bearing support system, control training system of pedestal and limbs, hammock and suspension system, weight support system and weight support sandbag or handle. The role of expansion board of hand is to make the flexed wrist and finger joint in extension position in case of wrist and finger injuries under bearing. Weight support system of sandbag and pulley can alleviate the bearing of limbs. Through increasing or decreasing the number of sandbags, the patients can be kept in pushing up position.
2. Design principle: Through frame support and weight support system, with the help of chest hammock of the patients, partial body weight of the patients are subtracted so that the patients can be kept in pushing up position using double upper limbs to support the trunk. The therapists can use Daoyin technique to guide the patients to push up and down with sudden change of position to create safe imminent danger state. The patients are encouraged to overcome the difficulties due to position change. The comprehensive effect can clear and activate the channels and collaterals, develop brain potential and recover motor function of upper limbs.

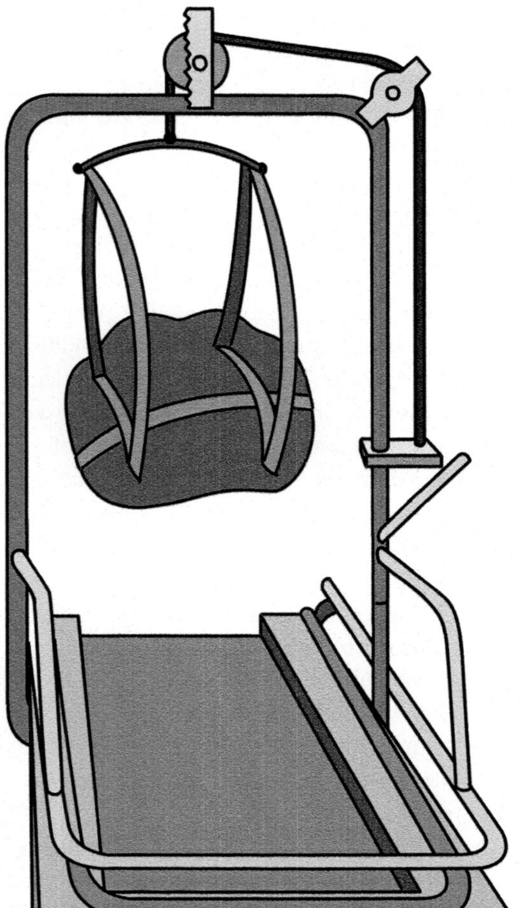

Fig. 19.28 Sketch map of Potential development training device of upper limbs

19.3.2.2 Operational Approach

1. Preparation before training: The patients wear hammock, put expansion board of hand on the injured hand and are in pushing up and down position. Two legs are on the sponge cushion of pedestal. This position can make the patients put their hands on the vertical line of weight support pulley on the middle of the top of braced frame and the hammock is connected with the hook of weight support system. The therapists stand in the injured side of the patients. According to exercise prescription, the therapists hang sandbag of weight support or exercise therapists can use hands to

hold the knob. According to the specific condition of the patients, the therapists give the proper assistance.

2. Training procedure includes pushing up and pushing down.
   (a) Pushing up training: The patients' elbow joints are in flexion position and they move the center of the body to paralyzed upper limb. The patients are guided to take a deep breath and expire slowly. After that, they concentrate on the breathing and hold their breath. They concentrate on triceps muscle of arm in the paralyzed side and feel the contraction of triceps muscle of arm during the slow pushing up. When the patients cannot push up themselves, exercise therapists help the patients. When the angle of elbow extension is no less than 90°, exercise therapists can decrease the assistive force suddenly according to the condition and use the words "push up, or you will fall and hold on, or you will bump" to create imminent danger atmosphere and encourage the patients to push up by themselves.
   (b) Pushing down training: The patients' elbow joints are in straight position. The patients are guided to take a deep breath and expire slowly. After that, they concentrate on the breathing to push down themselves slowly. They concentrate on triceps muscle of arm in the paralyzed side and feel the contraction of triceps muscle of arm during the slow pushing down. When the patients cannot push down themselves, exercise therapists help the patients. When the angle of elbow extension is no more than 90°, exercise therapists can decrease the assistive force suddenly according to the condition and use the words "hold on, or you will fall and hold on, or you will bump" to create imminent danger atmosphere and encourage the patients to keep in this position for 6 s.
   (c) Training time and therapy course: The training time is 20–30 min (once or twice a day) and there are 60 times in one therapy course.
3. Clinical indications, contraindications and announcements.

   Indications: This device is suitable for the stable patients with motor dysfunction [12] of upper limbs in acute and chronic phase after CNS injury, bone and joint, muscle injuries, such as hemiplegia, cerebral palsy, children cerebral palsy, incomplete paraplegia, peripheral nerve injury, joint and muscle dysfunction. It is also suitable for the patients whose motor function of upper limbs cannot be improved after traditional rehabilitation method.
   (d) Contraindications: The unstable patients in acute phase; the uncontrolled severe hypertension or diabetes mellitus; severe heart disease and pulmonary dysfunction with low cardiovascular response.
   (e) Considerations: The weak patients of long-term bed should do the acclimatization training before this training to increase the stress ability of cardiovascular stress. When the patients can stand erectly and the blood pressure is stable after 30 min, the patients can do this training. The training should be step by step. The training can be regulated through weight support and training time. It is forbidden to increase training intensity without a purpose. During the training, the therapists should activate the enthusiasm of the patients and atmosphere and use encouraging words. It is forbidden to use rebuke and critical words.

19.3.2.3 Potential Development Training Device of Lower Limbs

The device is used for the application of Daoyin technique to develop CNS potential of autonomic movement of lower limbs, promote CNS plasticity and functional reorganization and recover lost motor function as much as possible.

Essential Structure and Design Principle

1. Essential structure includes weight support system, sandbag, frame support system, scale pedal and hammock (Fig. 19.29). Sandbag and weight support system can decrease bearing of

limbs. Through increasing or decreasing the number of sandbag, the amount of weight support can be adjusted. Hammock have the weight support and protective effect through suspension function of the root of thigh and waist. Through sudden postural change, the therapists use Daoyin speech to create a safe dangerous state. With the increase of the training difficulties, the training can develop the motor ability of lower limbs and conduction speed. There are footprints in the scale pedal with three marks such as 60 (outside), 80 (middle) and 100 (the center of the circle). Through goal and motive mechanism, the patients can do control training of lower limbs.
2. Design principle: Through the weight support and protection effects of the device, the patients are able to stand up. The therapists can use Daoyin technique to guide the patients to squat up, squat down and control the lower limbs with sudden postural change to create safe dangerous state and encourage the patients to overcome the difficulties due to postural change. Scale pedal provides the training condition of goal and motive mechanism. The comprehensive effects can clear and activate the channels and collaterals, develop brain potential and recover motor function of lower limbs.

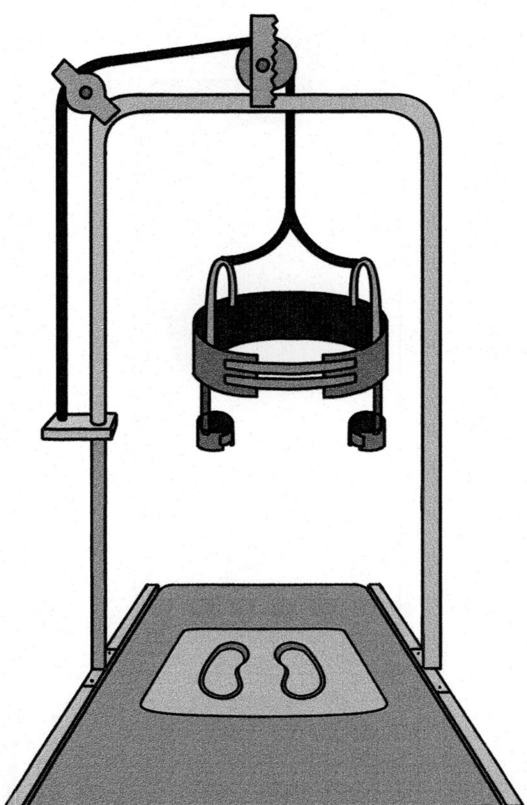

Fig. 19.29 Sketch map of potential development training device of lower limbs

Operational Approach

1. Preparation before training: The patients wear hammock and hang sangbag according to the amount of weight support. According to the specific condition, the therapists stand in one side, the front or the back of the patients. The patients use two hands to grasp the handrail in the lateral wall of potential training device.
2. Training procedure includes squat up, squat down and control ability training of lower limbs.
   (a) Squat up training: The patients are in kneeling-squatting position and try to move the center of the body to paralyzed side. The patients are guided to take a deep breath and expire slowly. After that, the patients concentrate on taking a deep breath and hold their breath. The patients concentrate on the quadriceps femoris in the paralyzed side and feel the contraction of quadriceps femoris during the standing up. If the patients cannot stand up by themselves, exercise therapists should help them. When the angle of knee extension is no less than 90°, exercise therapists can decrease the assistive force suddenly according to the condition and use the words “stand up, or you will fall and hold on, or you will bump” to create imminent danger atmosphere and encourage the patients to keep in this position for 6 s and stand up by themselves.
   (b) Squat down training: Exercise therapists guide the patients to concentrate on taking a deep breath and hold their breath. During the slow squat down process, they move the center of the body to lower

limbs in the paralyzed side and feel the tension of quadriceps femoris. If the patients cannot squat down by themselves, exercise therapists should help them. When the angle of knee joint flexion is no more than 90°, exercise therapists can decrease the assistive force suddenly according to the condition and use the words "hold on, or you will fall and hold on, or you will bump" to create imminent danger atmosphere and encourage the patients to keep in this position for 6 s.

(c) Control ability training of lower limbs: under the weight support and protection condition, the patients put two foots on the center of the circle and move the center of the body to healthy side. The therapists guide the patients to try to flex hip and knee, elevate injured limbs, put foot in the injured side on the center of the circle and complete these movements.

(d) The training time and therapy course: The training time is 30 min (once or twice a day) and there are 60 times in one therapy course. At the end of one therapy course, the therapists should re-evaluate the training effect and decide whether to do the next training or not.

3. Clinical indications, contraindications and considerations.

(a) Indications: This device is suitable for the stable patients with motor dysfunction of lower limbs [13] in acute and chronic phase after CNS, bone and joint, muscle injuries, such as hemiplegia, cerebral palsy, children cerebral palsy, incomplete paraplegia, peripheral nerve injury, joint and muscle dysfunction. It is also suitable for the patients whose motor function of lower limbs cannot be improved after traditional rehabilitation method.

(b) Contraindications: The unstable patients in acute phase; the uncontrolled severe hypertension or diabetes mellitus; severe heart disease and pulmonary dysfunction with low cardiovascular response.

(c) Considerations: The weak patients of long-term bed should do the acclimatization training before this training to increase the stress ability of cardiovascular stress. When the patients can stand erectly and the blood pressure is stable after 30 min, the patients can do this training. The training should be step by step. The training can be regulated through weight support and training time. During the training, the therapists should activate the enthusiasm of the patients and atmosphere and use encouraging words. It is forbidden to use rebuke and critical words.

Except for potential development training device mentioned above, there are a series of training equipment such as potential development training device of the trunk (Fig. 19.30), potential development training device of tibialis anterior muscle (Fig. 19.31), potential develop-

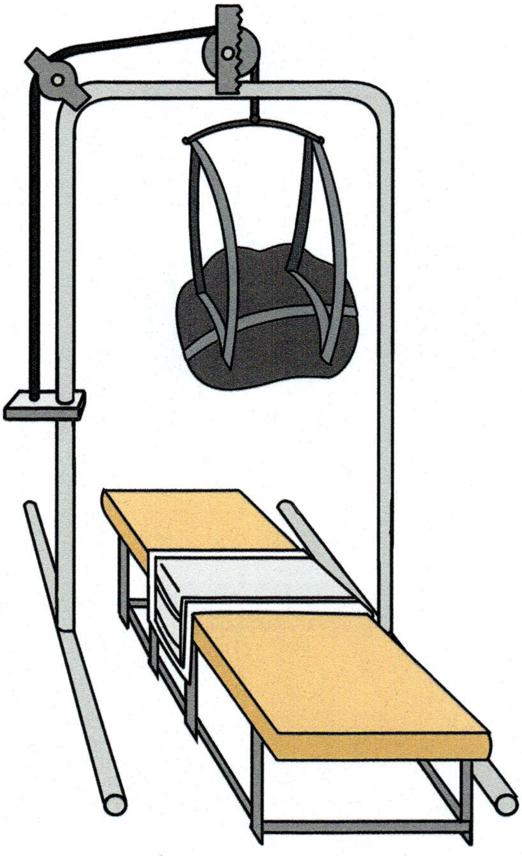

Fig. 19.30 Sketch map of potential development training device of the trunk

ment training device of hamstring muscle (Fig. 19.32), potential development training device of balance (Fig. 19.33) and potential development training device of walking (Fig. 19.34). The training should be guided by six-step Daoyin technique of guiding collaterals through meridians or normal method. With the increase of training difficulty, the training can clear and activate the channels and collaterals, develop brain potential, increase the control ability of brain and conduction speed of nerve.

19.3.2.4 Abnormal Gait Rectification Weight Support and Walking Training Device

According to rehabilitation therapeutic principle of neurological training, we developed special training equipment to rectify abnormal gait and remodel normal gait. For the patients with mild symptoms, they do the training according to the three-stage rehabilitation method. When they do the third stage training, the device can be used for the assistive device. For the severe patients with children cerebral palsy, they do rehabilitation training according to standing in early period and walking development, the device can be used for potential development training and walking training to increase the excitability of walking center of sacral cord in order to recover walking and standing ability. For the patients with severe hemiplegia or motor dysfunction of limbs, they do rehabilitation training according to standing in early period and walking development. Their purpose is to recover assistive standing and walking function through abnormal gait rectification weight support and walking training in the early phase. That whether motor pattern is abnormal or not is not the key point.

Essential Structure and Design Principle

1. Essential structure: Abnormal gait rectification weight support and walking training device is composed of bearing, weight sup-

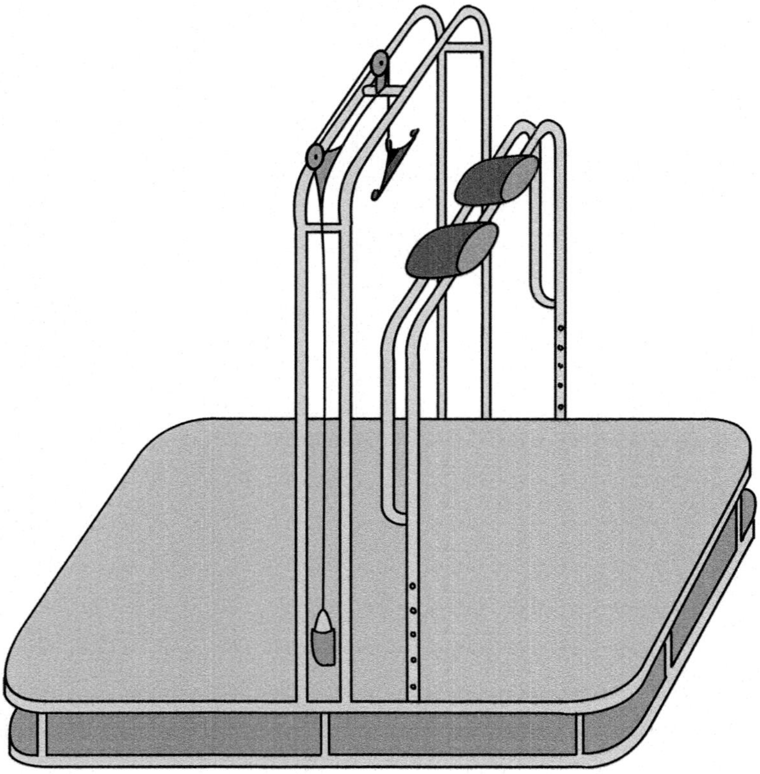

Fig. 19.31 Sketch map of potential development training device of tibialis anterior muscle

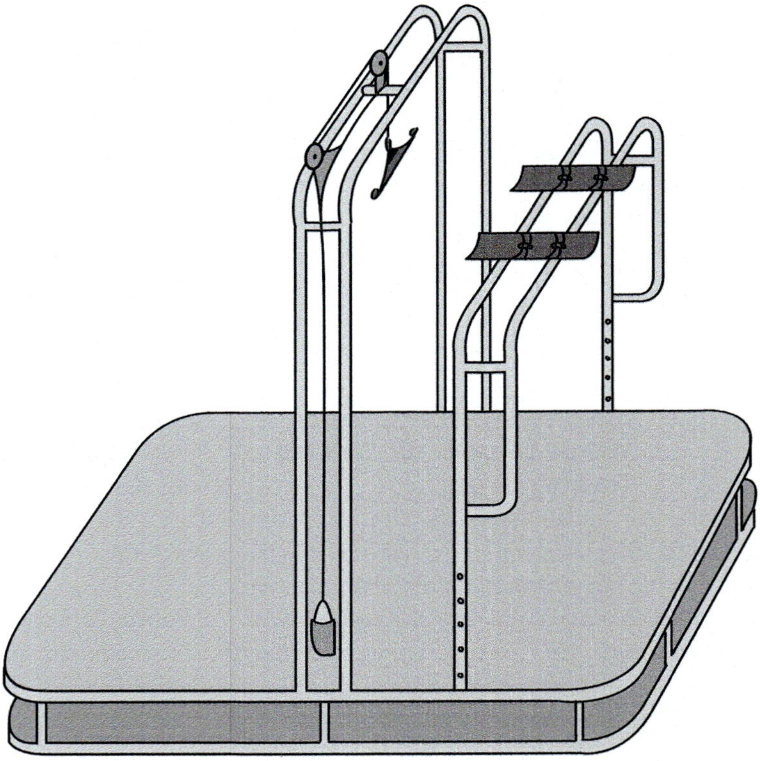

Fig. 19.32 Sketch map of potential development training device of hamstring muscle

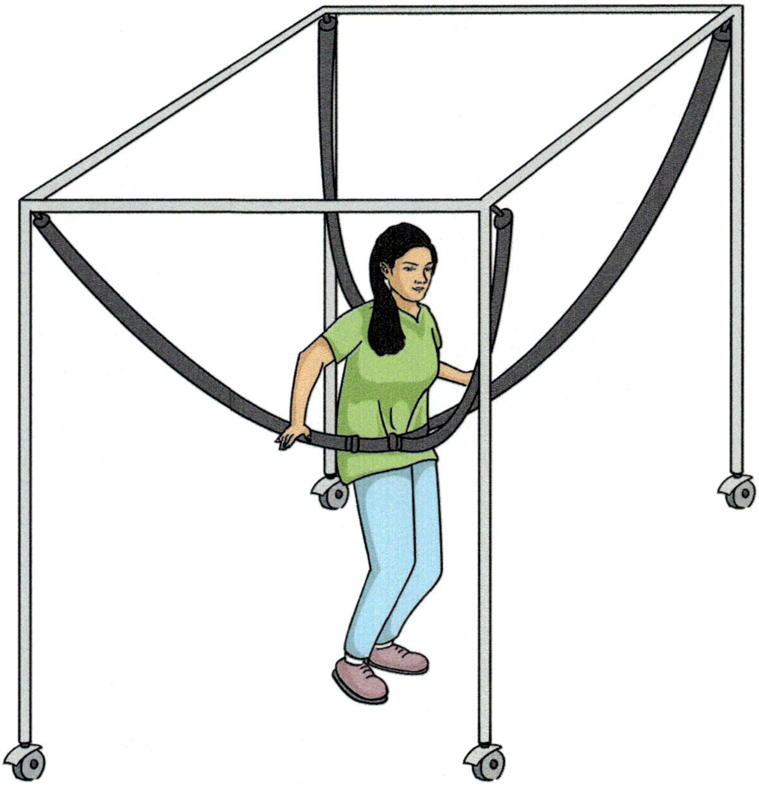

Fig. 19.33 Sketch map of potential development training device of balance

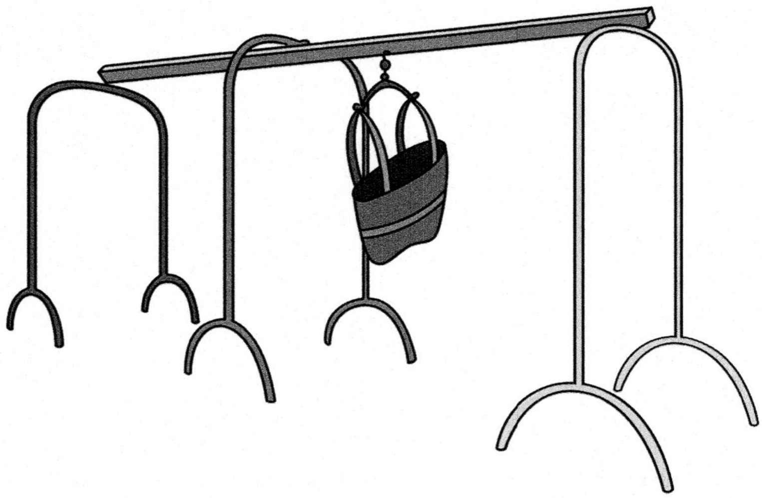

Fig. 19.34 Sketch map of potential development training device of walking

port and protection system, abnormal gait rectification system and normal gait training system (Fig. 19.35).

(a) Bearing, weight support and protection system is composed of bearing frame, weight support winch, pulley, handrail and weight support hammock. Bearing frame is a rectangular frame (180 cm × 150 cm) that is made from double curved hot drawing welded steel tube. The diameter is 36 mm and the wall thickness is 4 mm. There are two layers and the space is 50 cm. In the middle of the frame, two U-shaped tubes are welded in parallel (190 cm × 150 cm). In the middle of the top of two U-shaped tube, fixed pulley and its back plate are welded. Fixed pulley and winch are welded separately in one corner of the top of U-shaped tube and the midpoint of the wall on the same side. Steel wire (diameter is 3 mm) connects hammock connecting rod in frame and weight support winch on the lateral wall. At the bottom of rectangle frame, four universal wheels are fixed. In the middle of the front, handrail is fixed and the height is adjustable. The back is connected to dismountable protection bar. Weight support hammock is divided into swimsuit type and waistcoat type. The stress parts of swimsuit type are iliac region and chest-back. Hammock connects two thighs in waistcoat type. The stress parts are chest-back and pelvis. According to the specific condition of the patients, the patients select the proper type. The dressing

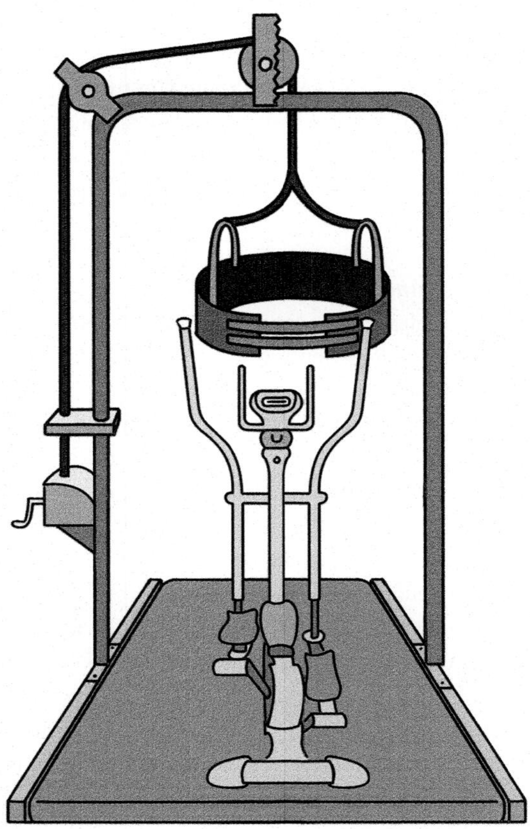

Fig. 19.35 Sketch map of abnormal gait rectification, weight support and walking training device

should be comfortable without oppression of local soft tissue and affecting joint motion.

(b) Abnormal gait rectification system: the therapists select elastic band with different width and thickness to produce elastic rectification band of lower limbs abduction and foot dorsiflexion with different elasticity. Abduction band of lower limbs can prevent excessive adduction of lower limbs in walking. One end is connected to steel tube in upper layer of bearing frame and the other end is connected to the inferior of knee joint through nylon thread gluing. Elastic band of foot dorsiflexion can prevent foot drop and strephenopodia. One end is connected to the top of bearing frame and the other end is connected to the front of injured foot. The tightness of rectification band cannot affect walking in adduction of lower limbs and foot drop.

The training should be done on the gait and footprint training footpath.

Design Principle

1. Through weight support and suspension of the device, the patients can be kept in standing position. The device can provide safe condition to prevent falling down and bumping. The patients use two hands to grasp the handrail so that they can walk stably. Rectification band of foot drop and lower limbs adduction can rectify lower limbs adduction, foot drop and strephenopodia through elastic recoil. During walking, the patients can use their own force to rectify lower limbs adduction, foot drop and strephenopodia. If they are not rectified completely, elastic band can keep the normal gait. With the help of gait and footprint training footpath, the patients can do the training with a purpose.
2. Operational approach.

   Preparation before training the patients can wear hammock in sitting or standing position. According to exercise prescription, the amount of weight support can be adjusted. According to the specific condition of the patients, the therapists stand in one side, the front or the back of the patients. The patients use two hangs to grasp the front handrail. According to the degree of lower limbs adduction and foot drop [14], the tightness of the rectification band is adjusted so that the patients can walk with the affection of lower limbs adduction and foot drop.
3. Training procedure.
   (a) Auxiliary power walking training: Exercise therapists move training device forward and the patients practice stepping forward with the movement of the training device.
   (b) Autonomous power training: The patients move training device forward and practice stepping forward at the same time.
   (c) Disassembled slow movement training of gait of Daoyin technique: exercise therapists use six-step Daoyin technique in traditional Chinese medicine to guide the patients to do disassembled gait training on the basis of regulation of mind and breath.
   (d) Control ability training of lower limbs: Under the condition of weight support and protection, the patients are guided to do the training of hip flexion, foot dorsiflexion and hip abduction in situ. The specific procedures are as follows: the therapists are in standing position, move the center of the body to one side and guide the patients to flex hip joint as quick as possible on the basis of regulation of mind and breathing. If there is adduction of lower limbs, the patients are guided to abduct hip joint, dorsiflex ankle joint and then put the heel of the foot on the footprint of the footpath. The purpose of this training is to increase the speed and flexibility of limbs. The patients are asked to relax, not to exert excessive force in case of excessive associated reaction. The patients should shorten the time of completing the training gradually.
4. The training time and therapy course: The training time is 30 min (once a day) and there

are 30 times in one therapy course. At the end of one therapy course, the therapists should re-evaluate the training effect and decide whether to do the next training or not.

With the increase of myodynamia of hip flexor, hip abductor, tibialis anterior muscle and peroneus longus and brevis of the patients, autonomous dominant ability, control ability of limbs and walking ability, the patients should reduce the amount of weight support and traction force of rectification band gradually. After that, they can walk independently without weight support, traction and hand.

5. Clinical indications, contraindications and announcements.
   (a) Indications: This device is suitable for the stable patients with severe motor dysfunction of lower limbs in acute and chronic phase who cannot do normal weight support walking training after CNS injury, such as hemiplegia, cerebral palsy, children cerebral palsy, incomplete paraplegia, peripheral nerve injury, joint and muscle dysfunction. It is also suitable for the patients who are difficult to do normal weight support walking training because of adduction of lower limbs or foot drop due to muscle spasm or paralysis.
   (b) Contraindications: The unstable patients in acute phase; the uncontrolled severe hypertension or diabetes mellitus; severe heart disease and pulmonary dysfunction with low cardiovascular response.
   (c) Announcements: the weak patients of long-term bed should do the acclimatization training before this training to increase the stress ability of cardiovascular stress. When the patients can stand erectly and the blood pressure is stable after 30 min, the patients can do this training. The training should be step by step. The training can be regulated through weight support and training time. During the training, the therapists should activate the enthusiasm of the patients and atmosphere and use encouraging words. It is forbidden to use rebuke and critical words.

19.3.2.5 Stride, Gait and Shifting of Weight Support Training Device

According to the rehabilitation therapeutic principle of neurological training, stride, gait and shifting of weight support training device is developed, which is the basis of gait training.

Essential Structure and Design Principle

Essential structure of stride, gait and shifting of weight support training device is composed of two parts (Fig. 19.36).

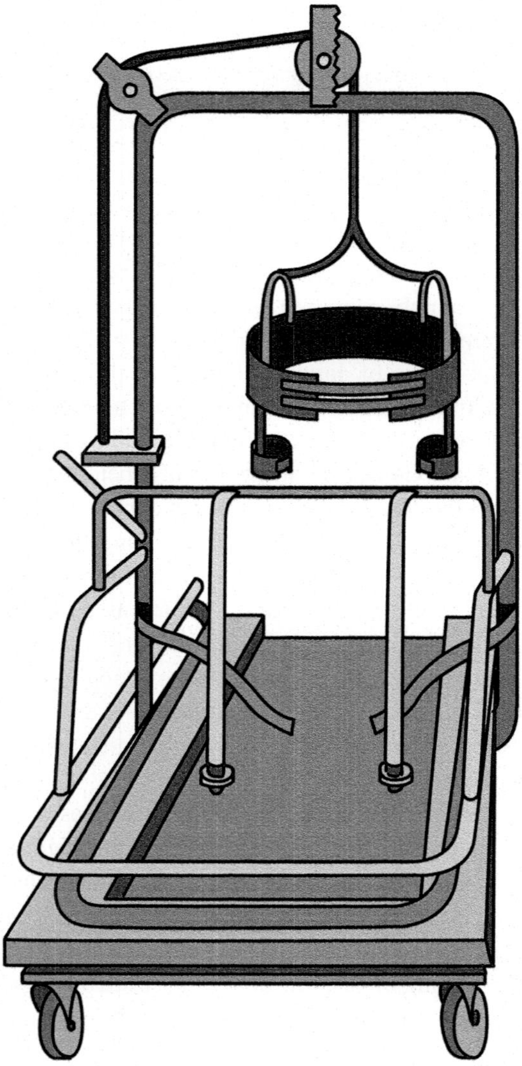

Fig. 19.36 Sketch map of stride, gait and shifting of weight support training device

1. Essential structure is composed of weight support and training system.
   (a) Weight and frame support system: It can reduce the bearing of limbs. The patients can use manual pulley to adjust the amount of weight support and use suspension hammock to elevate trunk and waist to protect them and make them in standing position.
   (b) Stride, gait and shifting of weight support training system: During movement, it can rotate like an oval and adjust resistance through control system in machine. With the increase of training difficulty, the patients can do the training of control ability of limbs and conduction speed of nerve.

Design Principle

Stride, gait and shifting of weight are the basic training of gait training. There are several elements to form normal gait. Consistent stride: the stride of limb in the healthy side is bigger than that of limb in injured side in the patients with hemiplegia because of short bearing time due to weak force of injured limbs, which induces abnormal gait. Consistent bearing time: short bearing time of injured limb may lead to abnormal gait. Consistent stride width: when there is adductor tension or spasm and contracture of lower limbs, adduction in the steeping forward of injured limbs can lead to abnormal gait because the stride width is different between healthy limb and injured limb. Consistent leg speed: because it is difficult to start stepping forward of injured limbs, the leg speed is different between two sides, which is manifested as abnormal gait.

On the basis of previous training such as neural potential development and motor program reestablishment, before gait training, the patients should do the basic movement training such as stride, gait and shifting of weight and focus on the training of stride width in the stride training. Shifting of weight is that during the process of stepping forward, the patients should make the stepping forward leg without load bearing so that the leg can reach the required height as soon as possible.

According to different stature of different people, stride, gait and shifting of weight device can be divided into five grades with different stride and stride width. Only after the center of weight is transferred, the patients can do the training of stride and gait according to goal and motive mechanism. The training should be guided by six-step Daoyin technique of guiding collaterals through meridians or normal method. With the increase of training difficulty, the training can clear and activate the channels and collaterals, develop brain potential, increase the control ability of brain and conduction speed of nerve.

Operational Approach

1. Operation procedure: Quick start—the therapists press the ST/STOP button and start the training. During the training, the therapists can use upward and downward arrow to adjust the resistance. Set goal: the therapists press MODE button and select manual function. Display frame (the lower part) of resistance grade blink automatically. The therapists can use upward and downward arrow to select training grade (1–16) and press ST/STOP button for the training.

   Auxiliary instructions: computer on board can record nine users' training data. The therapists can set individual training goal and store it for the next training. The therapists can set the goals of time, distance or quantity of heat. The control program of heart rate can adjust the resistance automatically to increase or decrease the training amount of the patients in order to reach the setting goal of heart rate.
2. Training procedure: Retentive fitness or warm-up: the 10 min after the beginning, the patients can increase training intensity gradually. Aerobic exercise: the patients can do mild exercise persistently for a long time (35–60 min). There is a little sweat after training, but there is no gasp in any case. Endurance and aerobic exercise is the consistent intensive training (20–40 min). Stride and shifting of weight training: on the basis of regulation of mind and breath, the patients are guided to move the center of weight to one side and then move it to the other side when the body is moved forward. If

necessary, the patients can use upper limbs to pull the rod for help. The training can be done in circles. The patients feel the shifting of weight and stepping forward.

3. The training time and therapy course: The training time is 30 min (once a day) and there are 30 times in one therapy course. At the end of one therapy course, the therapists should re-evaluate the training effect and decide whether to do the next training or not.
4. Clinical indications, contraindications and announcements.
   (a) Indications: This device is suitable for the patients with motor dysfunction of lower limbs in acute phase, especially for rehabilitation training of gait, stride and shifting of weight of the patients with obsolete hemiplegia, incomplete paraplegia, peripheral nerve injury and joint and muscle dysfunction after the other methods are invalid.
   (b) Contraindications: The unstable patients in acute phase; the uncontrolled severe hypertension or diabetes mellitus; severe heart disease and pulmonary dysfunction with low cardiovascular response, dizziness and blood pressure decrease in standing position.
   (c) Announcements: During training, the patients should concentrate and wear sports shoes. During the training, after the patients complete all the movements of shifting of weight, they should move the center of weight to the other side. The training should be step by step. It is forbidden to increase the training intensity suddenly. During the training, the therapists should activate the enthusiasm of the patients and atmosphere and use encouraging words. It is forbidden to use rebuke and critical words.

19.3.3 Training Device

Neurological training appliances and devices are not equipped with the objective indexation display function of the effect of six-step Daoyin technique of guiding collaterals through meridians. Therefore, they cannot be used for the training with a purpose and are not suitable for the training of motor program reestablishment. Because there is no definite surpassing goal, goal and motive mechanism cannot enhance the training effects of neural potential development and motor program reestablishment.

Corollary equipment of neurological training is developed to solve the problems mentioned above. It can display curve, sound or digit of Daoyin technique on the screen through different ways and increase the functions of therapeutic item selection, training method mechanism explanation, setting of surpassing goal, Daoyin technique automatic speech instruction, main and collateral channels instruction, data storage and analysis.

This kind of equipment is developed to alleviate the labour intensity of the therapists, increase the training effect of rehabilitation technique of neurological training and increase the clinical application value of rehabilitation training of neurological training to a new level.

On the basis of training device, this kind of equipment is developed to add the real-time detection and display function of effect of Daoyin technique. According to the effect of Daoyin technique, it can be manifested as the strength of motor program signal from brain to muscle, the intensity of muscle contraction, the strength of resistance, the size of joint motion. After that, through biofeedback mechanism [15], the patients are guided to do the training with a purpose. Therefore, there are many kinds of equipment. According to the clinical application of neurological training, they can be used for the training of neural potential development, motor program reestablishment, motor pattern remodeling, balance, stride, gait and shifting of weight, speech recognition, sphincter, virtual reality training device.

In this chapter, we only introduce the major training device used for motor function rehabilitation and introduce the common training device of speech recognition.

The common characteristics of neurological training device.

1. Six step Daoyin technique in traditional Chinese medicine is used. According to the pathway of main and collateral channels, Qi is guided from meridians to collaterals or from collaterals to meridians, which is the method of guiding collaterals through meridians.
2. It is equipped with the functions of real-time detection and digital display of the effect of Daoyin technique. It can detect and display the consistent curve, sound, number or image in digit.
3. Different therapeutic items and surpassing goals can be set, just like practicing archery towards target to increase accuracy and practicing jumping with transverse bar to increase the jump height. Therefore, the patients are guided to do the training with a purpose through biofeedback and goal and motive mechanism.
4. Data storage and auto-analysis.
5. Animation spot instruction of meridian point and automatic speech Daoyin function can guarantee the correctness of Qi in main and collateral channels. One of the key techniques of guiding collaterals through meridians or guiding meridians through collaterals is to guarantee Qi guided by six-step Daoyin technique to go through correct main and collateral channels. Both exercise therapists and the patients know little about correct main and collateral channels. Qi in the correct main and collateral channels is the basis to implement the method of guiding collaterals through meridians correctly. On the basis of meridian points animation developed previously and key meridian points, animation spot blink technique is used in virtual human body. The spot speed is synchronized with automatic speech instruction of Daoyin technique. Flicker is used to mark the pathway and meridian point to guarantee the correctness and uniformity of the pathway, which provides condition for the standard application of the technique of guiding collaterals through meridians.
6. Weight support and protection function: Weight support system of the equipment can help the patients to stand up and complete the uncompleted movements at ordinary times. It can prevent the falling down and bump of the patients, which is good for the training safety.

19.3.3.1 Basic Neurological Training Device of Neurological Training

This kind of equipment can extract some kind of signal and display the instant effect of Daoyin technique. Therefore, the patients can do the training with a purpose. It is the important and essential part of all kinds of training device.

1. Neurological training device of guiding collaterals through meridians: Neurological training devices of guiding collaterals through meridians give out motor program signal to agonistic muscle and antagonistic muscle of joint motion through Daoyin technique and clearing and activating the channels and collaterals. The intensity of this signal is real-time objective indicator of the degree of clearing and activating the channels and collaterals and is the promoter of clearing and activating the channels and collaterals. It can be used for the training of CNS potential development, single joint movement and motor program reestablishment of associated movement in which multiple joints are involved. It can also be assembled in other neurological training device. With objective indicator of instant effect of various kinds of trainings, the patients can do the training with a purpose.
   (a) Design principle: Motor program is biological drive signal given out from CNS cells to the muscles (agonistic muscle and antagonistic muscle) of joint motion proportionally and sequentially. The coordinated and orderly movement can complete the instruction of some kind of actual functional movement. In traditional opinion, the received electrical signal in muscle contraction is generated by muscle contraction itself. Our experiment demonstrated that electromyographic signal is motor program signal [16], which is driven by the drive signal from CNS to muscle. It

is generated before muscle contraction, but not generated by muscle contraction itself. This provides scientific basis for the training of motor program signal detection, display and reestablishment. Therefore, only developing neural potential and activating CNS cells are not enough. Some methods should be used to make the cells work coordinately and orderly so that the lost motor function can be recovered.

Neurological training device (Fig. 19.37), electrical signal detection and reception system is used to detect the control signal from CNS to agonistic muscle and antagonistic muscle and display it on fluorescent screen in a continuous curve. Therefore, the Daoyin technique effect is clear. The therapists and the patients can observe the progress and shortcoming of the therapy. According to the requirements, computer program allows the therapists to set therapeutic items with different degree of difficulty. The patients should have continuous, definite, new surpassing goal and improved direction. Through goal and motive mechanism, feedback condition can be adjusted and the patients are guided to do the training with a purpose. The method can activate the enthusiasm of the patients to do active movement of limbs. With the cooperation of expiration and inspiration, the patients can control the limbs movement gradually. Many clinical control studies verified that this kind of technique has good therapeutic effect. This method is used as the key technique to form new kind of rehabilitation method.

(b) Characteristics: On the basis of the general characteristics of training device, neurological training device has the following characteristics.

High sensitivity: Neurological training device can extract motor program signal of cortex motor center from the skin surface of muscle and display motor program signal of agonistic muscle and antagonistic muscle in different colored curves. The therapists can use computer program to set different therapeutic items and surpassing goals. Through goal and motive mechanism, motor program of coordinated movement in cortex motor center can be trained.

The guarantee of standard application of Daoyin technique of guiding collaterals through meridians: There are several functions such as automatic speech instruction cooperated with Daoyin technique of guiding collaterals through meridians,

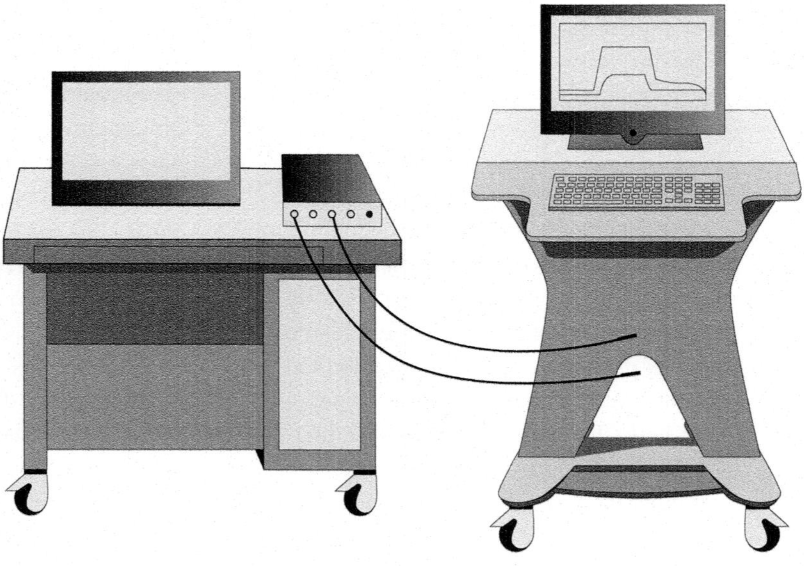

Fig. 19.37 Sketch map of neurological training device of guiding collaterals through meridians

therapeutic mechanism demonstration of motor program reestablishment and animation spot instruction of meridian points to guarantee the correctness, standardization and normalization of main and collateral channels.

The equipment has four leads that can be used for single and combined application. It is suitable for single joint movement motor program reestablishment training of multiple joint associated movements.

(c) Operational approach: we use knee extension as an example. In a warm, quiet and lucifugal room, the patients lie, semi-sit or sit before the neurological training device. Surface reception electrode is pasted. The placement of quadriceps femoris electrode: the first surface electrode is placed on 6 cm above patella, skin surface of the belly of quadriceps femoris. Twelve centimeter upward the first electrode, the second electrode is placed. The ground electrode is placed between the two electrodes. Surface electrode is connected to the first lead of biofeedback device through wire. The placement of hamstring muscles electrode: the first surface electrode is placed 2 cm above popliteal space, skin surface of the belly of hamstring muscles. Six centimeter upward the first electrode, the second electrode is placed. The ground electrode is placed between the two electrodes. The surface electrode is connected to the third lead of biofeedback device through wire. The therapists use six-step Daoyin technique of guiding collaterals through meridians in traditional Chinese medicine to encourage the patients to do knee extension in sitting position, standing position and walking actively for 15 min separately. If the patients cannot extend knee actively, the patients can do knee extension training with help. The patients are in kneeling-squatting position, move the center of weight to injured side and is encourage to stand up by themselves with the help of exercise therapists and lower limb in healthy side. When the patients are able to walk, they can do motor program reestablishment training of knee extension in walking. The initial data is the highest signal from motor center to quadriceps femoris and hamstring muscles at the first time. The highest signal is used as the base point to make two elevation lines. Daoyin technique is used to guide the patients to make the signal surpass the baseline in the next training of quadriceps femoris. The signal intensity of hamstring muscles is lower than the baseline except for this signal of hamstring muscles. During therapy, when the signal of quadriceps femoris almost reaches the summit, the therapists say the words “hold on, or you will fall and higher, or you will bump” to create the imminent dangerous condition to make the patients feel dangerous. Therefore, the signal of quadriceps femoris can surpass the baseline as much as possible. Meanwhile, the patients don’t increase or decrease the signal intensity of hamstring muscles. After that, the new highest point is the baseline. The same method is used to guide the patients to try to make the signal of quadriceps femoris surpass new baseline and the signal of hamstring muscles lower than the new baseline. The rest can be done in the same manner and the training can be done repeatedly.

(d) The training time and therapy course: The training time is 50 min (once a day) and there are 30 times in one therapy course. At the end of one therapy course, the therapists should re-evaluate the training effect and decide whether to do the next training or not.

(e) Indications, contraindications and announcements.

Indications: This device is suitable for the patients with motor dysfunction of in acute and chronic phase such as obsolete hemiplegia, incomplete paraplegia, children cerebral palsy, incomplete paraplegia, facial paralysis, peripheral nerve injury, joint and muscle dysfunction. Especially the other therapeutic methods are invalid.

Contraindications: The patients are in acute phase, which affect the salvage. It is not suitable for the patients who are not allowed to do exercise after surgery of bone, joint or muscle injury or with unhealed wound.

Announcements: the patients should concentrate on the training. During training, the patients should focus on the intensity and proportion of motor program signal, but not on the range of joint motion and strength of muscle contraction. The training should be step by step and it is forbidden to increase anti-resistance without a purpose. The anti-resistance time should not be more than 6 s. This kind of training is not the training to enhance myodynamia, but the training of developing brain potential through muscle contraction dominated by brain. The degree of muscle contraction is the external manifestation and objective indicator of the intensity of motor program signal. Long-term muscle contraction can lead to fatigue, which cannot manifest the motor program signal and its strength. Therefore, the patients cannot do the training of motor program reestablishment. During the training, the therapists should activate the enthusiasm of the patients fully, activate training atmosphere, use encouraging words and avoid using scolding words.

19.3.3.2 Myodynamia Guided Device of Guiding Collaterals Through Meridians

The signal source of neurological training device is the change of myodynamia (traction).

1. Design principle: When Daoyin technique is used to guide the patients to do active movement training, the signal from brain to agonistic muscle should be strong and the contraction force should be strong so that active movements of joint can be completed. At this time, it can manifest the driven ability of brain to agonistic muscle in joint motion. This is the objective indicator of effect of Daoyin technique. Through real-time detection and display of myodynamia and biofeedback, the patients can do the training of neural potential development with a purpose.
2. Basic structure: The intensity of myodynamia can be tested through tension sensor, mainly the intensity of agonistic muscle contractility. Therefore, myodynamia guided device of guiding collaterals through meridians is single channel. It can real-timely detect the intensity of myodynamia and display it in curve or digit. The surpassing goal can be set with this. Through biofeedback and goal and motive mechanism, central neural potential is developed to increase the active contraction and myodynamia of muscles (Fig. 19.38).
3. Operational approach of myodynamia guided device: operational approach, therapy time, therapy course, therapeutic item, indications, contraindications and announcements of myodynamia guided device of guiding collaterals through meridians are the same as these of neurological training device of guiding collaterals through meridians. However, myodynamia guided device is only used for the training of potential development, but not for the training of motor program reestablishment and motor pattern remodeling.

19.3.3.3 Muscular Tension Guided Device of Guiding Collaterals Through Meridians

The signal source of muscular tension guided device is the muscular tension change of agonistic muscle and antagonistic muscle in joint motion.

1. Design principle: When Daoyin technique is used to guide the patients to do active movement training, the signal from brain to agonistic muscle should be strong and the contraction force should be strong so that active movements of joint can be completed. At this time,

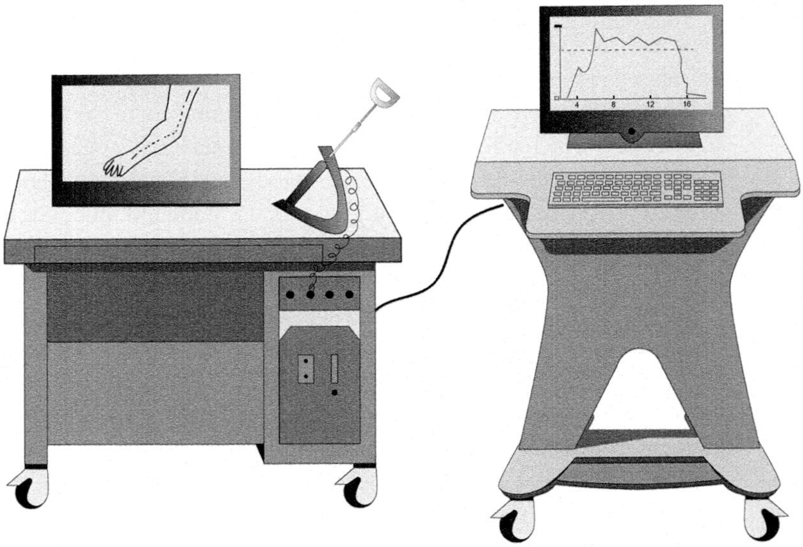

Fig. 19.38 Sketch map of myodynamia guided device of guiding collaterals

strong contractility of agonistic muscle leads to increase of muscular tension (hardness increases). Antagonistic muscle must relax or slightly contract so that the muscular tension is small. It can manifest whether the motor program that dominates joint is normal or not from the other side. This is the objective indicator of effect of Daoyin technique. It can real-timely detect and display the change of muscular tension and the patients can do the training of neural potential development and motor program reestablishment.

The change of muscular tension can be received by the reception electrode on the skin surface of the muscle and then is conducted to the computer through pressure sensor. After analysis and processing, the data is showed on the screen in curve or digit.

2. Basic structure: Except for using reception pressure as signal source, the other designs are the same as these of neurological training device (Fig. 19.39).
3. Operational approach, therapy time, therapy course, therapeutic item, indications, contraindications and announcements of muscular tension guided device of guiding collaterals through meridians are the same as these of neurological training device of guiding collaterals through meridians.

19.3.3.4 Virtual Reality Training Device of Neurological Training

It is the reception equipment for actual bioelectricity signal. Because of high sensitivity, it is easy to be influenced by external signals such as cellphone signal and automobile engine signal. Actual signal detection of training effect cannot be increased for a long time. If the actual signal cannot be increased for a while, the patients, the patients and their family may lose the confidence of further therapy and give it up. Rehabilitation equipment of neurological training is developed according to virtual reality human body training. It can simulate motor program signal and elevation. Daoyin technique is used for the training of active joint motion of actual resistance to develop brain potential and reestablish motor program.

1. Design principle: Virtual human body and animation technique are used to explain the relationship between CNS and motor function of limbs and the pathway and mechanism of motor function recovery after CNS injury with dub. Animation technique is used to simulate the motor program signal of various kinds of movements. According to goal and motive mechanism, simulated agonistic

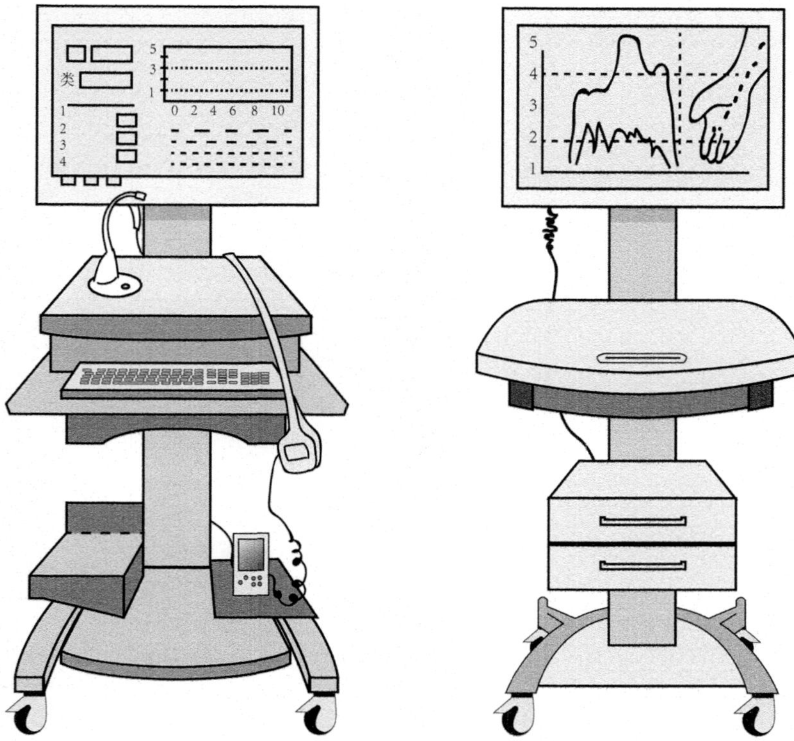

Fig. 19.39 Sketch map of muscular tension guided device of guiding collaterals through meridians

muscle signal intensity is set. According to the step by step mechanism, simulated motor program and elevation are arranged from weak to strong. Dynamic image of reestablishment training of simulated motor program signal is made or recorded separately. Six-step Daoyin technique in traditional Chinese medicine of guiding collaterals through meridians is made for dub. Vista software programming management program is used for the operating personnel to call all kinds of training package.

2. Essential structure: Virtual reality training device or system of neurological training is composed of five parts (Fig. 19.40).
    (a) Mechanism explanation of virtual therapy: Animation dub technique is used to explain why CNS injury can lead to motor dysfunction of limbs and the mechanism of recovering motor function. The anatomical structure and basic functional orientation of CNS, what is motor program signal and how to complete limbs movements. Although CNS cells are lack of regeneration ability, through developing neural potential and activating reserved conduction pathway, the functions of the injured cells can be replaced and the lost motor functions can be recovered through motor program reestablishment. Active movement, willpower and emergent state are the good conditions to develop neural potential. Six-step Daoyin technique in traditional Chinese medicine of guiding collaterals through meridians is used to guide the patients to develop neural potential through active movement and creating safe imminent dangerous state. Only practicing the archery towards target can increase the accuracy. The simulated motor program signal curve of different intensity and proportion of all joint motions are the reference for the patients to reestablish motor program in joint motion.

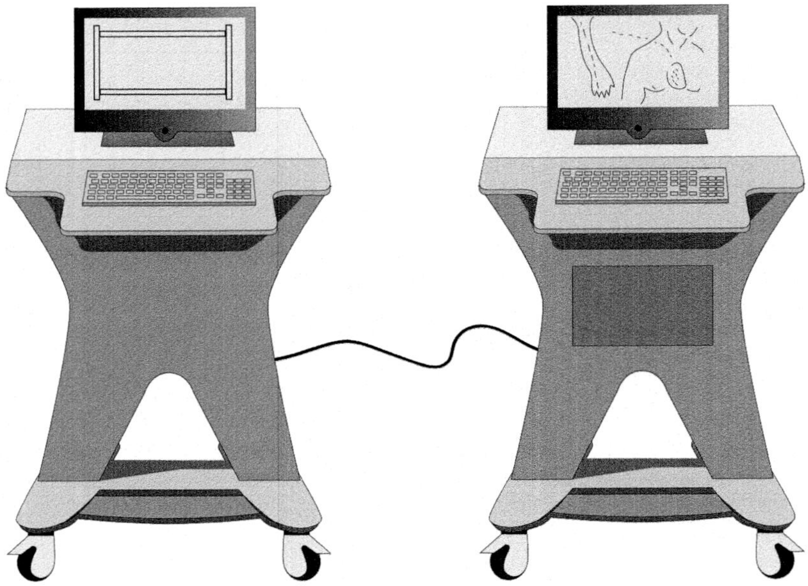

Fig. 19.40 Sketch map of virtual reality training device of guiding collaterals through meridians

(b) The therapists should know the actual movement defect and simulate normal joint motions. Video is used to know actual motor dysfunction. According to the fact that people are not familiar with their own voice and motor pattern, camera is used to record the joint motion of motor dysfunction. The video is played on the screen real-timely. The therapists simulate normal joint motion and establish therapeutic mission and target. The patients are asked to do the same movement of identical joints in healthy side to find out the movement difference in injured side and establish preliminary training mission and target.

(c) Simulation video and virtual animation are used to explain the mission, target and mechanism of the therapy. Through simulation video of normal motor pattern of identical joint with dub, the training mission and target are further explained to the patients. Virtual animation is used to explain the training of neural potential development, motor program reestablishment and recovery of joint motor function.

(d) Hardware structure: These software are installed in the hard disk of the computer. Training screen is used to display mechanism animation and training curve. Operational screen is used for the therapists to choose therapeutic items.

(e) Auxiliary function: Background music selection: the program is equipped with different kinds of music such as slow, light and passion to activate therapeutic atmosphere and encourage the enthusiasm of the patients. Therapeutic items selection: The movement of all parts such as face, upper limbs, trunk and lower limbs, the joint motion such as elbow extension, wrist flexion and foot dorsiflexion and mechanism demonstration are established into a database and stored. Vista software is used to make a management platform. According to therapeutic requirements, the therapists select the therapeutic item and press the automatic start. Storage and analysis: the training item, degree and progress of the patients can be stored. Virtual training is not the real data so that it can only be used for the inquiry of training condition, but not the analysis data of training effect.

3. Operational approach.
   (a) Therapeutic items selection: According to the actual condition of the patients, the therapists select the therapeutic item and press automatic start for the training.
   (b) Background music selection: According to the personal favorite of the patients, they select slow, light or passional music to activate therapeutic atmosphere and encourage the enthusiasm of the patients.
   (c) Autonomous joint motion and anti-resistance training under actual instruction: according to the joint motion such as elbow extension or flexion and the actual movement ability of the patients, the therapists select the corresponding intensity of motor program signal and start the animation video. According to the dub, when the video signal curve increases, the therapists exert resistance on the orientation of joint motion so that the patients can find out the signal orientation. Through anti-resistance, the training of neural potential development and motor program reestablishment can be done.
   (d) The training time and therapy course: The training time is 50 min (once a day) and there are 30 times in one therapy course. At the end of one therapy course, the therapists should re-evaluate the training effect and decide whether to do the next training or not.
   (e) Clinical indications, contraindications and announcements.

      Indications: It is suitable for the training of all kinds of motor dysfunction after CNS injuries such as hemiplegia, cerebral palsy, paraplegia, children cerebral palsy and facial paralysis, the training of limbs motor dysfunction induced by bone and joint injuries.

      Contraindications: The patients with unhealed bone, joint and muscle injuries after surgery who affect the rescue in acute phase.

      Announcements: Before training, the immerse technique should be used so that the patients can devote themselves into therapeutic environment, which is the premise of guaranteeing the therapy. The cooperation between the therapists and the patients is very important. If the cooperation is not good, the training of the patients may be not synchronized with video signal curve. Therefore, the patients may wrongly think that the simulated signal is false and the therapy is invalid. Before therapy, the therapists explain the therapeutic mechanism to the patients in fact and seek the patients' recognition, which are very important. The therapy should be step by step. The training amount and the degree of anti-resistance should be increased gradually.

19.3.3.5 Training Device of Motor Function Training

It is mainly used for recovering the lost motor function. According to three-stage rehabilitation method of neurological training, except for neurological training device of guiding collaterals through meridians used for motor program reestablishment, it can be used for the neural potential development of upper limbs, lower limbs, trunk, tibialis anterior muscle, hamstring muscles, stride, gait and shifting of weight and walking balance training device. It can be modified on the basis of equipment and it is added with signal detection and display function. In addition, there is training device used for motor pattern remodeling.

1. Neural potential development training device of guiding collaterals through meridians includes potential development training device of upper limbs (Fig. 19.41) and lower limbs (Fig. 19.42). The role is to recover the functions of undead nerve cells in injure area. Normal nerve cells around injured area can replace the injure cells and the conduction pathway and reflex arc between neurons or between nerve and muscle are reestablished to recover lost autonomous motor function.

   In order to meet the requirements mentioned above, potential development equip-

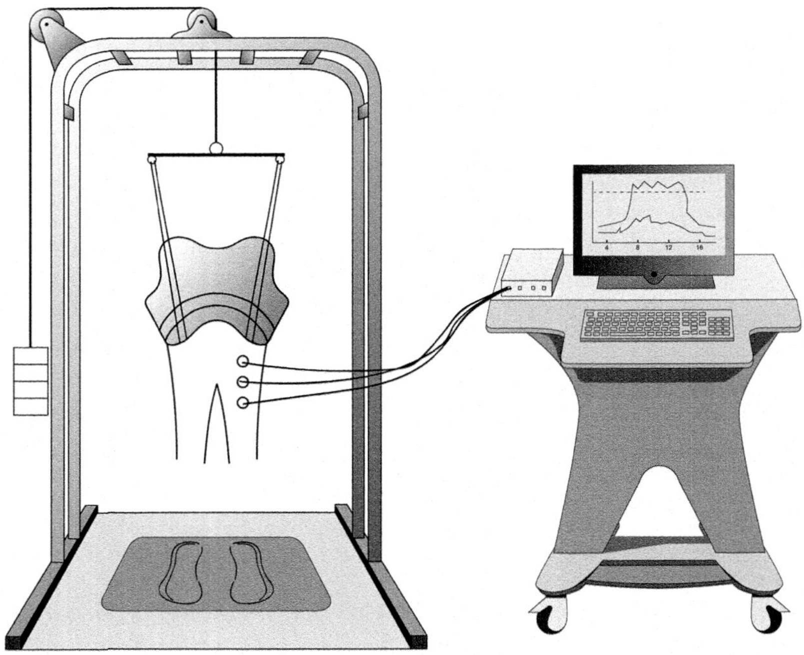

Fig. 19.41 Sketch map of lower limbs neural potential development training device of guiding collaterals through meridians

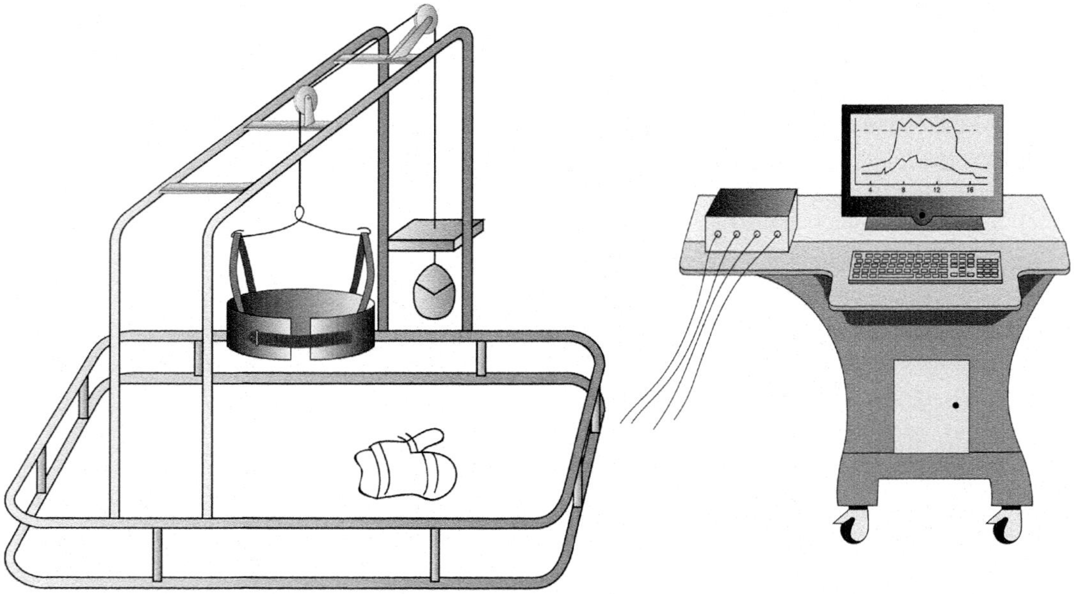

Fig. 19.42 Sketch map of upper limbs neural potential development training device of guiding collaterals through meridians

ment of neurological training of guiding collaterals through meridians includes the following basic structure and function.

(a) Weight support and protection system is composed of bearing frame, pedestal, weight support and protection system and weight support sandbag. It can reduce the partial weight of the patients so that they can complete the required movement. According to the functional improvement, the amount of weight support should be decreased. The training should be from easy to difficulty and step by step. Because of suspension effect of weight support system on human body, it can prevent the falling down or bump. The method and words are used to create safe imminent dangerous state. Because the patients know there is no danger, it can eliminate the fear and tension of the patients. Comprehensive effect can create safe imminent dangerous state good for neural potential development.
(b) Digital display and feedback system of Daoyin technique effects: it can detect, analyze and display motor program signals in continuous curve or sound to show the Daoyin technique effect real-timely. According to the actual condition of the patients, new surpassing goal is set. Through goal and motive mechanism and biofeedback, six-step Daoyin technique of guiding collaterals through meridians is used to develop CNS potential and promote plasticity and functional reorganization in order to recover lost motor function.
(c) Animation spot instruction of meridian points and automatic speech instruction: On the basis of important acupuncture points, animation spot and synchronous tracking Daoyin technique tape, conduction pathway and real-time position of flicker of light spot are good for correct and standard application of the technique of guiding collaterals through meridians. Therefore, the technique of guiding collaterals through meridians can be used to clear and activate the channels and collaterals and increase training effect.
(d) The training time and therapy course: The training time is 30 min (once or twice a day) and there are 60 times in one therapy course. At the end of one therapy course, the therapists should re-evaluate the training effect and decide whether to do the next training or not.
(e) Clinical indications, contraindications and announcements are the same as these of upper and lower neural potential development training device of guiding collaterals through meridians.

2. Lower limbs motor pattern remodeling training device of guiding collaterals through meridians: Developed neural potential development and reestablished motor program are not equal to recovered motor function. Actual application training is required to transfer developed potential and established motor program into actual daily life ability, which is a process of motor pattern remodeling. Not only the method of motor pattern remodeling is required, but also corollary equipment of motor pattern remodeling is required.

   This equipment has the following characteristics. Weight support and protection; it can extract program signal of CNS motor pattern, display it real-timely and set surpassing goal; animation spot instruction and Daoyin technique automatic speech instruction of guiding collaterals through meridians; it can prevent unnecessary joint motion in limbs movements and promote remodeling of normal motor pattern effectively; result storage and automatic analysis; it is easy to operate (Fig. 19.43).

   Therapy course, indications, contraindications and announcements of motor pattern remodeling training device of guiding collaterals through meridians are the same as these of abnormal gait rectification weight support and walking training device.

3. Sphincter ani training device of guiding collaterals through meridians. This training device (Fig. 19.44) is specially developed for

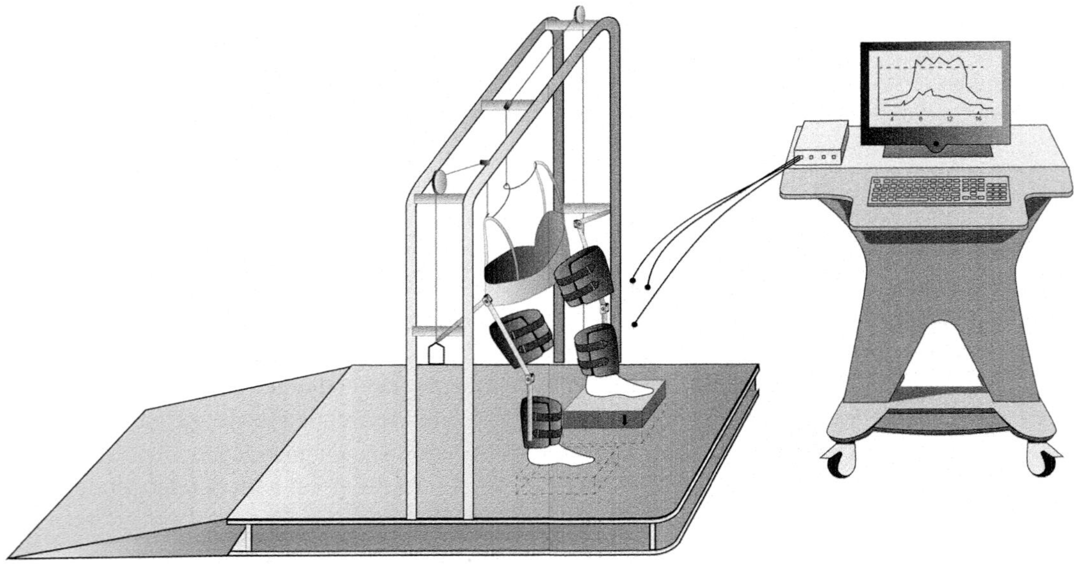

Fig. 19.43 Sketch map of motor pattern remodeling training device of guiding collaterals through meridians

Fig. 19.44 Sphincter ani training device of guiding collaterals through meridians

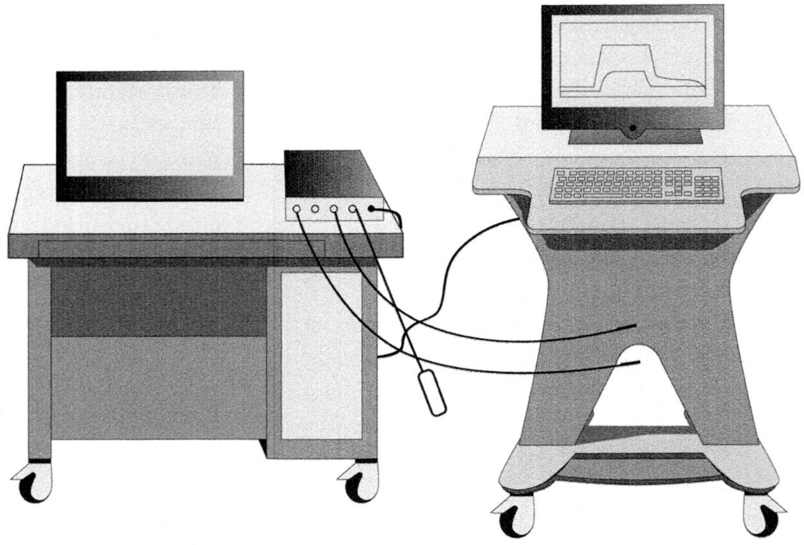

gatism. The characteristics are as follows. Tailor-made cylinder probe with round head is placed into anus and there is signal reception electrode in probe. There are sphincter ani and anal tube muscle electrodes (three electrodes in each group). When anal tube muscle (agonistic muscle) contracts and sphincter ani (antagonistic muscle) relaxes, it is suitable for the patients with difficult defecation short of power. When sphincter ani (agonistic muscle) contracts and anal tube muscle (antagonistic muscle) relaxes, it is suitable for rehabilitation training of the patients with fecal incontinence.

Specific operational approach, indications, contraindications and announcements refer to the second segment of Chap. 17.

19.3.4 Training Robot

In clinical rehabilitation practices of neurological training, the author found that the therapeutic effect of this technique not only depends on correct assessment and formulation of therapeutic schedule, but also is related to correct application of active movement, proper anti-resistance, safe imminent dangerous state and passional encourage guided by Daoyin technique. However, even if a sophisticated rehabilitation doctor or the therapists can master these techniques, it is difficult to encourage the patients and create safe imminent dangerous state for neural potential development.

In addition, one therapist can treat one patient with passion. If one therapist is asked to treat more than eight patients, he cannot be full of passion. Moreover, the therapists may be full of passion in one day but cannot be full of passion every day, even the basic passion for maintaining the therapy. On the other hand, rehabilitation therapy is the one-to-one bare-handed operation technique. Treating one patient at least requires one therapist. For the severe patients who totally lose motor function, they usually require two or more therapists and auxiliary personnel to complete it. Besides, over fatigue or operation miss of the therapists during training is one of the causes of accident injuries of the patients.

Because of various shortcomings, rehabilitation technique of neurological training cannot be applied correctly. The therapy occupies too many manpower resources. The labor intensity is strong. The number of the patients is small. It may induce accident of the patients and directly affect the effect and clinical application of rehabilitation training of neurological training, which is an urgent problem in the development process of rehabilitation technique of neurological training. The purpose of rehabilitation training of neurological training robot is to overcome the shortcoming of clinical application of neurological training and give play to the therapeutic effect of the method.

According to the theory of rehabilitation technique, training procedure, training types and training part of neurological training, we developed a series of rehabilitation training of neurological training robots to promote CNS plasticity that is in accordance with training requirements of active motor function and use the motor dysfunction as the training target. The robot can give play to the effect of the method of rehabilitation training of neurological training, overcome the shortcoming of the technique, guarantee the safety and correctness of this technique, highlight the characteristics of rehabilitation technique in traditional Chinese medicine, increase efficiency and therapeutic effect and improve life quality of the disabled.

19.3.4.1 Basic Functions of Rehabilitation Training of Neurological Training Robot

In order to meet the requirements of different training functions and body parts, rehabilitation training robot of neurological training is equipped with the following functions.

1. The training is automatic after starting: The training is done automatically according to technical requirements of neural potential development, motor program reestablishment and motor pattern remodeling of neurological training.
2. Entire active movement: Rehabilitation training robot of neurological training is designed for the training of entire active movement. It changed the passive movement training way that robot helps people to do exercise, which goes against CNS potential development. It is good for CNS potential development and functional reorganization.
3. It can meet the technology application requirements of the method of guiding collaterals through meridians or guiding meridians through collaterals and normal six-step Daoyin technique in traditional Chinese medicine.
4. It can detect motor program signal, resistance signal, joint angle signal or analog signal and show the effect of Daoyin technique in a curve, digit or sound real-timely.
5. Animation spot flicker of main and collateral channels and acupuncture point, synchronized six-step Daoyin technique automatic speech instruction tracking display

6. It is with automatic anti-resistance and the resistance is adjustable. The therapists can set therapeutic item and condition and select therapeutic item.
7. It is with man-machine conversation, wired or wireless manipulation, data storage and analysis.

19.3.4.2 The Kinds of Rehabilitation Training Robot of Neurological Training

According to training technique and training part, rehabilitation training robot of neurological training can be divided into three kinds. There are two types in each kind. According to the source of biofeedback signal, the robot is divided into actual motor program signal and virtual motor program signal.

In addition, every type includes normal method and six-step Daoyin technique in traditional Chinese medicine of guiding collaterals through meridians, which are immersed into every type. The combination forms a series of rehabilitation training robot of neurological training with different functions, which meets the requirements of rehabilitation training.

1. Rehabilitation training robot of potential development of neurological training: There are three kinds and six types. Rehabilitation training robot of potential development of neurological training is divided into upper limbs, lower limbs and the trunk. The common characteristics are as follows: weight support and protection facility includes bearing frame, mechanical weight support device and protection device. Robot can be connected to the safety belt the patients wear to protect the patients away from accident. It can keep the training safely and adjust the amount of weight support automatically. High sensitivity of motor program signal: new type of motor program signal device increases the accuracy of extracting motor program signal and broadens therapeutic range. Function of creating imminent dangerous state automatically: Through software setting, robot can reduce support suddenly for 1–2 s when the patients do the training of potential development to create imminent dangerous state without support or assistance. Record can automatically encourage the patients to overcome difficulty and develop potential better.
2. Rehabilitation training robot of motor program reestablishment of neurological training: There are three kinds and six types. It can detect motor program signal from CNS to muscles real-timely. Automatic speech and animation six-step Daoyin technique instruction and resistance are good for recovering autonomous coordinated motor function in the training of motor program of all joints. It includes rehabilitation training robot of motor program reestablishment of single joint, rehabilitation training robot of motor program reestablishment of coordinated multiple joints and rehabilitation training robot of motor program reestablishment of walking. Every kind of rehabilitation training robot can be divided into actual and virtual motor program signal types. Two types of signals can be immersed into equipment.
3. Rehabilitation training robot of motor pattern remodeling of neurological training: There are three kinds and six types. It can do the training of upper limbs, lower limbs and balanced motor pattern remodeling. They have the following common characteristics: Active movement system of movement adjustment includes bearing frame, automatic weight support adjustment, providing resistance automatically, stride or grasping with upper limbs. It can restrain unnecessary movements in the motor pattern remodeling system effectively.

19.3.4.3 Rehabilitation Training Robot of Shoulder and Elbow of Neurological Training

Rehabilitation training robot of shoulder and elbow of neurological training is the automatic equipment specially used for the active movement training of shoulder and elbow, which belongs to the exoskeleton type robot system with the common characteristics of rehabilitation training robot of neurological training.

1. Design principle: This type of rehabilitation training robot of neurological training is composed of training software, exoskeleton system and control system.
   (a) Training software includes: explanation of rehabilitation therapy mechanism of neurological training, six-step implement tape of guiding collaterals through meridians, animation flicker spot automatic tracking and display system of the pathway of main and collateral channels, motor program signal detection and display system and virtual reality training system.
   (b) Exoskeleton system includes seat, support system of upper limbs and resistance providing system.
   (c) Control system includes operation interface, training items selection, resistance setting, surpassing goal setting, data storage and analysis, music selection.

      After the therapists select the therapeutic item and increased resistance through operation interface, on the basis of regulation of mind and breath, the patients are guided by Daoyin technique tape instruction and do extension and flexion autonomous movements of shoulder or elbow joint according to the pathway of main and collateral channels displayed by animation spot of human body. The system can exert selected resistance on the orientation of joint motion in proper time. The system use six-step Daoyin technique to encourage the patients to make the motor program signal surpass goal continuously until it is close to or reach the actual training level of the therapists. Therefore, it can develop potential, reestablish motor program and recover lost motor function.
2. The basic structure of exoskeleton is composed of seat, support frame of upper limbs and training system of shoulder and elbow.

The seat is with high back to maintain the patients in a comfortable sitting position. Support frame of upper limbs is composed of lattice framing of aluminium alloy, artificial shoulder joint, elbow joint, wrist and hand. Its role is to keep upper limbs in suspension function position to provide enough support for the forearm so that the patients can do training of shoulder and elbow joint. The upside of lattice framing of aluminium alloy is connected to artificial shoulder and elbow joint to allow protraction, rear protraction, adduction, abduction and rotation of the shoulder. The middle artificial elbow joint allows flexion and extension of elbow joint in physiological range (shoulder joint: 0–360°; elbow joint: 0–180°). Lattice framing in forearm is equipped with retractor device that is suitable for the patients with different arm length. Wrist and hand is equipped with handle for joint motion and anti-resistance training.

The anti-resistance force of joint motion is provided by electromagnetic clutch that is installed in the back of seat (the shoulder part of support frame of upper limbs). The strength of resistance provided by electromagnetic clutch is controlled by the computer software with different grade. The resistance in the same grade is not the equivalent resistance, which means the strength of resistance is increased with the increase of the angle of joint motion. It can also provide equivalent resistance, which means the strength of resistance is constant regardless of the angle of joint motion.

When the patients do the training of shoulder joint, electromagnetic clutch provides setting resistance. When the patients do extension and flexion training of elbow joint, electromagnetic clutch generates resistance to the arm through steel wire in the extension and flexion of elbow joint, which is good for the anti-resistance training of the patients. It can develop neural potential gradually, promote CNS plasticity and functional reorganization and realize the anticipated goal of rehabilitation through repeated training (Fig. 19.45).

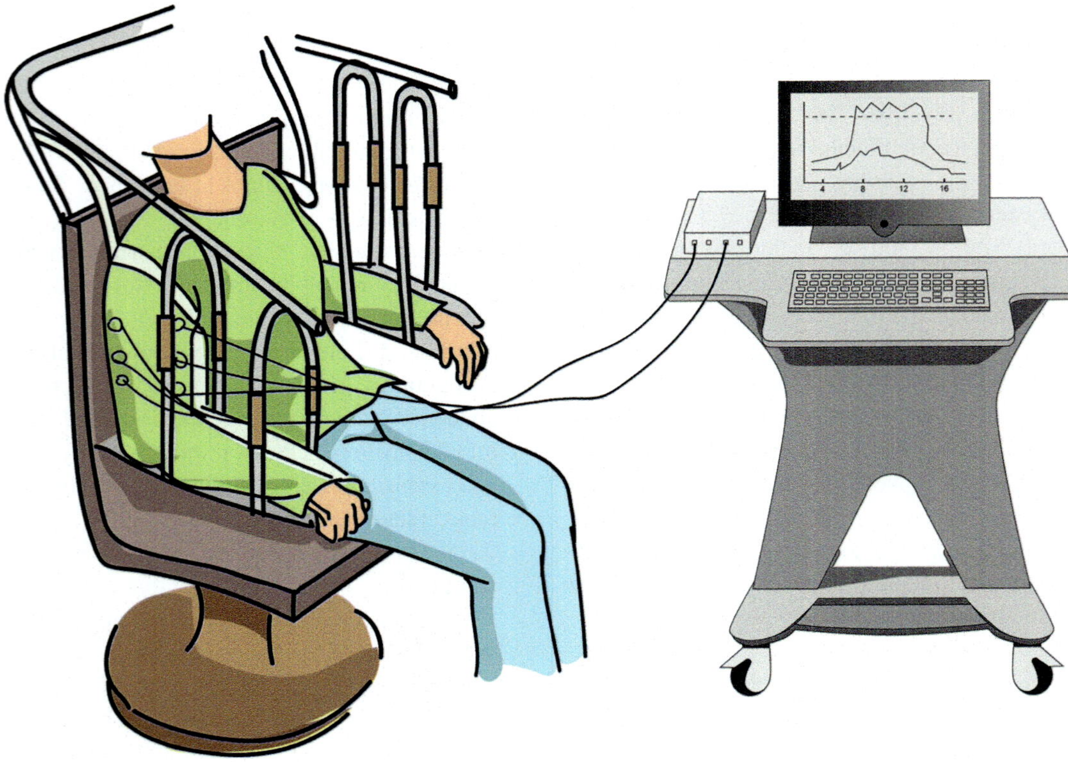

Fig. 19.45 Sketch map of rehabilitation training robot of shoulder and elbow joints of neurological training

3. Operational approach: For example, in the virtual reality training of elbow extension, the patients sit in the seat of the robot, put upper limbs in the mechanical arm of the robot and use fixing belt to fix it. Before training, the therapists select training item and the strength of resistance force and press the starting button. Remote manipulation is also available. The robot starts to autoplay six-step voice guidance of guiding collaterals through meridians and use flickering animation spot to track and display guided Qi, pathway of main and collateral channels and acupuncture points in virtual human body. Meanwhile, there is simulated motor program signal curve on the screen. At this moment, resistance device installed in mechanical arm can exert selected resistance to the patients automatically. Because of the characteristics of resistance device, the bigger the range of elbow extension of the patients is, the stronger the imposed resistance is. The patients must give out the stronger signal to enhance muscle contraction for anti-resistance. The patients should make motor program signal of agonistic muscle surpass the previous intensity and make the signal of antagonistic muscle lower than the previous intensity. After that, the patients enter into the relaxation process of activating collaterals.
4. The training time and therapy course: The training time is 50 min (once a day) and there are 30 times in one therapy course. At the end of one therapy course, the therapists should re-evaluate the training effect and decide whether to do the next training or not.
5. Clinical indications, contraindications and announcements.
   (a) Indications: It is suitable for motor dysfunction of shoulder and elbow joints after CNS injuries such as hemiplegia, cerebral palsy, paraplegia, children cerebral palsy. It is also suitable for the motor dysfunction of shoulder and elbow induced by bone, joint and muscle inju-

ries such as scapulohumeral periarthritis and brachial plexus injury.

(b) Contraindications: After surgery of shoulder and elbow joints, the patients with unhealed bone, joint and muscle injuries in acute phase affect rescue.

(c) Announcements: The patients sit well, put upper limb in correct position and fix it in case of prolapse and accident injury. After the training begins, the therapists are required to instruct the patients in detail. After the patients are familiar with the training, they can do self-training, but the medical staff should make an inspection and exam the training to rectify the mistake and deficiency in the training. For the patients with severe symptoms and cognition impairment, the therapists should accompany the patients for the training.

References

1. Liming W. The advanced medical equipment are the important condition for a hospital to rise the medical level. Inform Med Equip. 2002;1(1):32–3.
2. Yuqin Y, Xiaosheng H. Recent advance in molecular imaging tracing endogenous neural stem cells involved in neurogenesis. Chin J Neuromed. 2014;13(6):639–42.
3. Qingchun G, Tinghuai W, Wang T. The application of biofeedback in the rehabilitation of stroke. Foreign Med. 2002;10(5):363–6.
4. Hu C, Dingfang C. Endogenous neural stem cells and neural regeneration after cerebral ischemia. Foreign Med. 2002;10(5):367–9.
5. Wenbin Z, Xiaoke C, Guorui L, et al. Functional magnetic resonance imaging in the evaluation of cerebral reorganization in patients with space-occupying lesions in motor cortex. Chin J Postgrad Med. 2006;29(10):18–20.
6. Haihong ZHAO, Jianfei HUO, Zheng W, et al. Research on the effectiveness of the training method and device for lower limb motor pattern remodeling. Chin Med. 2013;8(7):921–3.
7. Lianghua T, Xuejun L, Zongpei L. Treatment experience in 189 cases of limb joint adhesion. J Trad Chin Orthop Traumatol. 2000;12(1):57.
8. Bingyao C, Siwei Y, Gong J. Recovery of spontaneous motor function after incomplete spinal cord injury. Chin J Trauma. 2002;18(1):55–6.
9. Bo Y, Jianming J, Wenjing H, et al. The effects of lower limb strength on balance. Chin J Phys Med Rehabil. 2006;28(7):466–8.
10. Yang J. Development of human potential. Chin Health Hum Res. 2006;5:58–9.
11. Bo Z, Huan Z, Yiwan W, et al. Antagonistic muscle massage combined with rehabilitation training to treat 35 patients with upper extremity flexion spasm after stroke. Zhej J Trad Chin Med. 2015;50(10):741–2.
12. Sheng B, Linhong J, Shurong J, et al. Robot-aided arm training methods based on neurological rehabilitation principles for stroke and brain injury patientd. Chin J Phys Med Rehabil. 2006;28(8):523–7.
13. Tusong W. Effect of comprehensive rehabilitation therapy on lower extremity dysfunction in stroke hemiplegic patients. Chin J Phys Med Rehabil. 2008;30(1):42–3.
14. Yong Y. Early rehabilitation intervention for foot drooping in hemiparetic patients. Med J Chin People's Health. 2009;21(13):1585–91.
15. Qingcun G, Tingkui W. Application of biofeedback in the rehabilitation of stroke. Foreign Med. 2002;10(5):363–6.
16. Rencheng W. Fractal analysis of surface EMG signals. Chin J Med Instrum. 1999;23(3):125.